MINIMALLY INVASIVE CANCER MANAGEMENT

F.L. Greene, B.T. Heniford
(Eds.)

Minimally Invasive Cancer Management

Second Edition

With 199 Figures and 37 Tables

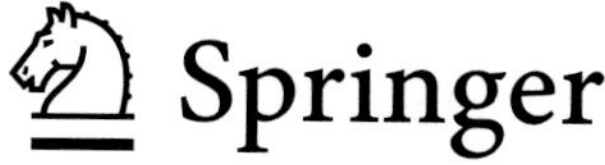

Frederick L. Greene
Chairman
Department of Surgery
Carolinas Medical Center
Charlotte
NC 28203
USA
frederick.greene@carolinashealthcare.org

B. Todd Heniford
Chief
Division of GI and Minimal
Access Surgery
Carolinas Medical Center
Charlotte
NC 28203
USA
todd.heniford@carolinashealthcare.org

ISBN 978-1-4419-1237-4 e-ISBN 978-1-4419-1238-1
DOI 10.1007/978-1-4419-1238-1
Springer New York Dordrecht Heidelberg London

Library of Congress Control Number: 2010929053

Printed on acid-free paper

Springer is part of Springer Science+Business Media (www.springer.com)

Foreword to the Second Edition

Dr. Greene and his colleagues present the second edition of their text, *Minimal Access Cancer Management.* Minimal access surgery is an area where the editors have taken a genuine leadership role. It is now firmly established that minimal access surgery has a major role to play in the management of the patient with malignancy. The primary benefits to diagnosis and staging are now accepted and recognized. It is extremely important to realize that minimal invasive surgery, and for that matter other forms of ablation, are techniques that utilizes technical advances brought from other areas of optics, instrumentation, and usable alternative energy sources. In the first edition the authors' goal was to provide "a repository for cognitive and technical information." This has now been achieved. In the management of the cancer patient, one might hope we are moving further from technical and discipline-based approaches to disease-based processes. The inevitability of this is reinforced by the intelligent patient and physician having already worked it out! One might argue that medical care has progressively moved to disease management rather than discipline-based management as is seen in cardiovascular, trauma, and burn centers.

This current monograph addresses the technical issues with great skill and emphasis. As with the first edition, however, there is still an opportunity to place this technique into the greater perspective of overall patient care. In particular, a greater emphasis on the evaluation of minimized morbidity and the characterization of benefits to patients and society in terms of financial cost have yet to be adequately addressed. It is clear that the advent of minimally invasive surgery has helped open surgery, not just in the development of technically useful instrumentation. How many times have I struggled to suture the vena cava, only now to place an angulated stapler with precision and safety?

Minimally invasive approaches have also influenced the management of patients as we focus on diminishing the size of the incision, even in open surgery. Certainly, the awareness that after minimally invasive procedures patients can leave the hospital earlier has influenced practice to discharge patients sooner than one might have in the past. Conversely, when the products of the operation and the hospital stay are dependent on the associated complications, as in pancreatectomy or major intra-abdominal procedures, the influence of the minimally invasive technique is less evident.

The chapter on pancreatic cancer highlights this dilemma. An appropriate emphasis is placed on the significant potential benefits of diagnostic laparoscopy, endoscopic ultrasound, and palliation with detailed technique. In resection, focus is on distal pancreatectomy initially for benign or low-risk malignancy with similar morbidity to the open technique. For more extensive resections, the technique is described, but no comment on benefit or even a comparison to open operative procedures is provided.

The editors appropriately illustrate the future possibilities, but again, this is very much a promissory note for new technologies that are relatively unproven. If the therapeutic modality can be proven to be efficacious, then, of course, minimizing the morbidity of its application would be a crucial advantage for the minimally invasive approach. There can be little doubt that large debulking procedures, which at best have had minimal significant impact on survival, will disappear. In this, the editors are correct; more precise diagnosis of systemic disease will limit the need for major surgical approaches to the primary tumor. I would have liked to have seen a greater emphasis on our ideas on disease management, such that techniques, whether minimally invasive or maximally invasive, would just become a part of the surgical oncologist's armamentarium.

As this second edition comes to press, we ask for the third edition with its associated validation of the approaches for overall delivery of healthcare, both for the individual patient and for the society as a whole. It does seem clear that we are comfortable that "how" you do the procedure is far less important than that the "correct" procedure be done for the "correct" reasons. The present edition confirms the technological advances. We look forward to the validation that in therapeutic resection for malignancy, the benefits of a minimally invasive approach are real, tangible, and cost-effective.

Murray F. Brennan, MD
Benno C. Schmidt Chair in
Clinical Oncology
Memorial Sloan-Kettering Cancer Center

Foreword to the First Edition

This extraordinarily well organized monograph represents a successful effort to encompass and amalgamate two rapidly advancing fields. The first is the long delayed maturation of surgical oncology as an independent discipline, which is reflected by the vigor of its society and by appropriate recognition, both by other oncologic specialties, and more importantly, by the surgical world as a whole. Furthermore, there has been a literally logarithmic increase in both the availability and appropriateness of minimally invasive methods for the perfection of diagnosis and treatment of many diseases, but especially neoplastic ones. This book represents a marriage of remarkable advances and imaging precision with the refinement of a whole variety of minimally invasive techniques.

There remain major concerns and issues vis-à-vis dissemination of cancer and implantation by especially the pneumoperitoneum used so much as part of minimal access abdominal surgery. It is difficult to define the full extent of these concerns, and whether they are simply mechanically, or indeed, immunologically mediated. In any case, the issue of the port site implantation needs to remain in the front rank of concerns by the growing numbers of surgical oncologists who practice well developed minimal access work.

The exciting advances in the pages that follow, however, must not distort the fundamental priorities of the surgical approach to cancer. The first is to be reminded that surgery is the ultimate curative endeavor, with far and away the largest proportion of patients with cancer cured by surgical means than *all* others combined. Furthermore, surgeons always need to be reminded that the palliative approach to cancer requires the most mature and precise judgment, and it is both quality and quantity of life that factor into the outcome of that ultimate equation. It is perhaps with that latter admonition that one need always be reminded that more traditional open techniques are always both ethical and judgmental fall-back positions of acceptable merit, when attempting minimal access palliation.

Over the past four decades, there has been a huge waxing and waning of surgical influence in the care of the cancer patient. This book is a further step toward strengthening the surgeon's role. Clearly at the end of World War II, the surgical care of the patient with neoplastic disease involved both definitive diagnosis and virtually the only treatment that was available, with the exception of radiation therapy for gynecological cancer. For a number of reasons for which many of us may be blamed, the surgeon's role in this important disease process shrunk precipitously with the advent of sophisticated radiation therapy, the alleged wonders of multi-modality treatment schemes, and sequential in-combination chemotherapy. It was only within the last few years of the century that the ethical and important role of surgeons in the overall management of the cancer patient began to be appreciated again. This is both a political and ethical issue, and requires that surgeons stand up most of all for their patients, and to a lesser degree, for their discipline, in practicing and reinforcing the primary role of the surgeon in cancer care. The marriage described in this tome takes that to a new and more significant level, and will serve the patients of the future, as well as it will its readers.

Hiram C. Polk, Jr., MD
Ben A. Reid Senior Professor and Chair
Department of Surgery
University of Louisville

Preface to the Second Edition

Since writing the preface to the first edition of *Minimally Invasive Cancer Management* in August 2000, we have entered a new century and the utilization of minimal access techniques for cancer management has been expanded significantly. Approaches to gastrointestinal malignancy of the foregut and colon have been incorporated into the management strategies for cancer patients. Throughout the world laparoscopic techniques are now applied not only for diagnosis and surveillance but also for extirpation of cancer. Tumor ablation, especially in the management of metastatic lesions of the liver, has taken on a greater importance and the opportunity to apply radiofrequency and microwave techniques through percutaneous approaches is now possible.

This second edition of *Minimally Invasive Cancer Management* serves as a compendium to catalog these new techniques that have created excitement in cancer management throughout the first decade of the twenty-first century. As is true with any monograph, the world of oncology and surgery continues to change and more applications for management continue to appear even as the completed second edition manuscripts go to press. Hopefully this monograph, in association with the peer reviewed literature, will enhance the reader's knowledge in these areas.

As is true with the first edition, the second edition could not have become reality without the supreme efforts and professional involvement of our editorial staff at Springer. I particularly want to recognize Portia Bridges for her marvelous editorial leadership and her ability to continue the process to its completion. In addition, Paula Callaghan and the staff at the New York office have been particularly supportive and it has been a pleasure again to work with our publishing colleagues at Springer.

I am mindful that the time and effort of creating this second edition could not be possible without stealing time from family, friends and the residents with whom we work on a daily basis. It is my hope that this second edition of *Minimally Invasive Cancer Management* is a suitable tribute to them for their support and patience.

April 2010 Frederick L. Greene, MD

Preface to the First Edition

The management of cancer continues to present challenges to the surgeon, especially in this era of heightened technology created by the introduction of minimal access approaches to the intraluminal, intrathoracic, and intraabdominal compartments. As newer technology abounds through ultrasound, energy systems, robotics, and continued reduction in size of instrumentation, the application for the cancer patient appears to be unlimited. It is with this sense of excitement that we undertook the task of bringing together information to create a monograph that would serve as a repository for cognitive and technical information relating to these approaches in our patients with cancer. Despite the newer modes of conveying information through the Internet and other types of cybertechnology, our colleagues at Springer recognized the importance of having a traditional monograph serve as a vehicle for conveying this information. In selecting our authors, we attempted to invite those who have had the experience, vision, and creativity not only to enhance the technology but also to effectively record their successes on paper.

The editorship of a textbook is a labor of love. This labor was made more pleasurable by the unfailing continued assistance and creative force shown by Laura Gillan and Terry Kornak, our senior editor and supervising production editor, respectively, at Springer. At every turn, Laura and Terry supported our direction and served as cheerleaders to assure that our efforts would be timely as well as useful to our surgical and oncology colleagues. We also appreciate the work of Cara Anselmo and, later, Carol Wang, who served as able assistants to Ms. Gillan.

Finally, we give full kudos to our families from whom we purloined additional time to ensure the success of this effort. We dedicate this book to our wives and children because of their understanding of our great desire to add to the betterment of our patients through our clinical and academic pursuits.

August 2000

Frederick L. Greene, MD
B. Todd Heniford, MD

Contents

Part I

Introductory Issues

Contributors

Maurice E. Arregui, MD
Program Director, St. Vincent/Indiana University Fellowships in Advanced Laparoscopy, Endoscopy and Ultrasound, Department of Surgery, Indiana University, St. Vincent Hospital, Indianapolis, IN 46260, USA

Anton J. Bilchik, MD, PhD, FACS
Clinical Professor, David Geffen School of Medicine, University of California, Los Angeles; Medical Director, California Oncology Research Institute, Santa Monica, CA 90403, USA

Juliane Bingener, MD
Associate Professor of Surgery, Division of General Surgery, Mayo Clinic, Rochester, MN 55905, USA

Kevin C. P. Conlon, MA, MCh, MBA, FRCSI, FACS, FRCS (Hon) (Glas), FTCD
Professor of Surgery, University of Dublin, Trinity College, Dublin, Ireland

Jill R. Dietz, MD
Director, Breast Cancer Program and Breast Surgery Fellowship, Women's Health Institute, Cleveland Clinic Foundation, Cleveland, OH 44195, USA

Maria M. Gonzalez, BS
Cancer Research Manager, Center for Cancer Prevention and Treatment, St. Joseph Hospital, Orange, CA 92868, USA

Frederick L. Greene, MD
Chairman, Department of Surgery, Carolinas Medical Center, Charlotte, NC 28203, USA

Nicholas A. Hamilton, MD
Resident, Department of General Surgery, Barnes–Jewish Hospital, Washington University School of Medicine, St. Louis, MO 63110, USA

Paul D. Hansen, MD, FACS
Program Director, Hepatobiliary and Pancreatic Cancer, Department of Surgery, Providence Portland Hospital, Portland, OR 97210, USA

B. Todd Heniford, MD
Chief, Division of GI and Minimal Access Surgery, Carolinas Medical Center, Charlotte, NC 28203, USA

John G. Hunter, MD
Mackenzie Professor and Chair, Department of Surgery, Oregon Health and Science University, Portland, OR 97239, USA

David A. Iannitti, MD
Chief, Hepatic-Pancreatico-Biliary Surgery, Clinical Associate Professor of Surgery, Department of Surgery, University of North Carolina, Chapel Hill; Carolinas Medical Center, Charlotte, NC 28203, USA

Kent W. Kercher, MD, FACS
Chief, Minimal Access Surgery, Clinical Associate Professor of Surgery, Department of General Surgery, Carolinas Medical Center, University of North Carolina School of Medicine, Charlotte, NC 28203, USA

Seigo Kitano, MD, PhD, FACS
Professor, Department of Surgery I, Oita University Faculty of Medicine, Yufu, Oita, 879-5593, Japan

Keith A. Kuenzler, MD
Assistant Professor of Surgery, Director, Minimally Invasive Pediatric Surgery, Department of Pediatric Surgery, Morgan Stanley Children's Hospital of NY – Presbyterian, Columbia University Medical Center, New York, NY 10031, USA

Virginia R. Litle, MD
Associate Professor of Surgery, Department of Surgery, University of Rochester School of Medicine and Dentistry, Rochester, NY 14642, USA

John H. Marks, MD
Co-Director, Marks Colorectal Surgical Associates; Assistant Professor of Clinical Surgery, MCP-Hahnemann University; Senior Investigator, Lakenau Institute for Medical Research; Department of Surgery, Lakenhau Hospital, Wynnewood, PA 19096, USA

John B. Martinie, MD, FACS
Department of General Surgery, Carolinas Medical Center, Clinical Assistant Professor, University of North Carolina, School of Medicine, Charlotte, NC 28203, USA

David P. Mason, MD
Staff Surgeon, Department of Thoracic Surgery, Cleveland Clinic, Cleveland, OH 44195, USA

Brent D. Matthews, MD
Chief, Section of Minimally Invasive Surgery, Department of General Surgery, Barnes–Jewish Hospital, Washington University School of Medicine, St. Louis, MO 63110, USA

Sudish C. Murthy, MD, PhD
Staff Surgeon, Department of Thoracic and Cardiovascular Surgery, Cleveland Clinic, Cleveland, OH 44195, USA

R. Wendel Naumann, MD
Director of Minimally Invasive Surgery in Gynecologic Oncology, Department of Obstetrics and Gynecology, Carolinas Medical Center, Charlotte, NC 28203, USA

Heidi Nelson, MD
Fred C. Anderson Professor of Surgery, Department of Colon and Rectal Surgery, Mayo Clinic, Rochester, MN 55904, USA

Kyle A. Perry, MD
Minimally Invasive Surgery Fellow, Department of Surgery, Oregon Health and Sciences University, Portland, OR 79239, USA

Jeffrey H. Peters, MD
Professor and Chairman, Department of Surgery, Strong Memorial Hospital, University of Rochester, Rochester, NY 14642, USA

Ajita S. Prabhu, MD
Fellow, Division of Gastrointestinal and Minimally Invasive Surgery, Department of General Surgery, Carolinas Medical Center, Charlotte, NC 28203, USA

Rashmi P. Pradhan, MD
Breast Fellow, Women's Health Institute, Cleveland Clinic Foundation, MGM Medical College, Cleveland, OH 44195, USA

Thomas W. Rice, MD
Daniel and Karen Lee Chair Thoracic Surgery, Professor of Surgery, Cleveland Clinic Lerner College of Medicine, Cleveland Clinic, Cleveland, OH; Head, Section of Thoracic Surgery, Department of Thoracic and Cardiovascular Surgery, Cleveland Clinic, Cleveland, OH 44195, USA

Steven S. Rothenberg, MD
Chief of Pediatric Surgery and Chairman, Department of Pediatrics, The Rocky Mountain Hospital for Children, Denver, CO; Clinical Professor of Surgery, Columbia University College of Physicians and Surgeons, Denver, CO 80111, USA

Jonathan C. Salo, MD
Division of Surgical Oncology, Department of General Surgery, Carolinas Medical Center, Charlotte, NC 20284, USA

Carol B. Sheridan, MD
Fellow, St. Vincent/Indiana University Fellowship in Advanced Laparoscopy, Endoscopy and Ultrasound, Department of Surgery, Indiana University, St. Vincent Hospital/Clarian North Hospital, Indianapolis, IN 46260, USA

Norio Shiraishi, MD
Associate Professor, Department of Surgery I, Oita University Faculty of Medicine, Yufu, Oita, 879-5593, Japan

David Sindram, MD, PhD
Department of General Surgery, Carolinas Medical Center, Charlotte, NC 28203, USA

Stephen M. Smeaton, MD
Department of General Surgery, Carolinas Medical Center, Charlotte, NC 28203, USA

James D. Smith, MB, BCh, BAO, MRCSI
Specialist Registrar, Professorial Surgical Unit, Trinity Centre for Health Sciences, Adelaide and Meath Hospitals incorporating the National Children's Hospital, Tallaght, Dublin 24, Ireland

Alexander Stojadinovic, MD
Vice Chairman, Department of Surgery, Walter Reed Army Medical Center, Washington, DC 20307, USA

Jang Wen Su, MBBS, MRCSED, MMed (Surgery), FRCSCTH, FAMS
Department of Thoracic and Cardiovascular Surgery, Cleveland Clinic, Cleveland, OH 44195, USA

Lee L. Swanstrom, MD
Clinical Professor of Surgery, Department of Surgery, Oregon Health Sciences University, Portland, OR 97210, USA

Chris M. Teigland, MD, FACS
Chairman, McKay Department of Urology, Carolinas Medical Center, Charlotte, NC; Clinical Professor of Surgery, University of Carolina at Chapel Hill, Charlotte, NC 28207, USA

Michael B. Ujiki, MD
Laparoscopic Management of Hepatobiliary Cancer, Department of Surgery, NorthShore University Health System, Evanston, IL 60201, USA

R. Matthew Walsh, MD
Professor of Surgery, Lerner College of Medicine, Case Western University, Cleveland, OH; Vice-Chairman, Department of General Surgery, Cleveland Clinic, Cleveland, OH 44195, USA

Thomas J. Watson, MD
Associate Professor of Surgery, Chief of Thoracic Surgery, Division of Thoracic and Foregut Surgery, Department of Surgery, University of Rochester Medical Center, Rochester, NY 14642, USA

Tonia M. Young-Fadok, MD, MS, FACS, FASCRS
Chair, Division of Colon and Rectal Surgery, Mayo Clinic, Phoenix, AZ 85054, USA

Part I

Introductory Issues

Indications and General Oncologic Principles

Frederick L. Greene

Contents

The cleaner and gentler the act of operation, the less pain the patient suffers, the smoother and quicker the convalescence, the more exquisite his healed wound, the happier his memory of the whole incident. (Moynihan [1])

Oncologic Principles

Before 1987, the laparoscope was considered an instrument that allowed only intraabdominal inspection and biopsy of lesions. With the introduction of laparoscopic cholecystectomy in the mid-1980s, the endoscopic technique has become an important method of performing minimal access surgical resection and lymph node staging, with application of other intraabdominal therapy such as thermal ablation of liver metastases. Laparoscopic staging has been applied to upper and lower gastrointestinal malignancies as well as tumors involving the pancreatobiliary tract. Although important in preoperative staging of abdominal cancer, the laparoscope has an even more important potential use in the identification of patients who will not benefit from open celiotomy for extirpation of tumor or bypass. Preoperative laparoscopic staging for esophageal and gastric cancer may identify patients with lymph node metastases whose disease would be understaged using traditional imaging techniques of computed tomography and percutaneous ultrasound.

The role of minimal access surgery for resection of malignant neoplasms has been widely debated and remains an area of controversy for surgical oncologists. The key issue is to ensure safe, complete oncologic resections and at the same time provide the additional benefits of the minimal access approach. The slow progress and acceptance of minimal access cancer surgery may be related to limitations in the

F.L. Greene, B.T. Heniford (eds.), *Minimally Invasive Cancer Management*,
DOI 10.1007/978-1-4419-1238-1_1,

skill, training, and experience in minimal access procedures specific to surgical oncology. Institutions dedicated to cancer management and training of surgical oncologists have now begun to embrace minimal access procedures for surgical resection [2]. Because of major recent advances in systemic, regional cytotoxic, and biologic therapy, as well as nonresectional ablation techniques, the strict separation of curative and palliative surgical intervention has been somewhat obscured. Metastasectomy and cytoreductive surgery often include patients in whom the intent is less likely cancer cure and more centered on the intent to prolong life with cancer and improve quality of life. It is in this context that minimal access surgical approaches may have a significant role by way of providing less traumatic and debilitating surgery when life span is limited and surgery is likely non-curative.

The management of cancer is a primary focus not only for the general surgeon but also for surgeons in many specialty areas. Despite the significant improvements in multimodality treatment over the last several decades, the extirpation of solid tumors continues to be the primary method of treating patients with cancer. Currently, neoadjuvant applications of chemotherapy and radiation are used to shrink tumor size or to "sterilize" the systemic circulation before removal of bulk tumors [3]. The improvement in the cancer patient is still dependent on the ability to remove solid cancers, because the consequence of leaving residual tumor in place is incurability. The primary indication for any diagnostic modality is to obtain information that may provide pathologic certainty and data relating to the stage of the cancer. The sixth edition of the *Tumor, Node, Metastasis (TNM) Staging Manual* [4] as well as the newly released seventh edition [5] developed by the American Joint Committee on Cancer in concert with the International Union Against Cancer (UICC) provides staging strategies that relate to most solid tumors.

Indications for Diagnostic Laparoscopy

Diagnostic laparoscopy is used in the evaluation of patients with primary abdominal malignancy or metastatic tumors that involve abdominal solid organs. The ability of current radiographic and isotopic studies to identify small areas of tumor is considerable; however, the false-negative rate of these studies warrants recommending intraabdominal evaluation prior to open celiotomy. Laparoscopic diagnostic techniques have been used predominantly to assess hepatocellular tumors [6], pancreatic neoplasms [7], esophageal cancers [8], gastric cancers [9], and non-solid tumors such as Hodgkin's lymphoma, which may primarily involve the abdomen. A primary indication for diagnostic laparoscopy is to identify patients who may not benefit from major open abdominal operations, and patients likely to have small metastases or cytology positive for cancer, which increases the likelihood of early recurrence and a poor survival. Very poor outcomes have generally occurred in patients with adenocarcinoma of the pancreas, which supports the conclusion that most patients with tumor outside of the pancreas do not benefit from extensive operations and organ extirpation. Studies have shown that positive cytology is apparent in these patients by the time pancreaticoduodenectomy is considered [10]. Similar results have been reported in patients with gastric adenocarcinoma [11]. The continued use of diagnostic laparoscopy will no doubt lead to further knowledge about the natural history and the primary methods of dissemination of abdominal tumors. The absolute role for the laparoscope as a diagnostic tool will be confirmed by well-designed, randomized, prospective studies, which most likely will conclude that endoscopic evaluation provides information that cannot be obtained even by current radiographic imaging. Further subsets of patients will be identified who may benefit from systemic chemotherapy especially when cytology is positive for cancer or when small peritoneal implants of tumor are identified prior to open exploration.

Although laparoscopy is not considered a primary modality of staging for most abdominal tumors, endoscopic staging is built on the sound principles gained during the era when exploratory laparotomy was the diagnostic and staging mainstay for the surgeon. Preoperative imaging continues to improve rapidly with technology developments. Currently surgeons can precisely judge the local, regional, and metastatic behavior of specific cancers with an abundance of studies. Modern clinical staging relies on high-grade functional and anatomic imaging studies such as multi-slice CT, endoscopic ultrasonography (EUS), MRI, and PET imaging alone or in combination with CT. The role of laparoscopy in the staging of gastrointestinal cancers continues to be debated as these radiologic and nuclear medicine techniques improve. Laparoscopy can also be augmented with intraoperative ultrasound to assess the liver parenchyma and to map local tumor characteristics. The intellectual case for staging laparoscopy can be made for cancers where other imaging modalities may understage disease by missing metastatic implants due to location, size, or inability to delineate a tumor's local extent. Initially, staging laparoscopy was described primarily in patients with esophageal, gastric, and pancreatic primaries. Diagnostic laparoscopy has also been useful in the staging of gallbladder cancer or establishing a diagnosis in cases of peritoneal disease with an unknown primary. There are currently no evidence-based medical (EBM) guidelines, such as a Cochrane analysis, to guide surgeons in this decision. The best evidence available to surgeons in real time is the National Comprehensive Network Practice Guidelines (NCCN), which are consensus documents updated yearly which outline cancer-specific algorithms that cover from workup through treatment [12].

The definitive role of diagnostic laparoscopy with or without ultrasonography is evolving as other non-invasive examinations such as CT, EUS, and PET/CT progress in their resolution and detection. Diagnostic laparoscopy has a role where there is a significant chance of peritoneal implants or surface hepatic lesions that are not well imaged with current techniques. Gastric and gallbladder cancers represent the "best case" examples for the role of laparoscopy in staging of these malignancies. One of the most difficult problems involves scheduling issues. If laparoscopic evaluation is performed as the first portion of a planned resection and is found to preclude a resection, then a large block of operating room time remains unused. On the other hand, if laparoscopy is performed as a stand-alone procedure on a separate day preceding the resection, the patient has to undergo two general anesthetics and incur increased cost. Diagnostic laparoscopy, whenever performed, can be an important staging tool, especially in advanced cases where identification of patients with metastatic disease can save the patient a prolonged recovery and the health-care system the cost of an unnecessary laparotomy.

The laparoscopic technique to diagnose an abdominal tumor should be used when pathologic information is needed and staging of a solid organ or visceral tumor is required to plan overall treatment. Newer modalities of radiologic and isotopic diagnoses must be used in conjunction with laparoscopic methods to assure that patient risk is diminished and overall cost is justified. Consideration of laparoscopy is often made at the conclusion of a workup involving multiple studies including CT, magnetic resonance imaging, percutaneous ultrasound, and PET scanning. The better approach is to consider using laparoscopic diagnosis and staging in the initial patient workup. Diagnostic laparoscopy has risks similar to any procedure requiring general anesthesia or local–regional anesthetic. A complete history, including recent symptoms and pertinent cardiac and pulmonary complaints, is required to assure that patients undergoing diagnostic laparoscopy are not placed at inappropriate risk during this procedure. Since the application of pneumoperitoneum creates specific cardiopulmonary and metabolic effects (see Chapter 3), careful review of the patient's history and a physical examination are important before undergoing diagnostic laparoscopy.

Successful technique in laparoscopic resection of abdominal cancer must be built on a strong foundation of interpretation and skill in diagnostic laparoscopy. Because these techniques are currently performed using pneumoperitoneum with carbon dioxide insufflation, the consequences of resection in this unusual environment must be understood (see Chapter 3). Because of the relatively recent introduction of laparoscopic resection, the physiologic and oncologic ramifications are not yet fully known. Laparoscopic surgical treatment of abdominal and chest malignancies requires the same dedication to clean removal of organs and tissues as open surgery. Unfortunately, no universal standard has been developed for the appropriate resection of cancers using open celiotomy techniques. Standards relating to lymph node clearance, mesenteric dissection, creation of appropriate margins from the borders of solid and luminal cancers, and anastomotic techniques have not been delineated for the majority of cancers.

Surgeons are taught to be gentle in tumor handling to avoid dissemination of cells into the venous circulation. Concepts of "no touch" have reiterated that vascular control of tumor outflow may be important prior to mobilization of gross disease. There is no doubt that in the treatment of patients with gastrointestinal malignancy, appropriate recognition of draining lymphatic tissue is essential and that resection of draining lymph nodes will at least facilitate accurate overall staging. In the past, surgeons were taught that en bloc removal of cancer and contiguous tissue is important when cancer is in contact with adjacent structures. The literature suggests that overall stress to the patient caused by en bloc removal of the cancer, blood loss, and the potential need for transfusion may compromise the patient's immune system to a greater extent [13]. The avoidance of substantial blood loss during traditional open surgery is a well-established principle.

It is mandatory that the instrumentation used by the laparoscopic oncologic surgeon helps avoid perforation and subsequent spillage of tumor cells. Enhanced magnification and visualization of tumor planes help greatly with operations that require fascial dissection. Because soft tissue of the abdomen or chest wall may be contaminated by malignant cells, specimens removed during laparoscopic surgical procedures must be placed in an appropriate receptacle such as an impervious bag prior to removal. Current concern about the presumed risk of port-site recurrence following laparoscopic procedures indicates that this oncologic principle may not be consistently applied [14].

Various management concerns for patients with cancer apply equally to open and laparoscopic operations. Since it is known that most patients with cancer are hypercoagulable, appropriate prophylaxis against deep venous thrombosis is important [15]. Pneumatic compression stockings are essential in patients undergoing laparoscopic surgery, because creation of pneumoperitoneum retards venous outflow from the lower extremities [16]. In addition, the nutrition of cancer patients as it relates to wound healing, immunocompetence, and hypoalbuminemia is important in both groups of patients. Appropriate use of enteral and peripheral nutrition supplementation is mandatory in patients with tumor cachexia. Establishment, if possible, of a normal serum albumin is crucial before a patient undergoes a major cancer operation using general anesthesia.

Immunologic Consequences of the Surgical Approach

Prior to the laparoscopic era, it had been well established that major open surgery is associated with the temporary suppression of a variety of cells that are involved with both innate and specific immunity including lymphocytes, neutrophils, monocytes, and macrophages. In addition, interactions between cells and other cellular functions are negatively influenced by open surgical trauma. Further, the ability to mount a positive response to a delayed-type hypersensitivity (DTH) recall antigen challenge is suppressed after surgery [17].

The relative contribution of each part of an abdominal procedure (abdominal wall access incision versus intraabdominal dissection and resection) to the post-surgical immunosuppression had not been assessed prior to the advent of advanced laparoscopic methods. The results of recent studies suggest that the method of entry into the abdomen is an important determinant of postoperative immune function. Minimally invasive methods, for a variety of immune parameters, have been shown to be associated with significantly better preserved function when compared to the equivalent open procedure. Of note, in many cases the differences are small and short lived, on the order of a day, and sometimes less for several variables. For a number of parameters no differences have been noted.

What is it about abdominal surgery that causes temporary suppression of the immune system? There are probably a number of contributing factors. There is evidence that the overall length of an abdominal wall incision is an important factor. Others [18], based on the results of a murine study, believe that the exposure of the abdominal cavity to air is the cause of the immunosuppression after open surgery. These latter investigators believe that small amounts of lipopolysaccharide (LPS) in the air cause immunosuppression by stimulating bacteria in the intestine to elaborate LPS which then translocates across the bowel wall after which it is absorbed systemically.

The controversy surrounding laparoscopic surgery for cancer has led to studies that have significantly increased our understanding of a surgical procedure's impact on the body. This will hopefully lead to new perioperative pharmacologic therapies that will lessen the deleterious immunologic effects of all types of surgery. An example of this type of approach is to administer immunostimulatory agents perioperatively to cancer patients. Such treatment in small animal studies has been shown to be associated with significantly lower tumor recurrence and metastases rates [19]. Mels et al. [20] in a small randomized trial of 16 open surgery patients demonstrated that perioperative doses of GMCSF (granulocyte–macrophage colony stimulating factor) were associated with significantly better preserved postoperative DTH responses and HLA-DR expression on monocytes than placebo. GMCSF is usually used as a bone marrow rescue agent in chemotherapy patients. A similar randomized human study of perioperative immunomodulation carried out at Columbia University in the setting of colorectal cancer has been published [21]. GMCSF was given daily for 3 days before surgery and then for the first four postoperative days (PODs) to patients undergoing minimally invasive surgery. The goal was to up-regulate immune function perioperatively and also to determine the impact of this treatment. The drug was well tolerated and was not associated with any discernible complications. Unlike the Mels study, the Columbia study did not demonstrate significantly better immune function after GMCSF treatment as measured by serial DTH responses, number of DR+ monocytes, an array of Th1/Th2 cytokines, or plasma IFN-γ levels. One possible reason for these findings may be that it was much harder to demonstrate immune benefits for the GMCSF group, because the immune function of the control patients (all laparoscopic patients) was better preserved than in the open surgery control of the Mels study, which demonstrated more dramatic decreases in the immune parameters followed. An unexpected and noteworthy finding of this GMCSF study was that it clearly demonstrated that GMCSF results in significantly higher soluble VEGF-receptor 1 levels and a significantly higher angiopoietin 1/angiopoietin 2 ratio on POD5 than in the control group. Further, post-GMCSF blood on POD5 was shown to significantly decrease endothelial cell proliferation and invasion in in vitro cultures. These results suggest that angiogenesis is inhibited by GMCSF.

Vascular endothelial growth factor (VEGF) is a potent inducer of angiogenesis, which is critical for wound healing, and plays a crucial role in the early steps in angiogenesis. It is logical to anticipate that plasma levels increase after major surgery. VEGF has also been shown to facilitate and to promote tumor growth. It has been demonstrated that many tumors, including colonic adenocarcinoma, cannot grow beyond 2–3 mm in size without the development of new blood vessels. When groups of cancer patients were evaluated pre-resection, their mean serum and plasma VEGF levels were significantly greater than the mean values of control populations without tumors [22, 23]. The height of the elevation for some tumors, including colon, correlates with the stage of disease and/or prognosis in some series.

What impact does surgery have on blood VEGF levels? A postoperative increase in plasma VEGF levels may facilitate tumor growth early after surgery. Early postoperative plasma VEGF levels were studied in the setting of both open and minimally invasive colorectal resection for cancer and for benign indications [24]. In the open cancer patients, a significant and stepwise increase was noted on POD1 and POD3 compared with preoperative levels. In the laparoscopic patients, on POD3 a significant VEGF increase was also noted over baseline. Notably the mean laparoscopic value, although increased, was significantly lower than that noted in the open group at the same timepoint. No increase was noted on POD1 in the closed group. Although the benign colorectal resection group's baseline VEGF levels were lower than the cancer group, their response to surgery was very similar: a steady increase in the open group and a delayed and blunted increase in the laparoscopic group.

An additional study [25] assessed plasma VEGF levels for the first postoperative month after laparoscopic colorectal resection for benign (30 patients) and malignant disease (49 patients). In the cancer patients, VEGF levels continued to rise and peaked during the third postoperative week. Significant elevations were noted from POD3 through the fourth postoperative week. Similar, yet lower and less persistent elevations were noted in the patients with benign disease (values peaked during the second week). To date, this is the first surgery-related plasma protein alteration that has been demonstrated to persist for this length of time. Whether levels for open colorectal resection patients would be similar remains to be shown. Although it is possible that open patients will manifest even greater plasma VEGF elevations, it is more likely that open patients will demonstrate similar elevations. Thus, the transient, 1- to 2-day delay in VEGF increase observed after closed surgery may be of little significance in light of the long duration of the effect.

Minimally invasive surgery is associated with less-marked perturbations of the immune system. It is desirable to maintain baseline immune function and status; thus laparoscopic surgery may be preferable to open methods from this vantage point. Better clinical data with regard to short-term or long-term outcome measures are needed that demonstrate advantages for the minimally invasive patients.

Lower wound infection rates and morbidity rates have been reported by some investigators [26]; these results may be the clinical reflection of better preserved immune function. The shorter length of stay may also, in some way, be related; however, this has not been proven and would be difficult to demonstrate.

Specific Organ Sites

Pancreatic Malignancy

Laparoscopy for staging of pancreatic malignancy is considered a category 2B recommendation as defined by NCCN consensus based on lower level evidence including clinical experience [27]. This opinion was based on a literature review of primarily small, clinical, single institution reports. In these studies laparoscopy was reported to be helpful in identification of peritoneal implants or surface studding on the liver or intestinal serosa. Many surgeons consider tumor location (body or tail lesions), significant CA 19-9 elevations, and large primaries as an indication for laparoscopy, because the potential to identify unresectable patients is greater in this subset of patients. Peritoneal washings for cytologic examination have been performed by multiple groups [10], but there is no consensus as to whether this should be done routinely if laparoscopy is performed. Although positive cytologic washing indicates M1 disease (stage IV) [4], there is disagreement whether this indicates an absolute reason to avoid resection [28]. Ultrasonography is advocated as an additional modality to gain more information regarding the location and relationship of the primary cancer to surrounding vascular structures.

Gastric Cancer

Laparoscopic evaluation of gastric cancer is also considered a category 2B recommendation in the NCCN practice guidelines [29]. It is recommended for patients prior to resection or referral for chemoradiation protocols. Gastric cancer has a greater likelihood of peritoneal implants than other cancers and this may explain why many centers use laparoscopy in the operative staging algorithm of these patients. A series from Memorial Sloan Kettering [9] examined the role of laparoscopy in detection of unknown peritoneal disease in patients with advanced gastric cancers with no evidence of metastatic disease on preoperative imaging. More than one-third (37%) of the patients were found to have unsuspected metastatic disease at the time of laparoscopy and were not resected.

Esophageal Cancer

Initially there was great enthusiasm for laparoscopy in the staging of esophageal malignancies, but some of the enthusiasm waned after the development of endoscopic ultrasound with ability to use fine needle aspiration (FNA) to definitively determine nodal status. In the most recent NCCN practice guideline, there is no mention or recommendation of laparoscopy in the document [30]. This is counter to the opinion held by the group at the University of Pittsburgh which has the largest United States experience in minimally invasive esophagectomy. They compared EUS with FNA to laparoscopic staging with examination of the peritoneum, liver capsule, stomach, and lesser sac [31]. Results demonstrated that 17% of patients were found to have metastatic disease at the time of laparoscopy that was not suspected. Laparoscopy was able to correctly stage patients who had suspicious nodes on imaging, but could not be biopsied by EUS. Their conclusion was that staging laparoscopy should be performed in patients who are being considered for neoadjuvant protocols and in those referred directly for resection.

Gallbladder Cancer

Patients who are found to have incidental cancers at the time of cholecystectomy that are T1b (invasion of muscle layer) or greater on pathologic exam should be strongly considered for diagnostic laparoscopy prior to definitive resection [32]. Gallbladder cancer has a proclivity to seed the peritoneum, surgical wounds, and laparoscopic port sites and can be overlooked in working up advanced cases. Peritoneal seeding from spillage of gallbladder contents can also lead to the finding of extensive seeding throughout the peritoneal cavity at the time of operation. The current NCCN practice guideline recognizes this finding and recommends strong consideration of laparoscopy before resection [33].

General principles in minimal access oncologic surgery eventually are directed to the specific tumor sites. Discussions regarding diagnostic and therapeutic issues by tumor site appear in Parts II–IV of this volume. The treatment of neoplastic lesions of specific organ sites differs from treatment of corresponding benign lesions with regard to the extent of resection and the consequences of shedding malignant cells during dissection.

Currently the most common use of minimal access techniques in cancer management is in the resection of colorectal cancer. Isolated reports [34, 35] of colonic resection led to single [36] and multi-institutional [37, 38] studies, which have attempted to develop algorithms and specific treatment plans. Anatomic studies in animals [39] have laid the groundwork for standardized human dissection [40]. These studies have shown that laparoscopic right hemicolectomy, sigmoid resection, and abdominal perineal removal of rectal cancer can be performed safely and to the same extent as open operations [37]. The short-term follow-up in these patients reveals an initial improved quality of life, lower rate of postoperative complications, reduction in postoperative pain, quicker return to eating, and a reduced length of hospital stay following laparoscopic colorectal procedures [41]. Traditional oncologic parameters such as the extent of nodal dissection and distance from tumor margins appear to be met in several reports of laparoscopic colon cancer management [37, 41]. Five-year follow-up has been reported in well-done clinical trials, which support the safety and efficacy of laparoscopic resection of colon cancer [41]. Relapse rates are similar to open resection techniques.

The oncologic benefits noted by the above reports do not lessen the importance of placing patients on well-structured, randomized studies to fully assess the possible laparoscopic-associated, long-term risks to the cancer patient. Franklin et al. [41] performed a prospective, but not randomized, study comparing recurrence rates after 193 laparoscopic resections with those after 224 open resections of colorectal cancer. No significant differences were identified after stratifying patients according to tumor stage. Similar results were reported in patients treated in the Clinical Outcomes of Surgical Therapy (COST) Study Group [37]. The authors reported locoregional and systemic recurrence rates of 3.5 and 10.1%, respectively, after a follow-up extending to 3 years. In these patients, trocar-site metastases were observed in four patients (1.08%).

In contrast to the feasibility of laparoscopic resection of colorectal cancer, attempts at resection of pancreatic cancer have not supported the routine application of this technique. Although not proven as an oncologic risk, the length of operative and anesthesia times required to accomplish such an undertaking may outweigh the benefits of improved pulmonary function and reduced abdominal wall trauma observed with laparoscopic surgery. Cuschieri [42] recognized the mismatch between the advantage of laparoscopic access and the complexity of the intervention necessary for pancreatoduodenectomy and concluded that laparoscopic resection offers no substantial benefit to the patient.

Surgeons using laparoscopic techniques for diagnosis and treatment of cancer must be skilled in using both the open and laparoscopic techniques. The need for conversion from a laparoscopic to an open operation is common and may, in fact, create an oncologic risk in these patients. The decision as to which patients should undergo laparoscopic and which should undergo open operations remains in the purview and surgical judgment of the operating surgeon.

References

1. Moynihan B (1920) The ritual of a surgical operation. Br J Surg 8:27
2. Are C, Brennan MF, D'Angelica M et al (2008) Current role of therapeutic laparoscopy and thoracoscopy in the management of malignancy: a review of trends from a tertiary care cancer center. J Am Coll Surg 206:709–718
3. Evans DB, Varadhachary GR, Crane CH et al (2008) Preoperative gemcitabine-based chemoradiation for patients with resectable adenocarcinoma of the pancreatic head. J Clin Oncol 26:3496–3502
4. Greene FL, Page DL, Fleming ID et al (eds) (2002) AJCC cancer staging manual, 6th edn. Springer, New York, NY
5. AJCC (2009) Cancer staging manual, 7th edn. Springer, New York, NY
6. John TG, Greig JD, Crosbie JL, Miles WF, Garden OJ (1994) Superior staging of liver tumors with laparoscopy and laparoscopic ultrasound. Ann Surg 220:711–719
7. Conlon KC, Dougherty E, Klimstra DS, Coit DG, Turnbull AD, Brennan MF (1996) The value of minimal access surgery in the staging of patients with potentially resectable peripancreatic malignancy. Ann Surg 223:134–140
8. Krasna MJ, Flowers JL, Attar S, McLaughlin J (1996) Combined thoracoscopic/laparoscopic staging of esophageal cancer. J Thorac Cardiovasc Surg 111:800–807
9. Burke EC, Karpeh MS, Conlon KC, Brennan MF (1997) Laparoscopy in the management of gastric adenocarcinoma. Ann Surg 225:262–267
10. Warshaw A (1991) Implications of peritoneal cytology for staging of early pancreatic cancer. Am J Surg 161:26–30
11. Ribeiro U Jr, Gama-Rodrigues JJ, Safatle-Ribeiro AV et al (1998) Prognostic significance of intraperitoneal free cancer cells obtained by laparoscopic peritoneal lavage in patients with gastric cancer. J Gastrointest Surg 2:244–249
12. National Comprehensive Network. Clinical practice guidelines in oncology. http://www.nccn.org. Accessed August 21, 2008
13. Busch OR, Hop WC, Hoynck van Papendrecht MA, Marquet RL, Jeekel J (1993) Blood transfusions and prognosis in colorectal cancer. N Engl J Med 328:1372–1376
14. Vukasin P, Ortega AE, Greene FL et al (1996) Wound recurrence following laparoscopic colon cancer resection. Results of the American Society of Colon and Rectal Surgeons Laparoscopic Registry. Dis Colon Rectum 39:S20–S23
15. Beebe DS, McNevin MP, Crain JM et al (1993) Evidence of venous stasis after abdominal insufflation for laparoscopic cholecystectomy. Surg Gynecol Obstet 176:443–447
16. Caprini JA, Arcelus JI, Laubach M et al (1995) Postoperative hypercoagulability and deep-vein thrombosis after laparoscopic cholecystectomy. Surg Endosc 9:304–309
17. Whelan RL, Franklin M, Holubar SD et al (2003) Postoperative cell mediated immune response is better

preserved after laparoscopic versus open colorectal resection in humans. Surg Endosc 17:972–978
18. Watson RW, Redmond HP, McCarthy J, Burke PE, Hayes DB (1995) Exposure of the peritoneal cavity to air regulates early inflammatory responses to surgery in a murine model. Br J Surg 82:1060–1065
19. Heys SD, Deehan DJ, Eremin O (1994) Interleukin-2 treatment in colorectal cancer: current results and future prospects. Eur J Surg Oncol 20:622–629
20. Mels AK, Statius Muller MG, van Leeuwen PA et al (2001) Immune-stimulating effects of low-dose perioperative recombinant granulocyte-macrophage colony-stimulating factor in patients operated on for primary colorectal carcinoma. Br J Surg 88:539–544
21. Kirman I, Belizon A, Balik E et al (2007) Perioperative sargramostim (recombinant human GM-CSF) induces an increase in the level of soluble VEGFR1 in colon cancer patients undergoing minimally invasive surgery. Eur J Surg Oncol 33:1169–1176
22. Werther K, Christensen IJ, Brunner N, Nielsen HJ (2000) Soluble vascular endothelial growth factor levels in patients with primary colorectal carcinoma. The Danish RANX05 Colorectal Cancer Study Group. Eur J Surg Oncol 26: 657–662
23. Karayiannakis AJ, Syrigos KN, Zbar A (2002) Clinical significance of preoperative serum vascular endothelial growth factor levels in patients with colorectal cancer and the effect of tumor surgery. Surgery 131:548–555
24. Belizon A, Balik E, Feingold DL et al (2006) Major abdominal surgery increases plasma levels of vascular endothelial growth factor: open more so than minimally invasive methods. Ann Surg 244:792–798
25. Belizon A, Horst P, Balik E et al (2008) Persistent elevation of plasma VEGF levels during the first month following minimally invasive colorectal resection. Surg Endosc 22:287–297
26. Neuhaus SJ, Watson DI (2004) Pneumoperitoneum and peritoneal surface changes: a review. Surg Endosc 18: 1316–1322
27. National Comprehensive Cancer Network. Pancreatic cancer guidelines. Clinical practice guidelines in oncology. http://www.nccn.org. Accessed 21 Aug 2008
28. Ferrone CR, Haas B, Tang L et al (2006) The influence of positive peritoneal cytology on survival on patients with pancreatic adenocarcinoma. J Gastrointest Surg 10: 1347–1353
29. National Comprehensive Cancer Network. Gastric cancer guidelines. Clinical cancer guidelines in oncology http://www.nccn.org. Accessed 21 Aug 2008
30. National Comprehensive Cancer Network. Esophageal cancer guideline. Clinical practice guidelines in oncology. http://www.nccn.org. Accessed 21 Aug 2008
31. Kaushik N, Khalid A, Brody D, Luketich J, McGrath K (2007) Endoscopic ultrasound compared with laparoscopy for staging esophageal cancer. Ann Thorac Surg 83: 2000–2002
32. Gourgiotis S, Kocher HM, Solaini L, Yarollahi A, Tsiambas E, Salemis NS (2008) Gallbladder cancer. Am J Surg 196:252–264
33. National Comprehensive Cancer Network. Guidelines for hepatobiliary cancer. Clinical practice guidelines in oncology. http://www.nccn.org. Accessed 21 Aug 2008
34. Jacobs M, Verdeja JC, Goldstein DH (1991) Minimally invasive colon resection (laparoscopic colectomy). Surg Laparosc Endosc 1:144–150
35. Phillips EH, Franklin ME, Carroll BJ, Fallas MJ, Ramas R, Rosenthal D (1992) Laparoscopic colectomy. Ann Surg 216:703–707
36. Franklin ME, Rosenthal D, Norem RF (1995) Prospective evaluation of laparoscopic colon resection versus open colon resection for adenocarcinoma. A multicenter study. Surg Endosc 9:811–816
37. Fleshman J, Sargent DJ, Green E et al (2007) Laparoscopic colectomy for cancer is not inferior to open surgery based on 5-year data from the COST Study Group trial. Ann Surg 246:655–664
38. Veldkamp R, Kuhry E, Hop WC et al (2005) Colon cancer laparoscopic or open resection study group (COLOR). Laparoscopic surgery versus open surgery for colon cancer; short-term outcomes of a randomized trial. Lancet Oncol 6:477–484
39. Böhm B, Milsom JW, Kitago K, Brand M, Stolfi VM, Fazio VW (1995) Use of laparoscopic techniques in oncologic right colectomy in a canine model. Ann Surg Oncol 2:6–13
40. Nelson H, Petrelli N, Carlin A et al (2001) Guidelines 2000 for colon and rectal surgery. J Natl Cancer Inst 93:583–596
41. Franklin ME, Rosenthal D, Abrego-Medina D et al (1996) Prospective comparison of open vs. laparoscopic colon surgery for carcinoma. Five year results. Dis Colon Rectum 39:S35–S46
42. Cuschieri A (1994) Laparoscopic surgery of the pancreas. J R Coll Surg Edinb 39:178–184

Chapter 2

Cancer Biology Relating to Minimal Access Management

Jonathan C. Salo

Contents

The introduction of laparoscopic colon resection for colon carcinoma in the 1990s was accompanied by a series of case reports of port site recurrences which appeared to occur with alarming frequency [1–8]. These reports tempered the initial enthusiasm for laparoscopic colectomy for colon cancer. They also prompted several lines of laboratory and clinical investigation, including animal experiments which attempted to replicate the cancer biology of laparoscopic cancer surgery, prospective accumulation of data regarding laparoscopic colon resection, and finally the organization and execution of several large-scale randomized clinical trials comparing laparoscopic and open resection for colorectal cancer.

After the initial series of case reports, the American Society of Colon and Rectal Surgeons laparoscopic registry of a series of 480 patients reported a port site recurrence rate of 1.1% [9], which was more in line with the expected wound recurrence rate after open colon resection. Subsequently, a number of large randomized trials were organized which compared laparoscopic resection with open resection for colon carcinoma. A recent meta-analysis of these trials concluded that there was no detectable difference between the two groups in terms of overall survival, cancer-specific survival, or local recurrence after a minimum of 3 years of follow-up [10]. Although some uncertainty exists regarding the equivalence of laparoscopic and open resection for rectal cancer (as opposed to colon cancer), the initial concerns about laparoscopic surgery being inherently unsafe for cancer surgery resection appear to not be borne out in these clinical trials.

Although the controversy regarding the suitability of laparoscopy for resection of colon carcinoma has been settled, there remains a need for tools and approaches to evaluate the application of new technology to cancer surgery. Settling the controversy regarding laparoscopic resection for colon carcinoma

F.L. Greene, B.T. Heniford (eds.), *Minimally Invasive Cancer Management*,
DOI 10.1007/978-1-4419-1238-1_2,

required the execution of several large (and time consuming and expensive) randomized clinical trials. In the evaluation of cancer treatment, tumor recurrence and survival are the most important endpoints, but can require substantial follow-up time to acquire sufficient data to draw comparative conclusions. As new technology for cancer surgery becomes available, it will be important to establish reliable clinical prognosticators which can serve as intermediate endpoints which can shorten the 'development cycle' of advances in clinical care. Equally important will be the development of robust animal models which will help guide the development of new therapies and explain mechanisms of cancer treatment and recurrence.

This chapter will review some of the animal studies which have attempted to develop experimental models of minimally invasive cancer surgery and will review clinical studies which have examined the interaction between cancer biology and minimally invasive surgery.

Systemic Effects of Minimally Invasive Surgery

As early as the 1950s, laparotomy was shown to increase the growth of tumors at distant sites in experimental animals. Fisher et al. [11] found that rats injected intraportally with carcinoma cells were resistant to hepatic metastasis, even up to 5 months after inoculation. If similarly treated mice were subjected to repeated laparotomy at 3 months, however, they were all found to develop hepatic tumors within several weeks of surgery. In that same era, carcinoma cells were implanted into the flank of rats subjected to sham laparotomy or control animals. The rats treated with laparotomy after tumor inoculation were more likely to have tumor take (62% vs. 32%) and had shorter survival [12]. Similar experiments showed that both thoracotomy and laparotomy increased the development of lung metastases in rats after intravenous inoculation [13]. Subsequent experiments suggested that some of this effect may be mediated by the systemic effects of pain generated by the laparotomy. Experiments in rats suggested that reducing the pain of surgery with spinal anesthesia mitigated the promotion of tumor at a distant site [14]. Similar effects were found in a murine hepatic metastasis model, in which spinal anesthesia reduced tendency for laparotomy to promote liver metastasis after intravenous injection of EL4 thymoma cells [15].

With the advent of laparoscopic cancer surgery, the promotion by laparotomy of tumor growth at distant sites was investigated further to determine whether laparoscopy might mitigate these adverse systemic oncologic effects. Several animal studies have compared the systemic effects of laparoscopy compared with laparotomy on the promotion of tumor growth at a distant site. C3H mice received an intradermal injection of the MMC mouse mammary carcinoma in the dorsal skin followed by either anesthesia alone, carbon dioxide insufflation, air insufflation, or laparotomy [16]. While there was no difference in tumor size between the two insufflation groups and the anesthesia-alone control group, the animals treated with laparotomy had tumors 1.5 times larger than the other groups at 12 days. These experiments were repeated with CT26 colon carcinoma in BALB/c mice and B16 melanoma in C57BL/6 mice with similar results [17]. A model of laparoscopy in the presence of pulmonary metastases used the intravenous injection of CT26 colon carcinoma cells in BALB/c mice. After tumor injection, mice were treated with a 3 cm laparotomy, carbon dioxide insufflation, or anesthesia alone. The lung weight and number of pulmonary metastases were significantly greater in the laparotomy group than the insufflation or anesthesia-alone groups. The carbon dioxide insufflation group had growth of tumor similar to that of the anesthesia control. A model of pulmonary metastatic disease evaluated the effects of open and laparoscopic colon resection in A/J mice [18]. Mice were subjected to anesthesia alone followed by either open cecal resection or laparoscopic cecal resection with carbon dioxide pneumoperitoneum. After surgery all mice received a tail vein injection of TA3-Ha mammary carcinoma cells and pulmonary metastases were evaluated 14 days later. Both the laparoscopic and the open resection groups had more metastases than the anesthesia control, but the open resection group had significantly more metastases than the laparoscopic resection group. A model of laparoscopy in the context of 'spontaneous' pulmonary metastases used B16 melanoma in C57BL/6 mice. In this model, excision of the tumor once it had become palpable resulted in the formation of pulmonary metastases 15 days later. After tumor excision, mice were treated with laparotomy, carbon dioxide insufflation at 4–6 mmHg, or anesthesia alone. The number of pulmonary metastases was higher in the insufflation group than the control group, but the laparotomy group had more metastases than the insufflation group [19]. BALB/c mice inoculated intravenously with 4T1 mammary carcinoma cells were then treated with carbon dioxide insufflation or laparotomy. Significantly more tumor grew in the laparotomy group than the insufflation group [20]. In all, these animal studies have suggested an advantage of laparoscopy over laparotomy as evidenced by enhanced tumor growth at distant sites due to laparotomy and an improvement in these adverse effects by laparoscopy. Attempts have been made to explain these differences based upon systemic cytokines, systemic growth factors, and systemic immune responses.

Effects of Minimally Invasive Surgery on Systemic Cytokines

Laparotomy, and to a lesser extent laparoscopy, stimulates an acute phase response mediated by the elaboration of tumor necrosis factor-alpha (TNFα (alpha)) and interleukin-1 beta (IL-1β (beta)) from macrophages and monocytes at the site of tissue injury. This transient release of cytokines is followed by a more sustained release of interleukin-6 (IL-6), which increases postoperatively beginning within 1 h after surgery, with a peak between 2 and 4 h, followed by normalization within a few days. IL-6 serves as a growth factor for B cells and stimulates the production of hepatic acute phase proteins, including C-reactive protein (CRP). CRP is produced by the liver and activates the complement cascade and stimulates phagocytosis by tissue macrophages and neutrophils. The initial cytokines trigger a cascade of additional cytokines which can last for up to several weeks after surgery [21]. The magnitude of the systemic acute phase response appears to be related to the magnitude of the surgical intervention [22].

Multiple clinical studies have examined the hypothesis that laparoscopy may be associated with a less dramatic acute phase reaction than open surgery. Several clinical studies have examined serum IL-6 levels after open compared with laparoscopic colectomy. Delgado et al. [23] found serum IL-6 to be significantly higher at 4, 12, and 24 h after open compared with laparoscopic colectomy. A report from Hong Kong comparing cytokines in laparoscopic vs. open colectomy found significantly higher levels of IL-6 after open colectomy, which peaked at 2 h after surgery [24]. IL-1β was also elevated in the open resection group compared with the laparoscopic resection group. Several similar reports confirm a blunted postoperative peak in IL-6 after open compared with laparoscopic colectomy [25–28].

Serum CRP levels are elevated after surgery and appear in many studies to be less elevated after laparoscopic colectomy compared with open colectomy [23–26] while other studies have failed to show differences in these cytokines [29–31]. Serum CRP was significantly more elevated after open distal gastrectomy than laparoscopic-assisted distal gastrectomy at postoperative days 2, 10, and 40 [32]. Although several studies have shown a blunted acute phase response in patients undergoing laparoscopic resection compared with open surgery, it remains unclear what relationship, if any, this has relative to the biology of cancer establishment and growth.

The differences in acute phase proteins between laparoscopy and open surgery have spawned a variety of lines of investigation in animals and patients which might link these changes to the risk of cancer growth or recurrence. The insulin-like growth factor 'axis' is a complex of two growth factors (IGF-I and IGF-II), the activity of which is modulated by a family of six circulating growth factor binding proteins. Epidemiologic evidence links increased levels of IGF-I and insulin-like growth factor binding protein 3 (IGFBP-3) to an increased risk of colorectal cancer. IGFBP-3 appears to inhibit the growth of a variety of cell lines both in vitro and in vivo [33]. Patients after open colon resection were found to have decreased levels of IGFBP-3 on the second postoperative day, which was not found in a group of patients undergoing laparoscopic surgery [34]. A study in human IGFBP-3 transgenic mice subjected to surgical intervention similarly found a decrease in IGFBP-3 levels in the laparotomy group which was not found in the pneumoperitoneum group [35]. The hypothesis has thus emerged that the decrease in IGFBP-3 levels after laparotomy may increase the amount of bioavailable IGF-I so that it might promote tumor growth in the immediate perioperative period.

Vascular endothelial growth factor (VEGF) is mitogenic for capillary endothelial cells in human and animal tumors and is the primary factor in angiogenesis, an essential step in carcinogenesis. Blockade of VEGF with agents such as bevacizumab has shown clinical efficacy in colorectal carcinoma and other gastrointestinal cancers. Serum VEGF is elevated after open surgery [36], and postoperative elevations are detectable for as long as 4 weeks after surgery [37]. A study of postoperative serum VEGF levels compared laparoscopic and open surgery in patients with benign colonic disease, colorectal cancer, and morbid obesity undergoing gastric bypass. Preoperative VEGF levels were elevated in the colorectal cancer patients compared with those with benign disease. All patient groups had elevated serum VEGF on postoperative day three. In open surgery patients, serum VEGF was elevated on postoperative day one but no elevation in VEGF was found at that same time in laparoscopic surgery patients [38].

Another element of the process of angiogenesis is endothelial progenitor cells derived from bone marrow that are critical to the formation of the new blood vessels required for the formation of metastatic foci [39]. Circulating endothelial progenitor cells have been found to be increased in the peripheral blood of patients with cancer [40]. In a murine model using C57BL/6 mice, laparoscopy was compared with laparotomy and control animals and the number of circulating endothelial progenitor cells was found to be higher in the laparotomy group [41]. In another model, 3LL Lewis lung tumors were implanted and then excised after laparotomy or laparoscopy, and the tumors homogenized and examined for the presence of endothelial progenitor cells. The laparotomy group had a larger percentage of endothelial progenitor cells within the tumors compared with the laparoscopy group [42].

In a search for mechanisms of how laparotomy promotes the growth of tumor at distant sites, investigators at Columbia University found that the serum of mice undergoing laparotomy caused much increased tumor cell proliferation in vitro of CT-26 murine colon carcinoma cells compared with serum from mice undergoing abdominal insufflation [43]. Fractionation of the serum of laparotomy-treated mice identified the mitogenic agent as platelet-derived growth factor (PDGF). Anti-PDGF antibody, when added to the serum of mice subjected to laparotomy, abrogated the in vitro mitogenic activity [44]. PDGF is known to complement the activity of VEGF in the formation of new blood vessels and can indirectly upregulate the expression of VEGF. PDGF is now under investigation as a target of anti-cancer therapies [45]. Taken together, the overexpression of PDGF after laparotomy is a plausible, yet unproven, mechanism by which the surgical stress of laparotomy may systemically promote tumor growth. It is yet untested whether laparoscopy may reduce serum PDGF levels compared with laparotomy.

In summary, minimally invasive surgery appears to elicit a blunted postoperative acute phase reaction compared with open surgery. The significance of this observation for cancer biology in these patients is not clear, but the findings of decreased levels in minimally invasive surgery patients of growth factors known to be associated with carcinogenesis are suggestive that further research may uncover a systemic benefit of minimally invasive surgery for patients with cancer.

Effects of Minimally Invasive Surgery on Systemic Immunity

The stress of surgery also can profoundly affect the components of cell-mediated immunity. The cellular immune system is comprised of complex interactions between B cells, neutrophils, T cells, macrophages/monocytes, dendritic cells, and NK cells. The delayed-type hypersensitivity reaction (DTH) is a nonspecific test of immune function which measures the cutaneous inflammation resulting from the injection of foreign antigen [46]. The DTH response appears to be dependent upon a complex interaction of immune effectors which predominantly includes the cellular (rather than humoral) immune system and is a significant prognosticators of cancer survival [47, 48]. Laparoscopy has been associated with better preservation of DTH responses both in animals [49–52] and in humans [53].

B Cells and Neutrophils

B cells secrete antibody and are important in anti-bacterial defenses and in conjunction with macrophages in antibody-dependent cellular cytotoxicity. Several studies have failed to show a difference in B cell numbers in peripheral blood after laparoscopic vs. open surgery [29, 54, 55].

Neutrophils are responsible for bacterial cell killing through phagocytosis and are an early component of acute inflammation and responses to infection. They migrate to sites of inflammation by following gradients of inflammatory cytokines such as interleukin-8 and interferon-γ (IFNγ (gamma)). A comparison between laparoscopic and open cholecystectomy patients showed increase in white blood cell count in the open surgery group which was accompanied by increases in neutrophil chemotaxis and superoxide release [56]. A clinical study of open surgery compared with laparoscopic surgery showed that neutrophil function declined significantly on the first postoperative day but had recovered by postoperative day six. The laparoscopic group did not have the same decline in postoperative neutrophil function [57].

T Cells

T cells are comprised of two subsets: CD8+ cytotoxic T cells and CD4+ helper T cells. CD8+ cytotoxic T cells recognize peptide fragments presented by the MHC class I cell surface receptor, which is present in most all cells. Helper T cells recognize peptide fragments presented by the MHC class II surface receptor HLA-DR and are further divided into the Th1 and Th2 subsets, which each elaborate a distinct subset of cytokines. Th1 cells secrete interleukin-2 (IL-2), IFNγ (gamma), and interleukin-12, which favors cell-mediated immunity, particularly the function of cytotoxic T cells. Th2 cells secrete interleukin-4, interleukin-5, interleukin-10, and interleukin-13 and favor humoral immunity and are generally suppressive of cytotoxic T cell function. The relationship between Th1/Th2 balance and cancer biology is complex, but most experimental models suggest that a Th1 response is preferable for tumor immunity. Perhaps the best evidence for the importance of the Th1/Th2 balance in tumor biology comes from gene array analysis of immune cells infiltrating colorectal cancer specimens. Based upon clusters of gene expression, patients whose tumors had a predominantly Th1 immune infiltrate had a better prognosis. The degree of Th1 vs. Th2 infiltrate was overall a stronger prognosticator for survival than the tumor stage [58].

Surgical trauma shifts the T cell balance from Th1 to Th2 immunity [59, 60]. Patients undergoing open cholecystectomy showed a reduction in IFNγ (gamma), while IFNγ (gamma) production increased in the laparoscopic cholecystectomy group, suggesting that laparoscopic cholecystectomy favors a Th1 response [61]. Another study of laparoscopic vs. open cholecystectomy showed decrease in the Th1 cytokines IL-2, IFNγ (gamma), and TNFα (alpha) in the open surgery group but no decrement in the laparoscopic surgery group [59]. Patients undergoing open distal gastrectomy were noted to have a decline in IFNγ (gamma) production (Th1) and increase in IL-4 production (Th2). Those treated with laparoscopic distal gastrectomy showed an increase in IFNγ (gamma) production without a change in IL-4 production [62]. Laparoscopic colectomy patients were found to have an increase in Th1 cytokines postoperatively, but not in the open or minilaparotomy groups [63]. In summary, these studies all suggest that laparoscopic surgery preserves a Th1 response among peripheral blood T helper cells.

Monocytes/Macrophages and Dendritic Cells

Peripheral monocytes and dendritic cells are responsible for the degradation of foreign proteins and the 'presentation' of short peptide fragments via the MHC class I receptor for the education of CD8+ cytotoxic T cells and via the MHC class II receptor HLA-DR for the education of CD4+ helper T cells. Dendritic cells are a small fraction of the cellular immune system with potent facility for activation of T cells through the expression of co-stimulatory molecules and secretion of lymphokines. The impact of laparoscopic vs. open surgery on HLA-DR expression on peripheral blood monocytes is inconsistent across studies. Hewitt compared laparoscopic and open colectomy patients and found that HLA-DR positive cells declined in both groups postoperatively with no differences between them [29]. In a comparison between laparoscopic and open surgery, HLA-DR expression in peripheral blood monocytes declined in both groups but recovered by postoperative day 7 in the laparoscopic group but not in the open group [55]. When laparoscopic cholecystectomy was compared with open cholecystectomy, a decrease in HLA-DR was seen in monocytes in both groups, with faster recovery of HLA-DR expression in the laparoscopic group [59]. Antigen presentation function, however, appeared similar between the two groups, as measured by the ability of peripheral monocytes to present bacterial superantigen to autologous T cells.

Natural Killer Cells

Natural killer (NK) cells are cytotoxic cells which recognize and kill transformed and infected cells. While CD8+ cytotoxic T cells rely on the MHC class I molecule for binding to target cells, NK cells selectively target cells which have down-regulated MHC class I expression, presumably to escape CD8+ cytotoxic cell recognition [64]. Natural killer cell reactivity is an important prognosticator for a variety of cancers. Peripheral NK cytotoxicity predicts recurrence in patients with colorectal cancer [65, 66] Intratumoral natural killer cells as assessed by immunohistochemistry are a strong prognosticator for colorectal cancers [67, 68] and for gastric cancer [69, 70].

In an animal model of NK activity in tumors, C57BL/6 mice with B16 melanoma injected in the flank received either laparotomy, insufflation, or anesthesia alone. Increase in flank tumor growth in the laparoscopy and laparotomy groups were observed at 48 h, but by 96 h tumors in the insufflation and laparoscopy groups were similar in size, but significantly larger in the laparotomy group. In these mice, splenocyte NK activity in the laparotomy group was significantly depressed at 48 and 96 h relative to the laparoscopy and anesthesia-alone groups [71]. Subsequent studies from the same investigators found that treatment of mice subjected to laparotomy with an immunostimulant appeared to ameliorate perioperative immunosuppression and improve survival in the treated mice [72].

In a comparative study of laparoscopic and open colectomy performed by Hewitt et al., NK cytotoxicity was found to decline in the postoperative period, but no differences were seen between the laparoscopic and open groups [29]. In a study of laparoscopic and open colectomy by Wichmann et al., NK cell counts declined in the postoperative period, but were significantly higher in patients undergoing laparoscopic resection [54].

In summary, open surgery is accompanied by a decline in systemic natural killer activity and a shift from Th1 to Th2 immunity. Both of these changes are assumed to be deleterious from the standpoint of cancer biology. The fact that these changes are blunted by minimally invasive surgery suggests a mechanism by which a minimally invasive approach may be advantage from the standpoint of systemic anti-tumor immunity.

Intraperitoneal Oncologic Effects

Laparoscopy is known to exert profound effects on the peritoneal cavity. In an attempt to understand the process of port site recurrence (PSR), a variety of studies have examined the effects of laparoscopy and its components on the growth of intraperitoneal tumor in animal models. These studies have been conducted in a wide variety of conditions with different controls and have reached a variety of diverging conclusions.

These studies have typically inoculated experimental animals with intraperitoneal tumor cells and then subjected them to a variety of surgical interventions including pneumoperitoneum with a variety of gases, laparoscopy with either gas insufflation or 'abdominal lift' technique, laparotomy, or anesthesia alone. Several studies have shown greater tumor growth after laparoscopy compared with laparotomy or anesthesia-alone controls [73–75] while several others have come to the opposite conclusion [76–83] while other studies have not shown a difference [84, 85]. The results from these animal studies must be viewed from the perspective that the rate of intraperitoneal and port site recurrence is not detectably different between open and laparoscopic colon resection.

The theoretical effects of laparoscopic surgery on intraperitoneal tumor recurrence are related to mechanical factors, factors related to the port site wounds, and effects of the pneumoperitoneum on tumor cells, the peritoneal cavity, and the peritoneal immune system.

Tumor Cell Shedding from the Primary Tumor

The first step in the pathogenesis of intraperitoneal tumor recurrence is the shedding of tumor cells from the operative specimen. Laparoscopic surgery differs from open surgery in the greater reliance on instruments for retraction and manipulation of the tumor and surrounding tissue. An illustrative clinical scenario is when an unsuspected gallbladder carcinoma is removed via laparoscopic cholecystectomy. Small series have shown a high rate of peritoneal and port site recurrence after laparoscopic cholecystectomy in this situation [5, 86–88] which has been reported to occur in up to 10 of 21 patients. By contrast, wound recurrences did not occur in any of 89 patients in whom a gallbladder harboring gallbladder carcinoma was removed via open technique [89]. A clinical study of laparoscopic cholecystectomy (for benign disease) has shown the appearance of gallbladder mucosal cells in the peritoneal cavity at the end of surgery in 6 of 15 patients [90]. These observations may shed light on a mechanism for port site metastasis of gallbladder carcinoma after laparoscopic cholecystectomy. They also suggest that careful handling of the tumor is important in clinical laparoscopic cancer surgery.

The effect of tumor manipulation on port site recurrence has been studied in several animal models. Mice were injected with CT26 tumor cells under the splenic capsule, forming a tumor within 7–10 days. A splenectomy was then performed with or without prior crushing of the spleen to simulate intraoperative trauma to the tumor. Subsequent to the splenectomy, half of the animals were subjected to carbon dioxide pneumoperitoneum. The mice with crushing of the tumor had significantly more tumor recurrences at the port site, and the incidence of tumor growth was independent of subsequent pneumoperitoneum [91]. The same investigators then compared open resection to laparoscopic resection with carbon dioxide pneumoperitoneum. They found that over the course of four experiments, the incidence of port site recurrence remained constant in the open surgery group, but declined in the laparoscopic group. This suggests that with experience, there may have been less traumatic handling of the tumor resulting in less shedding of tumor cells, with a resulting lower incidence of intraperitoneal recurrence [92, 93]. A rat model used the rectal administration of Tc-99m pertechnetate for intraluminal labeling of the colonic mucosal cells. Studies confirmed that the radioactivity was confined to the bowel lumen. A resection of the cecum was performed either intracorporeally or extracorporeally. Half of the animals underwent traumatic manipulation of the cecum prior to resection. Contamination of the port sites was then measured by excision of the port sites and counting their radioactivity. Manipulation of the cecum was found to dramatically increase the rate and intensity of contamination of the port sites [94]. A similar experimental model used GW-39 human colon carcinoma cells injected into the omentum of hamsters. Different groups were subjected to tumor bivalve, crush, strip, or excision, followed by pneumoperitoneum. All of the tumor manipulation groups showed higher rates of port site recurrence than the control groups without tumor manipulation. The addition of subsequent pneumoperitoneum did not affect the rate of port site recurrence [95]. In summary, tumor manipulation appears to be a major determinant of intraperitoneal tumor metastasis in animal models and may be a more important factor than pneumoperitoneum in these models.

Tumor Cell Dissemination Within the Peritoneal Cavity

The dissemination of tumor cells within the peritoneal cavity is another step in the pathogenesis of port site recurrence. There are several possibilities for the route of tumor cell transport from the local tumor area to the port site and other areas within the abdomen. Surgical instruments, which are in direct contact with the tumor, can become contaminated with tumor cells and disseminate them within the peritoneal cavity and to port sites. In a pig model, human HeLa cells were radioactively labeled with 51Cr. Contamination of the port wounds was measured by excising the port wounds and counting radioactivity [96]. The magnitude of port site contamination increased with greater numbers of tumor cells seeded into the peritoneal cavity. Both ports and instruments were found to be contaminated with tumor cells, and the surgeon's port was more likely to be contaminated than the assistant's port or the camera port [97]. The degree of contamination of the port sites was related to the amount of activity of the instruments. Pneumoperitoneum did not appear to play a role in the magnitude of contamination of port sites or instruments, as similar levels were noted with gasless laparoscopy. A similar porcine model [98] with real-time gamma counter imaging showed that tumor cells became widely distributed throughout the abdominal cavity with or without carbon dioxide insufflation. Tumor cell contamination was found in 4 of 10 instrument washings but in only of 30 filters used to capture cells from the exhausted carbon dioxide.

In a clinical study, the peritoneal fluid, trocars, instruments, and carbon dioxide samples were analyzed from 12 patients undergoing staging laparoscopy for pancreatic cancer [99]. PCR was used to detect low levels of mutant k-ras from tumor cells and found tumor cells in 6 of 12 peritoneal samples, four of 12 trocars, and four of 11 instrument washings. Significantly, no mutant DNA was found in any of the 12 carbon dioxide samples.

While tumor manipulation appears to contribute to intraabdominal tumor contamination, several case reports exist in which port site recurrence occurred without any manipulation of the tumor. These cases include port site metastasis after laparoscopic cholecystectomy due to underlying undiagnosed cancers of the colon or pancreas [100–102]. Port site metastasis has been reported after diagnostic laparoscopy without any manipulation of the tumor [103], although in general the incidence of port site recurrence after staging laparoscopy is quite low [104].

Questions have been raised whether it is possible for tumor cells to be aerosolized by pneumoperitoneum, which might account for port site recurrences. This has been studied using in vitro, animal, and clinical models. Several in vitro models have failed to demonstrate aerosolization of tumor cells while the same models have shown contamination of instruments in the same experimental setup [105–107]. Several animal experiments have also failed to show evidence of aerosolization [96, 108, 109].

Local Surgical Factors in Port Site Recurrence

The propensity of recurrences within the port site raises the question of whether there is something inherent in the host environment of the port sites which makes it susceptible to tumor growth. The growth factors and angiogenic factors present in the healing wound of the port site may be an important factor in tumor take. The relationship between local trauma and port site metastasis was investigated in a rat model in which tumor cells were injected intraperitoneally and port incisions made in all four quadrants, followed by pneumoperitoneum. Half of the port incisions were crushed to simulate surgical trauma. Tumor growth was significantly higher at the port sites which had undergone additional trauma [110]. A porcine model used radioactively labeled human colon cancer cells injected into the peritoneal cavity, and then subjected the animals and port sites to variety of manipulations. The port site incisions were enlarged and filters placed surrounding the trocars themselves. Manipulation of the port resulted in more abdominal wall contamination with tumor cells, as did leakage around the port site [96]. Other local factors may influence the propensity for port site recurrence such as the manner of closure of the port site incisions. Rats were inoculated into a flank incision with rat mammary adenocarcinoma cells, and the tumors subsequently lacerated intraperitoneally. Animals were treated either with carbon dioxide pneumoperitoneum or with no pneumoperitoneum. Small incisions were made in each of three quadrants, and the incisions closed in one of three methods: skin alone; skin and fascia; or skin, fascia, and peritoneum. No differences existed in tumor growth between the pneumoperitoneum and the no-pneumoperitoneum groups. Closure of just the skin, when compared with closure of all three layers, resulted in significantly more tumor growth [111]. In a porcine model, a combination of maneuvers to reduce port site recurrence such as trocar fixation, peritoneal closure, and rinsing of instruments reduced the port site recurrence rate from 64 to 14% [112].

Effect of Pneumoperitoneum on Intraperitoneal Tumor Growth

Carbon dioxide pneumoperitoneum is used clinically for laparoscopic surgery as it is inexpensive, widely available, non-flammable, non-explosive, and highly soluble in plasma. The effect of pneumoperitoneum on intraperitoneal tumor growth has been examined in a variety of rodent and pig models. These experiments have typically relied upon the intraperitoneal inoculation of tumor cells followed by a variety of experimental surgical conditions. The experimental groups have typically compared anesthesia alone to pneumoperitoneum with carbon dioxide or a variety of alternate gasses such as helium or argon or air. Pneumoperitoneum using carbon dioxide has been shown to promote greater intraperitoneal tumor growth compared with anesthesia alone [79, 80, 113–115] and with gasless laparoscopy [73, 78, 116–119] while some studies have shown no differences [116, 120, 121].

In an effort to dissect the mechanisms of the effects of carbon dioxide pneumoperitoneum, comparisons have been made with helium, as a model inert gas. Carbon dioxide insufflation has been shown to result in greater intraperitoneal tumor growth than helium in several studies [74, 78, 122–127] while some studies have shown no difference between the two gases [116, 128, 129]. However, when helium was compared with argon and nitrogen, helium was found to have substantially less growth of intraabdominal tumor, raising the question of whether helium might have specific properties [130]. When helium was compared to carbon dioxide and air pneumoperitoneum, there was equivalent growth of intraperitoneal inoculated tumor in the carbon dioxide and air groups and significantly less in the helium group [131]. A similar study in which rats underwent partial hepatectomy for hepatocellular carcinoma found that helium was associated with less tumor growth than open surgery, carbon dioxide laparoscopy, or air laparoscopy. In this study, tumor growth was more rapid with air insufflation than carbon dioxide insufflation. In vitro studies suggest that helium, rather than serving as an inert agent, may have tumor suppressive properties [124].

Effect of Pneumoperitoneum on Peritoneal Mesothelial Cells

The peritoneum is lined by a single layer of mesothelial cells covered with microvilli and resting upon a basal lamina or basement membrane. Exposure of the basal lamina appears to be a critical step for the adherence and growth of tumor cells within the peritoneum [132–134]. Several animal models have examined ultrastructural changes to the peritoneal surface as a result of pneumoperitoneum which may affect the susceptibility of the peritoneum to support tumor growth. A study in nude mice examined the ultrastructural changes in the mesothelium in response to pneumoperitoneum as documented by electron microscopy [135]. Animals subjected to anesthesia did not differ from controls, but animals subjected to pneumoperitoneum exhibited characteristic changes in the mesothelium. Beginning within 2 h of release of pneumoperitoneum, the mesothelial cells retracted and rounded up, exposing large areas of the basal lamina. Peritoneal macrophages appeared after 2 h, and lymphocytes appeared at 24 h. By 48 h mesothelial cell regeneration had begun, which was largely completed by 96 h. The same group looked at tumor growth within their model [113] and injected melanoma cells intraperitoneally after pneumoperitoneum. Within the pneumoperitoneum group, melanoma cells were seen to adhere to the exposed basal lamina and form diffuse clusters of tumor growth over the next 96 h. The control group showed no evidence of peritoneal surface change and no evidence of tumor metastasis. A similar study in mice compared the ultrastructural changes induced by laparotomy or pneumoperitoneum [136]. While pneumoperitoneum induced a transient rounding up of mesothelial cells, laparotomy induced mesothelial cell detachment which persisted at 72 h. A similar study from another research group, however, using rats and a syngeneic colon carcinoma cell lines showed similar alterations, but only in 4 of 25 animals subjected to carbon dioxide pneumoperitoneum and in none of the control animals [137].

It is not known whether these ultrastructural changes in the mesothelium were related to the carbon dioxide itself, hydrostatic pressure, or the effects of cooling or desiccation. A similar study using a thoracoscopic model in pigs showed that insufflation with dry carbon dioxide resulted in more dramatic changes to the pleura than insufflation with humidified gas [138]. A comparison in rats between cold and heated carbon dioxide [139] showed that insufflation with cold carbon dioxide lead to desquamation of mesothelial cells with exposure of the basal lamina, while insufflation with heated carbon dioxide led to rounding up the mesothelial cells but no exposure of the basal lamina. In the original model of nude mice, heated carbon dioxide pneumoperitoneum mitigated the ultrastructural changes induced by cold pneumoperitoneum [140]. Other experiments have also demonstrated less tumor growth with warm pneumoperitoneum compared with cold [141] as well as less peritoneal injury with heated CO_2 compared with cold carbon dioxide [142]. Similar experiments undertaken in rats, however, showed ultrastructural changes in the peritoneum with both cold and dry carbon dioxide pneumoperitoneum and warm and humidified pneumoperitoneum, as well as gasless laparoscopy [143]. While it is difficult to reconcile these studies, they suggest that the observed phenomenon of pneumoperitoneum increasing the risk of port site recurrence (PSR) in animal models may be related to the tissue damage to the mesothelial layer of the peritoneum.

The pressure used for insufflation appears to have an effect on the biology of tumor growth in experimental models and might be expected to also be a variable in the trauma to the mesothelial layer. In a rat model of intraperitoneal tumor inoculation, rats were treated with either no insufflation or insufflation with pressures of 4, 10, or 16 mmHg. Rats treated with higher pressures had greater tumor growth, and this effect was present whether the insufflation was conducted with air or helium [144]. On the other hand, a nude rat model using carbon dioxide or helium did not show a difference in tumor growth between groups insufflated with a pressure of 4 or 8 mmHg [145]. A rat model of colon carcinoma found that tumor growth at a distant site was increased by pneumoperitoneum of 5, 10, or 15 mmHg but intraperitoneal tumor growth was increased by insufflation at 5 or 10 mm Hg but was suppressed at 15 mmHg [146].

While these experiments suggest that there are biologic differences between insufflation at different pressures, the application to clinical practice is not clear, as there is no clear way to determine what pressure in a rodent or pig model is comparable to levels of pneumoperitoneum used for humans in clinical practice.

Effect of Pneumoperitoneum on Peritoneal Immune Cells

The primary immune effector cells within the peritoneum are peritoneal macrophages, which change in number and function in response to inflammatory stimuli such as surgery or through the stimulation of surface toll-like receptors (TLR), which recognize the presence of microorganism. Macrophages provide several functions, from initiation of the immune response to degradation of cellular debris and antigen presentation [147]. Peritoneal macrophages harvested from rodents after pneumoperitoneum show decreased spontaneous release of TNFα (alpha) [73, 148], less phagocytic activity as evidenced by decreased clearance of intravascular carbon [149], and impaired ability to clear the intracellular parasite listeria monocytogenes [150] compared with anesthesia-alone controls. The impact of pneumoperitoneum on macrophage function may be mediated by direct effects or through acidification of the peritoneal environment [88, 151–155]. The change in pH appears responsible for much of the alteration of macrophage function seen during pneumoperitoneum in animal models [156, 157].

When macrophage function after pneumoperitoneum is compared with laparotomy, a more complex picture emerges. Laparotomy in A/J mice was associated with a greater decrease in macrophage function and number than carbon dioxide pneumoperitoneum or controls. The spontaneous production of TNFα (alpha) and nitrous oxide was increased, however, in the laparotomy group, perhaps as an indicator of immune activation due to the trauma of laparotomy [158]. In a similar model, laparotomy led to increased spontaneous TNFα (alpha) release, while leading to decreased phagocytosis and stimulated response to *Escherichia coli* [159].

The presence of endotoxin, also known as lipopolysaccharide (LPS), in the air has led to the hypothesis that some of the effects of laparotomy in experimental models might be due to the effects of endotoxin present when the peritoneal cavity is exposed to air. Endotoxin is derived from the cell wall of Gram-negative bacteria and is ubiquitous in the environment and in the air [160]. Endotoxin is known to be present in elevated quantities in the air of animal research facilities [161–163] and is difficult to measure and especially difficult to remove from experimental reagents. Endotoxin stimulates macrophage and dendritic cell activation and also has direct effects on tumor cell growth [164]. This hypothesis suggests that endotoxin in the air could affect peritoneal and systemic immune responses as well as peritoneal tumor growth.

This hypothesis is supported by several observations in animal models where exposure of the peritoneal cavity to air resulted in increased tumor growth and increased inflammatory response. Watson et al. examined the inflammatory response of peritoneal macrophages in CD-1 mice after insufflation with carbon dioxide, insufflation with air, laparotomy, or anesthesia alone. The spontaneous release of TNFα (alpha) and superoxide was greatest in the laparotomy group, followed by the air laparoscopy group, which were both greater than the carbon dioxide laparoscopy or control groups [165]. Moehrlen et al. [159] compared carbon dioxide insufflation with air insufflation in NMRI mice and found that the air group showed higher rates of migration of neutrophils into the peritoneal cavity and decreased neutrophil apoptosis.

In a model of resection of Morris hepatoma 3924A from rats, Schmeding et al. [124] compared resection via open technique vs. laparoscopy with carbon dioxide, helium, or room air. The highest rate of tumor recurrence was found in animals treated with laparoscopy with room air. Jacobi [80] compared growth of colon adenocarcinoma DHD/K12/TRb in BD IX rats and found that both laparotomy and air pneumoperitoneum resulted in similar intraperitoneal tumor growth, which was greater than tumor growth with carbon dioxide pneumoperitoneum or controls. Pidgeon et al. examined the effects of laparoscopy on the growth of lung metastases from 4T1 mammary carcinoma cells after intravenous tumor inoculation. Laparotomy was compared with air insufflation, carbon dioxide insufflation, and anesthesia alone. An additional treatment group consisted of an intraperitoneal injection of 10 μg of endotoxin. Tumor growth after carbon dioxide insufflation was similar to anesthesia alone, but was greater after air insufflation, open laparotomy, or treatment with endotoxin [20]. The same group showed that intraperitoneal endotoxin injection resulted in increased numbers of lung metastasis [166] and was accompanied by increased angiogenesis. In an elegant model, Luo inoculated CT26 colon carcinoma cells into BALB/c mice. The rate of pulmonary metastases was increased by the administration of endotoxin. Genetic modification of the tumor cells to inhibit their NF-κ (kappa) B activity, however, caused endotoxin to act to suppress tumor growth of the modified tumor cells, through increasing apoptosis [167].

The complexity of the interaction between the immune system, surgical intervention, and intraperitoneal tumor growth is exemplified by two reports from investigators at the University of Adelaide. They used a model of intraperitoneal injection of the DA mammary adenocarcinoma line in Dark Agouti rats. Tumor growth was measured by dividing the peritoneal cavity into six sectors and enumerating the number of sectors involved with tumor growth. The intraperitoneal injection of 400 mg of endotoxin 4 h prior to tumor inoculation lead to a significant increase in tumor growth [73], with all six sectors involved with tumor in all the animals treated with endotoxin. In another report, the same investigators pre-treated rats with either intraperitoneal endotoxin, cyclosporine (an immunosuppressant), or control 18 h prior to laparoscopy and tumor inoculation. In this experimental setup, the prior administration of endotoxin resulted in significantly less tumor growth, with a majority of peritoneal sectors being free of visible tumor growth [168].

While it is difficult to harmonize all relevant animal experiments into a unified theory of the biology of minimally invasive surgery, the majority of animal and clinical experiments suggest that laparoscopy is associated with a blunted acute phase reaction, preservation of systemic cellular responses, and decreases in intraperitoneal inflammation. The impact of these differences is still unclear from the standpoint of tumor biology. It is clear that the interaction between the host immune system and tumor biology is more complex than originally imagined in Burnet and Thomas's theory of immune surveillance [169]. For instance, tumor-associated macrophages can either inhibit tumor growth through cytotoxicity [170] or promote tumor growth [171] through the elaboration of cytokines such as epidermal growth factor [172] or angiogenic factors [173, 174]. While there is evidence that the immune system can protect the host from transformed cells [175], there is also emerging evidence that inflammation can serve to promote tumor growth [176–178].

Conclusion

In summary, despite the initial concerns about port site recurrence associated with laparoscopic cancer surgery, it is clear from well-designed clinical trials that laparoscopic resection for colon cancer is not associated with a detectable detriment to cancer outcomes. The Barcelona investigators, in fact, found a survival advantage to laparoscopic colon resection for their stage III patients [179], although this observation has not been made in any of the other large clinical trials. Animal experiments support the general principles of oncologic surgery of minimal manipulation of the tumor and careful surgical care of the port site incisions.

While the trauma of surgery is known to induce local and systemic host responses to injury, these effects appear to be less dramatic in minimally invasive surgery. The relative immunosuppression and acute phase reaction induced by open surgery appears to be mitigated by a minimally invasive approach. Laparotomy appears to be accompanied by the increase in systemic growth factors and angiogenic factors. It is yet unclear whether these elevations are clinically significant from an oncologic perspective and if so whether they can be mitigated by a minimally invasive approach.

There additionally appear to be effects of open surgery on peritoneal inflammation which are less dramatic in laparoscopic surgery. The precise impact of laparoscopy on the peritoneal host response is still unclear due to the complexities of the animal experimental models. The results of animal experiments are not yet sufficiently robust to determine whether these differences in peritoneal inflammation are a net benefit or detriment in reducing the risk of cancer recurrence. An attractive, but unproven, hypothesis is that by minimizing local inflammation and the systemic immunosuppression of open surgery, minimally invasive surgery may reduce the risk of cancer recurrence. Further research is needed to unravel the complex interactions between surgical trauma, tumor biology, and the host response of the extracellular matrix and immune effectors.

References

1. Cava A, Roman J, Gonzalez QA et al (1990) Subcutaneous metastasis following laparoscopy in gastric adenocarcinoma. Eur J Surg Oncol 16:63–67
2. Chapman AE, Levitt MD, Hewett P et al (2001) Laparoscopic-assisted resection of colorectal malignancies: a systematic review. Ann Surg 234:590–606
3. Clair DG, Lautz DB, Brooks DC (1993) Rapid development of umbilical metastases after laparoscopic cholecystectomy for unsuspected gallbladder carcinoma. Surgery 113:355–358
4. Curet MJ (2004) Port site metastases. Am J Surg 187: 705–712
5. Drouard F, Delamarre J, Capron JP (1991) Cutaneous seeding of gallbladder cancer after laparoscopic cholecystectomy. N Engl J Med 325:1316
6. Fusco MA, Paluzzi MW (1993) Abdominal wall recurrence after laparoscopic-assisted colectomy for adenocarcinoma of the colon. Report of a case. Dis Colon Rectum 36: 858–861

7. Wexner SD, Cohen SM (1995) Port site metastases after laparoscopic colorectal surgery for cure of malignancy. Br J Surg 82:295–298
8. Johnstone PA, Rohde DC, Swartz SE et al (1996) Port site recurrences after laparoscopic and thoracoscopic procedures in malignancy. J Clin Oncol 14:1950–1956
9. Vukasin P, Ortega AE, Greene FL et al (1996) Wound recurrence following laparoscopic colon cancer resection. Results of the American Society of Colon and Rectal Surgeons Laparoscopic Registry. Dis Colon Rectum 39:S20–S23
10. Kuhry E, Schwenk WF, Gaupset R et al (2008) Long-term results of laparoscopic colorectal cancer resection. Cochrane Database Syst Rev 4:CD003432
11. Fisher B, Fisher EN (1959) Experimental evidence in support of the dormant tumor cell. Science 130:918–919
12. Buinauskas P, McDOnald GO, Cole WH (1958) Role of operative stress on the resistance of the experimental animal to inoculated cancer cells. Ann Surg 148:642–645
13. Hattori T, Hamai Y, Harada T et al (1977) Enhancing effect of thoracotomy and/or laparotomy on the development of the lung metastases in rats after intravenous inoculation of tumor cells. Jpn J Surg 7:263–268
14. Bar-Yosef S, Melamed R, Page GG et al (2001) Attenuation of the tumor-promoting effect of surgery by spinal blockade in rats. Anesthesiology 94:1066–1073
15. Wada H, Seki S, Takahashi T et al (2007) Combined spinal and general anesthesia attenuates liver metastasis by preserving TH1/TH2 cytokine balance. Anesthesiology 106:499–506
16. Southall JC, Lee SW, Bessler M et al (1998) The effect of peritoneal air exposure on postoperative tumor growth. Surg Endosc 12:348–350
17. Southall JC, Lee SW, Allendorf JD et al (1998) Colon adenocarcinoma and B-16 melanoma grow larger following laparotomy vs. pneumoperitoneum in a murine model. Dis Colon Rectum 41:564–569
18. Carter JJ, Feingold DL, Kirman I et al (2003) Laparoscopic-assisted cecectomy is associated with decreased formation of postoperative pulmonary metastases compared with open cecectomy in a murine model. Surgery 134:432–436
19. Da Costa ML, Redmond P, Bouchier-Hayes DJ (1998) The effect of laparotomy and laparoscopy on the establishment of spontaneous tumor metastases. Surgery 124:516–525
20. Pidgeon GP, Harmey JH, Kay E et al (1999) The role of endotoxin/lipopolysaccharide in surgically induced tumour growth in a murine model of metastatic disease. Br J Cancer 81:1311–1317
21. Lin E, Calvano SE, Lowry SF (2000) Inflammatory cytokines and cell response in surgery. Surgery 127: 117–126
22. Cruickshank AM, Fraser WD, Burns HJ et al (1990) Response of serum interleukin-6 in patients undergoing elective surgery of varying severity. Clin Sci (Lond) 79:161–165
23. Delgado S, Lacy AM, Filella X et al (2001) Acute phase response in laparoscopic and open colectomy in colon cancer: randomized study. Dis Colon Rectum 44: 638–646
24. Leung KL, Lai PB, Ho RL et al (2000) Systemic cytokine response after laparoscopic-assisted resection of rectosigmoid carcinoma: a prospective randomized trial. Ann Surg 231:506–511
25. Schwenk W, Jacobi C, Mansmann U et al (2000) Inflammatory response after laparoscopic and conventional colorectal resections - results of a prospective randomized trial. Langenbecks Arch Surg 385:2–9
26. Braga M, Vignali A, Zuliani W et al (2002) Metabolic and functional results after laparoscopic colorectal surgery: a randomized, controlled trial. Dis Colon Rectum 45: 1070–1077
27. Ordemann J, Jacobi CA, Schwenk W et al (2001) Cellular and humoral inflammatory response after laparoscopic and conventional colorectal resections. Surg Endosc 15:600–608
28. Harmon GD, Senagore AJ, Kilbride MJ et al (1994) Interleukin-6 response to laparoscopic and open colectomy. Dis Colon Rectum 37:754–759
29. Hewitt PM, Ip SM, Kwok SP et al. (1998) Laparoscopic-assisted vs. open surgery for colorectal cancer: comparative study of immune effects. Dis Colon Rectum 41:901–909
30. Mehigan BJ, Hartley JE, Drew PJ et al (2001) Changes in T cell subsets, interleukin-6 and C-reactive protein after laparoscopic and open colorectal resection for malignancy. Surg Endosc 15:1289–1293
31. Dunker MS, Ten Hove T, Bemelman WA et al. (2003) Interleukin-6, C-reactive protein, and expression of human leukocyte antigen-DR on peripheral blood mononuclear cells in patients after laparoscopic vs. conventional bowel resection: a randomized study. Dis Colon Rectum 46:1238–1244
32. Jung IK, Kim MC, Kim KH et al (2008) Cellular and peritoneal immune response after radical laparoscopy-assisted and open gastrectomy for gastric cancer. J Surg Oncol 98:54–59
33. Alami N, Page V, Yu Q et al (2008) Recombinant human insulin-like growth factor-binding protein 3 inhibits tumor growth and targets the Akt pathway in lung and colon cancer models. Growth Horm IGF Res 18(6): 487–496
34. Kirman I, Cekic V, Poltoratskaia N et al (2005) Open surgery induces a dramatic decrease in circulating intact IGFBP-3 in patients with colorectal cancer not seen with laparoscopic surgery. Surg Endosc 19:55–59
35. Belizon A, Kirman I, Balik E et al (2007) Major surgical trauma induces proteolysis of insulin-like growth factor binding protein-3 in transgenic mice and is associated with a rapid increase in circulating levels of matrix metalloproteinase-9. Surg Endosc 21:653–658
36. Futami R, Miyashita M, Nomura T et al (2007) Increased serum vascular endothelial growth factor following major surgical injury. J Nippon Med Sch 74:223–229
37. Belizon A, Balik E, Horst P et al (2008) Persistent elevation of plasma vascular endothelial growth factor levels during the first month after minimally invasive colorectal resection. Surg Endosc 22:287–297
38. Belizon A, Balik E, Feingold DL et al (2006) Major abdominal surgery increases plasma levels of vascular endothelial growth factor: open more so than minimally invasive methods. Ann Surg 244:792–798
39. Rosenzweig A (2003) Endothelial progenitor cells. N Engl J Med 348:581–582

40. Mancuso P, Burlini A, Pruneri G et al (2001) Resting and activated endothelial cells are increased in the peripheral blood of cancer patients. Blood 97:3658–3661
41. Condon ET, Wang JH, Redmond HP (2004) Surgical injury induces the mobilization of endothelial progenitor cells. Surgery 135:657–661
42. Condon ET, Barry BD, Wang JH et al (2007) Laparoscopic surgery protects against the oncologic adverse effects of open surgery by attenuating endothelial progenitor cell mobilization. Surg Endosc 21:87–90
43. Lee SW, Gleason NR, Southall JC et al (2000) A serum-soluble factor(s) stimulates tumor growth following laparotomy in a murine model. Surg Endosc 14: 490–494
44. Lee SW, Gleason NR, Stapleton GS et al (2001) Increased platelet-derived growth factor (PDGF) release after laparotomy stimulates systemic tumor growth in mice. Surg Endosc 15:981–985
45. Homsi J, Daud AI (2007) Spectrum of activity and mechanism of action of VEGF/PDGF inhibitors. Cancer Control 14:285–294
46. Pietsch JB, Meakins JL, MacLean LD (1977) The delayed hypersensitivity response: application in clinical surgery. Surgery 82:349–355
47. Daly JM, Dudrick SJ, Copeland EM III. (1979) Evaluation of nutritional indices as prognostic indicators in the cancer patient. Cancer 43:925–931
48. Eilber FR, Morton DL (1970) Impaired immunologic reactivity and recurrence following cancer surgery. Cancer 25:362–367
49. Trokel MJ, Bessler M, Treat MR et al (1994) Preservation of immune response after laparoscopy. Surg Endosc 8: 1385–1387
50. Ueda K, Matteotti R, Assalia A et al (2006) Comparative evaluation of gastrointestinal transit and immune response between laparoscopic and open gastrectomy in a porcine model. J Gastrointest Surg 10:39–45
51. Gleason NR, Blanco I, Allendorf JD et al (1999) Delayed-type hypersensitivity response is better preserved in mice following insufflation than after laparotomy. Surg Endosc 13:1032–1034
52. Allendorf JD, Bessler M, Whelan RL et al (1997) Postoperative immune function varies inversely with the degree of surgical trauma in a murine model. Surg Endosc 11:427–430
53. Whelan RL, Franklin M, Holubar SD et al (2003) Postoperative cell mediated immune response is better preserved after laparoscopic vs. open colorectal resection in humans. Surg Endosc 17:972–978
54. Wichmann MW, Huttl TP, Winter H et al (2005) Immunological effects of laparoscopic vs. open colorectal surgery: a prospective clinical study. Arch Surg 140: 692–697
55. Bolla G, Tuzzato G (2003) Immunologic postoperative competence after laparoscopy versus laparotomy. Surg Endosc 17:1247–1250
56. Redmond HP, Watson RW, Houghton T et al (1994) Immune function in patients undergoing open vs. laparoscopic cholecystectomy. Arch Surg 129:1240–1246
57. Carey PD, Wakefield CH, Thayeb A et al (1994) Effects of minimally invasive surgery on hypochlorous acid production by neutrophils. Br J Surg 81:557–560
58. Galon J, Costes A, Sanchez-Cabo F et al (2006) Type, density, and location of immune cells within human colorectal tumors predict clinical outcome. Science 313:1960–1964
59. Brune IB, Wilke W, Hensler T et al (1999) Downregulation of T helper type 1 immune response and altered pro-inflammatory and anti-inflammatory T cell cytokine balance following conventional but not laparoscopic surgery. Am J Surg 177:55–60
60. Decker D, Schondorf M, Bidlingmaier F et al (1996) Surgical stress induces a shift in the type-1/type-2 T-helper cell balance, suggesting down-regulation of cell-mediated and up-regulation of antibody-mediated immunity commensurate to the trauma. Surgery 119:316–325
61. Di Vita G, Sciume C, Milano S et al (2001) Inflammatory response in open and laparoscopic cholecystectomy. Ann Ital Chir 72:669–673
62. Fujii K, Sonoda K, Izumi K et al (2003) T lymphocyte subsets and Th1/Th2 balance after laparoscopy-assisted distal gastrectomy. Surg Endosc 17:1440–1444
63. Evans C, Galustian C, Kumar D et al (2008) Impact of surgery on immunologic function: comparison between minimally invasive techniques and conventional laparotomy for surgical resection of colorectal tumors. Am J Surg 197(2):238–245
64. Trinchieri G (1989) Biology of natural killer cells. Adv Immunol 47:187–376
65. Tartter PI, Steinberg B, Barron DM et al (1987) The prognostic significance of natural killer cytotoxicity in patients with colorectal cancer. Arch Surg 122:1264–1268
66. Kondo E, Koda K, Takiguchi N et al (2003) Preoperative natural killer cell activity as a prognostic factor for distant metastasis following surgery for colon cancer. Dig Surg 20:445–451
67. Coca S, Perez-Piqueras J, Martinez D et al (1997) The prognostic significance of intratumoral natural killer cells in patients with colorectal carcinoma. Cancer 79: 2320–2328
68. Menon AG, Janssen-van Rhijn CM, Morreau H et al (2004) Immune system and prognosis in colorectal cancer: a detailed immunohistochemical analysis. Lab Invest 84:493–501
69. Ishigami S, Natsugoe S, Tokuda K et al (2000) Prognostic value of intratumoral natural killer cells in gastric carcinoma. Cancer 88:577–583
70. Ishigami S, Natsugoe S, Tokuda K et al (2000) Clinical impact of intratumoral natural killer cell and dendritic cell infiltration in gastric cancer. Cancer Lett 159:103–108
71. Da Costa ML, Redmond HP, Finnegan N et al (1998) Laparotomy and laparoscopy differentially accelerate experimental flank tumour growth. Br J Surg 85: 1439–1442
72. Da Costa ML, Redmond HP, Bouchier-Hayes DJ (2001) Taurolidine improves survival by abrogating the accelerated development and proliferation of solid tumors and development of organ metastases from circulating tumor cells released following surgery. J Surg Res 101:111–119
73. Mathew G, Watson DI, Ellis TS et al (1999) The role of peritoneal immunity and the tumour-bearing state on the development of wound and peritoneal metastases after laparoscopy. Aust N Z J Surg 69:14–18
74. Wenger FA, Jacobi CA, Kilian M et al (2000) The impact of laparoscopic biopsy of pancreatic lymph nodes with

helium and carbon dioxide on port site and liver metastasis in BOP-induced pancreatic cancer in hamster. Clin Exp Metastasis 18:11–14
75. Jones DB, Guo LW, Reinhard MK et al (1995) Impact of pneumoperitoneum on trocar site implantation of colon cancer in hamster model. Dis Colon Rectum 38:1182–1188
76. Allendorf JD, Bessler M, Kayton ML et al (1995) Increased tumor establishment and growth after laparotomy vs. laparoscopy in a murine model. Arch Surg 130: 649–653
77. Allendorf JD, Bessler M, Horvath KD et al (1999) Increased tumor establishment and growth after open vs. laparoscopic surgery in mice may be related to differences in postoperative T-cell function. Surg Endosc 13:233–235
78. Bouvy ND, Marquet RL, Jeekel H et al (1996) Impact of gas(less) laparoscopy and laparotomy on peritoneal tumor growth and abdominal wall metastases. Ann Surg 224:694–700
79. Bouvy ND, Marquet RL, Jeekel J et al (1997) Laparoscopic surgery is associated with less tumour growth stimulation than conventional surgery: an experimental study. Br J Surg 84:358–361
80. Jacobi CA, Ordemann J, Bohm B et al (1997) The influence of laparotomy and laparoscopy on tumor growth in a rat model. Surg Endosc 11:618–621
81. Lee SW, Gleason N, Blanco I et al (2002) Higher colon cancer tumor proliferative index and lower tumor cell death rate in mice undergoing laparotomy versus insufflation. Surg Endosc 16:36–39
82. Mutter D, Hajri A, Tassetti V et al (1999) Increased tumor growth and spread after laparoscopy vs. laparotomy: influence of tumor manipulation in a rat model. Surg Endosc 13:365–370
83. Takeuchi H, Inomata M, Fujii K et al (2004) Increased peritoneal dissemination after laparotomy versus pneumoperitoneum in a mouse cecal cancer model. Surg Endosc 18:1795–1799
84. Kuntz C, Kienle P, Schmeding M et al (2002) Comparison of laparoscopic versus conventional technique in colonic and liver resection in a tumor-bearing small animal model. Surg Endosc 16:1175–1181
85. Moreno EF, Nelson H, Carugno F et al (2000) Effects of laparoscopy on tumor growth. Surg Laparosc Endosc Percutan Tech 10:296–301
86. Fong Y, Brennan MF, Turnbull A et al (1993) Gallbladder cancer discovered during laparoscopic surgery. Potential for iatrogenic tumor dissemination. Arch Surg 128: 1054–1056
87. Wibbenmeyer LA, Wade TP, Chen RC et al (1995) Laparoscopic cholecystectomy can disseminate in situ carcinoma of the gallbladder. J Am Coll Surg 181:504–510
88. Sandor J, Ihasz M, Fazekas T et al (1995) Unexpected gallbladder cancer and laparoscopic surgery. Surg Endosc 9:1207–1210
89. Shirai Y, Ohtani T, Hatakeyama K (1997) Tumor dissemination during laparoscopic cholecystectomy for gallbladder carcinoma. Surg Endosc 11:1224–1225
90. Doudle M, King G, Thomas WM et al (1996) The movement of mucosal cells of the gallbladder within the peritoneal cavity during laparoscopic cholecystectomy. Surg Endosc 10:1092–1094
91. Lee SW, Southall J, Allendorf J et al (1998) Traumatic handling of the tumor independent of pneumoperitoneum increases port site implantation rate of colon cancer in a murine model. Surg Endosc 12:828–834
92. Lee SW, Gleason NR, Bessler M et al (2000) Port site tumor recurrence rates in a murine model of laparoscopic splenectomy decreased with increased experience. Surg Endosc 14:805–811
93. Lee SW, Whelan RL, Southall JC et al (1998) Abdominal wound tumor recurrence after open and laparoscopic-assisted splenectomy in a murine model. Dis Colon Rectum 41:824–831
94. Polat AK, Yapici O, Malazgirt Z et al (2007) Effect of types of resection and manipulation on trocar site contamination after laparoscopic colectomy: an experimental study in rats with intraluminal radiotracer application. Surg Endosc 22(5):1396–1401
95. Halpin VJ, Underwood RA, Ye D et al (2005) Pneumoperitoneum does not influence trocar site implantation during tumor manipulation in a solid tumor model. Surg Endosc 19:1636–1640
96. Allardyce RA, Morreau P, Bagshaw PF (1997) Operative factors affecting tumor cell distribution following laparoscopic colectomy in a porcine model. Dis Colon Rectum 40:939–945
97. Allardyce R, Morreau P, Bagshaw P (1996) Tumor cell distribution following laparoscopic colectomy in a porcine model. Dis Colon Rectum 39:S47–S52
98. Hewett PJ, Texler ML, Anderson D et al (1999) In vivo real-time analysis of intraperitoneal radiolabeled tumor cell movement during laparoscopy. Dis Colon Rectum 42:868–875
99. Reymond MA, Wittekind C, Jung A et al (1997) The incidence of port-site metastases might be reduced. Surg Endosc 11:902–906
100. Neuhaus S, Hewett P, Disney A (2001) An unusual case of port site seeding. Surg Endosc 15:896
101. Siriwardena A, Samarji WN (1993) Cutaneous tumour seeding from a previously undiagnosed pancreatic carcinoma after laparoscopic cholecystectomy. Ann R Coll Surg Engl 75:199–200
102. Ugarte F (1995) Laparoscopic cholecystectomy port seeding from a colon carcinoma. Am Surg 61:820–821
103. Jorgensen JO, McCall JL, Morris DL (1995) Port site seeding after laparoscopic ultrasonographic staging of pancreatic carcinoma. Surgery 117:118–119
104. Shoup M, Brennan MF, Karpeh MS et al (2002) Port site metastasis after diagnostic laparoscopy for upper gastrointestinal tract malignancies: an uncommon entity. Ann Surg Oncol 9:632–636
105. Sellers GJ, Whelan RL, Allendorf JD et al (1998) An in vitro model fails to demonstrate aerosolization of tumor cells. Surg Endosc 12:436–439
106. Thomas WM, Eaton MC, Hewett PJ (1996) A proposed model for the movement of cells within the abdominal cavity during CO2 insufflation and laparoscopy. Aust N Z J Surg 66:105–106
107. Texler ML, King G, Hewett PJ (1998) Tumour cell movement during heating and humidification of insufflating CO2: an in vitro model. Aust N Z J Surg 68: 740–742

108. Whelan RL, Sellers GJ, Allendorf JD et al (1996) Trocar site recurrence is unlikely to result from aerosolization of tumor cells. Dis Colon Rectum 39:S7–S13
109. Wittich P, Marquet RL, Kazemier G et al (2000) Port-site metastases after CO(2) laparoscopy. Is aerosolization of tumor cells a pivotal factor? Surg Endosc 14: 189–192
110. Tseng LN, Berends FJ, Wittich P et al (1998) Port-site metastases. Impact of local tissue trauma and gas leakage. Surg Endosc 12:1377–1380
111. Burns JM, Matthews BD, Pollinger HS et al (2005) Effect of carbon dioxide pneumoperitoneum and wound closure technique on port site tumor implantation in a rat model. Surg Endosc 19:441–447
112. Schneider C, Jung A, Reymond MA et al (2001) Efficacy of surgical measures in preventing port-site recurrences in a porcine model. Surg Endosc 15:121–125
113. Volz J, Koster S, Spacek Z et al (1999) The influence of pneumoperitoneum used in laparoscopic surgery on an intraabdominal tumor growth. Cancer 86:770–774
114. Hopkins MP, Dulai RM, Occhino A et al (1999) The effects of carbon dioxide pneumoperitoneum on seeding of tumor in port sites in a rat model. Am J Obstet Gynecol 181:1329–1333
115. Wu JS, Brasfield EB, Guo LW et al (1997) Implantation of colon cancer at trocar sites is increased by low pressure pneumoperitoneum. Surgery 122:1–7
116. Lecuru F, Agostini A, Camatte S et al (2002) Impact of pneumoperitoneum on tumor growth. Surg Endosc 16:1170–1174
117. Mathew G, Watson DI, Rofe AM et al (1997) Adverse impact of pneumoperitoneum on intraperitoneal implantation and growth of tumour cell suspension in an experimental model. Aust N Z J Surg 67:289–292
118. Watson DI, Mathew G, Ellis T et al (1997) Gasless laparoscopy may reduce the risk of port-site metastases following laparascopic tumor surgery. Arch Surg 132: 166–168
119. Bouvy ND, Giuffrida MC, Tseng LN et al (1998) Effects of carbon dioxide pneumoperitoneum, air pneumoperitoneum, and gasless laparoscopy on body weight and tumor growth. Arch Surg 133:652–656
120. Ishida H, Murata N, Yamada H et al (2000) Influence of trocar placement and CO(2) pneumoperitoneum on port site metastasis following laparoscopic tumor surgery. Surg Endosc 14:193–197
121. Hubens G, Pauwels M, Hubens A et al (1996) The influence of a pneumoperitoneum on the peritoneal implantation of free intraperitoneal colon cancer cells. Surg Endosc 10:809–812
122. Neuhaus SJ, Watson DI, Ellis T et al (1998) Wound metastasis after laparoscopy with different insufflation gases. Surgery 123:579–583
123. Neuhaus SJ, Ellis T, Rofe AM et al (1998) Tumor implantation following laparoscopy using different insufflation gases. Surg Endosc 12:1300–1302
124. Schmeding M, Schwalbach P, Reinshagen S et al (2003) Helium pneumoperitoneum reduces tumor recurrence after curative laparoscopic liver resection in rats in a tumor-bearing small animal model. Surg Endosc 17: 951–959
125. Jacobi CA, Sabat R, Bohm B et al (1997) Pneumoperitoneum with carbon dioxide stimulates growth of malignant colonic cells. Surgery 121:72–78
126. Jacobi CA, Wenger F, Sabat R et al (1998) The impact of laparoscopy with carbon dioxide versus helium on immunologic function and tumor growth in a rat model. Dig Surg 15:110–116
127. Yokoyama M, Ishida H, Okita T et al (2003) Oncological effects of insufflation with different gases and a gasless procedure in rats. Surg Endosc 17:1151–1155
128. Ridgway PF, Smith A, Ziprin P et al (2002) Pneumoperitoneum augmented tumor invasiveness is abolished by matrix metalloproteinase blockade. Surg Endosc 16: 533–536
129. Dorrance HR, Oien K, O'Dwyer PJ (1999) Effects of laparoscopy on intraperitoneal tumor growth and distant metastases in an animal model. Surgery 126:35–40
130. Gupta A, Watson DI, Ellis T et al (2002) Tumour implantation following laparoscopy using different insufflation gases. ANZ J Surg 72:254–257
131. Neuhaus SJ, Ellis TS, Barrett MW et al (1999) In vitro inhibition of tumour growth in a helium-rich environment: implications for laparoscopic surgery. Aust N Z J Surg 69:52–55
132. Birbeck MS, Wheatley DN (1965) An Electron Microscopic Study of the Invasion of Ascites Tumor Cells into the Abdominal Wall. Cancer Res 25:490–497
133. Buck RC (1973) Walker 256 tumor implantation in normal and injured peritoneum studied by electron microscopy, scanning electron microscopy, and autoradiography. Cancer Res 33:3181–3188
134. Kiyasu Y, Kaneshima S, Koga S (1981) Morphogenesis of peritoneal metastasis in human gastric cancer. Cancer Res 41:1236–1239
135. Volz J, Koster S, Spacek Z et al (1999) Characteristic alterations of the peritoneum after carbon dioxide pneumoperitoneum. Surg Endosc 13:611–614
136. Suematsu T, Hirabayashi Y, Shiraishi N et al (2001) Morphology of the murine peritoneum after pneumoperitoneum vs. laparotomy. Surg Endosc 15:954–958
137. Ordemann J, Jakob J, Braumann C et al (2004) Morphology of the rat peritoneum after carbon dioxide and helium pneumoperitoneum: a scanning electron microscopic study. Surg Endosc 18:1389–1393
138. Mouton WG, Bessell JR, Pfitzner J et al (1999) A randomized controlled trial to determine the effects of humidified carbon dioxide insufflation during thoracoscopy. Surg Endosc 13:382–385
139. Erikoglu M, Yol S, Avunduk MC et al (2005) Electron-microscopic alterations of the peritoneum after both cold and heated carbon dioxide pneumoperitoneum. J Surg Res 125:73–77
140. Volz J, Koster S, Schaeff B et al (1998) Laparoscopic surgery: the effects of insufflation gas on tumor-induced lethality in nude mice. Am J Obstet Gynecol 178: 793–795
141. Nduka CC, Puttick M, Coates P et al (2002) Intraperitoneal hypothermia during surgery enhances postoperative tumor growth. Surg Endosc 16:611–615
142. Peng Y, Zheng M, Ye Q et al (2008) Heated and humidified CO(2) prevents hypothermia, peritoneal injury, and

intra-abdominal adhesions during prolonged laparoscopic insufflations. J Surg Res 151(1):40–47
143. Hazebroek EJ, Schreve MA, Visser P et al (2002) Impact of temperature and humidity of carbon dioxide pneumoperitoneum on body temperature and peritoneal morphology. J Laparoendosc Adv Surg Tech A 12:355–364
144. Wittich P, Mearadji A, Marquet RL et al (2004) Increased tumor growth after high pressure pneumoperitoneum with helium and air. J Laparoendosc Adv Surg Tech A 14:205–208
145. Agostini A, Robin F, Jais JP et al (2002) Impact of different gases and pneumoperitoneum pressures on tumor growth during laparoscopy in a rat model. Surg Endosc 16: 529–532
146. Jacobi CA, Wenger FA, Ordemann J et al (1998) Experimental study of the effect of intra-abdominal pressure during laparoscopy on tumour growth and port site metastasis. Br J Surg 85:1419–1422
147. Jackson PG, Evans SR (2000) Intraperitoneal macrophages and tumor immunity: a review. J Surg Oncol 75:146–154
148. Neuhaus SJ, Watson DI, Ellis T et al (2000) Influence of gases on intraperitoneal immunity during laparoscopy in tumor-bearing rats. World J Surg 24:1227–1231
149. Gutt CN, Heinz P, Kaps W et al (1997) The phagocytosis activity during conventional and laparoscopic operations in the rat. A preliminary study. Surg Endosc 11:899–901
150. Chekan EG, Nataraj C, Clary EM et al (1999) Intraperitoneal immunity and pneumoperitoneum. Surg Endosc 13:1135–1138
151. Hanly EJ, Aurora AR, Fuentes JM et al (2005) Abdominal insufflation with CO_2 causes peritoneal acidosis independent of systemic pH. J Gastrointest Surg 9:1245–1251
152. Kuebler JF, Vieten G, Shimotakahara A et al (2006) Acidification during carbon dioxide pneumoperitoneum is restricted to the gas-exposed peritoneal surface: effects of pressure, gas flow, and additional intraperitoneal fluids. J Laparoendosc Adv Surg Tech A 16:654–658
153. Kuntz C, Wunsch A, Bodeker C et al (2000) Effect of pressure and gas type on intraabdominal, subcutaneous, and blood pH in laparoscopy. Surg Endosc 14:367–371
154. Wong YT, Shah PC, Birkett DH et al (2004) Carbon dioxide pneumoperitoneum causes severe peritoneal acidosis, unaltered by heating, humidification, or bicarbonate in a porcine model. Surg Endosc 18:1498–1503
155. Wildbrett P, Oh A, Naundorf D et al (2003) Impact of laparoscopic gases on peritoneal microenvironment and essential parameters of cell function. Surg Endosc 17: 78–82
156. Kos M, Kuebler JF, Jesch NK et al (2006) Carbon dioxide differentially affects the cytokine release of macrophage subpopulations exclusively via alteration of extracellular pH. Surg Endosc 20:570–576
157. Hanly EJ, Aurora AA, Shih SP et al (2007) Peritoneal acidosis mediates immunoprotection in laparoscopic surgery. Surgery 142:357–364
158. Iwanaka T, Arkovitz MS, Arya G et al (1997) Evaluation of operative stress and peritoneal macrophage function in minimally invasive operations. J Am Coll Surg 184: 357–363
159. Moehrlen U, Ziegler U, Boneberg E et al (2006) Impact of carbon dioxide versus air pneumoperitoneum on peritoneal cell migration and cell fate. Surg Endosc 20: 1607–1613
160. Rylander R, Bake B, Fischer JJ et al (1989) Pulmonary function and symptoms after inhalation of endotoxin. Am Rev Respir Dis 140:981–986
161. Borm PJ, van Hartingsveld B, Schins PF et al (1999) Priming of cytokine release and increased levels of bactericidal permeability-increasing protein in the blood of animal facility workers. Int Arch Occup Environ Health 72:323–329
162. Lieutier-Colas F, Meyer P, Larsson P et al (2001) Difference in exposure to airborne major rat allergen (Rat n 1) and to endotoxin in rat quarters according to tasks. Clin Exp Allergy 31:1449–1456
163. Pacheco KA, McCammon C, Thorne PS et al (2006) Characterization of endotoxin and mouse allergen exposures in mouse facilities and research laboratories. Ann Occup Hyg 50:563–572
164. Pikarsky E, Porat RM, Stein I et al (2004) NF-kappaB functions as a tumour promoter in inflammation-associated cancer. Nature 431:461–466
165. Watson RW, Redmond HP, McCarthy J et al (1995) Exposure of the peritoneal cavity to air regulates early inflammatory responses to surgery in a murine model. Br J Surg 82:1060–1065
166. Harmey JH, Bucana CD, Lu W et al (2002) Lipopolysaccharide-induced metastatic growth is associated with increased angiogenesis, vascular permeability and tumor cell invasion. Int J Cancer 101:415–422
167. Luo JL, Maeda S, Hsu LC et al (2004) Inhibition of NF-kappaB in cancer cells converts inflammation- induced tumor growth mediated by TNFalpha to TRAIL-mediated tumor regression. Cancer Cell 6:297–305
168. Neuhaus SJ, Watson DI, Ellis T et al (2000) The effect of immune enhancement and suppression on the development of laparoscopic port site metastases. Surg Endosc 14:439–443
169. Burnet FM (1970) The concept of immunological surveillance. Prog Exp Tumor Res 13:1–27
170. Chen JJ, Lin YC, Yao PL et al (2005) Tumor-associated macrophages: the double-edged sword in cancer progression. J Clin Oncol 23:953–964
171. Mantovani A, Romero P, Palucka AK et al (2008) Tumour immunity: effector response to tumour and role of the microenvironment. Lancet 371:771–783
172. Goswami S, Sahai E, Wyckoff JB et al (2005) Macrophages promote the invasion of breast carcinoma cells via a colony-stimulating factor-1/epidermal growth factor paracrine loop. Cancer Res 65:5278–5283
173. Parajuli P, Singh SM (1996) Alteration in IL-1 and arginase activity of tumor-associated macrophages: a role in the promotion of tumor growth. Cancer Lett 107:249–256
174. Sunderkotter C, Steinbrink K, Goebeler M et al (1994) Macrophages and angiogenesis. J Leukoc Biol 55: 410–422
175. Dunn GP, Bruce AT, Ikeda H et al (2002) Cancer immunoediting: from immunosurveillance to tumor escape. Nat Immunol 3:991–998
176. Baniyash M (2006) Chronic inflammation, immunosuppression and cancer: new insights and outlook. Semin Cancer Biol 16:80–88

177. Coussens LM, Werb Z (2002) Inflammation and cancer. Nature 420:860–867
178. Lin WW, Karin M (2007) A cytokine-mediated link between innate immunity, inflammation, and cancer. J Clin Invest 117:1175–1183
179. Lacy AM, Delgado S, Castells A et al (2008) The long-term results of a randomized clinical trial of laparoscopy-assisted versus open surgery for colon cancer. Ann Surg 248:1–7

Pneumoperitoneum: Metabolic and Mechanical Effects

Frederick L. Greene

Contents

Historical Concepts

The history of the application of pneumoperitoneum is fascinating from the aspect of both diseases treated with this concept and the development of abdominal air insufflation from a technical standpoint [1]. The name George Kelling is woven into the modern use of pneumoperitoneum for patients undergoing laparoscopy. Kelling, like many of his contemporary colleagues, considered that pneumoperitoneum might have therapeutic use. He advocated the use of this technique, which he called *lufttamponade*, for the treatment of patients with significant intestinal and intraabdominal bleeding. Kelling placed a cystoscope into the abdominal cavity of animals to identify organ ischemia, which may be secondary to aggressive instillation of intraabdominal room air.

Kelling's creation of pneumoperitoneum evolved from the work of Robert Simons of Bonn, Germany. Simons, working in the 1870s, introduced increasing amounts of gas into the abdominal cavities of animals and showed that pneumoperitoneum did not create an inflammatory response in the peritoneal lining [1]. A few years later, George Wagner of Berlin used various gases to create pneumoperitoneum and showed that the gas could be easily absorbed in most situations [1]. Early treatment using pneumoperitoneum was directed toward abdominal tuberculosis and showed some success in treating this disease process. Although Kelling was an ardent supporter of pneumoperitoneum, he could never encourage a patient to be treated using this technique.

Fortuitously, Hans Christian Jacobaeus of Sweden was able to use intraabdominal endoscopy in patients who were treated for tuberculosis. His initial patient population was restricted to those who manifested ascites. Jacobaeus was the first to instill air into the abdominal cavity as a presumed therapeutic

F.L. Greene, B.T. Heniford (eds.), *Minimally Invasive Cancer Management*,
DOI 10.1007/978-1-4419-1238-1_3,

application. He postulated that "the entry of air into the peritoneum should exert a favorable influence on healing" [1]. The use of carbon dioxide to create pneumoperitoneum developed in the 1930s as it was realized that an inert gas might be more appropriate for abdominal instillation. Rapid clearance through the peritoneal lining and the concomitant use of electrocautery were recognized as additional advantages of carbon dioxide pneumoperitoneum.

Current Concepts

Carbon dioxide pneumoperitoneum is the mainstay for the creation of an appropriate environment for diagnostic and therapeutic laparoscopy. As more advanced laparoscopic procedures are undertaken, the consequences of establishing carbon dioxide pneumoperitoneum become potentially greater, especially in patients with abdominal malignancy. The systemic effects of the creation of pneumoperitoneum depend primarily on the level of intraabdominal pressure created; therefore, the current trend is toward operating at lower pressures. Cardiopulmonary effects of pneumoperitoneum are directly related to insufflation pressures, and the incidence of arrhythmia may be heightened due to compression of the heart by elevation of the diaphragm [2]. In addition, acidemia caused by absorption by carbon dioxide increases the opportunity for abnormal cardiac rhythms because of the lowering of the arrhythmia threshold, a consequence of a lowered pH [3, 4]. These cardiopulmonary consequences occur in patients with benign and malignant lesions. Although a variety of gases have been used to create pneumoperitoneum, carbon dioxide continues to be effective for use in laparoscopic diagnostic and therapeutic procedures in cancer patients.

Carbon dioxide insufflation during laparoscopy has been shown to dampen the systemic stress response to surgery and to suppress peritoneal macrophage functions. Using peripheral blood neutrophils from healthy volunteers, Shimotakahara and colleagues [5] showed that exposure to 100% CO_2 completely blocked spontaneous and IL-8-induced migration of neutrophil function. This effect was more than would be expected from hypoxia alone. The effect on neutrophil function seems to be induced from acidification secondary to CO_2. In view of these findings, the ability to control infection as a potential complication of laparoscopic procedures is of concern. This may be a greater hazard as natural orifice transluminal endoscopic surgery (NOTES) is promulgated.

A number of animal studies have supported the concept that cellular dispersion occurs during peritoneal insufflation with resultant contamination of abdominal port sites by neoplastic cells [6–8]. Various studies have also compared the insufflation gas used and have generally shown that cellular dispersion may occur whether air, carbon dioxide, or another inert gas is used [8]. Ikramuddin et al. [6], using groups of patients with benign and malignant disease, concluded that aerosolization of cells may only be important when peritoneal carcinomatosis is present. These authors supported the continued use of pneumoperitoneum in the management of patients with abdominal malignancy. Lee et al. [9] showed that traumatic handling of neoplastic tissue might be more contributory than the effects of pneumoperitoneum in causing cellular dispersement.

The effects of pneumoperitoneum were studied by Mathew et al. [10] using a novel parabiotic rat model. They showed that carbon dioxide insufflation had a significant effect on tumor dissemination during laparoscopy, which led to port-site metastases. These authors further reported that tumor growth was not stimulated during gasless laparoscopy. A criticism of most animal studies, however, is that the laboratory environment may not replicate the clinical setting. The gas leak produced and the number of tumor cells used in these studies may not truly mimic the conditions in laparoscopic oncologic procedures.

An additional factor that might contribute to peritoneal implantation of tumor inoculum is the effect of carbon dioxide on cellular function of peritoneal cells. Evrard and coworkers [11] in France showed that peritoneal lymphocytes were neither destroyed nor locally impaired by a carbon dioxide challenge. Although a small reduction in cellular immunity was noted, this was observed to be transient. Their model studied the effect of carbon dioxide over a short time (1 h), leaving one to speculate as to the consequences of carbon dioxide insufflation in longer, more complex oncologic procedures. Jung et al. [12] studied the immunologic effects in the peritoneum in patients undergoing both open and laparoscopic-assisted gastrectomy for early gastric cancer. They studied serum and peritoneal fluid to report levels of tumor necrosis factor (TNF), interleukin (IL)-6, and IL-10. They reported reduced peritoneal immunologic activity in the patients undergoing laparoscopic resections for gastric cancer and discussed a concern regarding the use of laparoscopic procedures in this group of patients.

Environmental Effects

A potential downside of the creation of pneumoperitoneum is that "cold gas" is insufflated into the abdominal cavity and creates a hypothermic setting in patients who undergo prolonged laparoscopic techniques. Only recently has the application of gas warmers been advocated to assure that normothermia is maintained. At present, it is unknown whether hypothermic conditions adversely affect cancer patients. Clearly, stress may be increased in hypothermia, and therefore a greater reduction of immune competence may result. Unfortunately, an inadequate number of studies have been done to fully understand the hypothermic effect. The operating surgeon, however, must realize that techniques to counteract the hypothermia created by prolonged pneumoperitoneum must be used. Full discussion with anesthesia personnel should include methods of warming the patient during prolonged laparoscopic procedures.

Little has been studied regarding the consequences of hypothermia in the surgical patient. It is known that the infection rate and blood loss may be consequences of hypothermia, especially in those undergoing open colectomy [13]. It is known that peritoneal instillation of carbon dioxide is a major contributor in producing a hypothermic state, especially if the patient is not warmed appropriately during general anesthesia [14]. A study by Figueredo and Canosa [15] assessed 36 patients undergoing cholecystectomy by either the open or laparoscopic approach. Although there were no major differences in mean body temperature between patients in the open and laparoscopic groups, a trend toward lower body temperature was directly proportional to the length of the operative time in the laparoscopic group. These authors point out that during the laparoscopic procedures, heat loss occurs mainly by convection, which they defined as "the gain or loss of heat due to flows of a fluid (liquid or gas), when it circulates through a surface at a different temperature" [15]. The use of pneumoperitoneum, therefore, affects temperature regulation through the exposure of cool gas to the warm surface of the abdominal cavity. In addition, the velocity at which the gas is introduced into the abdomen is also directly related to the degree of hypothermia produced. It is anticipated that as laparoscopic procedures (especially in cancer patients) become more complex and lengthy, the effect of instilling cool (21°C) carbon dioxide into a warm abdominal cavity may be even greater. Studies to assess the metabolic consequences of hypothermia and to analyze this variant for its potential role in port-site recurrence are needed.

Further environmental effects may be noted as a consequence of pneumoperitoneum and reflect the mechanical forces exerted by expansion of the peritoneum. Volz et al. [16] in Germany reported that in a group of mice undergoing 6 mmHg pressure for an interval of 30 min, a definable, structural change occurred in the mesothelial cell lining of the parietal peritoneum. More specifically, after inspection of the cell lining using transmission electron microscopy, expansion of the intracellular clefts occurred and lasted for at least 12 h following the application of pneumoperitoneum (Figs. 3.1, 3.2, 3.3, 3.4). Eventually, a reparative process occurred manifested by the accumulation of macrophages and lymphocytes within the

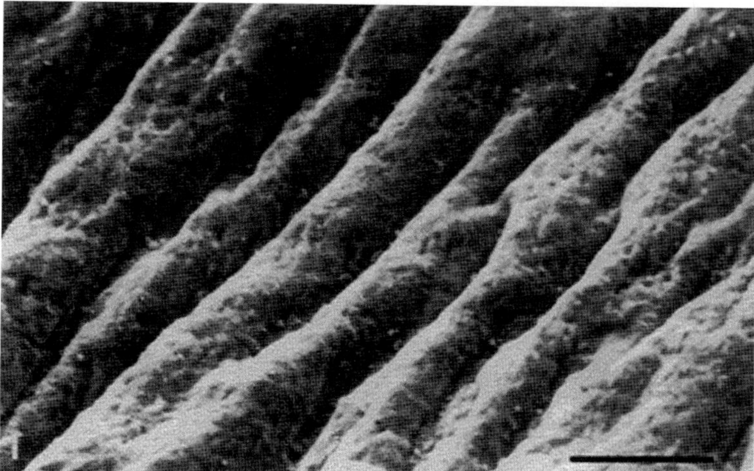

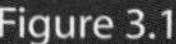
Figure 3.1

Normal peritoneal mesothelial lining in mice model. Magnification ×170 (from Volz et al. [16]. Reprinted with kind permission from Springer Science + Business Media)

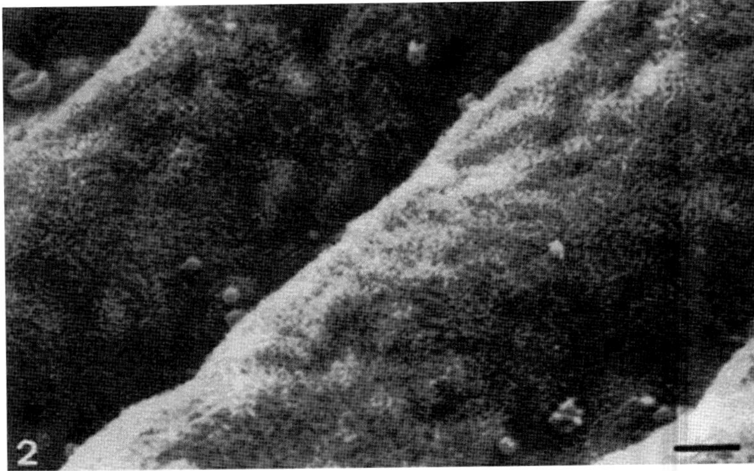

Figure 3.2

Normal peritoneal mesothelial lining in mouse model. Magnification ×710 (from Volz et al. [16]. Reprinted with kind permission from Springer Science + Business Media)

intracellular spaces. The importance of these observations is that tumor implantation associated with pneumoperitoneum may be a consequence of direct cellular disruption of the peritoneal lining. Alteration of the peritoneal surface may be an important consequence of pneumoperitoneum, creating an environment for widespread and earlier dissemination in the patient with cancer. It is unclear whether this is a pure mechanical consequence or secondary to the acidic medium created by introducing carbon dioxide into the abdominal cavity. If the chemical environment proves to be the more important consequence, the use of gases other than carbon dioxide may have a greater benefit for the cancer patient.

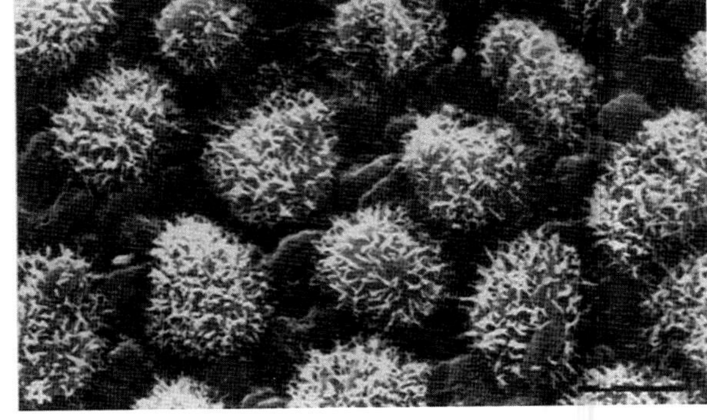

Figure 3.4

Peritoneal lining 2 h after CO_2 application at 6 mmHg for 30 min. Intercellular clefts and the underlying basal lamina are clearly visible. Magnification ×1,310 (from Volz et al. [16]. Reprinted with kind permission from Springer Science + Business Media)

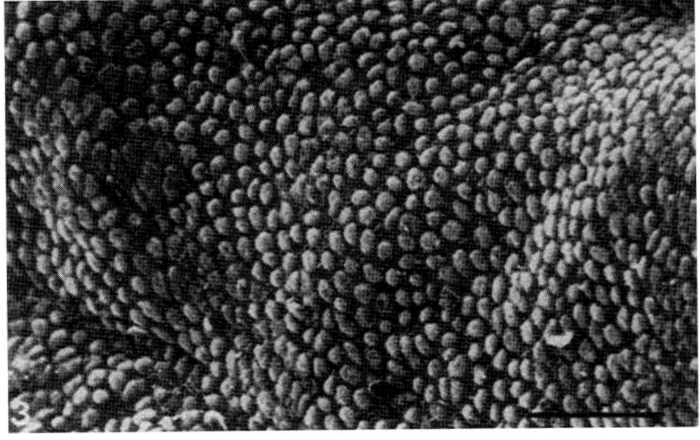

Figure 3.3

Peritoneal lining 2 h after CO_2 application at 6 mmHg for 30 min. Magnification ×170 (from Volz et al. [16]. Reprinted with kind permission from Springer Science + Business Media)

Intravascular Effects

A potentially detrimental consequence to the cancer patient may be hypercoagulability caused by pneumoperitoneum. A little known but potentially far-reaching effect is that endogenous arginine vasopressin levels are increased in direct proportion to increased intraabdominal pressure [17]. This elevation of endogenous vasopressin increases splanchnic vascular tone, and procoagulants such as factor VIII and von Willebrand factor are elevated secondary to the rise in arginine vasopressin levels [18]. Since cancer patients are presumed to be hypercoagulable, a secondary consequence of creating a pneumoperitoneum may be to heighten thrombogenic coagulation parameters in the patient. It is important, therefore, to keep the intraabdominal pressure as low as possible to decrease the vasopressin response. In addition, use of systemic anticoagulation for prophylaxis of deep venous thrombosis and the appropriate application of stockings and compression boots to the lower extremities are very important in cancer patients undergoing laparoscopic procedures.

Immunologic Alterations

There is probably no group of patients undergoing major operative procedures that are more at risk for the consequences of surgical trauma on the immune mechanisms than the cancer patient. The effects of general anesthesia and abdominal wall manipulation used during open and laparoscopic surgery reduce the patient's ability to maintain an effective immune system. This is especially important because of the overwhelming effect of the malignant process on the immune mechanism prior to the surgical procedure. It is very difficult to separate the overall consequences of pneumoperitoneum from those of other events that involve patients undergoing laparoscopic operations. In general, it has been shown that when compared with traditional operations, patients undergoing laparoscopic procedures have greater protection of the immune mechanisms [19]. Most of these studies, however, have been performed on animals with intact immune mechanisms and in patients without malignancies [19, 20]. It is reasonable to assume that patients who have immune compromise because of cancer have a response different from the normal population. A great concern is that the addition of pneumoperitoneum may reduce the immune competence, which is already reduced in patients with cancer. Currently, however, this fear has not been substantiated.

Mechanical Effects

A number of anecdotal reports of abdominal wall tumor implants after laparoscopic surgical procedures have intimated that laparoscopic intervention or, more pointedly, the addition of pneumoperitoneum has led to these port-site implants [9, 17]. A number of studies have suggested that pneumoperitoneum may be the mediator of a cellular diaspora caused by increased abdominal pressure at the time of tumor manipulation [21, 22]. There continues to be no evidence that a metabolic cause of this phenomenon has resulted from creation of a pneumoperitoneum in the cancer patient. Current estimates reveal port-site recurrence rates of approximately 1% in patients undergoing laparoscopic resection of colorectal cancer [23].

Aerosolization of cells by the pneumoperitoneum during laparoscopic procedures has not been confirmed. The local wound environment may play an important role in the mediation of trocar-site recurrence, and various strategies have been proposed to reduce or inhibit the growth of neoplastic cells in these areas [24, 25]. Treatment of the potential tumor implantation sites before the application of pneumoperitoneum has been advocated because of the continuous effects of increased abdominal wall pressure at the beginning of laparoscopic procedures and throughout the surgical event.

Conclusion

As we conclude this first decade of the 21st century, traditional, open surgical operations for abdominal malignancy are slowly being transformed to minimal access techniques. The use of carbon dioxide pneumoperitoneum remains a necessary adjunct even though mechanical lift devices have been developed to expand the abdominal space. While there have been advocates of mechanical lift who suggest a potential benefit for the cancer patient [26], the benefits of pneumoperitoneum outweigh any potential theoretical risks in this population of patients. It is clear that instillation of carbon dioxide may indeed create unwanted side effects such as increased intracranial pressure, especially in patients with brain metastases [27]. Therefore, it is important for the surgeon and anesthesiologist to understand the physiologic consequences of establishing increased abdominal wall pressure in patients with cancer.

The potential ramifications of the laparoscopic diagnosis and resection of abdominal tumors are in evolution. Thus far, there are no sequelae that indicate oncologically unsound practices as a consequence of establishing a pneumoperitoneum.

References

1. Litynski GS (1996) Anonymous highlights in the history of laparoscopy. Barbara Bernert Verlag, Frankfurt, pp 15–33
2. Andrus CH, Wittgen CM, Naunheim KS (1994) Anesthetic and physiological changes during laparoscopy and thoracoscopy: the surgeon's view. Semin Laparosc Surg 1: 228–240
3. Horvath KD, Whelan RL, Lier B et al (1998) The effects of elevated intraabdominal pressure, hypercarbia, and positioning on the hemodynamic responses to laparoscopic colectomy in pigs. Surg Endosc 12:107–114
4. Ho HS, Gunther RA, Wolfe BM (1992) Intraperitoneal carbon dioxide insufflation and cardiopulmonary functions. Laparoscopic cholecystectomy in pigs. Arch Surg 127: 928–933
5. Shimotakahara A, Kuebler JF, Vieten G, Kos M, Metzelder ML, Ure BM (2008) Carbon dioxide directly suppresses spontaneous migration, chemotaxis, and free radical production of human neutrophils. Surg Endosc 22: 1813–1817
6. Ikramuddin S, Lucas J, Ellison EC, Schirmer WJ, Melvin WS (1998) Detection of aerosolized cells during carbon dioxide laparoscopy. J Gastrointest Surg 2:580–584
7. Johnstone PA, Rohde DC, Swartz SE, Fetter JE, Wexner SD (1996) Port site recurrences after laparoscopic and thoracoscopic procedures in malignancy. J Clin Oncol 14: 1950–1956
8. Knolmayer TJ, Asbun HJ, Shibata G, Bowyer MW (1997) An experimental model of cellular aerosolization during laparoscopic surgery. Surg Laparose Endosc 7:399–402
9. Lee SW, Southall J, Allendorf J, Bessler M, Whelan RL (1998) Traumatic handling of the tumor independent of pneumoperitoneum increases port site implantation rate of colon cancer in a murine model. Surg Endosc 12:828–834
10. Mathew G, Watson DI, Ellis T, De Young N, Rofe AM, Jamieson GG (1997) The effect of laparoscopy on the movement of tumor cells and metastasis to surgical wounds. Surg Endosc 11:1163–1166
11. Evrard S, Falkenrodt A, Park A, Tassetti V, Mutter D, Marescaux J (1997) Influence of CO_2 pneumoperitoneum on systemic and peritoneal cell-mediated immunity. World J Surg 21:353–357
12. Jung IK, Kim MC, Kim KH, Kwak JY, Jung GJ, Kim HH (2008) Cellular and peritoneal immune response after radical laparoscopy-assisted and open gastrectomy for gastric cancer. J Surg Oncol 98:54–59
13. Kurz A, Sessler DI, Lenhardt R (1996) Perioperative normothermia to reduce the incidence of surgical wound infection and shorten hospitalization. N Engl J Med 334: 1209–1215
14. MacFadyen BV Jr. (1999) Hypothermia: a potential risk of CO_2 insufflation? Surg Endosc 13:99–100
15. Figueredo E, Canosa L (1997) Can hypothermia be evidenced during laparoscopic cholecystectomy? Surg Laparosc Endosc 7:378–383
16. Volz J, Köster S, Spacek Z, Paweletz N (1999) Characteristic alterations of the peritoneum after carbon dioxide pneumoperitoneum. Surg Endosc 13:611–614
17. Greene FL (1998) Pneumoperitoneum in the cancer patient: advantages and pitfalls. Semin Surg Oncol 15:151–154
18. Nussey SS, Bevan DH, Ang VT, Jenkins JS (1986) Effects of arginine vasopressin (AVP) infusions on circulating concentrations of platelet AVP, factor VIII C and von Willebrand factor. Thromb Haemost 55:34–36
19. Trokel MJ, Bessler M, Treat MR, Whelan RL, Nowyrod R (1994) Preservation of immune response after laparoscopy. Surg Endosc 8:1385–1388
20. Whelen RL, Franklin M, Holubar SD et al (2003) Postoperative cell mediated immune response is better preserved after laparoscopy vs. open colorectal resection in humans. Surg Endosc 17:972–978
21. Neuhaus SJ, Ellis T, Rofe AM, Pike GK, Jamieson GG, Watson DI (1998) Tumor implantation following laparoscopy using different insufflation gases. Surg Endosc 12:1300–1302
22. Reymond MA, Schneider C, Hohenberger W, Köckerling F (1998) The pneumoperitoneum and its role in tumor seeding. Dig Surg 15:105–109
23. Stocchi L, Nelson H (1998) Laparoscopic colectomy for colon cancer: trial update. J Surg Oncol 68:255–267
24. Goldberg JM, Maurer WG (1997) A randomized comparison of gasless laparoscopy and CO_2 pneumoperitoneum. Obstet Gynecol 90:416–420
25. Neuhaus SJ, Watson DI, Ellis T, Dodd T, Rofe AM, Jamieson GG (1998) Efficacy of cytotoxic agents for the prevention of laparoscopic port site metastases. Arch Surg 133:762–766
26. Watson DI, Mathew G, Ellis T, Baigrie CF, Rofe AM, Jamieson GG (1997) Gasless laparoscopy may reduce the risk of port-site metastases following laparoscopic tumor surgery. Arch Surg 132:166–168
27. Schöb OM, Allen DS, Benzel E et al (1996) A comparison of the pathophysiologic effects of carbon dioxide, nitrous oxide, and helium pneumoperitoneum on intracranial pressure. Am J Surg 172:248–253

Energy Sources in Laparoscopy

Ajita S. Prabhu, B. Todd Heniford

Contents

Introduction

The technological world of today revolves in large part around energy. By manipulating its many forms, our society has become more advanced than ever before. Surgery has indeed followed this upsurge in knowledge and equipment. The field of laparoscopic surgery in particular has generated and benefited from a plethora of technological advances involving energy. These instruments have improved the efficiency of operations and facilitated individual surgeon's ability to perform certain procedures. Taking advantage of these developments while avoiding potential complications is dependent on an understanding of and skill with the instrument. In all of surgery, this has been particularly true of instruments used for coagulation and hemostasis, beginning at the time that the first electrosurgery unit was put into practice in the 1920s. The intention of this chapter is to describe the basic physics and clinical use of the most commonly used energy sources in laparoscopic surgery.

Electrosurgery

The history of electrosurgery began approximately 5000 years ago. It is believed that the Egyptians treated tumors with cautery around 3000 BC [1]. One of the first to use electrosurgery via fulguration in the United States was a urologist, Edwin Beer, who removed urinary bladder tumors through an endoscope [2]. Dr. William T. Bovie, in collaboration with Dr. Harvey Cushing, however, was the true pioneer in electrosurgery. Dr. Cushing was a neurosurgeon who worked at Brigham and Women's Hospital, and Dr. Bovie was a biomedical engineer at Huntington Hospital. Dr. Cushing, like most neurosurgeons of his time,

F.L. Greene, B.T. Heniford (eds.), *Minimally Invasive Cancer Management*,
DOI 10.1007/978-1-4419-1238-1_4,

was very frustrated with uncontrolled bleeding and the subsequent high mortality rate of certain neurosurgical procedures. He had heard of the electrosurgical device, which could possibly provide safe and effective hemostasis. Working in conjunction, he and Dr. Bovie refined and advanced electrosurgical technology [3]. They performed the first neurosurgical procedure using electrocautery in 1926 [4]. This first procedure went well and generated tremendous interest. Dr. Cushing soon started to publish his series of successful cases and lectured extensively on the topic of electrosurgery [5].

Despite his not being the first to use electrical current for hemostasis, Dr. Cushing is generally given credit for its advancement due to his pursuit of the scientific understanding of the technology and his prolific discussions and publications [3]. These helped to educate other surgeons about the attributes of electrosurgery, which subsequently changed surgeons' perceptions and fears of the instrument. Interestingly, Dr. Cushing and Dr. Bovie received no financial gain from the development of the electrosurgical unit [6]. They worked with George Liebel, a businessman from Cincinnati, Ohio, and ultimately commercialized the electrosurgical device in the 1930s. Due to the skepticism associated with the instrument, however, the Dean of Harvard University discouraged Dr. Bovie from continuing his research. Many physicians and practitioners using electrosurgical energy at the turn of the century were considered charlatans. In fact, Dr. Ward, a surgeon of note at that time, wrote in *The American Journal of Surgery* in 1932, "An adequate surgical training is a prerequisite to the adoption of electrosurgery... It little behaves the novice to take up such a powerful weapon, dangerous in the hands of the unskilled" [7]. Interestingly, Harvard University refused to purchase the patent, which Dr. Bovie ultimately sold for $1.19 to the Liebel-Flarsheim Company [8].

Like most areas of surgery, the risk of surgical complications can be at least partially linked to the surgeon's fundamental knowledge of the subject. This has been related to the understanding of electrosurgery and its applicable biophysics [9]. The task of reducing any complication is usually enough to motivate surgeons; however, the influence of medical malpractice has given this issue a renewed importance. In particular, jury verdicts and settlements can help define the risks of electrosurgery in laparoscopy [10].

Electrosurgery Defined

The basics of electrosurgery begin with physics. Current, voltage, and resistance have a direct relationship. Current is defined as the flow or rate of flow of electrical charge. The values are expressed in amperes. The source of the current is the electrosurgical generator. Voltage is the electromotive force that "pushes" the current through resistance and is expressed in volts. Resistance, expressed in ohms and also referred to as impedance, is the property of a conductor that opposes the flow of an electrical current. During surgery the conductor is the patient. More specifically, the particular type of tissue upon which the surgeon is operating is the conductor, and each type of tissue (fat, muscle, liver, etc.) has its own basic properties that determine the resistance or impedance.

Another way to conceptualize this relationship is to compare electricity with water [11]. In this model electrons exist as molecules of water, and water pressure is then equivalent to voltage. When a volume of water at a defined pressure is pushed through a conduit over a time period, current is created. To define current in electrical terms means the passage of a quantity of electrons per area over time and this is measured in amperes. The relationship between current, voltage, and resistance is summed up by Ohm's law: current (I) = voltage (V) divided by the resistance (R). As the resistance increases, the voltage must also increase if the current remains the same. One additional application of this relationship is to define energy. Energy (power) is measured in watts: wattage (W) = voltage (V) multiplied by the current (I). This information can be applied and reproduced clinically by observing two electrosurgical phenomena:

(1) If an electrode is applied to fat, which has a high resistance (cautery does not function as efficiently as in fat), this increases the voltage if the wattage and current remain the same.
(2) When eschar coats the electrode tip, the resistance significantly increases, which subsequently increases the voltage for the same amount of power [3].

Applications of Electrosurgery

There is a difference between electrocautery and electrosurgery. Electrocautery is a direct current. The energy source is often a battery, which heats the surgical instrument. The "current" is then passed as heat from instrument to the tissue to which it is applied. On the other hand, electrosurgery is defined as alternating current. Electrical current is passed through the instrument and into the tissue. The tissue is heated by the conducted current resulting in a certain tissue effect [12].

Electrocution from a standard electrical outlet occurs at 110 V at 60 Hz cycles per second. This stimulation causes neuromuscular contraction and subsequently ventricular fibrillation that ultimately results in death. This effect appears to end at 100 kHz. Above this frequency, there is insufficient time for the ionic current to cause a depolarization of the cells, and the kinetic energy is dissipated as heat [13]. Electrosurgical generators today work in the 300–600 kHz range. To compare, radio and TV frequency operates at 550 kHz to 880 MHz.

Frequency affects temperature changes in the cell. As the temperature rises from 34 to 44°C, there are no visible external changes, but the biological effect is inflammation and edema. When the temperature range reaches 44–50°C, there are still no visible changes, but cellular processes cease as enzymatic activity is inactivated [14]. Between 50 and 80°C, coagulation of tissue occurs primarily because of protein denaturing. This appears as a blanching of the tissue. The tri-helical structure of collagen is disrupted and results in shrinkage. Additionally, the tissue desiccates as temperatures approach 100°C. The cell wall ruptures after the internal water reaches its boiling point of 100°C. At 200–300°C, the tissue will carbonize from dehydration. With continued heating of the tissue, the hydrocarbons combust resulting in vaporization [14].

Current density is another concept often mentioned in the context of electrosurgery. The basis of this concept is that the amount of heat generated is dependent on the amount of tissue contact the electrode receives. As the area of electrode contact increases (i.e., a larger tip on an electrocautery pencil), the current density decreases. This leads to decreased heat generation as the current is dispersed over a larger area. Essentially, when a large, flat tip is used on a cautery device, the heat generation decreases and, therefore, the visual display of the tissue effect is diminished. When the power setting is fixed, the current density decreases as the voltage increases.

Therapeutic Applications of Electrosurgery

The two forms are cutting and coagulation. The pure cutting form is also known as vaporization. This involves using a continuous sine wave, unmodulated and undamped. The current is of high frequency and of low voltage and results in rapid temperature rise with explosive vaporization [14]. The lateral thermal spread is minimal as is the depth of necrosis. Coagulation, on the other hand, uses short bursts of radio frequency sine waves with pauses between [11]. The percentage of time that the radiofrequency is on is described as the duty cycle. In the coagulation mode, the current is on typically 6% of the time period and off 94% of the time period [9]. To compare, the cutting setting would be considered to have a 100% duty cycle, because electrons are delivered 100% of the time. Most electrosurgical generators allow a blend setting. This function provides both cutting and coagulating effects at the same time. Blend 1 is typically a 50% duty cycle. Blend 2 is a 40% duty cycle with the current on 40% of the time. A very important concept to remember is that as the duty cycle diminishes, the voltage must increase to keep the power constant. A blended effect allows for cooling periods, which permit slow dehydration of cellular fluid and protein with the accompanying cell wall explosion and vaporization [9]. As the amperage is constant, the voltage is low based on a specific power. In the coagulation setting, the duty cycle has the current on for a short period of time, resulting in a low amperage current. Therefore, the voltage is significantly increased to maintain the same power setting given in the equation: W (wattage) = V (voltage) × I (current).

There are two types of coagulation: superficial or fulguration and deep or desiccation. Fulguration sprays electrical sparks to the tissue. This uses a high-voltage, low-current non-continuous (highly damped) waveform. This produces a superficial eschar with minimal depth of necrosis. This effect is seen when pressing the "coag" button and maintaining non-contact with the tissue. Desiccation ensues by making contact with the active electrode to the tissue. Then the "coag" or the "cut" button is depressed, and the energy is delivered to the tissue and converted to heat. This causes a deep necrosis and often a sticking eschar. Desiccation performed with cutting waveform results in greater depth of penetration and reduced charring. The tissue effects generated by electrosurgery are multifactorial depending on waveform, size of electrode, power setting, time of exposure, surgical technique, tissue type, and eschar formation.

Electrosurgery has two types of applications: monopolar and bipolar. The monopolar operation sends the current from the generator to the active electrode, the hand-piece, and from there directly into the tissue to which it is applied for the electrosurgical effect. The current then flows through the patient to the passive electrode, the grounding pad, and subsequently returns to the generator. In this fashion the electrosurgical effects occur only at the active electrode [9].

Bipolar has an active and a return electrode. The two arms of the circuit are part of a single surgical instrument, most often in the form of forceps. There is no need for a grounding pad to be applied to the patient as the current flows from one tip of the instrument to the other; only the tissue between the two electrodes is exposed to the electrical current [15]. Lower voltages are used to achieve the same tissue effect, because the poles are in close proximity to each other. Once the cells are dehydrated and charred, the current stops flowing and thus limits the process from damaging surrounding structures [16]. Hemostasis is obtained without unnecessary charring by using the cutting waveform in most modern bipolar units. Because of this arrangement, bipolar equipment has a more limited area of thermal spread compared with that of monopolar electrosurgery and produces less smoke. It also works well if saline or other fluid is in the surgical field, because the return electrode is very close to the active electrode. This same property also results in less electrical interference with implanted devices such as cardiac defibrillators or pacemakers. When compared with monopolar waveform application, bipolar has minimal risk of capacitive coupling, which will be discussed in detail later.

Monopolar and bipolar waveforms each have advantages and limitations. One main advantage of monopolar over bipolar electrosurgery is its ease of use. It also provides a greater penetration of current density, which can actually be an advantage for hemostasis in certain areas. Monopolar current often produces an area of coagulation twice that of bipolar current. An additional capability from coagulation and cutting is that the instrument can be used for blunt dissection. Saline solution offers a low resistance which results in poor monopolar function since much of the current is carried away; however, it works well in distilled water [17].

Argon Beam Coagulation

Argon beam coagulation is a sophisticated use of high-frequency electrosurgery [14]. Argon gas, which is inert and noncombustible, is ionized and used to conduct current via the argon plasma arc to targeted tissue [18]. The ionization process takes place as the surgical hand-piece activates a strong electric field in the background of flowing gas. Free electrons accelerate in the electric field to the point of ionizing the argon atom. This forms a multiplicative process resulting in an electron avalanche and forming plasma. This arcing causes wide, but superficial coagulation. This fulguration technique produces little smoke because of the reduced carbonization. The gas flow also blows blood from the field. There is minimal depth of penetration. In animal studies the effects of high power and prolonged (5 s) direct exposure to the argon beam still produced only superficial effects on bowel and bladder [19]. This is not a laser but only an electron channel to allow the delivery of monopolar current [20].

Complications

Complications using electrosurgery are well reported in the literature. In the 1970s the rates were reported as 2.3 per 1,000 procedures [21]. As laparoscopy has increased in popularity among general surgeons, the rates of injury have been described as 2–3.5 per 1,000 in laparoscopic cholecystectomy [17–22]. Thermal injury to the intestine resulting in eventual death has also been reported [23]. In 1993 the American College of Surgeons performed a survey during its annual meeting to define surgeon's perceptions about electrosurgical injury. The results of this study found that 18% of the more than 500 respondents had personally experienced an electrosurgical injury to their patients during laparoscopy. In addition, 54% of the respondents knew of another surgeon who had an experience with such a complication. This survey also revealed that 74% of the respondents use coagulation modes primarily during laparoscopic surgery [24]. Because the surgeon's view is limited to the area where the laparoscope is pointed, complications can occur outside the limited visual field. The incidence of these injuries appears to be decreasing as instrumentation has improved and the understanding of electrosurgery has improved.

Electrosurgical injuries outside the view of the laparoscope can occur for three reasons: direct coupling, insulation failure, and capacitive coupling [25].

Direct coupling usually results from unintended contact or electrical arc between the active electrode and a metal instrument or object. This contact energizes the object, which can include the laparoscope, grasper, or ligating clip and is often outside the field of vision. Current flow then may proceed from the newly energized metal instrument to any segment of bowel or other internal tissue touching the laparoscope or instrument at the same time [26]. This can also occur if the electrode is activated unintentionally resulting in an electrical current application to non-targeted tissue [27].

Insulation failure is equipment failure. These breaks in insulation can result in blow holes where current can spark to non-targeted and non-visualized tissue. Risk factors for this type of problem include repeated use of instrumentation, after cleaning/sterilization procedures, possibly a 5-mm instrument through a 10-mm port, and using high voltage [9, 27, 28]. The small and frequently undetectable breaks in electrode insulation are significantly more dangerous, because this allows for a higher current density and allows for a potentially serious injury to the patient [27].

Capacitive coupling occurs when current is transferred from the active electrode through intact insulation and into adjacent materials without direct contact. A capacitor exists when two conductors are separated by an insulation layer and have a difference in potential between them. When the active electrode is placed inside a trocar, this situation is created. Normally, the electrical current is dissipated from the trocar into the abdominal wall over the entire area of contact with the trocar, thus preventing injury. In the setting of a hybrid cannula (part plastic, part metal), the different materials can interfere with the transfer of the radiofrequency energy into the abdominal wall and subsequently to the passive electrode [20]. Longer instruments, thinner insulation, higher voltages, and narrow trocars are all factors that can increase the chance of injury.

One last site of electrical injury in the use of electrosurgery is the passive electrode or the grounding pad. When this pad is improperly applied, the current will seek another route of return to the generator, but this will likely be in the form of a contact point that promotes high current density, i.e., EKG leads, towel clips, stirrups, or head frames [9]. These types of injuries can be avoided by proper placement of the grounding pad, which includes contact with at least 20 cm^2 of body surface area, and avoidance of bony prominences, moist skin, and mechanical joints. Of course, this cannot compensate for manufacturing or quality defects, but it can minimize injury.

The best policy at present is to use the lowest possible power setting to achieve the desired surgical effect and to use the proper current waveform. Brief intermittent activation is preferred to prolonged activation for limiting incidence of stray current. In addition, if the expected tissue effect is not accomplished, assume defect in ground pad or capacitive or direct coupling. All metal or all plastic trocars are preferred over hybrids. Finally, an effort should be made to keep the activated electrode in the operative field at all times and to monitor the status of insulation of instruments.

Pacemakers and Electrosurgery

Surgeons should use caution when employing monopolar electrosurgical devices in patients with pacemakers or implantable cardioverter defibrillators. Monopolar electrosurgery may reset the pacemaker device or cause inappropriate sensing and/or therapeutic effects if used improperly. The pacemaker in a patient undergoing a surgical procedure requiring electrosurgery should probably be programmed to an asynchronous mode in order to avoid inhibition or oversensing of the device. Another option is to place a magnet over the pacemaker to obtain asynchronous pacing during periods of monopolar electrocautery [29]. The grounding pad should be placed as far as possible from the pulse generator and lead. If possible, short bursts of electrocautery on the lowest power setting should be used for the necessary effect. If there is doubt as to the correct action to take preoperatively, one can review the technical manual for the pacemaker, if it is available. Alternatively, a cardiologist can be consulted before the operation. Ideally, bipolar forms of electrocautery should be used in patients with pacemakers, because the energy is concentrated between the active and passive blade, and the energy does not pass through the patient [3]. Another alternative is ultrasonic energy.

Ultrasonic Energy

Harmonic

An alternative to or substitute for electrical energy sources (monopolar, bipolar electrosurgery) is the ultrasonic coagulating shears or the Harmonic device

(Ethicon Endo-Surgery, Cincinnati, OH). Few instruments developed over the last 20 years have facilitated a surgeon's ability to perform complex operations like the Harmonic device. Its impact was immediate and continues to have a dramatic impact on the implementation of minimally invasive surgery over many specialties. Ultrasonic coagulating shears are FDA approved to divide tissue and coagulate vessels of diameter up to 3 mm. The instrument was introduced in 1992 and became commercially available in 1993. Ultrasonic coagulating shears operate by converting electrical energy into mechanical vibrations. Electrical energy is transferred from a microprocessor-controlled generator to a transducer in the hand-piece [3]. The transducer contains a piezoelectric crystal which converts the electrical energy into vibrating ultrasonic wave energy at the same frequency [30]. This energy is delivered to the tip of the instrument to the active blade that will longitudinally vibrate rapidly over an excursion of 50–100 μm [31]. The frequency (55.5 Hz) is in a range that denatures collagen molecules, vaporizes cells, and provides both coagulation and cutting. As discussed earlier, collagen is denatured at a temperature of 80°C. The Harmonic device generates temperatures in this range and thus avoids the charring that can occur at higher temperatures. This results in a coaptive coagulation, which seals vessels by formation of a protein coagulum [32]. There is a cavitational effect of the ultrasonic devices, which provides additional tissue dissection by separating tissue layers with fluid vapors produced when the instrument is activated. The power level on the generator is used to modulate the cutting and coagulation effects, which are inversely related. Increasing the power setting from 1 to 5 increases the cutting speed (as does the blade excursion from 50 to 100 μm). Decreasing the power setting from 5 to 1 slows the cutting speed and provides improved hemostasis. A power setting of 3 (blade excursion of 70 μm) is the most versatile. Cutting speed is also a function of blade configuration, tissue tension, and grip force/pressure. A sharper blade increases cutting speed at the expense of more reliable hemostasis. Two additional factors are operator-dependent: a greater amount of tension on the tissue in apposition between the active blade and tissue pad and a firm grip on the ultrasonic coagulating shears handle achieves less coagulation with faster cutting [3].

There are multiple advantages to using an ultrasonic device or the Harmonic device in laparoscopy. Because this instrument operates at a lower temperature range than electrocautery, the tissue destruction is by vaporization instead of carbonization. This leads to less smoke production, greater visibility, and possibly less toxins to which the operating room personnel are exposed. The instrument produces a great deal of steam, which can lead to a very humid operative environment with frequent fogging of the laparoscope. As no electrical current is applied either to or through the patient, there is no risk of direct coupling or capacitative coupling injuries. One of the main advantages of this technology is the minimizing of lateral tissue injury. Since the effective operating temperatures are lower than those of electrosurgical instruments, the risk of adjacent thermal injury and resulting tissue destruction is decreased [3]. We have microscopically measured lateral thermal spread repeatedly in a laboratory setting and noted an average of 1.6–2.5 mm, but as much as 4 mm, of tissue necrosis [33, 34].

Although the decreased operating temperature is an advantage of the ultrasonic devices, it is by no means a "cold" instrument. The vibrating or active blade becomes very hot and remains so for several seconds after an application. After activating this instrument to transect tissue, the surgeon should not inadvertently touch bowel or other vital structures, which could induce a thermal injury and result in an immediate or delayed full thickness injury. Another limitation of the Harmonic device is that it should be reserved for vessels 3 mm or less in diameter. Bleeding may ensue if larger vessels are sealed or only partially transected using the instrument.

LigaSure

Another advance in energy sources is the LigaSure vessel sealing system (Valleylab, Boulder, Co) (Fig. 4.1). The impetus to develop this instrument was from surgeons demanding reliable, consistent, permanent vessel wall fusion with minimal thermal spread, and the formation of seal strengths comparable to existing mechanical techniques such as sutures and clips. The development of this technology was driven by several factors, including the inability of previous bipolar electrosurgical energy systems and ultrasonic thermal energy systems to reliably seal vessels greater than 2–3 mm in diameter, the time required for suture ligation, the tedium of laparoscopic intracorporeal suturing, and the expense of the endoscopic stapler for hemostasis during laparoscopic procedures. This electrothermal bipolar vessel sealer can seal vessels up to 7 mm in diameter. High current (4 amps) and low

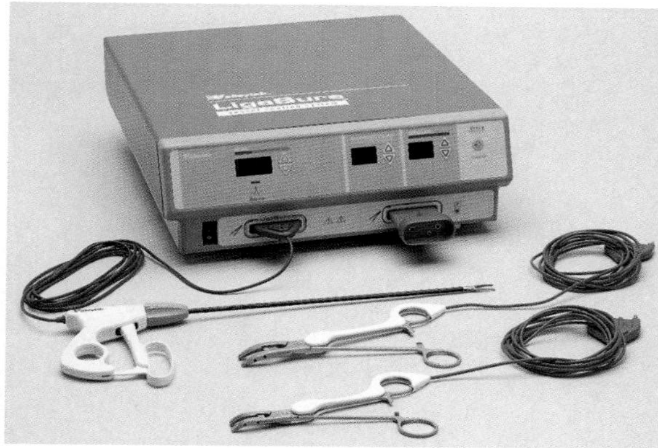

Figure 4.1

LigaSure vessel sealing system. (Copyright © 2009 Covidien. All rights reserved. Reprinted with permission of the Energy Based Devices and Surgical Devices Divisions of Covidien.)

voltage (<200 V) are used, as opposed to traditional electrosurgical instruments, which use low current and high voltage. Collagen and elastin within the vessel wall and surrounding connective tissue are denatured, and the pressure applied by the clamped instrument causes the denatured protein to reform while the vessel walls are in apposition. This results in a very strong and nearly translucent seal (Figs. 4.2 and 4.3). This seal can then be transected [35].

A unique feature of this technology is the feedback control. The initial radiofrequency resistance of the tissue in apposition is measured, and then the appropriate energy setting is used by the generator to deliver a pulsed energy wave. The resistance and subsequent energy delivery is repeated many times per second, allowing for constant feedback and adjustment of the energy dispensed, as well as a constant seal [36]. The instrument used has a ratcheted mechanism, much like other surgical clamps, that allows for a calibrated force to be applied to the targeted tissue area. The foot switch then activates the device, which sends out a precursor voltage scan. Subsequently as the radiofrequency energy is applied to the tissue, the temperature-dependent impedance is monitored until the seal is complete, at which point the device shuts off the energy delivery and emits an audible tone [37]. Seal strengths are comparable to mechanical ligation techniques such as sutures and clips and are significantly stronger than other energy-based techniques such as standard bipolar or ultrasonic coagulation [33, 35, 37, 38]. We have documented consistent burst strengths of the LigaSure's seals in excess of 550 mmHg, even in vessels of 7 mm or greater of size. The seals have proven to withstand more than three times normal systolic blood pressure [39]. In one study, the LigaSure device was noted to reduce operating time in open procedures compared to suture ligatures [35]. The use of the LigaSure device in laparoscopic surgery is still being defined but appears to have broad applications in all laparoscopic surgery as a useful energy source.

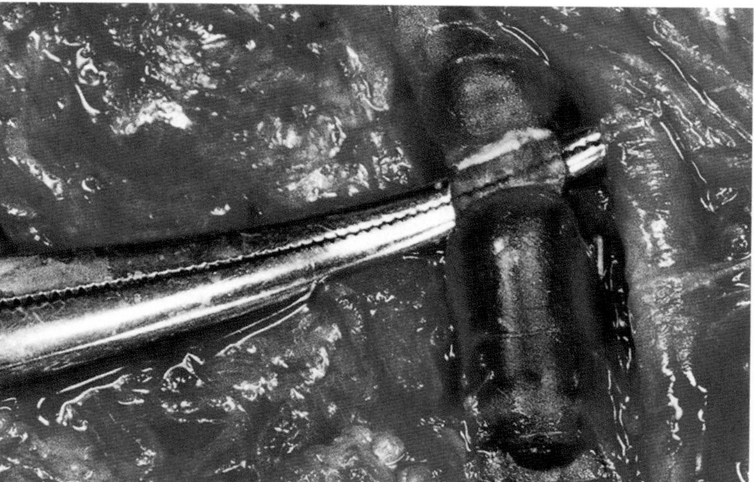

Figure 4.2

Translucent seal produced by LigaSure. (Copyright © 2009 Covidien. All rights reserved. Reprinted with permission of the Energy Based Devices and Surgical Devices Divisions of Covidien.)

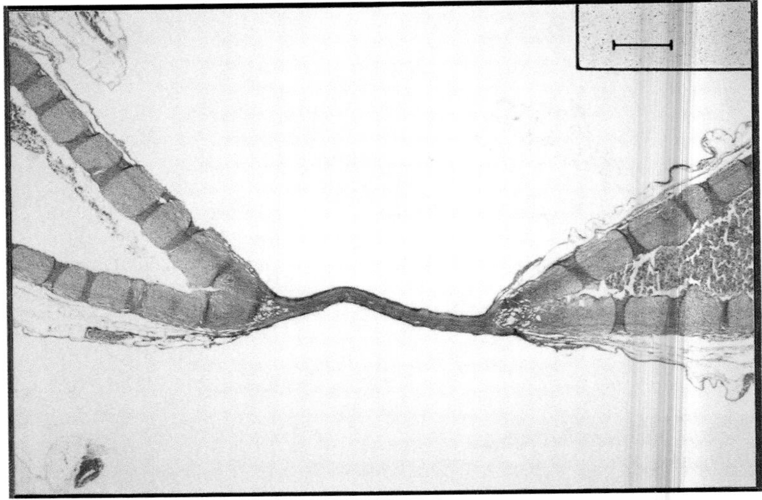

Figure 4.3

Histology sample of LigaSure seal.

EnSeal

The EnSeal Temperature Controlled Tissue Sealing Technology (Ethicon Endo-Surgery, Cincinnati, OH) is one of the newest devices available for sealing blood vessels. The 5 mm diameter shaft instrument delivers bipolar electrosurgical energy through a high-compression jaw with a tissue-dynamic energy delivery mechanism. Millions of nanometer-sized conductive particles direct the energy and control the temperature and heat in the tissue contained within the jaws of the device, thereby providing energy that turns off at approximately 100°C. The jaws provide a high uniform compression across the length of the jaw. An "I"-shaped blade (I-Blade^{TM} design) then advances as the tissue is being sealed, simultaneously cutting the sealed tissue [40]. This instrument is recommended and FDA approved for vessels of up to and including 7 mm in diameter.

A study documented burst pressures of 720 mmHg in vessels of 6–7 mm in size in a porcine model, which was a statistically significantly higher burst pressure than those documented in other comparable bipolar electrosurgical devices. However, even the lowest bursting pressures that were recorded were in the supraphysiologic range, which makes the clinical significance of these differences unclear [41]. Another potential advantage as noted in our study is no seal failures for the EnSeal device for 6–7 mm vessels [40].

Disadvantages, noted by Person et al. in the porcine model, were a shorter seal width of 1 mm (range 0.1–2.4 mm) than the LigaSure devices and a greater incidence of thermal injury to the smooth muscle in the vessel's media than both the LigaSure and Harmonic devices. Statistical analysis was not provided for these data [41]. Other disadvantages of the EnSeal device are the additional step to fire the built-in cutting mechanism and a longer seal time for vessels ≤7 mm (8.25 s) compared to several of the other electrosurgical and ultrasonic devices ($p < 0.05$) [40]. The EnSeal device is a novel system that has not been well described for clinical use.

Radiofrequency Energy

An additional instrument available for sealing vessels and tissue fluids in solid organ transaction is the TissueLink (Fig. 4.4) (TissueLink Medical, Inc,

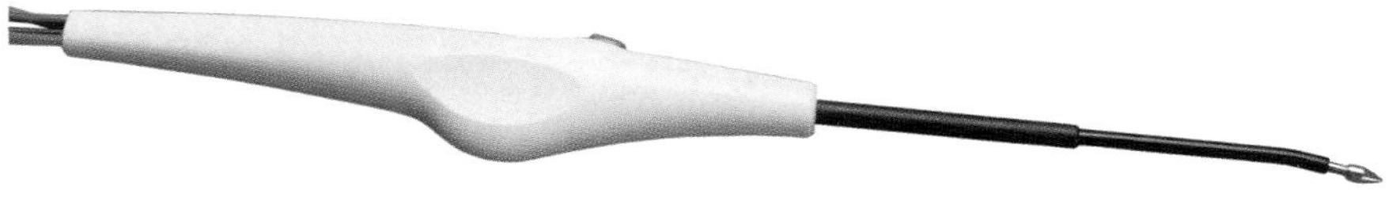

Figure 4.4

TissueLink device. (Courtesy of TissueLink Medical, Inc, Dover, New Hampshire)

Dover, New Hampshire), which employs radiofrequency energy. The device plugs into a standard operating room Bovie electrosurgical generator. The coagulation power is typically set between 90 and 100 W. A sterile liter of 0.9% saline is connected to the irrigation tubing and adjusted for a drip rate of 4–8 cc/min. Radiofrequency energy is applied through a low-volume saline drip, which cools the tip of the device, creating a "wet electrode" that seals tissue without charring. The thermal energy results in denaturing of protein in vessel walls and shrinks collagen, thereby sealing blood vessels [42]. Surgeons can use the device as a sort of cutting tool to section through tissues, can close particular vessels, or can "paint" and seal a large surface. This instrument is FDA approved for soft tissue surgeries. Multiple studies have demonstrated reduced blood loss in liver transaction when using the TissueLink device [42–44], and there is potential for reduced incidence of bile leaks as well [42].

The TissueLink is not recommended for sealing structures more than 6 mm in diameter. Another disadvantage is that constant suction is required to clear the saline used for irrigation, and the use of the TissueLink device alone may result in a slower pace of tissue transaction. Its use in combination with ultrasonic dissectors or hydrojet may shorten parenchymal transection time [42].

Conclusion

Traditional monopolar and bipolar electrosurgeries remain very useful in laparoscopic surgery. The need for meticulous hemostasis and the tedium of vessel ligation in advanced cases have propelled the development of new energy source devices, which have proven to be remarkably helpful in both laparoscopic and open surgery. While each of these energy sources has improved the efficiency and safety of minimally invasive techniques, they can also be associated with distressing complications. An understanding of the biophysics of these tools, their spectrum of effectiveness, and methods of application can improve our ability to perform surgery in a safe and proficient manner.

References

1. Breasted JH (1930) The Edwin Smith surgical papyrus. University of Chicago Press, Chicago, IL
2. Beer E (1983) Landmark article May 28, 1910: removal of neoplasms of the urinary bladder. By Edwin Beer. J Am Med Assoc 250(10):1324–1325
3. Laparoscopy 101: a resource for resident education, module 2: Energy sources. In. Charlotte, NC; 2002. www.DanMartinMD.com/utlap07.htm.
4. O'Connor JL, Bloom DA, William T (1996) Bovie and electrosurgery. Surgery 119(4):390–396
5. Cushing H (1928) Electrosurgery as an aid to the removal of intracranial tumors. Surg Gynecol Obstet 47:751–784
6. Goldwyn RM (1979) Bovie: the man and the machine. Ann Plast Surg 2(2):135–153
7. Ward G (1932) Electricity in medicine; electrosurgery. Am J Surg 17:86–93
8. Pollack S (1991) Electrosurgery of the skin. Churchill Living-Stone, New York, NY
9. Wu MP, Ou CS, Chen SL et al (2000) Complications and recommended practices for electrosurgery in laparoscopy. Am J Surg 179(1):67–73
10. Perantinides PG, Tsarouhas AP, Katzman VS (1998) The medicolegal risks of thermal injury during laparoscopic monopolar electrosurgery. J Health Risk Manag 18(1): 47–55
11. Soderstrom RM (1994) Electrosurgical injuries during laparoscopy: prevention and management. Curr Opin Obstet Gynecol 6(3):248–250
12. Soderstrom RM (1997) Principles of electrosurgery as applied to gynecology. In: Rock J, Thompson JD (eds) Te Linde's operative gynecology, 8 edn. Lippincott-Raven, Philadelphia, PA, pp 321–326
13. Sittner W, Fitzgerald JK (1976) High frequency electrosurgery. In: Berci G (ed) Endoscopy. Appleton-Century-Crofts, New York, NY, pp 214–220
14. Shimi SM (1995) Dissection techniques in laparoscopic surgery: a review. J R Coll Surg Edinb 40(4):249–259
15. Ballantyne G, Leahy PF, Modlin IM (1994) Laparoscopic surgery. W.B. Saunders, Philadelphia, PA
16. Rioux JE, Cloutier D (1974) A new bipolar instrument for laparoscopic tubal sterilization. Am J Obstet Gynecol 119(6):737–739
17. Nduka CC, Super PA, Monson JR et al (1994) Cause and prevention of electrosurgical injuries in laparoscopy. J Am Coll Surg 179(2):161–170
18. Platt RC, Heniford BT (2000) Development and initial trial of the minilaparoscopic argon coagulator. J Laparoendosc Adv Surg Tech A 10(2):93–99
19. Gale P, Adeyemi B, Ferrer K et al (1998) Histologic characteristics of laparoscopic argon beam coagulation. J Am Assoc Gynecol Laparosc 5(1):19–22
20. Sutton C (1995) Power sources in endoscopic surgery. Curr Opin Obstet Gynecol 7(4):248–256
21. Loffer FD, Pent D (1975) Indications, contraindications and complications of laparoscopy. Obstet Gynecol Surv 30(7):407–427
22. Fletcher DR, Hobbs MS, Tan P et al (1999) Complications of cholecystectomy: risks of the laparoscopic approach and protective effects of operative cholangiography: a population-based study. Ann Surg 229(4): 449–457
23. Peterson HB, Ory HW, Greenspan JR et al (1981) Deaths associated with laparoscopic sterilization by unipolar

electrocoagulating devices, 1978 and 1979. Am J Obstet Gynecol 139(2):141–143
24. Tucker RD (1995) Laparoscopic electrosurgical injuries: survey results and their implications. Surg Laparosc Endosc 5(4):311–317
25. Saye WB, Miller W, Hertzmann P (1991) Electrosurgery thermal injury. Myth or misconception? Surg Laparosc Endosc 1(4):223–228
26. Rock JA, Thompson JD (1997) Te Linde's operative gynecology, 8 edn. Lippincott-Raven, Philadelphia, PA
27. Brill AI, Feste JR, Hamilton TL et al (1998) Patient safety during laparoscopic monopolar electrosurgery – principles and guidelines. Consortium on electrosurgical safety during laparoscopy. JSLS 2(3):221–225
28. Tucker RD, Voyles CR (1995) Laparoscopic electrosurgical complications and their prevention. Aorn J 62(1):51–53, 55, 58–59 passim; quiz 74–77
29. AORN Recommended Practices Commitee. Recommended practices for electrosurgery. Aorn J 2005;81(3):616–618, 621–626, 629–632 passim.
30. Park AE, Mastrangelo MJ Jr., Gandsas A et al (2001) Laparoscopic dissecting instruments. Semin Laparosc Surg 8(1):42–52
31. Kunde D, Welch C (2003) Ultracision in gynaecological laparoscopic surgery. J Obstet Gynaecol 23(4):347–352
32. Amaral JF (1994) The experimental development of an ultrasonically activated scalpel for laparoscopic use. Surg Laparosc Endosc 4(2):92–99
33. Harold KL, Pollinger H, Matthews BD et al (2003) Comparison of ultrasonic energy, bipolar thermal energy, and vascular clips for the hemostasis of small-, medium-, and large-sized arteries. Surg Endosc 17(8):1228–1230
34. Goldstein SL, Harold KL, Lentzner A et al (2002) Comparison of thermal spread after ureteral ligation with the Laparo-Sonic ultrasonic shears and the Ligasure system. J Laparoendosc Adv Surg Tech A 12(1):61–63
35. Heniford BT, Matthews BD, Sing RF et al (2001) Initial results with an electrothermal bipolar vessel sealer. Surg Endosc 15(8):799–801
36. Heniford BT, Matthews B (2000) Basic instrumentation for laparoscopic surgery. In: Greene FL, Heniford BT (eds) Minimally invasive cancer management. Springer, New York, NY, pp 36–44
37. Campbell PA, Cresswell AB, Frank TG et al (2003) Real-time thermography during energized vessel sealing and dissection. Surg Endosc 17(10):1640–1645
38. Carbonell AM, Joels CS, Kercher KW et al (2003) A comparison of laparoscopic bipolar vessel sealing devices in the hemostasis of small-, medium-, and large-sized arteries. J Laparoendosc Adv Surg Tech A 13(6):377–380
39. Landman J, Kerbl K, Rehman J et al (2003) Evaluation of a vessel sealing system, bipolar electrosurgery, Harmonic device, titanium clips, endoscopic gastrointestinal anastomosis vascular staples and sutures for arterial and venous ligation in a porcine model. J Urol 169(2):697–700
40. Newcomb WL, Hope WW, Schmelzer TM et al (2008) Comparison of blood vessel sealing among new electrosurgical and ultrasonic devices. Surg Endosc 23(1):90–96
41. Smaldone MC, Gibbons EP, Jackman SV (2008) Laparoscopic nephrectomy using the EnSeal tissue sealing and hemostasis system: successful therapeutic application of nanotechnology. JSLS 12(2):213–216
42. Geller DA, Tsung A, Maheshwari V et al (2005) Hepatic resection in 170 patients using saline-cooled radiofrequency coagulation. HPB (Oxford) 7(3):208–213
43. Xia F, Wang S, Ma K et al (2008) The use of saline-linked radiofrequency dissecting sealer for liver transection in patients with cirrhosis. J Surg Res 149(1):110–114
44. Di Carlo I, Barbagallo F, Toro A et al (2004) Hepatic resections using a water-cooled, high-density, monopolar device: a new technology for safer surgery. J Gastrointest Surg 8(5):596–600

Biopsy and Staging: Technical Issues

James D. Smith, Kevin C. P. Conlon

Contents

Rationale

In the last decade cancer management has become more and more complex. Increasingly, evidence-based medicine has shown a benefit for neo-adjuvant chemotherapy and radiotherapy, prior to definitive surgery, in certain stages of cancer. This has led to the realization that resection alone may not be of benefit for the cohort of patients with high risk of recurrence. Accurate pre-operative staging of cancer has become essential for optimal patient care. Traditionally, patients were subjected to open exploration often for staging purposes. If unresectable disease was found, palliative resection or bypass procedures would be performed for symptomatic control. With the advent of endoscopic stenting of the gastrointestinal tract and biliary system for esophageal, gastric, and pancreatic cancers, symptomatic control for patients can now be obtained without need for open exploration. With this, exploratory laparotomy for cancer staging has become undesirable as it leads to increased patient morbidity and mortality [1, 2]. Therefore, the ability to identify unresectable disease can lead to a reduction in unnecessary laparotomies and, with this, reduced patient morbidity and better use of operating theatre time.

Non-invasive radiological techniques have also improved significantly in recent times, such as the development of multi-slice contrast-enhanced CT scanning, MRI, and PET [3]. These developments along with the increased availability of endoscopic ultrasound have led to significant improvements in pre-operative staging for gastrointestinal and intra-abdominal malignancies. However, there is still a cohort of patients who develop early metastatic disease despite "curative" surgery and of patients who are found to be inoperable at laparotomy [4]. Laparoscopic staging offers an adjunct to traditional pre-operative staging techniques in trying to identify this cohort of

F.L. Greene, B.T. Heniford (eds.), *Minimally Invasive Cancer Management*,
DOI 10.1007/978-1-4419-1238-1_5,

patients. It leads to increased accuracy of staging and facilitates optimal cancer management.

Although laparoscopy has increased morbidity compared to traditional staging techniques and carries the logistical issues of a second operation, the reduction of unnecessary laparotomies and identification of patients better served by other treatment modalities outweighs these concerns. Laparoscopy can identify patients with small metastatic liver deposits, occult peritoneal carcinomatosis, or circulating peritoneal cancer cells leading to a change in patient management [5].

Laparoscopic staging can be performed as a separate elective procedure or just prior to open operation. Although this adds a further procedure to a patient's pre-operative staging investigations, laparoscopy allows for more efficient use of operating room time as it reduces the incidence of unnecessary laparotomies due to more accurate staging. This constitutes better use of resources and leads to improved cost-effectiveness [5].

Operating Room Setup

As with any surgical procedure, appropriate setup of the operating theatre is essential for efficient, safe, and effective staging laparoscopy. The patient is placed supine on the operating table with both arms tucked in by the patient's side. The patient may be strapped in, or a compressed sand bag used, to prevent patient movement with tilting of the operating table. The surgeon generally stands on the right-hand side of the table with his assistant and camera operator on the opposite side. The monitors are placed above the operating field at shoulder level; however, this can be altered to surgeons' preference.

A basic laparoscopic instrument set is generally adequate for the procedure (Fig. 5.1). This normally consists of

- scissors,
- dissector,
- two graspers (atraumatic and toothed),
- suction irrigation device,
- biopsy forceps.

These may be disposable or reusable according to the institution's preference. Also a laparoscopic liver retractor and punch biopsy needle may be necessary. The ports used may also be disposable or reusable but generally consist of a blunt umbilical port to facilitate the camera (5 or 10 mm depending on the camera size), 5 mm ports, and one 12 mm port to facilitate laparoscopic ultrasound where needed.

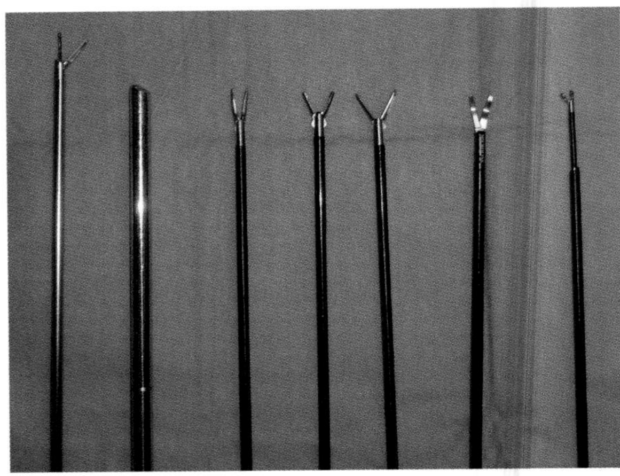

Figure 5.1
Standard laparoscopic set including SonoSurg, 30° laparoscope, and cup biopsy forceps (*far right*)

An oblique laparoscopic telescope or camera (30–45°) must be used as this facilitates visualization over the dome of the liver; however, this can be 5 or 10 mm. Encasing the laparoscope in warm water or the use of anti-fog solution can prevent fogging up of the laparoscope in the abdomen.

In the majority of cases cautery is sufficient for coagulation hemostasis; however, for more extensive dissection, the use of coagulating dissection instruments such as SonoSurg™ (Olympus) and harmonic scalpels along with argon beam coagulation may prove useful. A laparoscopic ultrasound device is also important for complete staging in certain malignancies such as pancreas cancer.

The patient is painted and draped as for a laparotomy and a bilateral subcostal incision is marked out prior to the creation of a pneumoperitoneum. The surface anatomy is distorted during a pneumoperitoneum and the ports can be placed through this marked incision as it would be the likely incision used for definitive surgery.

A Veress needle may be used to create a pneumoperitoneum; however, the authors prefer the modified Hasson technique as it is associated with a reduced incidence of visceral and vascular injury [6]. Ports can be placed along the bilateral subcostal incision and can range from two ports to four depending on the procedure and the level of retraction needed. If laparoscopic

Figure 5.2

Closure of a trocar port

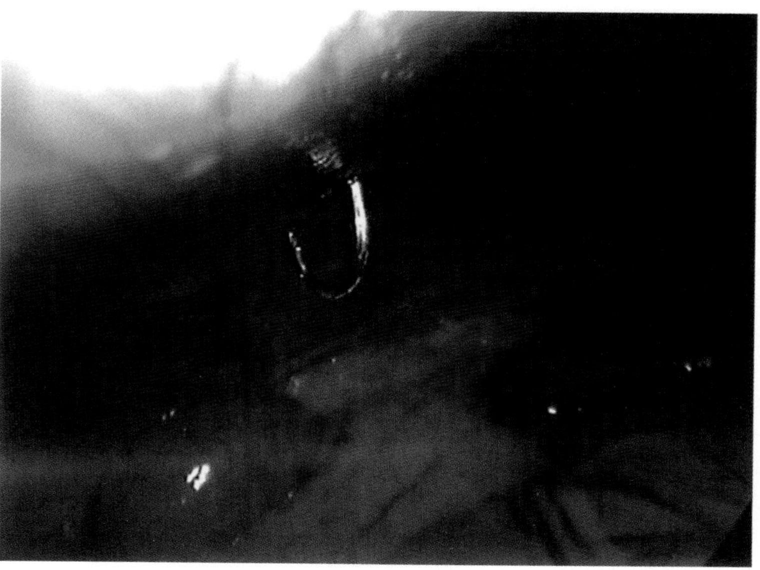

ultrasound is used, a 12 mm port must be placed in the right flank to facilitate the ultrasound probe. Port sites greater then 10 mm should be closed to prevent port site hernias (Fig. 5.2).

Technical Issues

Technically, staging laparoscopy should mimic open exploratory laparotomy where possible. The same principles of using the least invasive biopsy technique apply as with open surgery. The obvious limitations of laparoscopy, however, are lack of tactile sensation and no depth perception. These shortcomings can be compensated for by the use of intra-operative ultrasound and stereotactic imaging.

The biopsy techniques used laparoscopically mimic those performed in open surgery and from simplest to complex include the following:

- Peritoneal lavage for cytological analysis
- Fine needle aspiration
- Pinch or superficial biopsy
- Cup biopsy
- Core biopsy with or without laparoscopic ultrasound guidance
- Incisional/excisional biopsy
- Lymph node biopsy
- Sentinel node biopsy

We recommend an open technique for the creation of a pneumoperitoneum in all cases. An oblique-angled telescope is placed through the umbilical port. Trocars are placed in the right (12 and 5 mm) and left (5 mm) upper quadrants. A systemic examination of the peritoneal cavity is performed examining all four quadrants closely for metastatic disease. Adhesions are taken down where present. The primary tumor is assessed and local extent, size, and fixation are noted. Extension to contiguous organs such as the colon, duodenum, liver, spleen, and stomach are identified. Cytological washings are taken from the right and left upper quadrants after instillation of 200 ml of normal saline, prior to manipulation of the primary or metastatic tumor. (A third site in the pelvis increases the yield in gastric cancer.) The patient is then placed in a 20° reverse Trendelenburg position with 10° of left lateral tilt. Examination begins with visualization of the anterior and posterior surfaces of the left lateral segment of the liver and of the anterior and inferior surfaces of the right lobe. Palpation of the liver is achieved with the use of two closed grasping instruments (Fig. 5.3). The hilum of the liver is visualized and, by correctly positioning the 30° telescope, the foramen of Winslow is examined with the periportal lymph nodes. The patient is then placed in a 10° Trendelenburg position without lateral tilt and the omentum is retracted toward the left upper quadrant. This allows for the identification of the ligament of Treitz. The mesocolon is inspected, with particular attention paid to the mesocolic vein, which normally is quite visible. On completion of the mesocolic examination, the gastrohepatic omentum is incised, enabling visualization into the lesser sac and exposing the caudate lobe of the liver, vena cava, and celiac axis. Celiac, portal,

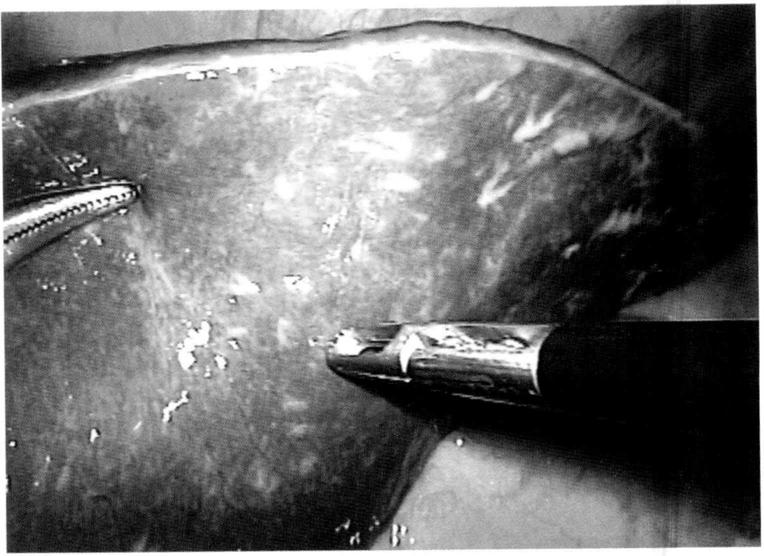

Figure 5.3

Examination of the under surface of the left lobe of the liver with two graspers demonstrating liver metastases

or perigastric nodes are inspected. The hepatic artery is identified and its course to the porta visualized. Within the lesser sac the "gastric pillar" can be seen and by retracting it laterally, the superior aspect of the pancreas can then be visualized down the splenic hilum.

One of the advantages that laparotomy has over laparoscopy is that the operating surgeon has a three-dimensional, as opposed to a two dimensional, view. Tactile sensation is also lost at laparoscopy. Laparoscopic ultrasound can be utilized to overcome these limitations. This is particularly advantageous in the staging of pancreas cancer [7].

The ultrasound probe is placed over the porta hepatis where the hepatic duct and portal vein can be visualized. The probe is then moved over the duodenum following the length of the bile duct and portal vein as it travels behind the pancreas and divides at its confluence into the splenic and superior mesenteric veins. Involvement of the veins can be assessed (Fig. 5.4). The superior mesenteric artery can be identified and assessed for tumor involvement. The probe

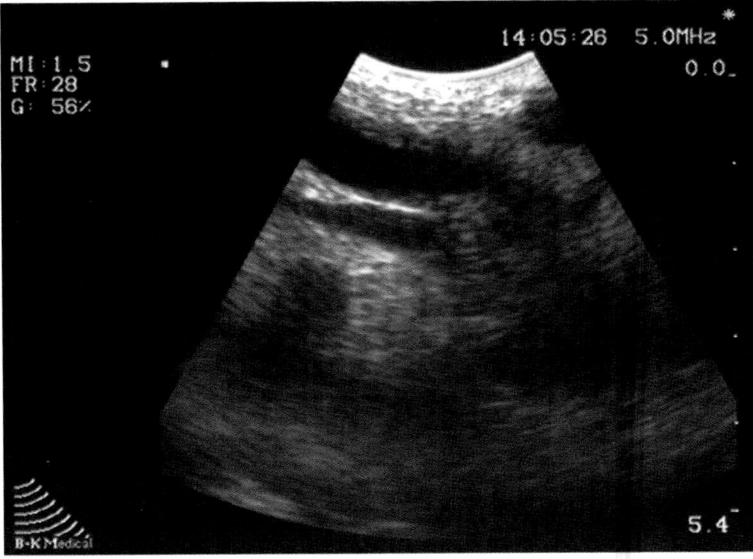

Figure 5.4

Laparoscopic ultrasound demonstrating tumor invading into the portal vein is then passed over the gastrohepatic omentum to aid visualization of the hepatic artery.

Often for gastrointestinal cancers such as esophageal and gastric cancers the left lateral lobe of the liver is elevated to expose the gastroesophageal junction with the patient placed in steep reverse Trendelenburg position. Here, the esophageal or gastric tumor can be inspected for extension into surrounding tissues.

In addition, for gastric cancers (Fig. 5.5) particular attention is paid to the perigastric nodes along the greater and lesser curvature and biopsies are performed if necessary. Following this, the porta hepatis and gastrohepatic ligaments can be inspected carefully. Next, the gastric tumor itself is inspected for extraserosal invasion and infiltration into surrounding structures. If the tumor is on the posterior stomach, then the lesser sac must be accessed to gain appropriate visualization.

For patients with hepatocellular cancers or colon cancer with liver metastases, when no metastatic disease is identified with inspection, a detailed laparoscopic ultrasound examination may be used to evaluate the deep hepatic parenchyma, portal vein, mesenteric vessels, celiac trunk, hepatic artery, entire pancreas, and even periportal and paraaortic lymph nodes. The addition of color flow Doppler can further assist in the assessment of vascular patency. This laparoscopic assessment for each tumor type can be performed within 25–40 min in experienced hands. For gastrointestinal cancers disseminated disease is determined by hepatic, serosal, peritoneal, or omental metastases which are seen and confirmed histologically.

Unresectability of pancreatic cancer is determined by the following:

- extrapancreatic extension of tumor (i.e., mesocolic involvement);
- celiac or high portal nodal involvement by tumor (Fig. 5.6);
- invasion or encasement of the celiac axis, hepatic artery, or superior mesenteric artery.

Patients who are found to have portal or mesenteric vein encroachment by tumor are considered potentially resectable and undergo exploratory laparotomy (Fig. 5.4).

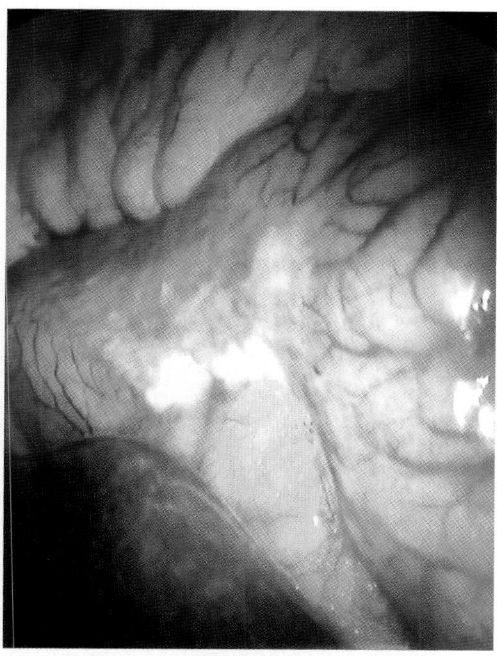

Figure 5.5

Gastric cancer located on the lesser curvature of the stomach

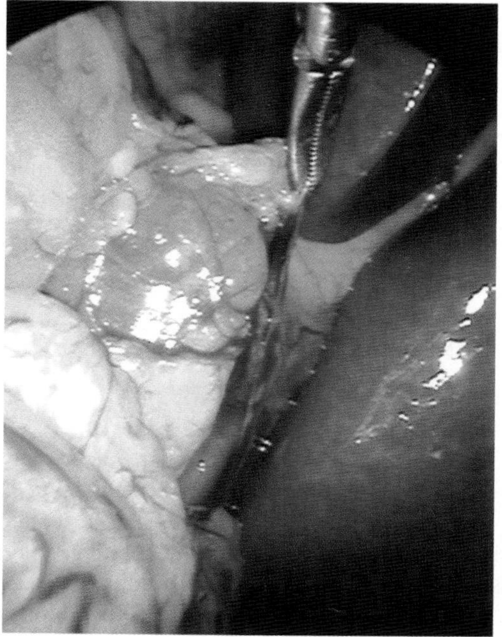

Figure 5.6

A pathological lymph node in the porta hepatis

Biopsy Techniques Following Standard Staging Laparoscopy

Peritoneal Lavage for Cytological Analysis

Peritoneal lavage for cytology should be performed in all staging laparoscopies for abdominal malignancies. The principle is that malignant cells easily exfoliate from primary tumors and may be picked up by this method, indicating the need for neo-adjuvant treatment.

Cytological analysis may also identify small volume peritoneal deposits or early peritoneal carcinomatosis which may be missed by direct visualization with the laparoscope. These patients may be better suited for palliative non-operative treatment modalities, as definitive oncological resections will be of limited benefit.

Informing the pathologist/cytologist of the procedure beforehand and discussing the clinical scenario often leads to better clinical yields and is advisable prior to undertaking the laparoscopy. Following peritoneal inspection and if no metastatic disease is found, peritoneal washings are taken from the RUQ, LUQ, and, in gastric cancers, the pelvis. The patient is positioned head down and tilted to the left. Approximately 200 ml of saline is placed in the LUQ of the abdomen. The abdomen is shaken. The saline is then aspirated and collected in a sterile container. The same procedure is repeated in the RUQ with the patient head down and tilted to the right. Finally, if indicated, the same procedure is repeated in the pelvis with the patient head down. The specimens should then be delivered to the cytopathologist for immediate analysis.

Fine Needle Aspiration Cytology (FNAC)

Laparoscopic FNAC is generally indicated if a cyst (generally hepatic or pancreatic) is identified on pre-operative imaging or at laparoscopy and there is uncertainty whether it represents malignant or benign disease. The majority of cysts, however, are generally amenable to less-invasive techniques such as CT-guided FNA or EUS-guided procedures. Where possible, with solid intraperitoneal lesions, biopsy techniques are superior as they give a greater diagnostic yield and are often easier with less associated complications than radiological techniques. Under direct vision, a 20 gauge needle attached to a suction device is used to aspirate the cyst. Alternatively, a spinal needle can be inserted into the peritoneal cavity under direct laparoscopic vision and then into the cyst. As with all cytology, a cytopathologist at hand with knowledge of the clinical question often delivers better results.

Pinch Biopsy/Scrape Biopsy

This technique, though not used often, is best utilized when on insertion of the laparoscope superficial lesions are identified on the surface of organs such as the liver, stomach, or bowel. The most common situation where this occurs is in peritoneal carcinomatosis which was previously undetected. Once identified, a full staging laparoscopy is rarely necessary as the diagnosis is often clear. Collection of multiple specimens is desirable where possible – particularly when no site for the primary tumor has been identified – as it allows the pathologist to use various stains in an attempt to find a primary site for the tumor.

Technically, the laparoscope can then be exchanged for an operating laparoscope or alternately only one further port may be necessary. Multiple lesions are forcibly peeled from the surface of non-essential organs if possible, often from the parietal peritoneum using forceps with serrated jaws.

Cup Biopsy

This is the preferred method in obtaining biopsies of superficial liver lesions identified at staging

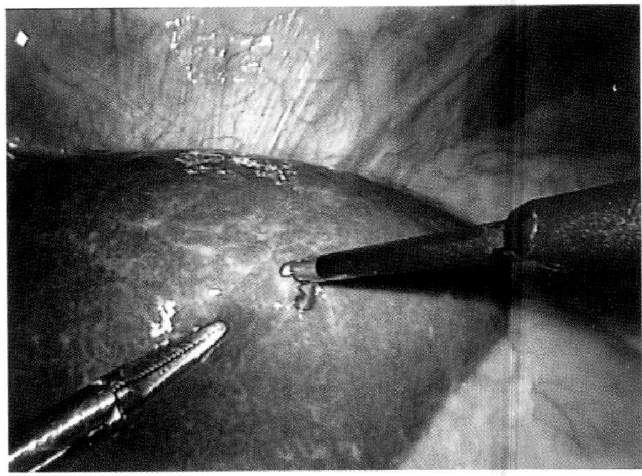

Figure 5.7

Laparoscopic biopsy forceps being used for biopsy of suspicious looking liver lesion

laparoscopy. For this we use a 5 mm biopsy forceps with a 2 mm cup as standard. This allows us to obtain adequate tissue for diagnostic purposes. Multiple samples may be taken to increase diagnostic yield. Figure 5.7 demonstrates this technique of liver biopsy. The cup is used to breech the liver capsule and a bite is taken out of the lesion. Further scoops can then be taken from the lesion and liver parenchyma as needed. Thorough hemostasis can easily be obtained with electrocautery or use of argon beam diathermy. It is important to avoid direct coupling or capacitance coupling which can lead to visceral injury. This incidence is reduced by limiting the gain of electrocautery to 30 W.

Core Biopsy and Laparoscopic Ultrasound Guidance

Laparoscopic core biopsy of intra-abdominal lesions is often indicated following failure of less-invasive radiological diagnostic techniques to obtain histological diagnoses necessary for treatment with neo-adjuvant, palliative, or primary chemoradiation. Laparoscopic core biopsy is also chosen when the tissue in question is close to important structures, such as tumors in the head of the pancreas, as it allows more direct visual control of the biopsy gun. A standard spring-loaded gun is preferable, with a 14 mm core allowing for generous tissue samples. Numerous passes are also preferable, giving the pathologist increased tissue to make an accurate diagnosis.

Following standard staging laparoscopy the lesion is isolated and exposed. To reduce the incidence of tumor seeding, the needle may be passed through a tight-sealing port so as to shield the abdominal wall from the contents of the biopsy. A blunt cautery-capable instrument should be ready in the non-dominant hand and positioned immediately adjacent to the biopsy site. Argon diathermy, where available, is particularly advantageous in controlling bleeding from the liver. The core needle is activated after feeling it pass well into the desired tissue. Immediately after removing the needle, the cautery-capable instrument is moved directly onto the needle puncture site and pressure is applied to achieve temporary hemostasis. These steps are repeated until enough tissue is obtained. The placing of a swab in the abdomen or suction often aids in the process of accurate placing of the biopsy needle particularly after the first pass. Laparoscopic ultrasound can be used to confirm the position of the needle of the core biopsy in the desired tissue to be biopsied.

Incisional Biopsy

Laparoscopic incisional biopsy of intra-abdominal malignancies or a retroperitoneal mass often follows after failed attempts at a tissue diagnosis from percutaneous or endoscopic methods. This method is generally used for masses for which excision is not a definitive treatment such as locally advanced unresectable disease or where there is doubt whether the mass is malignant (i.e., lymphoid mass).

Following standard staging laparoscopy the mass to be biopsied is isolated and exposed clearing other organs away where possible. For retroperitoneal biopsies mobilization and reflection of the colon medially may be necessary to expose the mass. Using scissors, while the non-dominant hand retracts, a generous piece of tissue can be excised. Cautery or argon beam coagulation can then be used for hemostasis at the biopsy site (the use of cautery for cutting may distort the histological architecture). The specimen should be placed in a bag for removal so as to prevent tumor seeding (Fig. 5.8). The incidence of tumor seeding, however, is low (<1%), which corresponds to wound recurrence at open surgery [8].

Excisional Biopsy

This technique is used where smaller lesions need to be biopsied and is generally reserved for masses with a low index of suspicion for malignant potential, such as a non-ulcerating lesion of the stomach unable to be excised endoscopically.

Following standard laparoscopy a flexible gastroscope is used intra-operatively to aid identification of the lesion. Mobilization of the stomach with division of the gastrocolic omentum and short gastric vessels may be necessary to gain adequate excision of the lesion. This can be done using a stapling device with vascular staples or coagulating instruments such as the harmonic scalpel or SonoSurg. A non-crushing bowel grasper can be placed over the duodenum to prevent insufflation of the small bowel. A figure of eight suture may be placed over the mass to aid retraction of the specimen. A generous wedge of stomach may then be excised using the endoscopic stapling device with intestinal staples. Multiple fires of the device may be necessary. Care must be taken not to narrow the lumen of the stomach too much and the gastroscope can be used to assess this. A laparoscopic bag should be used to retrieve the specimen, which should then be inspected to ensure that the lesion is excised with adequate margins.

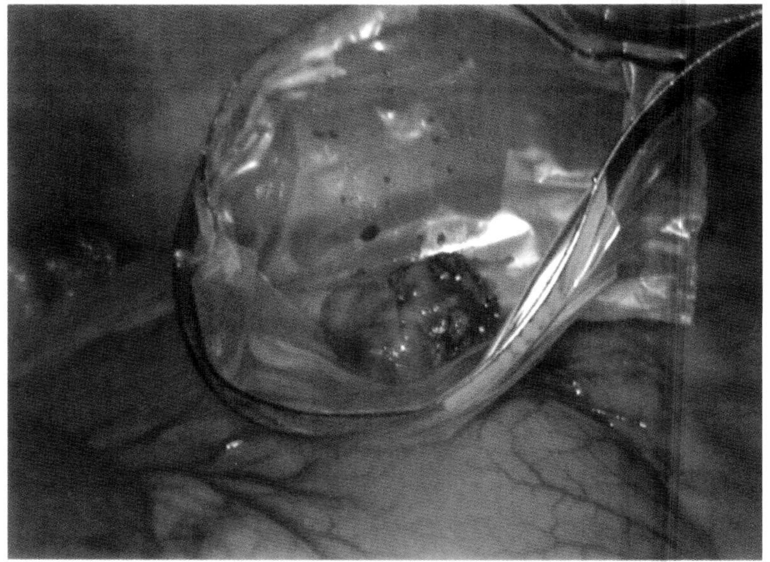

Figure 5.8

A biopsy specimen being removed through an endobag to prevent seeding of the tumor

Lymph Node Biopsy

Lymph node biopsies performed at laparoscopy are indicated where resectability of an intra-abdominal malignancy is in doubt, such as with celiac node involvement in pancreatic cancer. It may also be indicated in the diagnosis of lymphoma presenting with abdominal lymphadenopathy.

Following standard staging laparoscopy the lymph node in question is identified and isolated. This may necessitate dissection into the lesser sac or the retroperitoneum. The node should be handled gently, preferably with a Russian forceps to prevent damage to the node. The node should be excised whole where possible (Fig. 5.9). All feeding vessels including lymphatics should be clipped to aid hemostasis and prevent leakage of lymph. Again the specimen should be removed in a bag to limit tumor seeding. Where it is not possible to safely remove an entire node, a section or "pizza slice" of tumor can be excised. Argon beam coagulation or cautery must then be used for hemostasis.

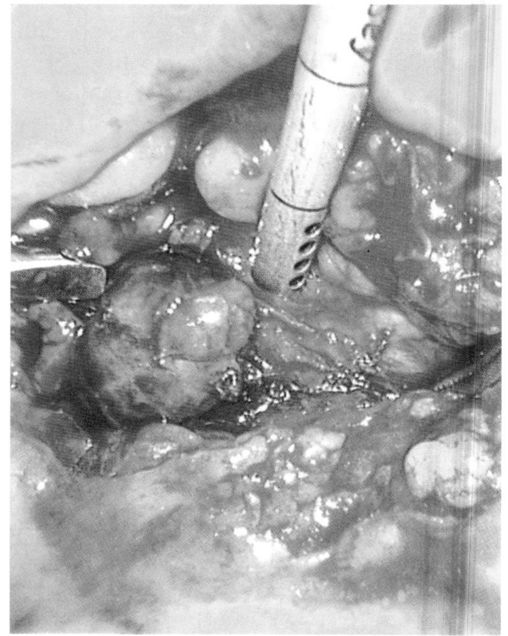

Figure 5.9

Retroperitoneal lymph node excision

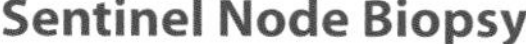

Sentinel Node Biopsy

While sentinel node biopsy is now standard treatment in breast cancer and melanoma, its use in GI cancer is currently being elucidated. Identifying sentinel nodes in esophageal and gastric cancers may reduce the need for radical lymph node dissection especially in early stage disease. A similar use can be found in colorectal cancers where sentinel node techniques can be used for lymph node staging in polyps with high-grade dysplasia or smaller cancers amenable to endoscopic or transanal resection. Identifying a sentinel node in colonic resections can facilitate more detailed analysis of key lymph nodes to identify micrometastatic disease which may be a predictor of tumor recurrence [9].

Sentinel nodes can be identified using either a dye, radiocolloid, or a combination of both. Radiocolloid should be injected sub-mucosally prior to surgery around the tumor endoscopically. A gamma probe can then be used laparoscopically to identify the node in question. When a dye technique is used it must be injected sub-mucosally using an endoscopic needle. The blue node can then be visualized in the lymph node drainage basin.

References

1. Moss AC, Morris E, Mac Mathuna P (2006) Palliative biliary stents for obstructing pancreatic carcinoma. Cochrane Database Syst Rev 2:CD004200, Review
2. Vitale GC, Davis BR, Tran TC (2005) The advancing art and science of endoscopy. Am J Surg 190(2):228–233, Review
3. Fernandez-del Castillo CC, Rattner DW, Warshaw AL (1995) Standards for pancreatic resection in the 1990s. Arch Surg 130:295–299
4. Geer RJ, Brennan MF (1993) Prognostic indicators for survival after resection. Am J Surg 165:68–72
5. Merchant NB, Conlon KC (1998) Laparoscopic evaluation in pancreatic cancer. Semin Surg Oncol 15:155–165
6. Hashizume M, Sugimachi K (1997) Needle and trocar injury during laparoscopic surgery in Japan. Surg Endosc 11(12):1198–1201
7. Minnard EA, Conlon KC (1998) Laparoscopic ultrasound enhances standard laparoscopy in the staging of pancreatic cancer. Ann Surg 228(2):182–187
8. Shoup M, Brennan MF, Karpeh MS, Gillern SM, McMahon RL, Conlon KC (2002) Port site metastasis after diagnostic laparoscopy for upper gastrointestinal tract malignancies: an uncommon entity. Ann Surg Oncol 9(7):632–636
9. Bilchik AJ, Trocha SD (2003) Lymphatic mapping and sentinel node analysis to optimize laparoscopic resection and staging of colorectal cancer: an update. Cancer Control 10(3):219–223

Ultrasound Techniques in Minimally Invasive Oncologic Surgery

Carol B. Sheridan, Maurice E. Arregui

Contents

Introduction

Ultrasound is an indispensable tool for the minimally invasive oncologic surgeon. The tactile sense which surgeons rely so much upon in cancer surgery is limited during laparoscopy, but that deficit can be filled, and frankly exceeded, by utilizing laparoscopic ultrasound (LUS) techniques. In addition, preoperative endoscopic ultrasound (EUS) provides the clinician with information for staging, delineates anatomic relationships to guide operative planning, and can provide a means for biopsy for tissue diagnosis. This chapter will introduce the application of perioperative and intraoperative ultrasound to the minimally invasive treatment of cancer.

Although the first use of operative ultrasound was in the early 1960s, it was the advent of real-time B-mode imaging by the 1980s that led to more widespread use of the technology in abdominal surgery. Hepatobiliary and pancreatic operations were among the first applications which benefited from the new modality. In the 1990s the field was advanced further by the introduction of color Doppler imaging and laparoscopic ultrasound probes. Radial and linear echoendoscopes were first developed in 1980. The initial report of direct EUS-guided fine-needle aspiration biopsy was in 1992 of a pancreatic head mass, and since that time this technology has been successfully utilized throughout the GI tract for cancer staging and biopsy [1].

Despite the rapid advances in ultrasound technology and the proven diagnostic and therapeutic advantages of ultrasound in the operating room, many surgeons lack formal training in its use. As with any surgical tool, there is a significant learning curve which must be overcome with opportunities for experience and mentorship. Although basic ultrasound training may be obtained by some in surgical residencies, advanced training and mastery will often require seeking out either courses offered by surgical

F.L. Greene, B.T. Heniford (eds.), *Minimally Invasive Cancer Management*,
DOI 10.1007/978-1-4419-1238-1_6,

societies or fellowships which include such training as part of their curriculum. Starting point for those surgeons interested in developing ultrasound skills is the American College of Surgeons, which offers a basic ultrasound course, and the Society of American Gastrointestinal and Endoscopic Surgeons, which has developed guidelines for training and credentialing surgeons in ultrasound.

Basic Equipment and Operating Room Setup for Laparoscopic Ultrasound

A laparoscopic ultrasound probe consists of a transducer, generally a side-viewing linear array, mounted at the end of a long 10 mm diameter shaft. This allows introduction of the probe through a 10–12 mm trocar. The tip should be flexible, ideally in four directions, in order to move the transducer both up and down and side-to-side to obtain the best contact with the surface being examined. Most probes operate at 5–10 MHz frequency. Higher frequency allows greater resolution at the expense of decreased penetration of tissue. In most situations, a 7.5 MHz frequency permits 6–8 cm penetration depth with the ability to detect lesions in the 1–4 mm range. Besides the standard real-time B-mode imaging, a machine with color Doppler capability is advantageous because vascular structures can be easily identified, facilitating interpretation of the anatomy. The LUS probe can be chemically sterilized so that it does not require a plastic sterile cover for use.

In our practice we find that placement of the probe through a trocar at the umbilicus provides the greatest freedom to examine all areas of interest in the abdominal cavity. During scanning, a 5 mm laparoscope is used through a trocar placed laterally on the abdominal wall to visualize the probe and guide its movement. The surgeon generally stands to the patient's right side and manipulates the probe with the right hand. The laparoscope may be controlled by the surgeon's left hand or by an assistant depending on trocar placement and the organ being examined. The ultrasound machine is controlled by a circulating nurse who must be familiar with its operation. In our operating rooms, the ultrasound images can be routed to one of the video monitors so that both the ultrasound image and the laparoscopic image are easily viewed by the surgeon (see Fig. 6.1). Digital recording capability is recommended for complete documentation of the exam.

Basic Techniques of Laparoscopic Ultrasound Examination

Organ-specific examination will be discussed in the subsequent sections, but there are general skills the laparoscopic ultrasonographer uses when scanning any target. The transducer may be placed directly on the surface of an organ, termed contact scanning, or just over the organ immersed in saline, termed stand-off scanning. Contact scanning works best on an organ with a smooth surface so that contact may be maintained. The normal liver and bowel wall permit good

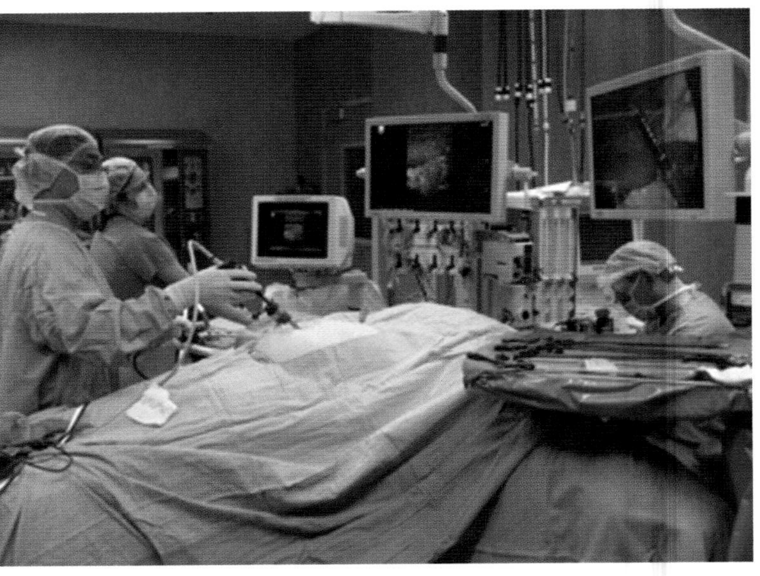

Figure 6.1

Typical operating room setup for laparoscopic ultrasound. Surgeon stands on patient's right, controlling the LUS probe with the right hand. Ultrasound and laparoscopic images are displayed on overhead OR video monitors

contact scanning. Contact scanning is also best suited for visualizing structures deep to the surface of an organ. Superficial characteristics are out of the focal distance of the transducer in a contact position and will not be well imaged. Stand-off scanning on the other hand places the probe further away from the surface of an organ, permitting good visualization of both irregular surfaces and superficial structures. Either technique is possible with the LUS probe.

Once placed, the probe is manipulated to view the organ of interest. Laparoscopic probes with four-way deflection permit similar movements used with handheld probes, including sliding, rocking, rotating, and tilting. Sliding and rocking are performed with hand motions in the same way as with an open probe; however, rotating and tilting require deflection of the probe tip. Depending on the probe, either wheels or levers control tip deflection and can be locked to maintain a desired tip position. Examination should always be performed in multiple planes to obtain a three-dimensional appreciation for the anatomy.

A systematic approach to scanning individual organs should be employed so that the exam is reproducible and nothing is missed. Like any laparoscopic skill, LUS has a learning curve. Integration of the laparoscopic view and ultrasound image and manipulation of the probe require practice. Acquiring laparoscopic ultrasound skill can be facilitated by initially gaining familiarity and comfort using handheld probes during open operations and by using ultrasound during common laparoscopic procedures such as cholecystectomy.

Laparoscopic Ultrasound for Hepatobiliary Neoplasms

Both the liver and the biliary tract are superbly imaged with intraoperative ultrasound. Intraoperative ultrasound of the liver can detect lesions too small to be picked up on preoperative CT or MRI or non-palpable lesions during open surgery. It is an essential tool for guiding laparoscopic resection or radiofrequency ablation. Ultrasound is not without its limitations, however, as some lesions may be isoechoic with the normal liver and therefore difficult to identify (see Fig. 6.2). Additionally, the cirrhotic liver is nodular and heterogeneous, potentially making neoplastic lesions more challenging to detect in this setting.

The classic application of ultrasound for the biliary tract has been evaluation of calculus disease. In experienced hands, LUS is as sensitive and specific as cholangiography for detecting common duct stones and is safe, low cost, and time saving. During intraoperative assessment of biliary neoplasms, ultrasound can provide accurate determination of resectability based on parenchymal invasion and vessel involvement. Inflammatory processes may limit ultrasound evaluation of the biliary system however. For example, tissue edema secondary to pancreatitis may obscure visualization of the distal common bile duct. The presence of pneumobilia can also interfere with imaging.

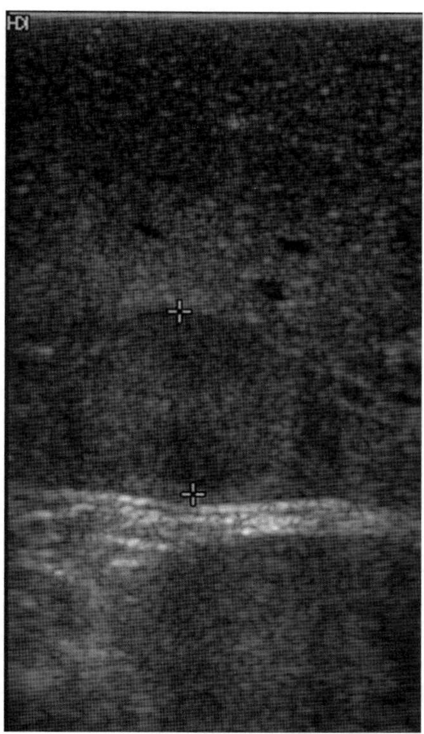

Figure 6.2
Lesions isoechoic to the normal liver parenchyma may be difficult to identify. The mass effect of this 1.5 cm lesion on the normal adjacent liver tissue in segment 7 helps the examiner recognize it

Techniques for Laparoscopic Ultrasound Exam of the Biliary Tree

The LUS probe is introduced through a periumbilical trocar, and a 5 mm laparoscope inserted through a right upper quadrant trocar is used to guide the probe movements. We start by placing the transducer obliquely over segment 4B (between the gallbladder and falciform ligament) to obtain a longitudinal view of the common bile duct. Color Doppler is used to clearly identify the portal vein behind the duct and the hepatic artery between the two structures, generally in a transverse view. The bile duct can be traced proximally toward the hilum and bifurcation of the hepatic duct and then distally toward the pancreas and duodenum. As the probe is brought caudally, the view of the common duct is lost as air interfaces below the liver edge. The probe should now be placed under the liver, longitudinally over the porta hepatis. Occasionally, with an enlarged liver, the edge may need to be elevated by an assistant in order to direct placement of the probe. Color Doppler should be used again to confirm the identity of the structures being examined. Care should be taken not to press downward with the transducer with any force during this portion of the exam because it may compress the bile duct and make it difficult to identify. The bile duct is again traced from the hilum toward the duodenum. The cystic duct is identified at this time. It is generally not possible to trace the common bile duct all the way down to the ampulla with the probe in the longitudinal orientation. Instead the transducer is rotated 90° to obtain a transverse view, and the duct followed once again from the porta hepatis down to the intrapancreatic portion of the duct (see Fig. 6.3). At the level of the pancreas, a transverse view through the duodenum is necessary to continue to examine the duct all the way to the papilla. This requires compression of the duodenum with the probe to minimize air artifact from the bowel lumen. An alternate technique, though rarely required, is instillation of fluid through a naso- or orogastric tube to distend the duodenum. In this view, the common duct can frequently be seen joining the pancreatic duct, and the bile duct should be seen all the way to its entry into the duodenal wall at the ampulla, which appears hypoechoic compared to the pancreas.

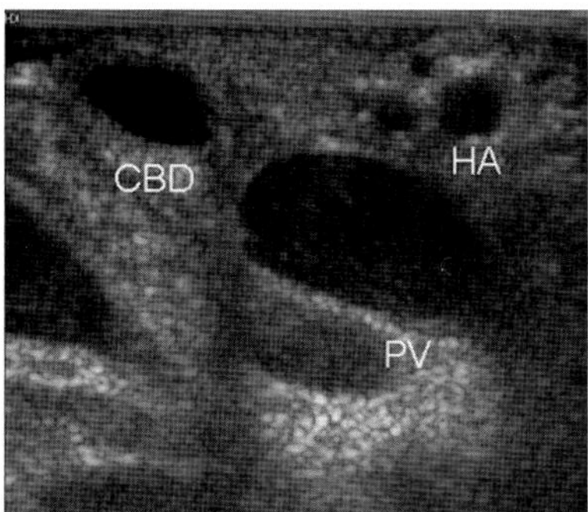

Figure 6.3

Transverse view of portal triad. This view of the common bile duct (CBD), hepatic artery (HA), and portal vein (PV) creates the 'Mickey Mouse' sign

Techniques for Laparoscopic Ultrasound Exam of the Liver

Port placement for the ultrasound probe and laparoscope may be the same as for examination of the biliary tree. If the patient has a relatively long distance between the xiphoid process and the umbilicus, the probe port may be better positioned above the umbilicus to facilitate exam of segments 7 and 8. Although we describe our preferred method of scanning the liver, many different approaches have been proposed. As long as the exam is done systematically with attention to anatomic detail, the surgeon's preferred method is acceptable.

We start our exam with the left hepatic lobe, identifying and examining segments 1 through 4. We initially place the transducer along the upper portion of the left side of the falciform ligament and adjust the depth of penetration to visualize the inferior vena cava and identify the caudate lobe adjacently. The probe is rocked side-to-side to see the entire segment. If imaging of the caudate lobe is impaired, for example, from a fatty liver, the probe may be moved below the left lateral segment and placed directly over the gastrohepatic ligament for closer inspection.

Next, keeping the probe to the left of the falciform ligament, segments 2 and 3 are examined. The left portal vein, distinguished from the hepatic veins by its hyperechoic wall, branches as it crosses to the left of the falciform ligament. The first, posterior branch will be to segment 2. The second, anterior branch will be to segment 3. The left hepatic vein may be identified by initially finding its junction with the IVC. Segment 2 will be posterior and superior to the left hepatic vein as it is followed out laterally; segment 3 will be anterior and inferior to it. The vascular structures can be quickly identified and then the segments scanned by sliding the probe back-and-forth over the liver surface. The probe is then moved to the right side of the falciform to examine segments 4A and 4B, which are bounded by the falciform and the middle hepatic vein, with a similar technique.

The right hepatic lobe, segments 5 through 8, is scanned next. Once again the vascular structures should be assessed first, followed by a complete examination of the parenchyma. Starting from the hilum, the right portal vein is followed first to its anterior branch. This divides into an anterior superior branch to segment 8 and an anterior inferior branch to segment 5. Segments 5 and 8 are located between the middle and right hepatic veins. The posterior branch of the right portal vein will likewise divide into a superior and inferior branch, supplying segment 7 and segment 6, respectively. Segments 6 and 7 are located posterior to the right hepatic vein. The substance of the right lobe is scanned in a back-and-forth manner, covering all four segments. To fully visualize segments 6 and 7 the transducer tip often needs to be flexed down and curved over the top and side of the exposed portion of the liver. Partial desufflation may also be used to bring the probe closer to the liver to complete the exam.

It is important to localize and document any lesions that are identified. Malignant hepatic lesions vary significantly in their appearance on ultrasound exam and frequently cannot be differentiated from benign lesions using ultrasound criteria alone. Any solid mass should be considered suspicious. Other malignant characteristics are a hypoechoic halo, mass effect on intrahepatic structures, invasion of hepatic vessels or ducts, and tumor thrombus [2] (see Fig. 6.4). Additionally, metastatic liver lesions from the same primary tumor tend to share and retain the same ultrasonographic appearance. An understanding of the hepatic vascular anatomy is crucial to correctly localize a lesion to a particular segment. When a lesion is identified, it should be scanned in multiple planes if possible and measurements made. Text documentation of the location as well as caliper measurements may be performed on the image by the technician operating the machine for the surgeon. Digital images should be printed or stored to a disk to become a part of the medical record.

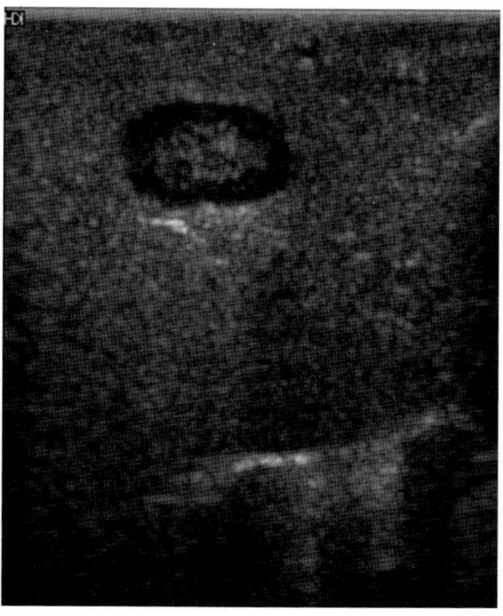

Figure 6.4

Liver lesion with features suspicious for malignancy. This GIST metastasis in segment 3 demonstrates the classic bull's-eye appearance of a malignant lesion

Specific Applications and Results of Laparoscopic Ultrasound for Hepatobiliary Tumors

Staging of Primary and Secondary Liver Tumors

In the late 1980s and early 1990s multiple studies supported that open intraoperative ultrasound was superior to preoperative imaging studies, including transabdominal ultrasound, CT, MRI, and angiography, in identifying liver lesions [3]. Not only did intraoperative ultrasound find lesions not appreciated preoperatively, but the new information changed the operative plan in 30–50% of cases. As laparoscopy became accepted, it was applied to staging of primary and secondary malignancies of the liver prior to resection or ablative therapies. Likewise, LUS was evaluated as an adjunctive tool in this setting. John et al. [4] reported their experience with laparoscopic staging with ultrasound of 43 patients with potentially resectable liver tumors in 1994. Thirty-three percent of these patients were found to have liver lesions not identified by laparoscopy alone and in 42% ultrasound added information beyond that obtained from laparoscopy that impacted resectability. In 2000, Jarnagin et al. [5] published a prospective non-randomized study of 186 patients with potentially resectable primary and secondary liver tumors; 104 laparoscopically staged patients were compared to 82 patients who had exploration without laparoscopy. They found that 83% of patients who were determined resectable laparoscopically and then underwent laparotomy had potentially curative resections, compared to 66% of those patients without staging laparoscopy. They also showed that laparoscopic staging reduces hospital stay and costs for unresectable patients. In the same year, Foroutani et al. [6] published their results of a prospective comparison of triphasic spiral CT vs. LUS for detection of primary and metastatic liver tumors. LUS detected all 201 lesions seen on CT as well as 21 additional tumors in 11 patients (20%). In all three of the above-mentioned studies, the majority of the tumors were secondary, most arising from metastatic colon cancer.

Among cirrhotic patients, LUS has proved especially useful in the diagnosis, staging, and treatment of hepatocellular cancer. Staging laparoscopy with ultrasound may be used to evaluate both patients with mild liver disease and HCC who may be candidates for resection and those with more advanced liver disease and HCC or equivocal findings for malignancy, who may be candidates for transplantation. Additionally, LUS-guided tumor ablation, most commonly radiofrequency ablation, is a therapeutic option for selected individuals. In a prospective study which included 68 Child's A and B cirrhotics with potentially resectable HCC who underwent laparoscopic staging with ultrasound, 15 (22%) were found to have additional malignant lesions not recognized on preoperative imaging. Only 3 of those 15 underwent the planned resection because the new lesion was in proximity to the original tumor. Seven of the 12 patients who were not resectable underwent laparoscopic ablative techniques instead [7]. In a study of patients with advanced liver disease and suspected HCC by Kim et al. [8], 12 of 18 patients were restaged (6 up-staged and 6 down-staged) as a result of staging laparoscopy and ultrasound. Of the six patients who were down-staged, four were able to receive transplants, and pathology of the explanted liver was consistent with the laparoscopic findings.

Ultrasound Guidance of Liver Biopsy, Ablation, and Resection

A major reason LUS is so useful in the evaluation of hepatic neoplasms is its application to safely and accurately perform biopsies. Simply visualizing a new lesion is frequently not sufficient to make a diagnosis. Our technique for LUS-guided liver biopsy is similar to others published in the literature [9]. Although periumbilical placement of the ultrasound probe port generally allows adequate ultrasound access to both lobes of the liver, port placement is also directed by lesion location if a biopsy is anticipated. Lesions in segments 6 and 7 may be best accessed by placing the patient in a partial lateral position so that the biopsy needle may transverse less parenchyma to reach the target. We generally use an 18 gauge cutting needle with an automatic firing mechanism to perform the biopsy. A 30° or 45° viewing laparoscope often provides the best view of the surface of the liver as well as the probe and needle entry site. The surgeon should control both the probe and the biopsy needle. An assistant is required to hold the laparoscope. It is important to be familiar with the firing mechanism of the biopsy needle before placement, especially the depth of penetration of the needle from the tip once it is loaded. Ideally the needle should enter the liver as close to the same plane as the longitudinal axis of the probe as possible. With the needle in the liver tissue, small rotations of the transducer will allow the surgeon to see the bright tip of the needle and it may then be advanced into the lesion under ultrasound guidance. Once the tip of the needle appears to be in a good position for biopsy and before firing, the probe may be adjusted to an angled plane with the needle to confirm that the needle has not skived through the target. After firing and removing the biopsy needle, pressure held with the ultrasound probe is often adequate to control bleeding; however, we frequently employ bipolar electrocautery on the biopsy site to assure hemostasis.

A number of ablative techniques directed against liver tumors can be performed laparoscopically, including cryoablation, ethanol injection, radiofrequency ablation, and microwave coagulation therapy. In these procedures, LUS is relied on for directing application of the therapy. Our preferred modality is radiofrequency ablation as it has a good safety profile, is applicable to both HCC and metastatic liver lesions, and, although level I evidence is lacking, it has been shown to be successful in prolonging survival and decreasing recurrence in select groups of patients [10]. In RFA, an electrode probe is placed in a lesion, the tip which is made up of an array of metal prongs is deployed, and then an alternating current is generated between the needle array and a grounding pad placed on the patient. The current causes heating of the surrounding tumor to 60–100°C leading to coagulation necrosis of the tissue. The end result is to create a thermal injury encompassing the lesion and 1 cm of normal parenchyma surrounding it. There are several important principles to ultrasound guidance of the RFA probe and performance of tumor ablation. First, precise probe placement is crucial to ablating the entire lesion and this depends completely on the ability of the surgeon to interpret the ultrasound image to assure the probe is in the right position. The probe should be directed in much the same way as is a biopsy needle. If the lesion can be encompassed by a single ablation, the probe is guided to its center and the prongs deployed (see Fig. 6.5). Viewing the deployed probe in longitudinal, transverse, and oblique views assures that the device is centered within the lesion. Passage of the probe needle through the lesion multiple times should be avoided as this can promote tumor cell seeding along the track. Second, if the lesion is large, multiple overlapping ablations will be required and must be planned out prior to getting started. Ablations should proceed from far to near the ultrasound transducer because the ablated tissue becomes hyperechoic, obscuring the view of the lesion (see Fig. 6.6). Last, at the end of the ablation, the ablated area should be scanned to observe for bleeding or hematoma formation. Finally, the track is also ablated as the probe is removed. This decreases the risk of tumor cell seeding and improves hemostasis.

Although it has not been widely adopted, likely secondary to the advanced skill set required and potentially increased technical difficulty, laparoscopic anatomic liver resections are being performed by some centers for both benign and malignant lesions. Based only on small series, laparoscopic liver resection appears to have acceptable morbidity and mortality and may be associated with the same advantages

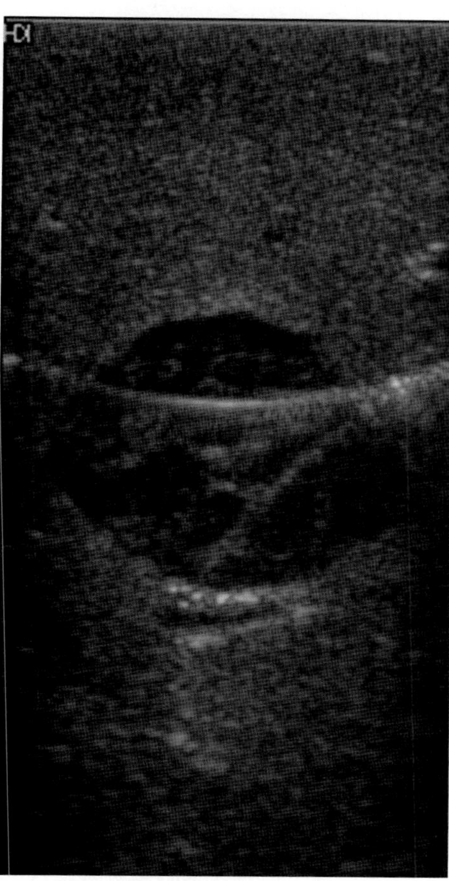

Figure 6.5

Pre-ablation image of lesion and RFA probe. The probe is deployed within the center of the lesion under ultrasound guidance

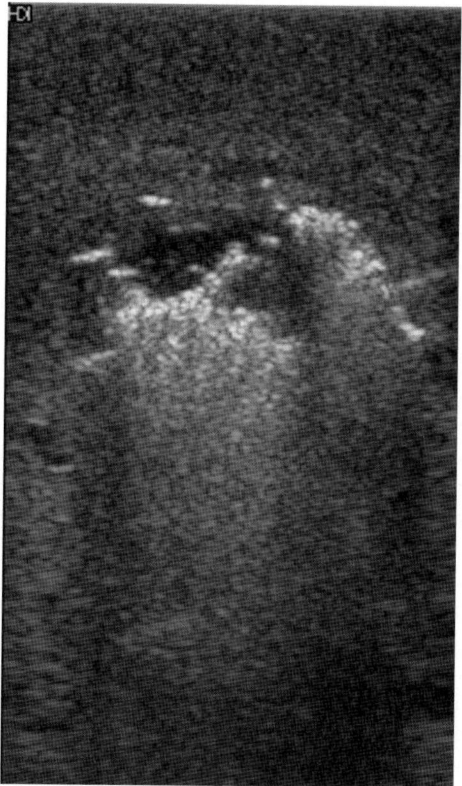

Figure 6.6

Lesion undergoing radiofrequency ablation. During ablation, the area of ablation becomes hyperechoic secondary to the formation of microbubbles within the tissues

that a laparoscopic approach brings other operations, including shorter hospital stays and decreased narcotic requirements. Not surprisingly, LUS is an essential tool in this endeavor and will continue to be influential in advancing minimally invasive hepatic therapies.

Techniques for Laparoscopic Ultrasound of the Pancreas

The entire pancreas is also easily accessible by an ultrasound probe placed through an umbilical trocar. The stomach and duodenum create a good acoustic window for viewing the gland as long as they are not excessively filled with air. Alternatively, the pancreas may be examined by direct contact scanning or standoff with saline within the lesser sac. Future procedures that will require opening the lesser sac should be considered before using this technique as entry into this plane may result in adhesions and obliteration of the space.

The pancreatic parenchyma may blend into the surrounding retroperitoneal fat, especially in older individuals. Orientation may be accomplished by identifying the vascular landmarks that surround the pancreas. It is frequently easiest to find the transverse view of the neck of the pancreas first, facilitated by identification of the portal vein/superior mesenteric vein seen below the pancreatic neck in a longitudinal direction (see Fig. 6.7). The pancreatic duct should be visible in this view, normally measuring no more than 3 mm in diameter. A very small decompressed duct, however, may be difficult to visualize. The gland may then be traced proximally toward the head and distally toward the tail by following the duct and maintaining it in a transverse view. Proximally, a complete view of the pancreatic head is accomplished by the lateral transduodenal view. This view permits examination of the ampulla and confluence of the common bile duct and pancreatic duct. When examining the pancreatic head, the uncinate process will be appreciated to the right and posterior to the superior mesenteric vein and portal vein. The uncinate process is typically less echogenic than the head of the pancreas and therefore can be confused for a hypoechoic neoplastic lesion if one is not familiar with the normal anatomic appearance (see Fig. 6.8). Other adjacent vascular structures that may help orient the ultrasonogapher, and often must be evaluated for local tumor invasion, are the celiac trunk, superior mesenteric artery, and splenic vessels. The celiac trunk is located cephalad to the body of the pancreas, the proximal SMA is posterior to the body of the gland, and the splenic vessels run longitudinally posterior to the body and tail of the pancreas. When examining the gland in a longitudinal orientation, the 'golf club sign' can be appreciated at the neck of the pancreas; the splenic vein is the shaft of the club, the portal vein is the head of the club, and the SMA is the golf ball (see Fig. 6.9).

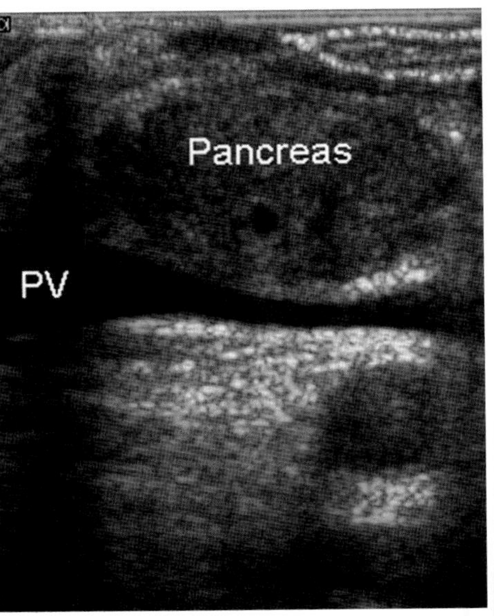

Figure 6.7

Transverse view of the pancreatic neck. The portal vein is seen below the pancreatic neck. The pancreatic duct is also visible in transverse view

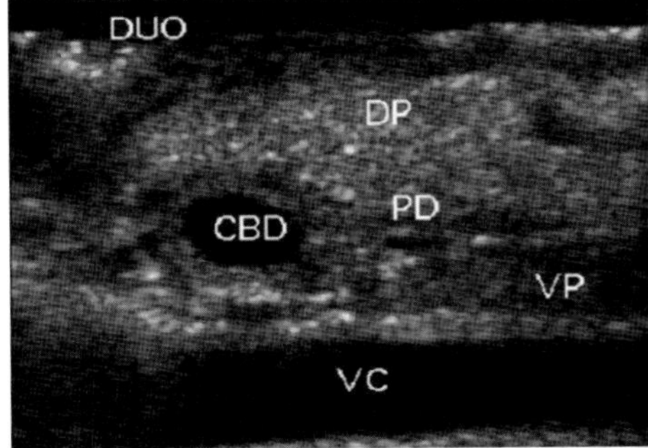

Figure 6.8

Normal appearing uncinate process. Note that the ventral pancreas (VP), or uncinate process, is hypoechoic compared to the dorsal pancreas (DP)

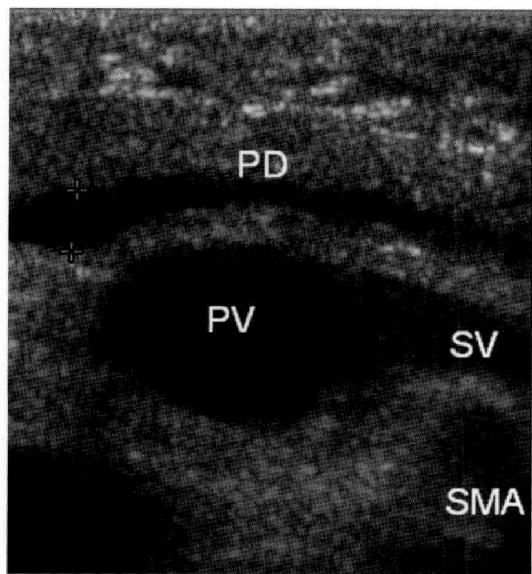

Figure 6.9

'Golf club sign.' In the longitudinal orientation over the neck of the pancreas, the splenic vein (SV), portal vein (PV), and superior mesenteric artery (SMA) create the appearance of golf club and ball

Specific Applications and Results of Laparoscopic Ultrasound for Pancreatic Neoplasms

LUS has been utilized in the workup and management of both benign and malignant pancreatic pathology. From an oncologic perspective, LUS has a role in staging pancreatic adenocarcinomas, localizing and resecting neuroendocrine tumors, and management of cystic pancreatic neoplasms.

Staging of Pancreatic Adenocarcinoma

Laparoscopic staging of pancreatic cancer has been championed by a number of pancreatic surgeons as a way to avoid unnecessary laparotomy in those patients who have locally advanced or metastatic disease which is not picked up with available preoperative imaging modalities. Modern high-quality CT scanning identifies unresectable patients with accuracy close to 100%, but a significant number of patients determined to be potentially resectable by CT scan will be found unresectable at exploration [11]. Based on recent literature, laparoscopic staging with ultrasound may avoid unnecessary laparotomy in at least 12%, and possibly up to 26%, of these patients [12, 13]. With respect to laparoscopic ultrasonography itself, a number of studies have demonstrated that it improves the accuracy of identifying unresectable tumors and support its routine use in laparoscopic staging of pancreatic cancer [14–16].

When performing a staging laparoscopy with ultrasound for pancreatic cancer, the steps remain essentially the same regardless of the location of the tumor within the gland. After visual inspection of all peritoneal surfaces, pelvis, root of mesentery, and surface of viscera and solid organs, the ultrasound exam is performed of the entire pancreas. Pancreatic adenocarcinomas are generally hypoechoic with respect to the pancreatic parenchyma. Compression by the tumor may cause distal pancreatic duct dilation. For pancreatic head tumors, special attention is made to the portal vein/superior mesenteric vein confluence to determine invasion. Color flow Doppler is used to determine patency if there is tumor encasement (see Fig. 6.10). The common bile duct should be identified and evaluated for obstruction. For body and tail tumors, evaluation of the splenic vessels and the celiac trunk is of greater importance. Splenic vein or artery invasion is not a contraindication to resection, but involvement of the celiac axis precludes resection. The retroperitoneal soft tissues, including the left adrenal gland and Gerota's fascia, and peripancreatic lymph nodes are inspected for signs of local invasion and metastasis. After inspection of the pancreas, the liver

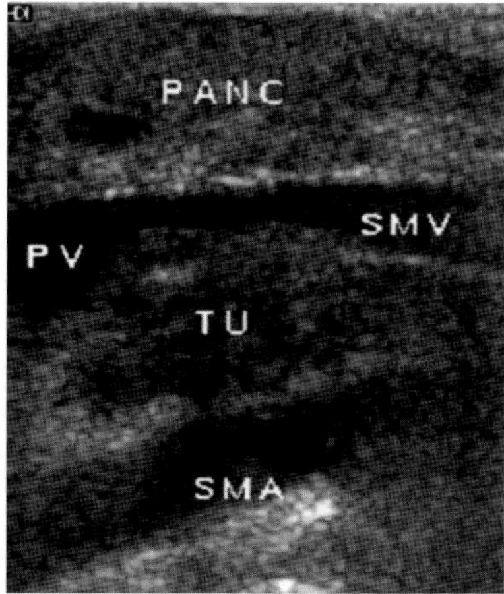

Figure 6.10

Tumor involvement of the portal vein/superior mesenteric vein confluence. Color flow Doppler is utilized to determine patency

is scanned for metastases. Investigation for aberrant vascular anatomy, including a replaced right hepatic artery, should be made and documented.

In our experience, >95% of patients determined resectable by staging laparoscopy will be successfully resected by pancreaticoduodenectomy. For those patients who have evidence of advanced disease which precludes resection, laparoscopic enteric and/or biliary bypass is an option utilized by some surgeons for patients with impending obstruction. We prefer endoscopic stenting in this population. Studies demonstrate less morbidity, and no significant difference in survival, for patients who undergo endoscopic stenting vs. surgical bypass for obstructing pancreatic tumors [11].

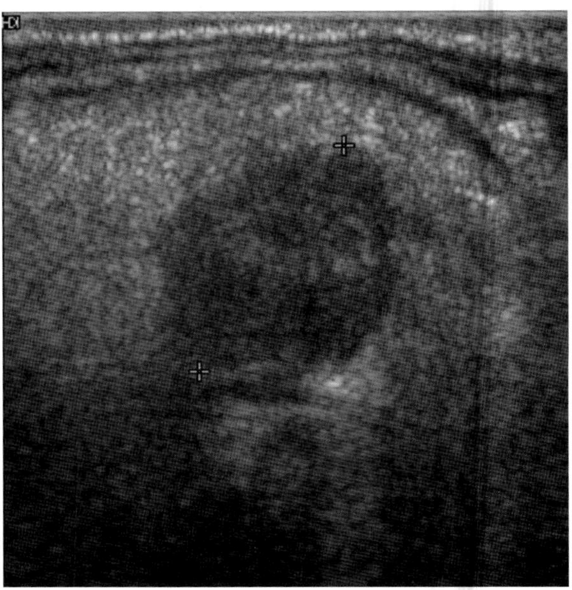

Figure 6.11

Non-functional neuroendocrine tumor of the distal pancreas. The patient underwent a laparoscopic distal pancreatectomy guided by LUS for this 1.6 cm non-invasive lesion

Localization and Resection of Pancreatic Neuroendocrine Tumors

Neuroendocrine tumors of the pancreas, otherwise known as islet cell tumors, are most commonly small, functional, benign tumors that are well-suited for minimally invasive resection. Because they are frequently subcentimeter in size, they can be difficult to localize with even high-quality CT or MRI scanning. Although the development of endoscopic ultrasound has allowed more of these lesions to be visualized preoperatively, EUS can be limited in visualizing small lesions in the tail of the pancreas. Therefore intraoperative ultrasound may still be considered the most sensitive modality to pinpoint their location. Benign, functional tumors like insulinomas appear as round hypoechoic lesions within the pancreas. With the aid of LUS, they can be enucleated, avoiding injury to the pancreatic duct and adjacent vascular structures [17]. Malignant neuroendocrine tumors of the pancreas, which are more frequently non-functioning, tend to be larger and more heterogeneous than their benign counterparts on ultrasound exam. Heterogeneity can arise from necrosis, calcification, or hemorrhage within the lesion. LUS may not be necessary for initial localization, but it can still be useful for determining resectability and guiding resection of these lesions (see Fig. 6.11).

Evaluation and Resection of Cystic Neoplasms of the Pancreas

Although LUS may selectively be applied to the management of pancreatic cystic neoplasms, it is EUS which has found an important application for the routine characterization of these tumors. Sonographic appearance is not diagnostic by itself, but can provide information regarding the nature of a cystic lesion. Simple cysts are uniloculated, round, and anechoic. Serous cystadenomas tend to be multiloculated or microcystic with a honeycomb appearance on ultrasound. They can be found anywhere within the gland (see Fig. 6.12). Simple cysts and serous cystadenomas are benign but may require excision if they are symptomatic. Mucinous cystadenomas are also multiloculated but have fewer septations giving a macrocystic appearance. They are more common in the body and tail of the pancreas. Intraductal papillary mucinous neoplasms (IPMN) appear as cystic dilatation of the main pancreatic duct or side branches. Both mucinous cystadenomas and IPMN have the potential for malignant degeneration and typically require resection.

Analysis of cyst fluid aspirated under ultrasound guidance provides additional information that can aid in diagnosis. Serous cyst fluid typically has low viscosity and a low CEA level. Mucinous cyst fluid has high viscosity and elevated CEA. Special staining for

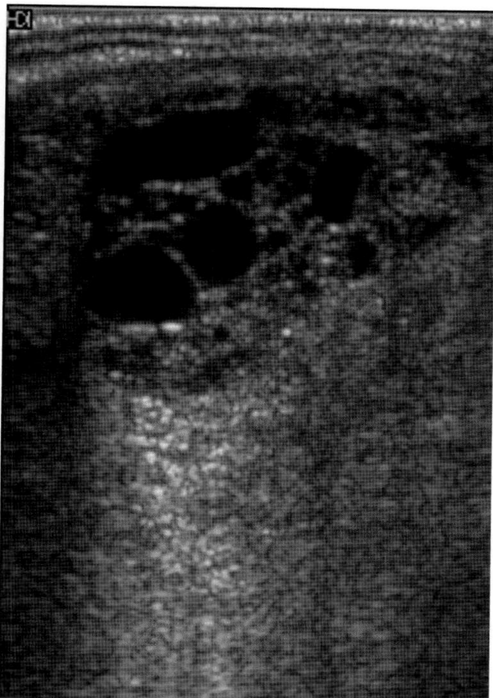

Figure 6.12

Giant multiloculated cystic lesion of the pancreatic tail. This lesion measured 20 cm × 15 cm × 10 cm and was determined to be a microcystic serous cystadenoma on final pathology

mucin is helpful. Additionally, molecular DNA analysis for mutations associated with pancreatic cancer is now frequently performed when the malignant potential of a lesion is in question.

Diagnostic laparoscopy with LUS may be applied to cystic pancreatic neoplasms which are not readily biopsied by EUS, especially lesions in the tail of the gland which have features suspicious for malignancy. LUS is also a useful guide for performing laparoscopic pancreatic resection for symptomatic or potentially malignant lesions. In the case of IPMN, LUS can help determine the line of resection at the level of normal appearing pancreatic duct.

Laparoscopic Ultrasound for Other Neoplasms

Every region of the abdominal cavity can be accessed with the ultrasound probe, and therefore any minimally invasive oncologic procedure may benefit from this tool. Applications for esophageal and gastric cancers, abdominal lymphomas, and other retroperitoneal and pelvic tumors are a few of the uses. Often included in the general application of LUS is evaluation of metastatic disease within lymph nodes. The next section will briefly describe general principles to applying ultrasound to lymph node evaluation and the final portion of the chapter will focus on a few more specific applications.

Techniques for Laparoscopic Ultrasound Examination of Lymph Nodes

Completion of an adequate lymphadenectomy is important for most gastrointestinal malignancies. A common application of an LUS lymph node examination is for staging upper GI cancers, where discovery of a metastatic node outside of the normal resection margins may determine a tumor unresectable. Alternatively, LUS may be used to guide lymphadenectomy. Lymph nodes which are in difficult locations to dissect out, for example, para-aortic and retroperitoneal locations or in previously operated on or radiated fields, can be evaluated and resected with the help of LUS.

Normal lymph nodes on ultrasound exam appear oblong in shape, are generally less than 1 cm in size, have indistinct borders, and have a hyperechoic hilum with a hypoechoic cortex. Metastatic infiltration causes the node to lose its hyperechoic center, enlarge, and become more rounded and discrete. However, it should be noted that inflammatory lymph nodes are enlarged and hypoechoic as well. Additionally, the average size of normal suprapancreatic and periportal lymph nodes is greater than 1 cm [18] (see Fig. 6.13). Ultrasound appearance is therefore not diagnostic for metastatic infiltration and must be confirmed with pathologic analysis of aspirated cells or excised tissue. Use of color flow Doppler helps identify lymph nodes and their relationship to nearby blood vessels and should be used when performing LUS-guided needle biopsies to prevent vascular injury.

Specific Applications of Laparoscopic Ultrasound to Other Neoplasms

Esophagus and Stomach

LUS has been applied to staging laparoscopy for both esophageal and gastric cancers. The addition of LUS

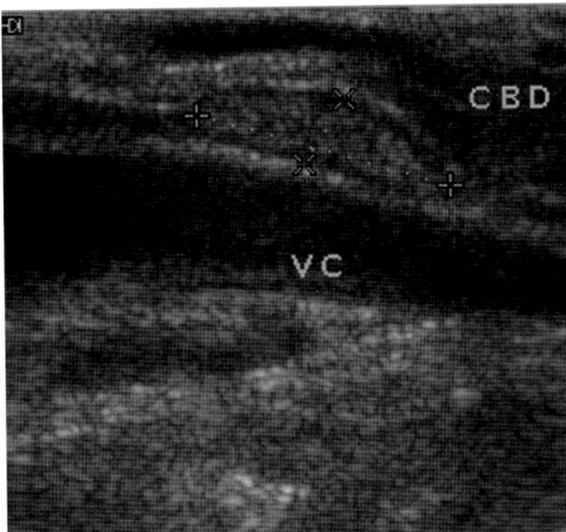

Figure 6.13

Normal periportal lymph node. The lymph node is oblong with a hyperechoic hilum and hypoechoic cortex, the borders of which are somewhat indistinct. Periportal lymph nodes are frequently greater than 1 cm in diameter

to staging increases the number of patients for whom unnecessary laparotomy can be avoided. Generally up to a quarter of patients with gastroesophageal cancer taken for staging will be found to have occult metastases. In a series of staging laparoscopy for esophageal cancer by Nguyen et al. [19], half of those found unresectable at laparoscopy were determined so based on advanced celiac axis nodal involvement, a finding dependent on the ultrasound evaluation alone. When applied to the staging of gastric cancer, LUS has the additional benefit of simultaneous evaluation of the depth of bowel wall invasion since the tumor is accessible to the probe. The normal five layers of the bowel wall visualized under EUS examination can be appreciated by a laparoscopic transducer as well.

Laparoscopic resection of gastric submucosal lesions is another area where LUS may find increased application. A large series of laparoscopically resected gastric gastrointestinal stromal tumors (GISTs) by Novitsky et al. [20] utilized LUS only for hepatic evaluation and relied on intraoperative endoscopy to guide gastric resection. Their results support that the laparoscopic approach is safe and effective for resection of gastric GISTs up to 8.5 cm in size. A subsequent case series has demonstrated that LUS can guide resection of gastric submucosal lesions including GISTs and proposes that it may be a simpler approach than intraoperative endoscopic guidance [21]. Certainly in experienced hands LUS can localize intramural lesions in the upper GI tract and would avoid the need for endoscopic insufflation which can impair the laparoscopic view.

Adrenal Gland and Kidney

The retroperitoneum is another area in which LUS can help guide the laparoscopic surgeon through a safe dissection. A laparoscopic approach to benign neoplasms of the adrenal gland is well accepted and increasingly is being applied to malignant tumors as well, albeit with caution. We routinely employ LUS to help in identification of the adrenal vein and avoid injury to adjacent structures during laparoscopic adrenalectomy [22]. Others have reported success applying LUS to guide laparoscopic partial adrenalectomies and nephrectomies [23, 24]. During partial adrenalectomy, LUS helps the surgeon resect the lesion with an adequate margin while sparing the blood supply to the remaining gland to preserve cortical function and avoid lifelong steroid replacement. When guiding partial nephrectomy, LUS defines the lesion's relationship both to the vasculature and to the collecting system.

Future of Ultrasound in Minimally Invasive Surgery

Ultrasound gives the surgeon back the information which he or she loses by not having his tactile sense within the operating field. Based on the many applications of ultrasound in the fields of minimally invasive surgery and oncology currently, the technology is certain to continue to grow. LUS as a tool in the surgeon's armamentarium is mainly limited by its learning curve. As long as surgeons are willing to take on the challenge of learning a new modality, the possibilities are wide open to advancing ultrasound techniques and relying on them to help our patients.

References

1. Yamao K, Sawaki A, Mizuno N, Shimizu Y, Yatabe Y, Koshikawa T (2005) Endoscopic ultrasound-guided fine-needle aspiration biopsy (EUS-FNAB): past, present, and future. J Gastroenterol 40:1013–1023

2. Adams RB (2005) Chapter 15: Intraoperative ultrasound of the liver. In: Machi J, Staren ED (eds) Ultrasound for surgeons, 2nd edn. Lippincott Williams and Wilkins, Philadelphia, PA, p 343
3. Thompson DM, Arregui ME (1998) Role of laparoscopic ultrasound in cancer management. Semin Surg Oncol 15:166–175
4. John TG, Greig JD, Crosbie JL, Anthony Miles WF, Garden OJ (1994) Superior staging of liver tumors with laparoscopy and laparoscopic ultrasound. Ann Surg 220:711–719
5. Jarnagin WR, Bodniewicz J, Dougherty E, Conlon K, Blumgart LH, Fong Y (2000) A prospective analysis of staging laparoscopy in patients with primary and secondary hepatobiliary malignancies. J Gastrointest Surg 4:34–43
6. Foroutani A, Garland AM, Berber E et al (2000) Laparoscopic ultrasound vs triphasic computed tomography for detecting liver tumors. Arch Surg 135:933–938
7. Montorsi M, Santambrogio R, Bianchi P et al (2001) Laparoscopy with laparoscopic ultrasound for pretreatment staging of hepatocellular carcinoma: a prospective study. J Gastrointest Surg 5:312–315
8. Kim RD, Nazarey P, Katz E, Chari RS (2004) Laparoscopic staging and tumor ablation for hepatocellular carcinoma in Child C cirrhotics evaluated for orthotopic liver transplantation. Surg Endosc 18:39–44
9. Santambrogio R, Bianchi P, Pasta A, Palmisano A, Montorsi M (2001) Ultrasound-guided interventional procedures of the liver during laparoscopy. Technical considerations. Surg Endosc 16:349–354
10. Garrean S, Hering J, Helton WS, Espat NJ (2007) A primer on transarterial, chemical, and thermal ablative therapies for hepatic tumors. Am J Surg 194:79–80
11. Stefanidis D, Grove KD, Schwesinger WH, Thomas CR Jr. (2006) The current role of staging laparoscopy for adenocarcinoma of the pancreas: a review. Ann Oncol 17:189–199
12. Thomson BN, Parks RW, Redhead DN et al (2006) Refining the role of laparoscopy and laparoscopic ultrasound in the staging of presumed pancreatic head and ampullary tumours. Br J Cancer 94:213–217
13. Bronfine BI, Arregui ME (2007) The role of laparoscopy with laparoscopic ultrasound for staging of pancreatic cancer in the ear of modern advanced imaging. Surg Endosc 21:S445
14. John TG, Greig JD, Carter DC, Garden OJ (1995) Carcinoma of the pancreatic head and periampullary region. Tumor staging with laparoscopy and laparoscopic ultrasonography. Ann Surg 221:156–164
15. Bemelman WA, DeWit LT, Van Delden OM et al (1995) Diagnostic laparoscopy combined with laparoscopic ultrasonography in staging of cancer of the pancreatic head region. Br J Surg 82:820–824
16. Minnard EA, Conlon KC, Hoos A, Dougherty EC, Hann LE, Brennan MF (1998) Laparoscopic ultrasound enhances standard laparoscopy in the staging of pancreatic cancer. Ann Surg 228:182–187
17. Spitz JD, Lilly MC, Tetik C, Arregui M (2000) Ultrasound-guided laparoscopic resection of pancreatic islet cell tumors. Surg Laparosc Endosc Percutan Tech 10:168–173
18. Koler AJ, Lilly MC, Arregui ME (2004) Suprapancreatic and periportal lymph nodes are normally larger than 1 cm by laparoscopic ultrasound evaluation. Surg Endosc 18:646–649
19. Nguyen NT, Roberts PF, Follette DM et al (2001) Evaluation of minimally invasive surgical staging for esophageal cancer. Am J Surg 182:702–706
20. Novitsky YW, Kercher KW, Sing RF, Heniford BT (2006) Long-term outcomes of laparoscopic resection of gastric gastrointestinal stromal tumors. Ann Surg 243:738–747
21. Santambrogio R, Montorsi M, Schubert L et al (2006) Laparoscopic ultrasound-guided resection of gastric submucosal tumors. Surg Endosc 20:1305–1307
22. Lucas SW, Spitz JD, Arregui ME (1999) The use of intraoperative ultrasound in laparoscopic adrenal surgery. The St. Vincent experience. Surg Endosc 13:1093–1098
23. Pautler SE, Choyke PL, Pavlovich CP, Daryanani K, Walther MM (2002) Intraoperative ultrasound aids in dissection during laparoscopic partial adrenalectomy. J Urol 168:1352–1355
24. Hoznek A, Salomon L, Antiphon P et al (1999) Partial nephrectomy with retroperitoneal laparoscopy. J Urol 162:1922–1926

Part II

Management of Foregut Cancer

Endoscopic Ablation of Barrett's Esophagus and Early Esophageal Cancer

Virginia R. Litle, Thomas J. Watson,
Jeffrey H. Peters

Contents

Introduction

Barrett's esophagus develops as a result of chronic, pathologic reflux of gastro-duodenal contents into the esophagus. The diagnosis is made upon the endoscopic finding of columnar lined epithelium in the distal esophagus associated with specialized intestinal metaplasia (IM) on histology [1, 2]. Barrett's esophagus is classified as non-dysplastic IM, low-grade dysplasia (LGD), or high-grade dysplasia (HGD). Population-based studies suggest that Barrett's esophagus is present in 1–2% of the US adult population [3] and is increasing in prevalence [4]. Screening upper endoscopy in patients undergoing colonoscopy has shown a remarkably high prevalence, varying from 7% to as much as 25% depending upon the population screened. In a general population of patients undergoing colonoscopy, Rex et al. reported that 6.8% were found to have esophageal intestinal metaplasia [5]. This prevalence was even higher (8.6%) among those patients who had concomitant GERD symptoms. In a predominantly white, males, non-GERD veteran population (>50 years of age) undergoing sigmoidoscopy, Gerson et al. reported a 25% prevalence of IM [6]. The cause of the epidemiologic increase in the detection of Barrett's esophagus is not entirely clear, but is likely related to the increase in the prevalence of and awareness of GERD, the eradication of Helicobacter pylori, a more liberal use of endoscopy, and/or the broad use of anti-secretory medications.

Risk of Progression to Dysplasia and Esophageal Adenocarcinoma

The significance of Barrett's esophagus and the driving force behind ablation therapy is its premalignant nature. The risk for a patient with non-dysplastic

F.L. Greene, B.T. Heniford (eds.), *Minimally Invasive Cancer Management*,
DOI 10.1007/978-1-4419-1238-1_7,

Barrett's esophagus to progress to esophageal adenocarcinoma has been reported to be 0.4–1.0% per patient per year [7, 8], a risk 30–125 times higher than the general population [9]. This fact along with the increasing prevalence of Barrett's esophagus has fueled a 300–500% rise in US esophageal cancer incidence over the last 30 years, an increase in incidence that surpasses that of all other cancers [10, 11].

Prospective prevalence and incidence studies of the development of dysplasia also reveal significant risk for neoplastic deterioration. At the initial diagnosis of Barrett's esophagus in 1,376 patients studied prospectively by Sharma et al. (Tables 7.1 and 7.2), a large proportion had already developed LGD (7.3%), HGD (3.0%), or adenocarcinoma (6.0%) [12]. Follow-up surveillance endoscopy was performed on 618 of the patients with non-dysplastic Barrett's over an average of 4 additional years. Sixteen percent (4% per year) progressed to LGD, 3.6% to HGD (approximately 1%/year), and 2% to adenocarcinoma (0.5% per year). Thus, the risk for a patient with non-dysplastic IM to progress to either HGD or adenocarcinoma, diagnoses which prompt a significant intervention, is 1.4% per patient per year. Stated differently, 1 in 71 patients with non-dysplastic Barrett's esophagus are at risk to have their esophagus removed every year due to the development of HGD or adenocarcinoma.

Table 7.1. Incidence of LGD, HGD, and cancer at primary diagnosis of Barrett's esophagus

New case diagnosis	Number	Percentage of cases
IM	1,376	100
LGD	101	7.3
HGD	42	3.0
Cancer	91	6.7

Table 7.2. Incidence of LGD, HGD, and cancer in non-dysplastic Barrett's patients

Diagnosis	Total	Percentage of risk in 4 years	Percentage of risk per year
Total IM patients	618	NA	NA
New LGD	100	16.1	4.3
New HGD	22	3.6	0.9
Cancer	12	2.0	0.5

Modified from Sharma et al. [12].

Rationale for Endoscopic Ablation of Barrett's Epithelium

Akin to the removal of premalignant polys in the colon, smoking cessation, and other interventions to minimize malignant risk, removal of premalignant esophageal epithelium is ideally desirable. Doing so however requires a technique for safe, effective (complete), and reproducible removal of all metaplastic tissue in a given patient. Achieving this goal has been quite elusive to date. Multiple endoluminal techniques that have been applied in an attempt to ablate or resect of Barrett's epithelium include (1) circumferential balloon-based radiofrequency ablation, (2) photodynamic therapy (PDT), (3) endoscopic mucosal resection (EMR), (4) laser ablation, (5) argon plasma coagulation (APC), (6) multipolar electrocoagulation (MPEC), and (7) cryotherapy. Each of these will be discussed below.

There are multiple challenges inherent in achieving safe, effective, and reproducible removal of Barrett's epithelium. Each of these factors must be considered when evaluating a technique for managing this disease: (1) access (the targeted portion of the esophagus is ~30–40 cm from incisors), (2) the corrugated nature of the esophageal lumen (an uneven epithelial target), (3) mucous and gastric contents affecting the ablative effect of any energy source, (4) esophageal motility which creates a moving ablation target, (5) an appropriate depth of injury to the muscularis mucosae, not into the submucosa, and (6) longevity.

Further, the ideal technique to achieve safe, effective, and reproducible ablation of Barrett's esophagus should (1) be feasible for an endoscopist skilled in interventional techniques to perform; (2) be capable of removing all Barrett's epithelium; (3) result in no sub-squamous IM (buried glands); (4) have a very low rate of complications, such as stricture formation, bleeding, or perforation; (5) and be well tolerated by the patient, thus enabling repeat therapy as needed for the lifetime of the patient for recurrent (new) or persistent disease.

Ackroyd et al. reported that the thickness of non-dysplastic IM (500±4 μm, range 390–590 μm) is similar to that of normal squamous epithelium (490±3 μm, range 420–580 μm) [13]. This narrow range and tight standard deviation for Barrett's thickness suggests that inter and intra-patient variability is small. Thus an ablation technique that repeatedly and uniformly penetrates at a minimum to the muscularis mucosae (~700 μm) and at a maximum to the top of the submucosa (~1,000–1,500 μm) should reliably and safely remove Barrett's epithelium.

Barrett's ablation includes both the "proactive" eradication of Barrett's esophagus, potentially leading in the long term to demonstration of a risk reduction for developing adenocarcinoma, and treatment of dysplastic and neoplastic epithelium which has already developed. Both are important end points.

Ablation Technology and Outcomes

Circumferential Balloon-Based Radiofrequency Ablation (RFA)

Radiofrequency ablation (RFA) using a balloon-based endoscopically guided technique (HALO^{360} System, BÂRRX Medical, Inc., Sunnyvale, CA) is among the most promising new endoscopic therapies for elimination of both non-dysplastic and dysplastic Barrett's epithelium. The device consists of a balloon with tightly spaced coils on its surface, which conduct high-frequency radio waves, generating heat (Fig. 7.1). The balloon, which is sized to match the diameter of the esophagus, is inflated, bringing the coils in apposition to the metaplastic tissue and serves to dilate the targeted portion of the esophagus to a standardized pressure (0.5 atm), transiently flattening the esophageal folds to a standardized tension or stretch. With the esophagus in slightly dilated state, a high-power, ultra-short burst of ablative energy (~300 ms) is applied to the epithelium, resulting in a uniform ablation depth to the muscularis mucosae (~1,000 μm) [14]. Dosimetry studies have calibrated the depth of injury to be deep enough to destroy the epithelium, but not to cause deep circumferential damage, which is associated with stricturing of the esophagus. The key features allowing uniform ablation, reproducible depth, and wide-field removal of the epithelium are (1) very high-power (300 W), (2) ultra-short energy delivery time (<300 ms), (3) tightly spaced bipolar electrode array (<250 μm between electrodes), (4) standardized wall tension with balloon dilation, (5) standardized energy density (Joules of energy delivered to each cm^2 of epithelium, J/cm^2), and (6) large surface area of electrode (>30 cm^2) [14].

In contrast to previous modalities of ablative therapies, RFA has been associated with a high rate of complete reversion to squamous epithelium. Cohort studies suggest that when the balloon-based device is utilized, followed by further treatments with a smaller, non-circumferential device to treat focal areas of remaining disease (Fig. 7.2), up to 97% of

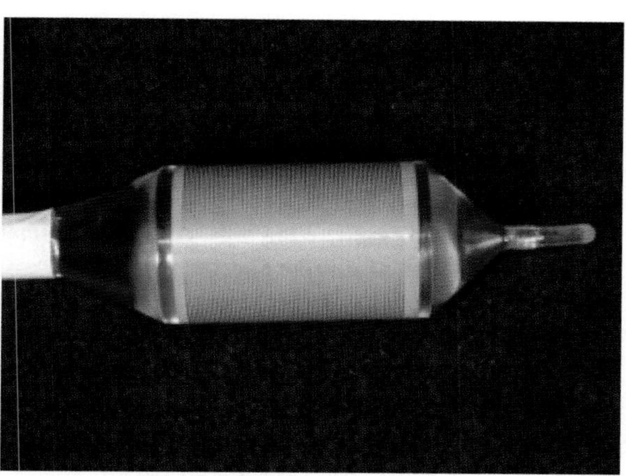

Figure 7.1

Balloon-based electrode (HALO^{360} Ablation Catheter, BÂRRX Medical, Inc., Sunnyvale, CA). Three cm length with 60 narrowly spaced circumferential electrode bands

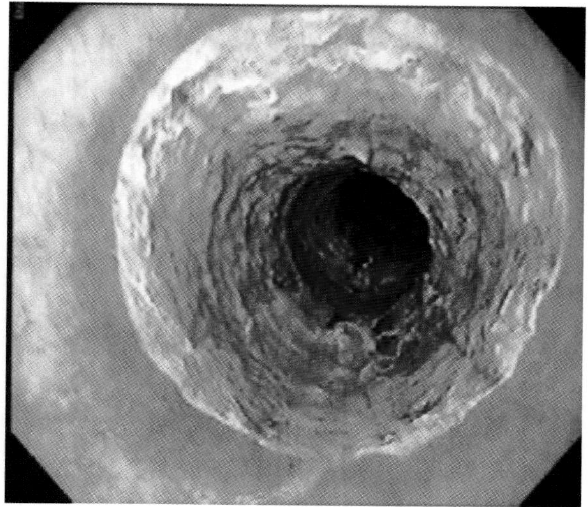

Figure 7.2

Endoscopic appearance after delivery of a single ablation with the HALO^{360} System using 12 J/cm^2 in human esophagus

subjects with non-dysplastic BE show complete reversion to squamous epithelium [15]. In contrast to previous ablative procedures which have been associated with stricture rates of 20% or more, the stricture rate of with this approach is low (0–1%). Other studies confirm this extremely low rate of strictures.

This high rate of complete response and excellent safety profile suggest that it is appropriate for the first time to consider extending ablative therapy to subjects with low-grade and non-dysplastic Barrett's epithelium. Although rates of disease progression are obviously lower, risks and costs associated with the treatment are also reduced. In a cost-benefit analysis assessing the cost-effectiveness of RFA in non-dysplastic disease, treatment was noted to be cost-effective compared to endoscopic surveillance. This was especially true if the interval of surveillance endoscopy could be altered, or if surveillance after ablation could be omitted.

Initial reports determined the appropriate energy dose and assessed the safety and efficacy of this device in animals and resected surgical specimens. In both the porcine model and the human esophagectomy patients, ablation depth was directly related to energy density delivered, with 8–12 J/cm^2 resulting in complete removal of epithelium (Fig. 7.3) [14]. There were no strictures and no significant submucosal injury within this energy density range. Deeper injury and subsequent stricture formation were evident at higher energy density settings (>20 J/cm^2). Evaluation in human subjects undergoing esophagectomy revealed similar findings with ablation performed 1–2 days prior to esophageal resection. Energy density settings of 10 and 12 J/cm^2 resulted in complete epithelial ablation in all areas of balloon electrode contact. The maximum depth of ablation was the muscularis mucosae, with no submucosal injury, thus corroborating the animal study findings in this energy density dose range [14].

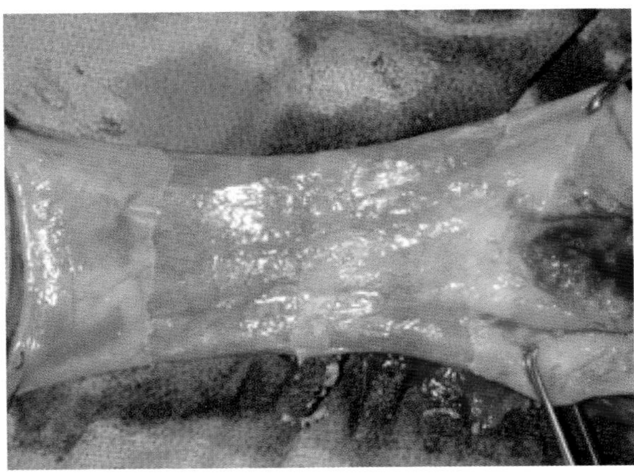

Figure 7.3

Resected human esophagus. Two separate ablation zones delivered with the HALO^{360} System at 10 J/cm^2. Squamous epithelium completely sloughed to the level of the muscularis mucosae

Dunkin et al. studied the effect of this device in a larger series of patients undergoing esophagectomy using 10 or 12 J/cm^2 delivered once (1×) or twice (2×). Complete removal of the esophageal epithelium without injury to the submucosa or muscularis propria was possible using the balloon-based electrode at 10 J/cm^2 (two overlapped applications in one treatment session, 2×) or 12 J/cm^2 (1× or 2×). A second application (2×) did not significantly increase ablation depth; therefore overlapping ablations zones did not portend a significantly deeper injury [16].

Smith et al. randomized applications of 10, 12, or 14 J/cm^2 and 2–6 times using histologic assessment of esophagectomy specimens as the outcome measure [17]. Subjects underwent endoluminal ablation of one or two circumferential 3 cm segments of the esophagus containing IM-HGD using the HALO^{360} System. Following esophagectomy, multiple sections from each ablation zone were evaluated using H&E and microscopy. Maximum ablation depth was the lamina propria or muscularis mucosae (mm) in 10/11 specimens. One section treated at the highest energy (14 J/cm^2, 4×) had edema in the submucosa. In the well-overlapped areas of treatment 91% (10/11) of specimens had no evidence of IM-HGD remaining. In one specimen the majority of IM-HGD was ablated, but small focal areas remained. In three specimens there was IM-HGD at the edge of the treatment zones where overlap of the multiple energy applications was incomplete. They concluded that complete ablation of IM-HGD in 91% of treatment zones, without excessively deep injury, was possible using this device [17].

Clinical studies utilizing RF ablation were first reported in 2005. Sharma et al. reported on the use of this device in a multi-center dosimetry trial in patients (n=32) with non-dysplastic IM (AIM-I). The procedure was performed using conscious sedation on an outpatient basis with a median procedure time of 24 min. Single applications of 8, 10, and 12 J/cm^2 energy densities were evaluated. The procedure was well tolerated and there were no strictures or buried

Table 7.6. Photodynamic therapy for clinically early esophageal cancer

References	Agent/other therapies	Clinical tumor stage (*n*)	Complete response (%)	Follow-up (months)	Esophageal cancer-specific survival (%)
Pech et al. [32]	ALA	T1 (21)	62	38	80 (both groups)
	ALA/ER/KTP/APC	T1 (10)	100	36	
Gossner et al. [31]	ALA	T1 (19)	53	17 (mean)	NA
Panjehpour et al. [37]	Porfimer sodium	T1 (3)	100	10 (mean)	NA
		T2 (4)	100		
Overholt et al. [36]	Porfimer sodium	"Early" (9)	44	59 (mean)	89
Corti et al. [46]	Porfimer sodium	T1 (30)	43	NA	NA
	Porfimer sodium	T2 (7)	28		
	Porfimer sodium/radiotherapy	T1 (30)	87		
		T2 (7)	57		
McCaughan et al. [68]	Porfimer sodium	T1 (7)	57	NA	71

T = tumor; NA = not available; ALA = 5-aminolevulinic acid; Endoscopic resection = ER; APC = argon plasma coagulation; KTP = potassium titanyl phosphate.

as the standard of care in appropriate risk patients.

PDT Ablation of Superficial Invasive Adenocarcinoma. Several authors have reported outcomes of PDT for superficial or "early" esophageal cancer in small series of patients (Table 7.6) [31, 32, 36, 37, 46]. Pech et al. have reported one of the larger series of patients with mucosal tumors treated with PDT using ALA. Twenty-six of the 32 patients (81%) required only one PDT treatment and endoscopic resection (ER) and laser ablation for visible lesions was added in 10 of the 32 patients. At a median follow-up of 3 years, 29% had developed recurrent or metachronous cancer, although only one (11%) ultimately succumbed to esophageal cancer [32]. It is important to note that PDT ablation of early cancers is commonly combined with EMT and/or argon plasma coagulation or laser ablation. At least one report added radiotherapy to PDT improving complete response to 82%, nearly double than that of PDT alone [46]. Interpretation of the data is confounded not only by additional treatment regimens but also by the extent of disease being treated. By example, Corti et al. included T*is* lesions, more traditionally classified as HGD, resulting in a 40% complete response rate for "early" cancer.

Further, PDT fulfills few (one) of the ideal criteria for endoscopic ablative therapy; it is minimally invasive. PDT is an expensive modality, requiring capital investment for the dye, and a high cost of the photosensitizing agent which can exceed $2,000 per treatment course. Two significant risks have been reproducibly associated with PDT including the risk of skin injury and esophageal stricture in approximately 30% of patients.

What is the role of PDT for ablation of BE, dysplasia, and mucosal cancer? Given the stricture rate associated with repeated PDT, the authors favor radioablation over PDT for ablation of BE and LGD. Patients with multifocal HGD confirmed by at least two pathologists who are good operative risks should be offered the option of esophagectomy and EMR with radioablation followed by endoscopic surveillance. The limitations of availability of PDT may soon make this option obsolete.

Cryotherapy

Cryotherapy is a promising new addition to the armamentarium for endoscopic ablation of Barrett's epithelium. The early and limited data derives from one small study in 11 patients [47]. The technique involves inserting a cryotherapy catheter through the working channel of the endoscope through which liquid nitrogen (–196°C) is applied onto the diseased esophagus circumferentially. Although data is very limited, initial advantages of cryoablation over other treatments such as laser, BarrX, and ER may include no perforation, bleeding, or stricture risks [47]. The complications again from this one small study did include chest pain and solid-food dysphagia at an incidence of 9%. At 6-month follow-up there were no buried glands identified at 6-month follow-up and the ablation rate of BE was 9 of 11 patients (78%) (Johnston). An attractive scientific advantage suggested from canine data is that cryotherapy can induce an auto tumor-specific immunity and have an added benefit to local endoscopic ablation of BE or dysplasia [48, 49].

Endoscopic Resection (ER)

Endoscopic ablative techniques are intended to destroy the targeted esophageal mucosa. While this strategy may be advantageous for metaplasia or neoplasia confined to the epithelium, a disadvantage is that a specimen is not retrieved for histologic assessment. Such a paradigm, therefore, risks leaving more deeply penetrating malignancy inadequately treated and prevents accurate pathologic staging. Endoscopic resection (ER), on the other hand, provides a specimen that allows not only a determination of the completeness of resection but also an assessment of the deep and lateral margins, the grade of tumor differentiation, and the presence of lymphovascular or venous invasion, all factors that have been shown to hold prognostic significance for esophageal neoplasia [50].

Endoscopic resection was initially developed in Japan for treatment of superficial squamous cell carcinomas of the esophagus [51, 52]. Following the Japanese experience, ER was adopted by physicians in the United States and Europe for excisional biopsy of small (less than 2 cm) mucosal irregularities or nodules in the setting of Barrett's esophagus (BE) as well as for potentially curative treatment of small, biopsy-proven, early esophageal adenocarcinomas.

ER, thus, has two potential applications: (1) The resected specimen can serve as a large biopsy to guide subsequent definitive therapy, observation of non-neoplastic disease, or esophagectomy for high-grade dysplasia (HGD) or invasive cancer with tailoring of the procedure based upon depth of tumor penetration [53]; (2) The procedure can be performed with curative intent (with or without adjunctive mucosal ablation of residual metaplasia/dysplasia) for tumors at low risk for metastatic spread to regional lymph nodes or distant sites.

When ER is being considered as curative therapy for esophageal neoplasia, the depth of tumor penetration, as assessed at the time of pathologic evaluation of the resected specimen, is critical in determining the potential for nodal spread. Multiple series from the surgical literature have evaluated outcomes after esophagectomy with regional lymphadenectomy for esophageal adenocarcinoma and have correlated the incidence of nodal metastasis with the depth of tumor invasion [54–61]. Tumors limited to the mucosa appear to have a limited potential for nodal disease, approximating 2–5% [58]. For adenocarcinomas penetrating the muscularis mucosa and involving the submucosa, the incidence of nodal metastasis appears to increase to the 20–30% range [54, 58]. Some series, however, would suggest that tumors invading into the superficial submucosa (SM1) have a low incidence of nodal metastasis, similar to disease limited to the mucosa, while deeper submucosal lesions (SM2–3) portend a worse prognosis [58, 59]. The data supporting this contention, however, is far too premature to allow definitive conclusions to be drawn. In addition, ER may not excise the entire submucosa, making determinations of relative submucosal depth of penetration difficult. Tumors involving the muscularis propria have an even higher chance of associated nodal spread, in the range of 45–80% [54, 55].

Thus, the prevailing opinion is that ER is appropriate as therapy with curative intent only for tumors limited to the mucosa. If the resected specimen demonstrates more deeply invading tumor, an esophagectomy with regional lymphadenectomy is indicated, assuming the patient has no contraindications to surgical intervention. Also, as HGD or intramucosal carcinoma (IMC) is frequently multifocal in nature [60], ER is typically used on discrete endoscopically identifiable abnormalities and combined with another endoscopic or surgical procedure to eliminate more widespread regions of metaplasia/dysplasia. Treatment adjuncts in such situations include esophagectomy, possible with minimally invasive [62] and/or vagal-sparing techniques [63], or endoscopic ablation of the residual pathologic epithelium.

ER Technique: The widely utilized terminology "endoscopic mucosal resection" (EMR) is a misnomer in that the resection plane utilizing the methods to be described typically is within the submucosa, often down to its interface with the muscularis propria. Thus, more than merely the mucosal layer generally is excised. The term "endoscopic resection" (ER) is a more accurate descriptor of the procedure.

A number of techniques have been described for performing ER. All share the basic principle of isolation of a defined segment of esophageal mucosa and excision using a snare cautery device. Differences relate to the use of submucosal injection of saline (with or without dilute epinephrine) to separate the esophageal mucosa from the underlying muscle layer and the manner in which the lesion subsequently is lifted and isolated for snare application.

Perhaps the simplest variant of ER is snare resection alone without elevation or submucosal injection. This technique is best applied to polypoid lesions of the esophageal mucosa, in that flat lesions cannot be snared without some form of mucosal elevation. A common resection method has been the use of submucosal injection of saline with dilute epinephrine (10–20 ml injection, 1:100,000 solution) to separate the mucosa from the underlying muscularis propria. The target lesion can then be aspirated into a specially designed cap (Olympus EMR-001, Olympus America, Center Valley, Pennsylvania) attached to the end of a standard flexible adult endoscope ("cap-assisted" ER). The cap is equipped with an inner groove that allows seating of a standard cautery snare. Once the mucosa is within the cap, the snare can be tightened around the base of the lesion and cautery applied, effectively amputating the specimen in the submucosal plane. Prior to application of cautery, the lesion should be gently "tugged" to give the operator a sense of mobility away from the muscularis and to prevent inadvertent full-thickness injury to the esophageal wall. The resected specimen typically remains within the cap and can be extracted as the endoscope is withdrawn. The procedure typically can be completed with a single passage of the endoscope.

A similar method, and perhaps the most widely performed, utilizes a variceal banding device with supplied cap system to isolate the target lesion. Various single-use multiband systems (Duette Multiband Mucosectomy System, Cook Medical, Bloomington, Indiana or Bard Six-Shooter, Bard Interventional Products, Billerica, Massachusetts) are commercially available. The technique involves "sucking" the mucosa into the cap (without prior submucosal injection) and applying a rubber band to the base of the elevated mucosa, creating a pseudopolyp ("suck and ligate" ER). The lesion is then excised either above or below the band using snare electrocautery. The excised specimen can be retrieved using any of a variety of devices such as a net or polypectomy grasper. Advantages of this technique compared to cap-assisted resection are that submucosal injection is not necessary and that the snare does not need to be seated in the cap, a process that may be time-consuming and difficult to master. Disadvantages of this method are the need to reintroduce the endoscope after banding to position the snare and the need to retrieve the free-floating specimen.

Specimen handling and subsequent pathologic assessment are key components of the ER procedure. The specimen can be tacked to a small piece of corkboard to preserve the margins and to allow intraoperative measurement of specimen diameters. The importance of an experienced pathologist cannot be overemphasized. If an expert in esophageal pathology is not available at the endoscopist's institution, consideration should be given to having the specimen sent to a center of excellence for review, particularly in that a high degree of interobserver variability exists in the grading of dysplasia and early esophageal neoplasia [64, 65] and the subtleties of pathologic evaluation may impact the subsequent course of treatment.

ER Risks: Bleeding and esophageal perforation are the most significant risks. The endoscopist must possess the experience to recognize these problems should they arise, as well as the expertise, tools, and facilities to manage them in a safe and effective manner. Most bleeding is self-limited and will resolve with observation. More brisk bleeding typically can be controlled with injection of dilute epinephrine, electrocautery, or application of endoscopic clips. Perforations require significant judgment and skill to treat in the most efficacious manner without excessive morbidity. Another potential complication of ER, particularly when performed in a circumferential fashion, is esophageal stricture, which is usually quite readily managed with serial dilations.

A less obvious potential complication is an incomplete resection. ER of a discrete lesion risks leaving either a positive deep or lateral resection margin. A deep margin involved with cancer is an absolute indication for proceeding with additional definitive therapy such as esophagectomy or combined chemoradiation. Similarly, tumor invading beyond the muscularis mucosa into the submucosa carries a significant risk of nodal metastatic spread and also should be addressed with a more definitive approach. Endoscopic resections, particularly for larger regions of disease, may be piecemeal in fashion. Some endoscopists may choose to resect large areas of metaplasia/dysplasia/neoplasia with multiple resections in one session or in multiple sessions. In such cases, the target lesions may be removed in fragments and margins may be not only violated but also impossible to determine on subsequent pathologic assessment. In addition, residual dysplasia/neoplasia is commonly left behind as islands, at the periphery of resection, or as occult synchronous lesions within residual metaplastic mucosa.

ER Outcomes: The largest experience with ER for early esophageal adenocarcinoma was reported in 2007 by Ell et al. from Wiesbaden, Germany [50]. Their series included 100 patients from a total of 667 referred with suspected intraepithelial neoplasia. Eligibility criteria to undergo ER are listed in Table 7.7. A total of 144 resections (1.47 per patient) were performed without major complications. Most tumors (69%) occurred in the setting of short-segment BE. Endoscopic resection was combined with either argon plasma coagulation (APC) for short-segment BE or photodynamic therapy (PDT) for long-segment BE in 49 patients. Only one-third of resections were proven histologically to be R0 at the lateral margins, though no resection specimen was found to have a positive deep margin. Complete local remission, defined as an R0 resection plus one normal follow-up endoscopy or an R1 or Rx (indeterminate) lateral resection margin plus two consecutive negative follow-up endoscopies, was achieved in 99 out of the 100 patients by a mean of 1.9 months and a maximum of 3 resections. Metachronous or recurrent disease occurred in 11% of patients during a mean follow-up period of 36.7 months, though repeat treatment with endoscopic resection was successful in all cases. The calculated 5-year survival was 98%, with no cancer-related deaths during the follow-up period.

A follow-up report to the Wiesbaden experience was published in 2008 [66]. Their cohort was increased to 349 patients with a mean follow-up of 63.6 months. Metachronous lesions were noted in 21.5% and subsequent esophagectomy was necessary in 3.7% for failed endoscopic control of neoplasia. Multiple risk factors for recurrent disease were found, including piecemeal resections, long-segment BE, lack of ablative therapy after ER, and multifocal neoplasia.

A point worthy of emphasis is the intensive surveillance protocol utilized by the Wiesbaden group subsequent to initial endoscopic therapy [50]. Follow-up endoscopies were planned at 1, 2, 3, 6, 9, and 12 months after treatment and then at 6-month intervals until the 5 year anniversary. Every second visit included an endoscopic ultrasound, computed tomography, and abdominal ultrasound. Annual checkups after 5 years included high-resolution endoscopy with biopsies, as indicated. With further study, the essential elements of this follow-up regimen undoubtedly will be defined, hopefully reducing some of the burden of the surveillance protocol.

ER in Combination with Radiofrequency Ablation for Early Carcinoma: A recent report from the Netherlands assessed outcomes in 44 patients with BE and dysplasia or early esophageal adenocarcinoma (EAC) [67]. Thirty-one patients first underwent ER, 16 with early EAC, 12 with HGD, and 3 with low-grade dysplasia (LGD). The worst histology remaining after any ER and prior to the first radiofrequency (RF) ablation was HGD in 32, LGD in 10, and no dysplasia in 2. A complete histologic eradication of all dysplasia, as well as complete endoscopic and histologic clearance of BE, was achieved in 98% after a median of one circumferential ablation session, two focal ablation sessions, and rescue ER in three patients. Complications occurred during ER in five patients, including four mild bleeding episodes managed with endoscopic techniques and one esophageal perforation treated with endoscopic clips and placement of a covered esophageal stent. Four patients (9%) developed dysphagia after ablation, improved after a median of three endoscopic dilatations; all had undergone widespread ER. After

Table 7.7. Eligibility criteria for endoscopic resection

(1) No evidence of more advanced tumor (>T1), lymph node involvement, or systemic metastasis on staging evaluation;
(2) Patient has opted against esophagectomy after being informed that surgical resection is the standard of care;
(3) Tumor deemed low risk for lymphatic or systemic spread:
  a. Lesion diameter <20 mm
  b. Macroscopically polypoid or flat without ulceration
  c. Well-differentiated or moderately differentiated adenocarcinoma
  d. Limited to the mucosa on the basis of staging procedures (e.g., endoscopic ultrasound) and proven on histologic examination of resected specimen
  e. No invasion of lymphatics or veins on histologic examination of resected specimen

Reprinted with permission from Watson [70].

a median follow-up of 21 months, no dysplasia had recurred. In 1,475 follow-up biopsies obtained from neosquamous epithelium, only one (0.07%) revealed buried glandular mucosa. These results demonstrate that stepwise circumferential and focal RF ablation, with or without adjunctive ER to assess and treat focal nodules, is safe and effective at eradicating dysplasia and BE at short- to medium-term follow-up. These data underscore the feasibility of ER in a highly select subgroup of patients referred with HGD or IMC and treated at a specialty center. In such situations, the outcomes at 5 years are excellent, with cure rates approximating those obtained via esophagectomy.

A few words of caution are in order, however, with regard to the applicability of this technique to the overall population of patients referred with esophageal neoplasia. Whether similar results can be obtained in the general community by non-specialty physicians/centers is not known. As HGD and IMC are frequently multifocal, the need to address potential residual neoplastic mucosa is apparent and the importance of close follow-up cannot be overemphasized. The presence of occult malignancies, particularly ones involving the submucosa with possible nodal metastases, must be considered. As many such patients are young with a long life expectancy, the possibility of new tumors arising beyond 5 years must be considered. Quality of life has not been assessed after ER and compared to esophagectomy. While the advantages of a less invasive approach to treatment of HGD/IMC are intuitive, less obvious is the potential for anxiety that comes with the need for serial endoscopic interventions and surveillance over a prolonged time period as well as the persistence of any anatomic or functional foregut derangements that led to the development of BE in the first place.

Endoscopic resection has arisen as a valuable tool in the armamentarium of physicians treating early esophageal neoplasia. As with all new procedures, the treating physician must possess an adequate understanding of the strengths and limitations of the technique in order to apply it in appropriate circumstances. Patient selection is critical and the exact indications for ER will continue to be elucidated as the available data mature. An expert team is desirable, consisting of endoscopists knowledgeable in assessment and treatment of esophageal disease, experienced esophageal surgeons, and dedicated pathologists. Given the commitment of resources and personnel necessary for optimal assessment and management, patients with such neoplasms are best treated in a specialty center. ER, in patients otherwise deemed appropriate candidates for esophagectomy, should be considered only in carefully selected cases.

References

1. Spechler SJ (2002) Barrett's esophagus. N Engl J Med 346(11):836–842
2. Peters JH, Hagen JA, DeMeester SR (2004) Barrett's esophagus. J Gastrointest Surg 8(1):1–17
3. Ronkainen J, Aro P, Storskrubb T et al (2005) Prevalence of Barrett's esophagus in the general population: an endoscopic study. Gastroenterology 129:1825–1831
4. Prach AT, MacDonald TA, Hopwood DA, Johnston DA (27 Sept 1997) Increasing incidence of Barrett's oesophagus: education, enthusiasm or epidemiology? Lancet 350(9082):933
5. Rex DK, Cummings OW, Shaw M et al (2003) Screening for Barrett's esophagus in colonoscopy patients with and without heartburn. Gastroenterology 125:1670–1677
6. Gerson LB, Shetler K, Triadafilopoulos G (2002) Prevalence of Barrett's esophagus in asymptomatic individuals. Gastroenterology 123:636–639
7. O'Connor JB, Falk GW, Richter JE (1999) The incidence of adenocarcinoma and dysplasia in Barrett's esophagus: report on the Cleveland Clinic Barrett's Esophagus Registry. Am J Gastroenterol 94:2037–2042
8. Drewitz DJ, Sampliner RE, Garewal HS (1997) The incidence of adenocarcinoma in Barrett's esophagus: a prospective study of 170 patients followed 4.8 years. Am J Gastroenterol 92:212–215
9. Provenzale D, Kemp JA, Arora S, Wong JB (1994) A guide for surveillance of patients with Barrett's esophagus. Am J Gastroenterol 89:670–680
10. American Cancer Society (2005) Cancer facts and figures 2005. American Cancer Society, Atlanta, GA
11. Ries LAG, Eisner MP, Kosary CL et al (eds) (2005) SEER Cancer Statistics Review, 1975–2002. National Cancer Institute, Bethesda, MD, http://seer.cancer.gov/csr/1975_2002/, based on November 2004 SEER data submission, posted to the SEER web site 2005
12. Sharma P et al (2001) Progression of Barrett's esophagus to high-grade dysplasia and cancer: preliminary results of the BEST trial. Gastroenterology 120:A16
13. Ackroyd R, Brown NJ, Stephenson TJ, Stoddard CJ, Reed MWR (1999) Ablation treatment for Barrett oesophagus: what depth of tissue destruction is needed? J Clin Path 52:509–512
14. Ganz RA, Utley DS, Stern RA, Jackson J, Batts KP, Termin P (2004) Complete ablation of esophageal epithelium with a balloon-based bipolar electrode: a phased evaluation in the porcine and in the human esophagus. Gastrointest Endosc 60(6):1002–1010
15. Sharma VK, Wang KK, Overholt B et al (2007) Balloon based circumferential endoscopic radiofrequency ablation of Barrett's esophagus: 1-year follow-up of 100 patients. Gastroint Endosc 65:185–195

16. Dunkin BJ, Martinez J, Bejarano PA et al (2006) Thin-layer ablation of human esophageal epithelium using a bipolar radiofrequency balloon device. Surg Endosc 20:125–130
17. Smith CD, Bejarano P, Melvin WS, Patti M, Muthusamy R, Dunkin BJ (2007) Endoscopic ablation of intestinal metaplasia containing high-grade dysplasia in esophagectomy patients using a balloon based ablation system. Surg Endosc 21:560–569
18. Sharma VK, McLaughlin R, Dean P, DePetris G, Moirano MM, Fleischer DE (2005) Successful ablation of Barrett's esophagus with low-grade dysplasia using BÂRRX bipolar balloon device: preliminary results of the ablation of intestinal metaplasia with LGD (AIM-LGD) Trial. Gastroint Endosc 61(5):AB143
19. Fleischer DE, Sharma VK, Reymunde A et al (2005) A prospective multi-center evaluation of ablation of non-dysplastic Barrett's esophagus using the BÂRRX bipolar balloon device: ablation of intestinal metaplasia trial (AIM-II). Gastroenterology 128(4):A236
20. Shaheen NJ, Sharma P, Overholt BF et al (2008) A randomized multicenter sham-controlled trial of radiofrequency ablation (RFA) for subjects with Barrett's esophagus (Be) containing dysplasia: interim results of the AIM dysplasia trial. Gastroenterology 134:A–37
21. Shaheen NJ, Goldblum JR, Sampliner RE et al (2008) Are biopsies after ablation for dysplastic Barrett's esophagus of adequate depth to detect glandular mucosa beneath the neo-squamous epithelium; Comparative histopathologic outcomes from a randomized controlled trial (AIM dysplasia trial). Gastroenterology 134:A–724
22. Lightdale CJ, Overholt BF, Wang KK et al (2008) Predictors and quantitative assessment of incomplete response after radiofrequency ablation for dysplastic Barrett's esophagus: analysis of randomized sham-controlled clinical trial (The Aim dysplasia trial). Gastrointest Endosc 67: AB–182
23. Pouw RE, Gondrie JJ, Van Vilsteren FG et al (2008) Stepwise circumferential and focal radiofrequency ablation of Barrett's esophagus with high grade dysplasia or early carcinoma. Gastroenterology 134:A844
24. Ganz RA, Overholt BF, Sharma VK et al (Jul 2008) Circumferential ablation of Barrett's esophagus that contains high-grade dysplasia: a US multicenter registry. Gastrointest Endosc 68(1):35–40. Epub 2008 Mar 19
25. Webber J, Herman M, Kessel D, Fromm D (1999) Current concepts in gastrointestinal photodynamic therapy. Ann Surg 230:12–23
26. Moghissi K, Dixon K (2003) Photodynamic therapy (PDT) in esophageal cancer: a surgical view of its indications based on 14 years experience. Technol Cancer Res Treat 2:319–326
27. Litle VR, Luketich JD, Christie NA et al (2003) Photodynamic therapy as palliation for esophageal cancer: experience in 215 patients. Ann Thor Surg 76:1687–1693
28. Bugelski PJ, Porter CW, Dougherty TJ et al (1981) Autoradiographic distribution of hematoporphrin derivative in normal and tumor tissue of the mouse. Cancer Res 41:4606–4612
29. Yuan J, Mahama-Reluc PA, Fournier RL, Hampton JA (1997) Predictions of mathematical models of tissue oxygenation and generation of singlet oxygen during photodynamic therapy. Radiat Res 148:386–396
30. Greenwald BD (2000) Photodynamic therapy for esophageal cancer: update. Chest Surg Clin North Am 10:625–637
31. Gossner L, May A, Sroka R et al (1999) Photodynamic destruction of high grade dysplasia and early carcinoma of the esophagus after the oral administration of 5-aminolevulinic acid. Cancer 86:1921–1928
32. Pech O, Gossner L, May A et al (2005) Long-term results of photodynamic therapy with 5-aminolevulinic acid for superficial Barrett's cancer and high-grade intraepithelial neoplasia. Gastrointest Endosc 62:24–30
33. Ortner M, Zumbusch K, Liebetruth J et al (1997) Photodynamic therapy of Barrett's esophagus after local administration of 5 aminolevulinic acid. Gastroenterology 112:A633
34. Overholt BF, Panjehpour M, Haydek JM (1999) Photodynamic therapy for Barrett's esophagus: follow-up in 100 patients. Gastrointest Endosc 49:1–7
35. Laukka MA, Wang KK (1995) Initial results using low-dose photodynamic therapy in the treatment of Barrett's esophagus. Gastrointest Endosc 42:59–63
36. Overholt BF, Panjehpour M, Halberg DL (2003) Photodynamic therapy for Barrett's esophagus with dysplasia and/or early stage carcinoma: long-term results. Gastrointest Endosc 58:183–188
37. Panjehpour M, Overholt BF, Haydek KH et al (2000) Results of photodynamic therapy for ablation of dysplasia and early cancer in Barrett's esophagus and effect on oral steroids on stricture formation. Am J Gastroenterol 95: 2177–2184
38. Wang KK, Wong Kee Song M, Nijhawan P, Nourbakhsh A, Anderson M, Balm R (1998) Clinical course of photodynamic therapy indirect esophageal strictures. Gastroenterology 114:G2894
39. Wolfsen HC (2002) Photodynamic therapy for mucosal esophageal adenocarcinoma and dysplastic Barrett's esophagus. Dig Dis 20:5–17
40. Wolfsen HC, Ng CS (2002) Cutaneous consequences of photodynamic therapy. Cutis 69:140–142
41. Malhi-Chowla N, Wolfsen HC, DeVault KR (2001) Esophageal dysmotility in patients undergoing photodynamic therapy. May Clin Proc 76:987–989
42. Ackroyd R, Brown NJ, Davis MF et al (2000) Photodynamic therapy for dysplastic Barrett's oesophagus: a prospective, double blind, randomized, placebo controlled trial. Gut 47:612–617
43. Sampliner R (2004) Endoscopic ablative therapy for Barrett's esophagus: current status. Gastrointest Endosc 59:66–69
44. Wang KK (1999) Current status of photodynamic therapy of Barrett's esophagus. Gastroint Endosc 49:520–523
45. Ferguson MK, Naunheim KS (1997) Resection for Barrett's mucosa with high-grade dysplasia: implications for prophylactic photodynamic therapy. J Thorac Cardiovasc Surg 114:824–829
46. Corti L, Skarlatos J, Boso C et al (2000) Outcome of patients receiving photodynamic therapy for early esophageal cancer. Int J Radiat Oncol Biol Phys 47(2):419–424
47. Johnston MH, Eastone JA, Horwhat JD et al (2005) Cryoablation of Barrett's esophagus: a pilot study. Gastrointest Endosc 62:842–848

48. Ablin RJ (2001) Cancer of the oesophagus: a possible role for cryosurgery. Eur J Surg Oncol 27:332–334
49. Grana L, Ablin RJ, Goldman S et al (1981) Freezing of the esophagus: histological changes and immunological response. Int Surg 66:295–301
50. Ell C, May A, Pech O et al (2007) Curative endoscopic resection of early esophageal adenocarcinomas (Barrett's cancer). Gastrointest Endosc 65:3–10
51. Inoue H, Endo M, Takeshita K et al (1992) A new simplified technique of endoscopic esophageal mucosal resection using a cap-fitted panendoscope. Surg Endosc 6:264–265
52. Takeshita K, Tani M, Inoue H et al (1997) Endoscopic treatment of early oesophageal or gastric cancer. Gut 40: 123–127
53. Maish MS, DeMeester SR (2004) Endoscopic mucosal resection as a staging technique to determine the depth of invasion of esophageal adenocarcinoma. Ann Thorac Surg 78:1777–1782
54. Rice TW, Zuccaro G Jr., Adelstein DJ et al (1998) Esophageal carcinoma: depth of tumor invasion is predictive of regional lymph node status. Ann Thorac Surg 65:787–792
55. Nigro JJ, Hagen JA, DeMeester TR et al (1999) Prevalence and location of nodal metastases in distal esophageal adenocarcinoma confined to the wall: implications for therapy. J Thorac Cardiovasc Surg 117:16–23
56. Van Sandick JW, Van Lanschot JJB, ten Kate FJW et al (2000) Pathology of early invasive adenocarcinoma of the esophagus or esophagogastric junction: implications for therapeutic decision making. Cancer 88:2429–2437
57. Stein HJ, Feith M, Mueller J, Werner M, Siewert JR (2000) Limited resection for early adenocarcinoma in Barrett's esophagus. Ann Surg 232:733–742
58. Buskens CJ, Westerterp M, Lagarde SM, Bergman JJ, ten Kate FJW, van Lanschot JJB (2004) Prediction of appropriateness of local endoscopic treatment for high-grade dysplasia and early adenocarcinoma by EUS and histopathologic features. Gastrointest Endosc 60:703–707
59. Liu L, Hofstetter WL, Rashid A et al (2005) Significance of the depth of tumor invasion and lymph node metastasis in superficially invasive (T1) esophageal adenocarcinoma. Am J Surg Path 29:1079–1085
60. Oh D, Hagen JA, Chandrasoma PT et al (2006) Clinical biology and surgical therapy if intramucosal adenocarcinoma of the esophagus. J Am Coll Surg 203:152–161
61. Altorki NK, Lee PC, Liss Y et al (2008) Multifocal neoplasia and nodal metastases in T1 esophageal carcinoma: implications for endoscopic treatment. Ann Surg 247:434–439
62. Fernando HC, Luketich JD, Buenaventura PO, Perry Y, Christie NA (2002) Outcomes of minimally invasive esophagectomy (MIE) for high-grade dysplasia of the esophagus. Eur J Cardiothorac Surg 22(1):1–6
63. Peyre CG, DeMeester SR, Rizzetto C et al (2007) Vagal-sparing esophagectomy: the ideal operation for intramucosal adenocarcinoma and Barrett's with high-grade dysplasia. Ann Surg 246(4):665–671
64. Ormsby AH, Petras RE, Henricks WH et al (2002) Observer variation in the diagnosis of superficial oesophageal adenocarcinoma. Gut 51:671–676
65. Montgomery E, Bronner MP, Goldblum JR et al (2001) Reproducibility of the diagnosis of dysplasia in Barrett esophagus: a reaffirmation. Hum Pathol 32(4):368–378
66. Pech O, Behrens A, May A et al (2008) Long-term results and risk factor analysis for recurrence after curative endoscopic therapy in 349 patients with high-grade intraepithelial neoplasia and mucosal adenocarcinoma in Barrett's oesophagus. Gut 57:1200–1206
67. Pouw RE, Gondrie JJ, Sondermeijer CM et al (2008) Eradication of Barrett esophagus with early neoplasia by radiofrequency ablation, with or without endoscopic resection. J Gastrointest Surg 12:1627–1637
68. McCaughan JS, Ellison EC, Guy JT et al (1996) Photodynamic therapy for esophageal malignancy: a prospective twelve-year study. Ann Thor Surg 62: 1005–1010
69. Overholt BF, Wang KK, Burdick JS et al (2007) Five-year efficacy and safety of photodynamic therapy with Photofrin in Barrett's high-grade dysplasia. Gastrointest Endosc 66:460–468
70. Watson TJ (2008) Endoscopic resection for Barrett's esophagus with high-grade dysplasia or early esophageal adenocarcinoma. Sem Thorac Cardiovac Surg 20(4): 310–319

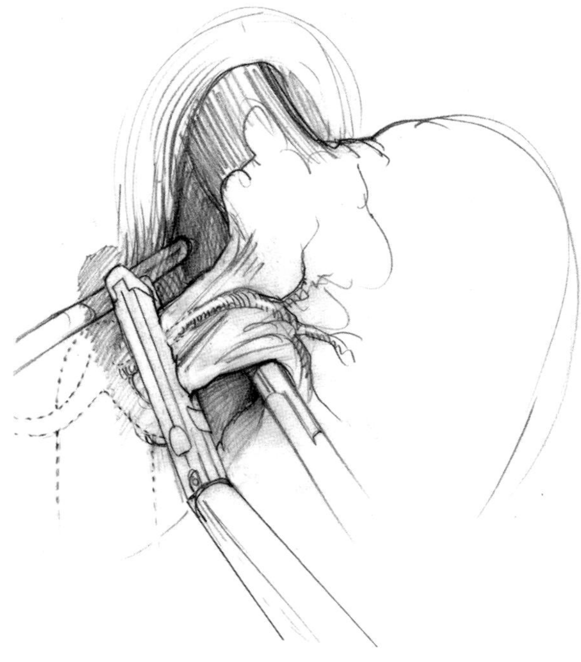

Figure 8.2

Division of left gastric artery and vein. The vessels are divided with a vascular stapler near the base of the left gastric artery to maximize the lymph node harvest. Used with permission from Hunter [71]

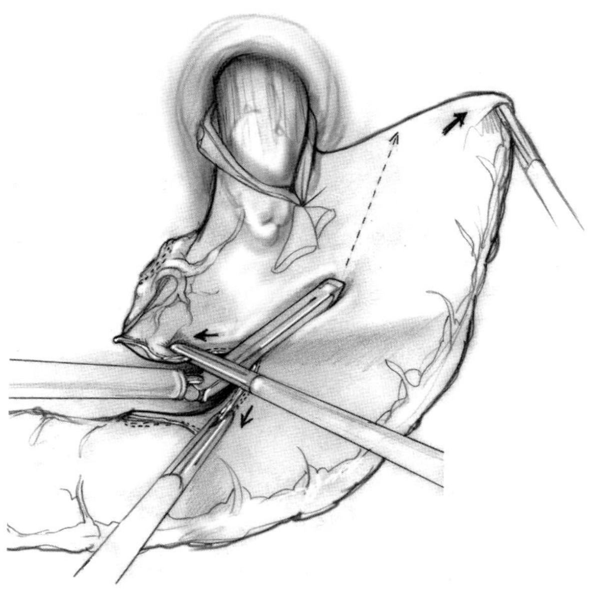

Figure 8.3

Creation of neoesophagus. A 5 cm gastric tube is created using serial firings of a laparoscopic stapler beginning on a point 6 cm proximal to the pylorus along the lesser curvature. Used with permission from Hunter [71]

posterior gastric artery is divided and all lymphatic tissue in this area is maintained with the specimen. The entire gastrocolic omentum is divided and the posterior gastric mobilization is continued until the gastroduodenal artery is visualized. A full Kocher maneuver is performed to mobilize the duodenum and allow the pylorus to be passed to the level of the esophageal hiatus without tension.

Creation of the Gastric Conduit and Distal Esophageal Mobilization

When the stomach is completely mobilized, a point 6 cm proximal to the pylorus is identified along the lesser curvature. The stomach is divided longitudinally using a laparoscopic stapler with 4.5 mm staple depth to create a neoesophagus 3–5 cm wide (Fig. 8.3). The distal margin of the specimen side is then resected and sent for frozen section analysis. The distal esophagus is circumferentially mobilized with its accompanying lymphatic tissue as high in the mediastinum as can be safely visualized. The planes for this dissection proceed along the bilateral pleurae, the pericardium, and the aorta.

Cervical Esophageal Exposure

A 5 cm incision is made along the anterior border of the sternocleidomastoid muscle and this muscle is retracted laterally. The carotid sheath is mobilized laterally and the fascia overlying the esophagus is opened along the length of the incision. Esophageal mobilization is the accomplished using blunt finger dissection as far distally as can be accomplished.

Esophageal Inversion

A retrograde inversion technique is used for patients with high-grade dysplasia. The specimen is divided using a laparoscopic stapler just below the gastroesophageal junction, and the gastric specimen is retrieved in a plastic bag. A vein stripper is passed distally through a cervical esophagotomy and retrieved laparoscopically via a small gastrotomy at the gastric staple line and withdrawn through the 15 mm trocar (Fig. 8.4). The anvil is attached and the gastrotomy is reinforced with a horizontal mattress suture. The vein stripper is returned to the abdominal cavity and withdrawn from the cervical incision, creating a distal-to-proximal inversion of the esophagus within the mediastinum (Fig. 8.5). This action places the mediastinal attachments on tension so that they can be divided under direct vision with all lymphatic tissue included within the inversion. This dissection is carried out as far cephalad as visualization allows, then the dissection is completed by blunt finger dissection, and the specimen is removed via the cervical incision (Fig. 8.6). The esophagus is divided at the level of the cervical gastrotomy and the proximal resection margin is sent for frozen section analysis.

Alternatively, an antegrade esophageal inversion is used for patients with invasive cancer. Two stay sutures are placed in the distal aspect of the cervical esophagus and the esophagus is divided with a stapler. A cervical esophagotomy is created and a vein stripper is passed distally until it can be seen abutting the gastric staple line. The incision for the 12 mm port site along the left costal margin is extended medially to allow exteriorization of the specimen along the vein stripper. A small gastrotomy is created and the vein stripper withdrawn. The anvil is attached to the cervical end of the vein

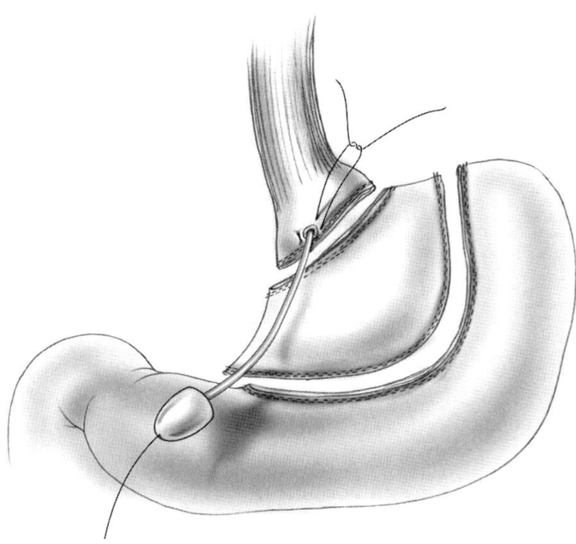

Figure 8.4

Preparation for retrograde esophageal inversion. The vein stripper passed from the cervical esophagotomy exits the stomach and is buttressed by a U stitch. Attachment of the anvil allows esophageal inversion. Used with permission from Hunter [71]

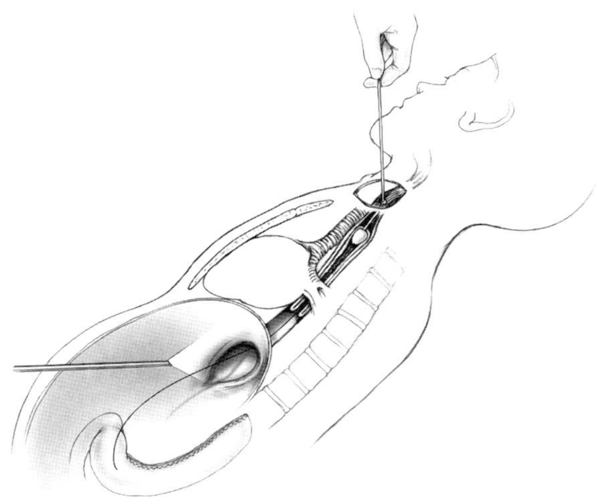

Figure 8.5

Esophageal inversion. Saggital view of the course of esophageal inversion as the mediastinal dissection is accomplished under direct vision. Used with permission from Hunter [71]

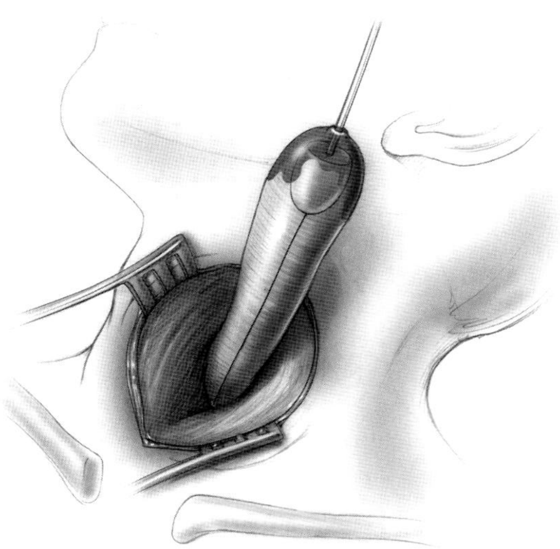

Figure 8.6

Specimen retrieval via cervical incision. The inverted esophagus is delivered through the cervical incision. Used with permission from Hunter [71]

stripper and the esophagotomy is reinforced with a mattress suture. A proximal-to-distal esophageal inversion is created by placing traction in the vein stripper from the abdomen, and the esophagus is removed via the abdominal incision. The proximal margin is sent for frozen section analysis and the laparoscopic trocar is replaced.

Esophageal Reconstruction

Whether antegrade or retrograde, a 60 mm silk suture is attached to the end of the vein stripper so that following specimen removal, the suture lies trough the mediastinum. The proximal end of the suture is tied to a 28-french chest tube which is guided through the mediastinum and into the abdominal cavity as the surgeon provides traction on the suture from below. The tip of the gastric conduit is sutured to the chest tube and gently pulled up through the posterior mediastinum. The stomach is pulled up into the cervical incision and a stapled end-to-side anastomosis is performed. The staple line on the lesser curvature is rotated posteriorly and the neoesophagus is elevated to skin level. A transverse gastrotomy is created and an end-to-side stapled anastomosis is created. A nasogastric tube is placed into the gastric conduit and passed to the level of the diaphragmatic hiatus, and the remaining gastrotomy is closed in two layers. A closed suction drain is placed alongside the anastomosis, and a laparoscopic jejunostomy tube is placed for enteral feeding and medication access.

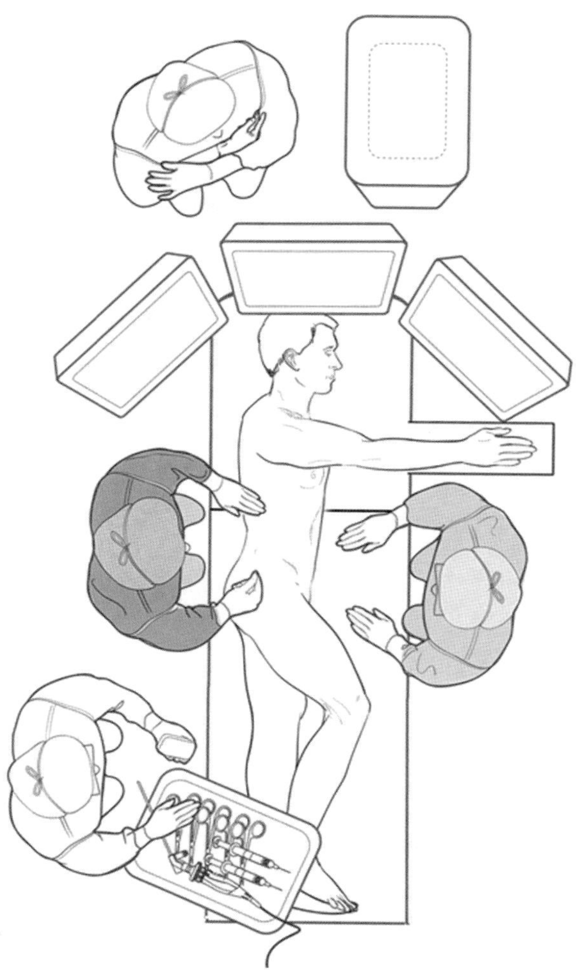

Figure 8.7

Patient position for thoracoscopic esophageal mobilization. Used with permission from Hunter [71]

Thoracoscopic–Laparoscopic Esophagectomy

Thoracoscopy

The patient is intubated with a double-lumen endotracheal tube and placed in the left lateral decubitus position. The surgeon stands on the right and the assistant on the left. Four ports are used: a 10 mm camera port in the 7th or 8th intercostal space at the midaxillary line, a 5 mm port in the 8th or 9th space at the posterior axillary line, a 10 mm port in the 4th intercostal space at the anterior axillary line, and a 5 mm trocar just posterior to the tip of the scapula (Fig. 8.7).

The inferior pulmonary ligament is divided and the mediastinal pleura opened to the level of the azygous vein to expose the esophagus. The azygous vein is divided with a vascular stapler and the esophagus is dissected circumferentially and encircled with a penrose drain for retraction. The esophagus is mobilized circumferentially from the level of the thoracic inlet to the diaphragm including all lymphatic tissue between the pleura, pericardium, and aorta (Fig. 8.8). Near the thoracic inlet, care is taken to avoid injury to the membranous trachea and recurrent laryngeal nerves. Following complete esophageal mobilization, a chest tube is placed, two-lung ventilation is resumed, and all port sites are closed.

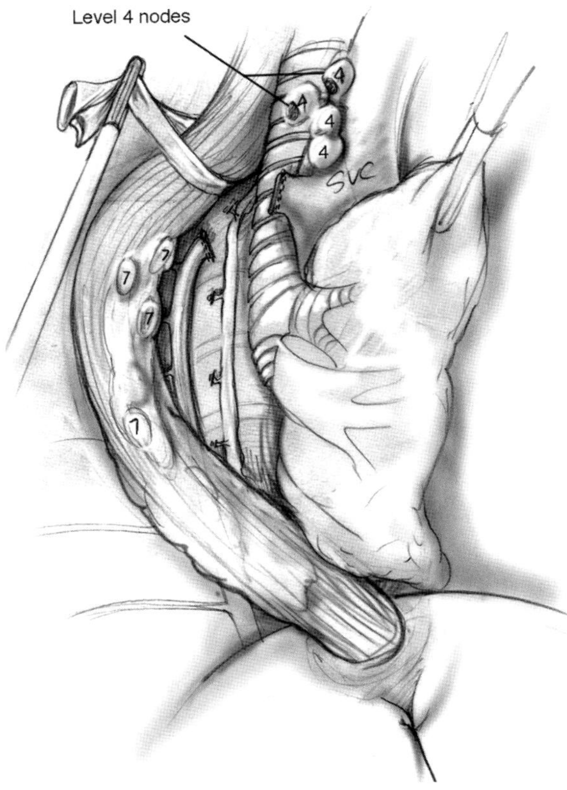

Figure 8.8
Completed thoracoscopic esophageal mobilization. Shown are the divided azygous vein and thoracic duct branches and clearance of lymphatic tissue to the level of the diaphragmatic hiatus. Used with permission from Hunter [71]

Laparoscopy

The patient is repositioned in the supine split-legged position and the neck and abdomen are prepared and draped. The port placement, gastric mobilization, and gastric conduit creation proceed as previously described for inversion esophagectomy. Following the creation of the neoesophagus and mobilization of the cervical esophagus, the tip of the gastric conduit is sutured to the distal end of the specimen and passed through the mediastinum as the specimen is removed via the cervical incision. After the gastric pull up is complete, an end-to-side esophagogastrostomy is created as previously described.

Choice of Approach

Endoscopic mucosal resection, LIE, and TLE represent complimentary approaches to esophageal cancer treatment with distinct advantages and disadvantages. EMR provides an approach that can reduce the morbidity and mortality for patients with early cancers, while improving the staging of these cancers without precluding subsequent esophageal resection if pathologic upstaging occurs.

Laparoscopic inversion esophagectomy is a safe approach to minimally invasive esophagectomy that can be performed in less time and with lower blood loss than TLE [50]. Further studies are required to evaluate the differences in morbidity following these approaches, as the single cavity approach may reduce postoperative pain, cardiac, and pulmonary complications. Currently we utilize this approach for patients undergoing esophagectomy for high-grade dysplasia and early cancers that are not amenable to EMR. LIE is, however, inappropriate for patients with upper esophageal tumors or bulky tumors that make inversion difficult or impossible, and these patients should be approached by TLE.

The ideal approach to patients with invasive cancers in the distal third of the esophagus, whether open or minimally invasive, remains controversial. Advocates of transthoracic approaches cite increased lymph node yield obtained by extended lymphadenectomy under direct vision, while others favor decreased perioperative morbidity offered by transhiatal approaches. A recent randomized controlled trial compared open transthoracic esophagectomy with extended lymph node dissection to transhiatal esophagectomy using an approach similar to the antegrade inversion esophagectomy described earlier and found no difference in 5-year survival [51]. Further comparative studies are required to confirm these findings and clarify the indications for TLE and LIE.

Palliation of Dysphagia

Dysphagia is the most common presenting symptom of esophageal cancer, but it does not occur until the lesion occupies 80–90% of the esophageal circumference. Thus, the majority of esophageal cancer patients present with unresectable locally advanced or metastatic disease. Palliation is an important goal of therapy in this group of patients, and several options exist.

Esophageal Dilation

The normal functional diameter of the esophagus is 25 mm, and dysphagia occurs at about 13 mm. Endoscopic balloon dilation can be used for transient relief by dilating malignant strictures up to 17 mm [52]. These dilations should be performed over a guidewire, because dilation without the use of a guidewire has been associated with increased risk of esophageal perforation [53]. Also, this approach is only used as a preliminary measure for immediate symptom relief because the results only last for 1–2 weeks.

Esophageal Stenting

Self-expanding metallic stents were introduced in the 1990s, allowing successful deployment in 90% of cases with reduced complication rates compared to previously available fixed diameter stents. These stents provide symptomatic relief to upward of 95% of patients [54, 55]. Major disadvantages include high cost, tumor ingrowth, and the 20–40% complication rate. Complications include chest pain, stent migration, fistulazation, airway obstruction, and hemorrhage [56–58]. More recently, self-expanding plastic stents have been introduced with the advantage that they can be repositioned or removed as necessary. More data are needed regarding the success rate of stent placement and rates of complications, especially stent migration.

Nd:YAG Laser

Laser recanalization of the esophageal lumen can be achieved in 90% of patients using the neodymium: yttrium aluminum garnet (YAG) laser [59, 60]. This technique can be accomplished with no systemic complications on an outpatient basis. Generally, this requires every other day treatments for approximately 1 week (three to four treatments). However, treatment must be repeated every 4–6 weeks, and complications may occur in 4–9% of cases [61]. Also, while this approach does well for mid-esophageal lesion, masses in the proximal esophagus or near the gastroesophageal junction are difficult to access [62].

Photodynamic Therapy

Photodynamic therapy (PDT) uses a photosensitizing agent in combination with non-thermal laser exposure to damage the microvasculature of the esophageal tumor, rendering it ischemic [63]. PDT is technically easier to perform than Nd:YAG laser treatment and can be used for patients with partially obstructing tumors that cannot be adequately treated with the Nd:YAG treatments. PDT is also preferred for patients with longer than 8 cm tumors located in the proximal or distal esophagus and completely obstructing lesions [64]. Advantages of this approach include avoidance of the globus sensation and gastroesophageal reflux associated with esophageal stent place in the proximal esophagus and across the gastroesophageal junction, respectively. Contraindications to PDT include porphyria or allergies to porphyrins and presence of an esophagobronchial fistula. This approach is also associated with 4–8 weeks of photosensitivity, during which patients must avoid sun exposure.

Palliative Chemotherapy and Radiation

Systemic chemotherapy with platinum-based chemotherapy has been shown to relieve dysphagia in 70% of patients and improve symptoms in 90% [65–68]. Radiation at doses of 30–37.5 Gy are used for palliation; however, this approach may be complicated by recurrent dysphagia due to stricture [69]. Intraluminal brachytherapy has also been used to successfully palliate dysphagia, but may be complicated by early post-procedure dysphagia due to tissue edema [70].

Palliation of dysphagia has a profound effect on the quality of life for patients with unresectable esophageal cancer. Currently there is no ideal method of symptom palliation, and these methods each work best in different circumstances. Therefore, thorough knowledge of the available treatment options allows esophageal surgeons to tailor the treatment regimen to the individual characteristics of each patient and provide the best symptom relief.

References

1. Gopal DV, Jobe BA (2002) Screening for Barrett's esophagus may not reduce morbidity and mortality due to esophageal adenocarcinoma – Commentary. Evid Based Oncol 3: 144–145
2. Spechler SJ (2002) Clinical practice: Barrett's Esophagus. N Engl J Med 346:836–842

3. Spechler SJ (2001) Screening and surveillance for complications related to gastroesophageal reflux disease. Am J Med 111:130S–136S
4. Jemal A, Siegel R, Ward E et al (2008) Cancer statistics, 2008. CA Cancer J Clin 58:71–96
5. el-Serag HB (2002) The epidemic of esophageal adenocarcinoma. Gastroenterol Clin North Am 31:421–440
6. Nigro J, DeMeester S, Hagen J et al (1999) Node status in transmural esophageal adenocarcinoma and outcome after en bloc esophagectomy. J Thorac Cardiovasc Surg 117: 960–968
7. Lagergren J, Bergstrom R, Lindgren A, Nyren O (1999) Symptomatic gastroesophageal reflux as a risk factor for esophageal adenocarcinoma. N Engl J Med 340: 825–831
8. Jobe BA, Enestvedt CK, Thomas CR Jr. (2006) Disease-specific multidisciplinary care: a natural progression in the management of esophageal cancer. Dis Esophagus 19: 417–418
9. Blazeby JM, Wilson L, Metcalfe C, Nicklin J, English R, Donovan JL (2006) Analysis of clinical decision-making in multi-disciplinary cancer teams. Ann Oncol 3:457–460
10. Birkmeyer JD, Siewers AE, Finlayson EV et al (2002) Hospital volume and surgical mortality in the United States. N Engl J Med 346:1128–1137
11. Kelsen DP, Ginsberg R, Pajak TF et al (1998) Chemotherapy followed by surgery compared with surgery alone for localized esophageal cancer. N Engl J Med 339:1979–1984
12. Swanstrom LL, Hanson P (1997) Laparoscopic total esophagectomy. Arch Surg 132:943–949
13. Luketich JD, Alvelo-Rivera M, Buenaventura PO et al (2003) Minimally invasive esophagectomy: outcomes in 222 patients. Ann Surg 238:486–495
14. Jobe BA, Kim CY, Minjarez RC, O'Rourke R, Chang EY, Hunter JG (2006) Simplifying minimally invasive transhiatal esophagectomy with the inversion approach: lessons learned from the first 20 cases. Arch Surg 141: 857–866
15. Esophagus. American Joint Committee on Cancer (1997) AJCC cancer staging manual, 5th edn. Lippincott-Raven Publishers, Philadelphia, pp 65–69
16. Ellis FH, Heatley GJ, Krosna MJ, Williamson WA, Balogh K (1997) Esophagogastrectomy for carcinoma of the esophagus and cardia: a comparison of findings and results after standard resection in three consecutive 8 year time intervals, using improved staging criteria. J Thorac Cardiovasc Surg 113:836
17. Iizuka T, Isono K, Kakegawa T, Watanabe H (1989) Parameters linked to ten-year survival in Japan of resected esophageal carcinoma. Japanese committee for registration of esophageal carcinoma cases. Chest 96:c1005–c1011
18. Korst RJ, Rusch VW, Venkatraman E et al (1998) Proposed revision of the staging classification for esophageal cancer. J Thorac Cardiovasc Surg 115:660–670
19. Puli RS, Reddy JBK, Bechtold ML, Antillon D, Ibdah JA, Antillon MR (2008) Staging accuracy of esophageal cancer by endoscopic ultrasound: a meta-analysis and systematic review. World J Gastroenterol 14:1479–1490
20. Takashima S, Takeuchi N, Shiozaki H et al (1991) Carcinoma of the esophagus: CT vs. MR imaging in determining resectability. Am J Roentgenol 156:297–302
21. Quint LE, Glazer GM, Orringer MB (1985) Esophageal imaging by MR and CT: study of normal anatomy and neoplasms. Radiology 156:727–731
22. Lehr L, Rupp N, Siewert JR (1988) Assessment of resectability of esophageal cancer by computed tomography and magnetic resonance imaging. Surgery 103:344–350
23. Luketich J, Schauer P, Meltzer C et al (1997) Role of positron emission tomography in staging the patient with esophageal cancer. Ann Thorac Surg 64:765–769
24. Luketich J, Freidman D, Weigel T et al (1999) Evaluation of distant metastases in esophageal cancer: 100 consecutive PET scans. Ann Thorac Surg 68:1133–1137
25. Suntharalingam M, Mougham J, Coia LR et al (1999) The national practice for patients receiving radiation therapy for carcinoma of the esophagus: results of the 1996–1999 patterns of care study. Cancer 85:2499–2505
26. Kelsen DP, Ginsberg R, Pajak TF et al (1998) Chemotherapy followed by surgery compared with surgery alone for localized esophageal cancer. N Engl J Med 339:1974–1984
27. Medical Research Council Oesophageal Cancer Working Group (2002) Surgical resection with or without preoperative chemotherapy in oesophageal cancer: a randomised controlled trial. Lancet 359:1727–1733
28. Ancona E, Ruol A, Santi S et al (2001) Only pathologic complete response to neoadjuvant chemotherapy improves significantly the long term survival of patients respectable esophageal squamous cell carcinoma: final report of a randomised trial of preoperative chemotherapy versus surgery alone. Cancer 91:2165–2174
29. Geh JI, Crellin AM, Glynne-Jones R (2001) Preoperative (neoadjuvant) chemoradiotherapy in oesophageal cancer. Br J Surg 88:338–356
30. Reynolds JV, Muldoon C, Hollywood D et al (2007) Long-term outcomes following neoadjuvant chemoradiotherapy for esophageal cancer. Ann Surg 245:707–716
31. Kodama M, Kakegawa T (1998) Treatment of superficial cancer of the esophagus: a summary of responses to a questionnaire on superficial cancer of the esophagus in Japan. Surgery 123:432–439
32. Soetikno R, Kaltenbach T, Yeh R, Gotoda T (2005) Endoscopic mucosal resection for early cancers of the upper gastrointestinal tract. J Clin Oncol 23:4490–4498
33. Ell C, May A, Pech O, Gossner L et al (2007) Curative endoscopic resection of early esophageal adenocarcinomas (Barrett's cancer). Gastrointest Endosc 65:3–10
34. Katada C, Muto M, Manabe T, Ohtsu A, Yoshida S (2005) Local recurrence of squamous-cell carcinoma of the esophagus after EMR. Gastrointest Endosc 61:219–225
35. Conio M, Repici A, Cestari R et al (2005) Endoscopic mucosal resection for high-grade dysplasia and intramucosal carcinoma in Barrett's esophagus: an Italian experience. World J Gastroenterol 11:6650–6655
36. Birkmeyer JD, Siewers AE, Finlayson EV et al (2002) Hospital volume and surgical mortality in the United States. N Engl J Med 346:1128–1137
37. Kelsen DP, Ginsberg R, Pajak TF et al (1998) Chemotherapy followed by surgery compared with surgery alone for localized esophageal cancer. N Engl J Med 339:1979–1984
38. Cuschieri A, Shimi S, Banting S (1992) Endoscopic oesophagectomy through a right thoracoscopic approach. J R Coll Surg Edinb 37:7–11

39. DePaula AL, Hashiba K, Ferreira EA, de Paula RA, Grecco E (1995) Laparoscopic transhiatal esophagectomy with esophagogastroplasty. Surg Laparosc Endosc Percut Tech 5:1–5
40. Law S, Fok M, Chu KM, Wong J (1997) Thoracoscopic esophagectomy for esophageal cancer. Surgery 122:8–14
41. Nguyen NT, Follette DM, Wolfe BM, Schneider PD, Roberts P, Goodnight JE Jr. (2000) Comparison of minimally invasive esophagectomy with transthoracic and transhiatal esophagectomy. Arch Surg 135:920–925
42. Nguyen NT, Roberts P, Follette DM, Rivers R, Wolfe BM (2003) Thoracoscopic and laparoscopic esophagectomy for benign and malignant disease: lessons learned from 46 consecutive procedures. J Am Coll Surg 197:902–913
43. Luketich JD, Alvelo-Rivera M, Buenaventura PO et al (2003) Minimally invasive esophagectomy: outcomes in 222 patients. Ann Surg 238:486–495
44. Avital S, Zundel N, Szomstein S, Rosenthal R (2005) Laparoscopic transhiatal esophagectomy for esophageal cancer. Am J Surg 190:69–74
45. Luketich JD, Nguyen NT, Schauer PR (1998) Laparoscopic transhiatal esophagectomy for Barrett's esophagus with high-grade dysplasia. JSLS 2:75–77
46. Sadanaga N, Kuwano H, Watanabe M et al (1994) Laparoscopy-assisted surgery: a new technique for transhiatal esophageal dissection. Am J Surg 168:355–357
47. Swanstrom LL, Hanson P (1997) Laparoscopic total esophagectomy. Arch Surg 132:943–949
48. Akiyama H, Tsurumaru M, Ono Y, Udagawa H, Kajiyama Y (1994) Esophagectomy without thoracotomy with vagal preservation. J Am Coll Surg 178:83–85
49. Jobe BA, Kim CY, Minjarez RC, O'Rourke R, Chang EY, Hunter JG (2006) Simplifying minimally invasive transhiatal esophagectomy with the inversion approach: lessons learned from the first 20 cases. Arch Surg 141:857–866
50. Perry KA, Enestvedt CK, Teicher N, Hunter JG (2008) Short term outcomes of minimally invasive esophagectomy: laparoscopic inversion esophagectomy versus combined laparoscopic-thoracoscopic approach (abstract). European Association of Endoscopic Surgeons, Stockholm
51. Omloo JM, Lagarde SM, Hulscher JB et al (2007) Extended transthoracic resection compared with limited transhiatal resection for adenocarcinoma of the mid/distal esophagus. Ann Surg 246:992–1001
52. Heit HA, Johnson LF, Siegel SR, Boyce HW Jr. (1978) Palliative dilation for dysphagia in esophageal carcinoma. Ann Intern Med 89:629–631
53. Hernandez LV, Jacobson JW, Harris MS (2000) Comparison among the perforation rates of Maloney, balloon, and Savary dilation of esophageal strictures. Gastrointest Endosc 51:460–462
54. Ellul JP, Watkinson A, Khan RJ, Adam A, Mason RC (1995) Self-expanding metal stents for the palliation of dysphagia due to inoperable oesophageal carcinoma. Br J Surg 82:1678–1681
55. Cowling MG, Hale H, Grundy A (1998) Management of malignant oesophageal obstruction with self-expanding metallic stents. Br J Surg 85:264–266
56. Ell C, May A (1997) Self-expanding metal stents for palliation of stenosing tumors of the esophagus and cardia: a critical review. Endoscopy 29:392–398
57. Morgan RA, Ellul JP, Denton ER, Glynos M, Mason RC, Adam A (1997) Malignant esophageal fistulas and perforations: management with plastic-covered metallic endoprostheses. Radiology 204:527–532
58. Mayoral W, Fleischer D, Salcedo J et al (2000) Nonmalignant obstruction is a common problem with metal stents in the treatment of esophageal cancer. Gastrointest Endosc 51:556–559
59. Buset M, Dunham F, Baize M, de Toeuf J, Cremer M (1983) Nd-YAG laser, a new palliative alternative in the management of esophageal cancer. Endoscopy 15:353–356
60. Alexander GL, Wang KK, Ahlquist DA et al (1994) Does performance status influence the outcome of Nd:YAG laser therapy of proximal esophageal tumors? Gastrointest Endosc 40:451–454
61. Bisgaard T, Wojdemann M, Heindorff H, Svendsen LB (1997) Nonsurgical treatment of esophageal perforations after endoscopic palliation in advanced esophageal cancer. Endoscopy 29:155–159
62. Mellow MH, Pinkas H (1984) Endoscopic therapy for esophageal carcinoma with Nd:YAG laser: prospective evaluation of efficacy, complications, and survival. Gastrointest Endosc 30:334–339
63. Marcon NE (1994) Photodynamic therapy and cancer of the esophagus. Semin Oncol 21:20–23
64. Lightdale CJ, Heier SK, Marcon NE et al (1995) Photodynamic therapy with porfimer sodium versus thermal ablation therapy with Nd:YAG laser for palliation of esophageal cancer: a multicenter randomized trial. Gastrointest Endosc 42:507–512
65. Ilson DH, Saltz L, Enzinger P et al (1999) Phase II trial of weekly irinotecan plus cisplatin in advanced esophageal cancer. J Clin Oncol 17:3270–3275
66. Ilson DH, Forastiere A, Arquette M et al (2000) A phase II trial of paclitaxel and cisplatin in patients with advanced carcinoma of the esophagus. Cancer J 6:316–323
67. Spiridonidis CH, Laufman LR, Jones J et al (1998) Phase I study of docetaxel dose escalation in combination with fixed weekly gemcitabine in patients with advanced malignancies. J Clin Oncol 16:3866–3873
68. Tebbutt NC, Norman A, Cunningham D et al (2002) A multicentre, randomised phase III trial comparing protracted venous infusion (PVI) 5-fluorouracil (5-FU) with PVI 5-FU plus mitomycin C in patients with inoperable oesophago-gastric cancer. Ann Oncol 13:1568–1575
69. O'Rourke IC, Tiver K, Bull C, Gebski V, Langlands AO (1988) Swallowing performance after radiation therapy for carcinoma of the esophagus. Cancer 61:2022–2026
70. Sur RK, Donde B, Levin VC, Mannell A (1998) Fractionated high dose rate intraluminal brachytherapy in palliation of advanced esophageal cancer. Int J Radiat Oncol Biol Phys 40:447–453
71. Hunter JG (2010) Atlas of minimally invasive surgical operations. Philadelphia, PA: McGraw-Hill

Laparoscopic Resection of Gastrointestinal Stromal Tumors

Ajita S. Prabhu, B. Todd Heniford

Contents

Gastrointestinal stromal tumors (GISTs) represent a rare but distinct histopathologic group of intestinal neoplasms of mesenchymal origin [1]. Historically, most of these tumors were classified as leiomyomas, leiomyoblastomas, and leiomyosarcomas due to the mistaken belief that they were of smooth muscle origin [1–3]; however, with the advent of electron microscopy and immunohistochemistry, a pleuropotential intestinal pacemaker cell, the interstitial cell of Cajal, was identified as the origin of GISTs [4]. These cells have myogenic and neurogenic architecture and are found within the myenteric plexus, submucosa, and muscularis propria of the gastrointestinal (GI) tract [4, 5]. The recent discovery and identification of the CD117 antigen, a c-kit proto-oncogene product, and CD34, a human progenitor cell antigen, in the majority of GIST have led to further delineation of the cellular characteristics of these neoplasms [6–8].

Although GISTs tumors are found throughout the gastrointestinal tract, the stomach is the site of occurrence in more than half of patients [2, 3, 9–11]. The most common symptoms of gastric GISTs are bleeding and abdominal pain; however, most patients are asymptomatic and the lesions are discovered incidentally during upper endoscopy performed for other reasons [12]. The potential for spread is difficult to predict due to the lack of clear clinical or pathologic signs of malignancy other than obvious metastasis at surgery. In addition, local recurrence or distant metastasis may not present until years after the initial diagnosis [9]. Surgical resection is required for cure of gastric GISTs. In the past, a 1–2 cm margin was believed to be necessary for an adequate resection [12, 13]; however, DeMatteo et al. demonstrated that tumor size and not negative microscopic surgical margins determine survival [2]. These findings support the local resection of GIST lesions, including both wedge and submucosal resections.

F.L. Greene, B.T. Heniford (eds.), *Minimally Invasive Cancer Management*,
DOI 10.1007/978-1-4419-1238-1_9,

Although the feasibility of minimally invasive resections of gastric GISTs has been established [11, 12, 14–18], this approach had previously been advocated to be limited to lesions <2 cm [10, 19]. We have since demonstrated that gastric GISTs $\geq$ 8 cm can be laparoscopically resected safely and with excellent long-term disease-free survival [20]. We offer the majority of our patients a minimally invasive approach for the resection of GISTs. Potential advantages to a laparoscopic resection include decreased analgesic requirements, improved cosmesis, and an earlier return to normal activity and self-reliance.

The operative approach depends on tumor location. All of the laparoscopic techniques are analogous to an open approach, although laparoscopic transgastric resection and endoscopically assisted endoluminal surgery are unique to minimally invasive surgery. Prior to the resection, a formal abdominal exploration is performed to rule out peritoneal seeding or hepatic metastasis. The diaphragm, peritoneum, and surface of the liver are examined. Following an abdominal exploration and regardless of the technique employed, open or minimally invasive, intraoperative ultrasound is performed. Intraoperative ultrasound provides distinctive anatomic detail of the liver for evaluation of metastatic deposits and provides real-time guidance for intraoperative biopsies of suspicious lesions [21]. During a laparoscopic approach, intraoperative ultrasound often provides anatomic details regarding the tumor's location as well as adjacent structures.

Preoperative Preparation

Patient selection including the diagnosis, location of the tumor, previous surgical history, and patient comorbidities can play a key role in a surgeon's successful implementation of a minimally invasive procedure. The patient's overall medical condition should be assessed and cardiopulmonary comorbidities are evaluated preoperatively as conducted for any major operation. In general, patients to undergo laparoscopy should be able to tolerate general anesthesia and a laparotomy. Key points in a patient's history should include the type and extent of previous abdominal operations, confirmation of the patient's diagnosis (if possible), and a review/discussion of the diagnostic studies completed to date. A lengthy dialogue concerning the operation proposed, the options, the risks, and the possible outcomes should be included in the preoperative encounter.

In the more immediate period prior to surgery, the patient should have no food or liquid by mouth for at least 8 h. If gastric dysmotility is diagnosed preoperatively, one should consider maintaining a clear liquid diet for a full day preceding the operation in an effort to reduce the chance of having retained solid material within the stomach. An H_2 receptor blocker or proton pump inhibitor is often given preceding surgery. As well, a broad-spectrum antibiotic is administered prior to the initial incision. Sequential compression devices are applied to the lower extremities to reduce the risk of deep venous thrombosis. After general anesthesia is established, a bladder catheter is placed and an orogastric tube is inserted. After the stomach has been aspirated, the orogastric tube is removed and the absence of other tubes, in the esophagus is confirmed with the anesthetist.

The setup in the operating room is the same for most upper gastrointestinal surgeries. The patient is in a supine position with arms abducted on arm boards. We use a split leg table in nearly all circumstances. This allows the surgeon to stand between the patients legs and directly face the stomach. This also allows for assistance to stand on the patient's left and right side very comfortably. Monitors are placed over the patient's shoulders bilaterally. The locations of the ports are demonstrated in Fig. 9.1. One assistant on the right maintains the liver retractor via the right subcostal port and holds the camera. The assistant on the left uses the most left lateral port for retraction. The assistant on the right side can be replaced by simply mounting a stationary liver retractor while the assistant on the left takes over the duties as camera operator. The surgeon primarily uses the upper midline and left mid-abdominal ports. The port in the left lateral rectus sheath is the primary operative port through which an endoscopic linear stapler is introduced. However, any port can be replaced with a 12 mm sleeve to allow a different angle in which to transect the stomach. The first port placed is usually in the midline, one-quarter to one-third of the distance between the umbilicus and the xiphoid, and is used for the camera. This port is typically not placed at the umbilicus unless the lesion in question is located in the distal one-half of the stomach. In our experience, an umbilical port tends to be somewhat low when the dissection is focused around the proximal stomach. The same can be stated for the other ports as well. When the lesion is in the distal portion of the stomach, all of the trocar positions can be moved slightly inferiorly to keep the ports from being directly over the operative site.

Figure 9.1

Trocar strategy for laparoscopic gastric wedge resections

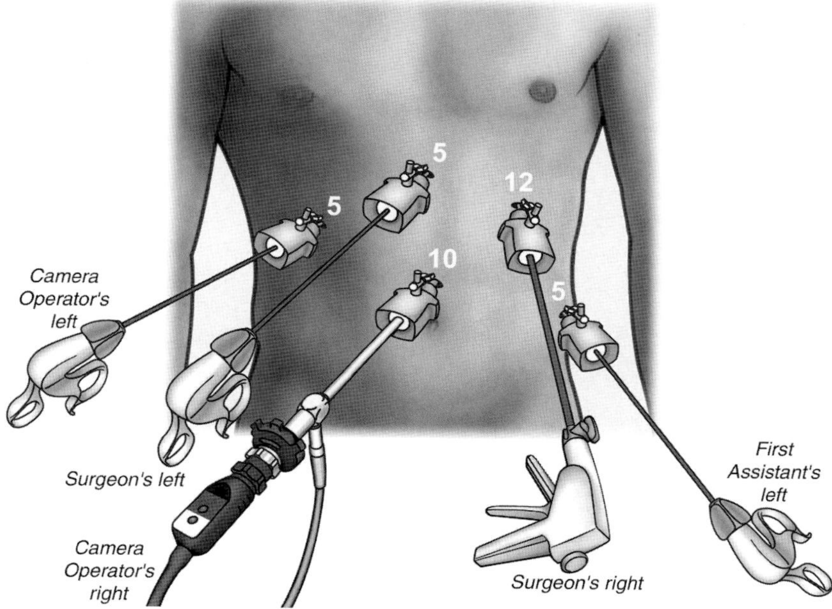

After insertion of the initial ports, the patient is placed in a steep Trendelenburg's position. The initial oral gastric tube and esophageal stethoscope are removed as soon as the stomach is noted to be decompressed. Stapling across a nasogastric tube is an embarrassing and troublesome event that most surgeons would like to avoid and forget. Intraoperative endoscopy has become an integral part of most of our laparoscopic gastric resections. It is used to identify the exact location of small lesions, evaluate/plan the extent of resection margins, and examine/test the reconstruction or gastric closure. The possibility of troublesome over insufflation of the small intestine with the loss of intraabdominal working space is uncommon. An experienced endoscopist and the judicious use of air insufflation are important. Occlusion of the duodenum with an atraumatic grasper can also reduce this problem. In all cases our specimens are placed in a retrieval bag. We believe this technique may help prevent tumor spread within the abdomen and/or trocar sites and may decrease bacterial contamination of the abdomen and port site.

Prior to the resection, a formal abdominal exploration is performed to rule out peritoneal spread or hepatic metastasis. The diaphragm, peritoneum, and surface of the liver are examined. Following a visual abdominal exploration, intraoperative ultrasound is performed for tumors with malignant potential. Intraoperative ultrasound provides distinctive anatomic detail of the liver for evaluation of metastatic deposits and provides real-time guidance for intraoperative biopsies of suspicious lesions. During a laparoscopic approach, intraoperative ultrasound can provide anatomic details regarding the primary tumor's location as well as adjacent vital (vascular) structures.

Local Excision Techniques by Location

Anterior Gastric Wall

Masses located on the anterior wall of the stomach are amenable to wedge resection utilizing a linear endoscopic gastrointestinal anastomosis (GIA) stapler. The locations of the ports are demonstrated in Fig. 9.2 [22]. If the tumor is extraluminal, it is usually visualized on initial inspection with the laparoscope. Those lesions that are intraluminal are often identified by a characteristic dimpling of the gastric serosal surface or by bimanual palpation of the stomach with laparoscopic instruments. As mentioned previously, intraluminal visualization by a flexible endoscope assists with tumor localization and may guide resection to ensure adequate margins and to safeguard against comprising the gastric inlet or outlet. After identifying the lesion, the short gastric vessels are ligated and divided as needed. Typically, this maneuver is performed with the assistant on the left retracting the omentum and gastrosplenic

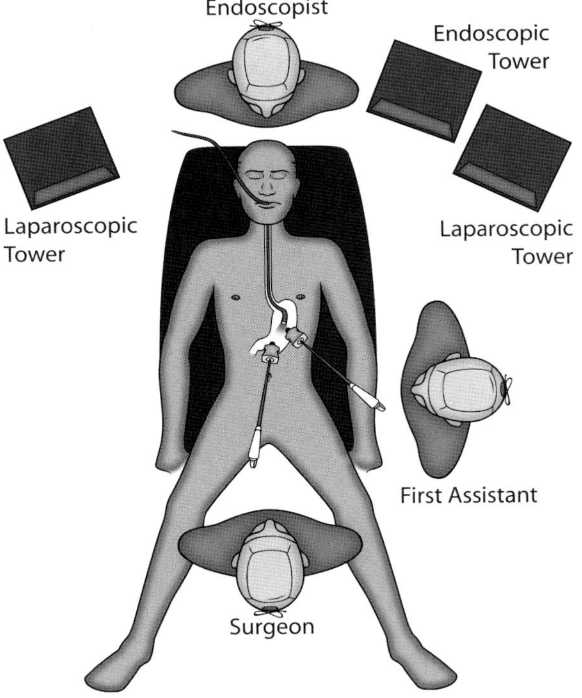

Figure 9.2

Trocar placement for laparoscopic resection of an anterior gastric wall gastrointestinal stromal tumor

ligament laterally, while the surgeon retracts the stomach medially and transects the vessels with ultrasonic coagulating shears.

Following this initial step, one must decide between one of two techniques to perform the gastric wedge resection. The simplest technique is to elevate the anterior gastric wall near the tumor with atraumatic bowel grasper and simultaneously sliding an endoscopic GIA stapler under the tumor. An adequate margin of uninvolved, normal stomach is included with the tumor as the gastric wall is divided with the stapler. An alternative method to elevating the anterior gastric wall with bowel graspers is to place two seromuscular sutures on each side of the lesion approximately 1–2 cm beyond the lesion to ensure that the stitches do not penetrate or perforate the tumor. The sutures are elevated simultaneously and the stapler is placed just under the sutures to resect the tumor and a small margin of normal stomach.

Another technique is to circumferentially excise the gastric tumor and a surrounding margin of normal tissue using ultrasonic coagulating shears. This technique is simplified by insufflating the stomach with a flexible endoscope, allowing the site where the stomach is to be opened to be determined by observing the tumor both endoscopically and via the laparoscope. Typically, the incision into the stomach is made 2 cm from the lesion to make certain that the tumor is not lacerated. This technique allows for a more precise excision of normal tissue at the margins of the tumor compared to the technique utilizing an endoscopic GIA stapler. The gastrotomy can be closed by laparoscopic intracorporeal suturing or by placing 2–4 full-thickness traction sutures along the cut edge of the gastrotomy and using an endoscopic linear stapler to re-approximate ("close") the gastrotomy.

Posterior Gastric Wall

There are two techniques to approach posterior gastric wall masses. One method entails creating an anterior gastrotomy over the lesion after it is endoscopically localized. As described previously, the location of the gastrotomy is determined by visual cues from the gastroscope and laparoscope while simultaneously palpating the gastric wall with laparoscopic graspers. Through the anterior gastrostomy, normal gastric tissue adjacent to the tumor is grasped with laparoscopic bowel grasper or, alternatively, traction sutures can be placed on each side of the tumor much as described for anterior gastric tumors. The tumor and a surrounding margin of normal stomach are elevated through the gastrotomy and resected by an endoscopic linear stapler. The staple line is examined for bleeding and any bleeding points are oversewn. The anterior gastrotomy is closed as previously described.

An innovative technique for posterior gastric wall masses less than 3–4 cm in greatest diameter is percutaneous intragastric resection. Laparoscopic intragastric or "endoluminal" surgery involves the placement of balloon- or mushroom-tipped laparoscopic trocars (2–10 mm) percutaneously into the stomach (insufflated by a flexible endoscope) similar to the placement of a percutaneous endoscopic gastrostomy tube. The pylorus may be occluded with a balloon-tipped nasogastric tube but infrequently needed. An angled laparoscope, positioned through one of the percutaneous gastric trocars, is preferred for visualization of the operative field, but a flexible endoscope can be used in combination with two working trocars. A dilute epinephrine solution (1:100,000) is injected

Recently, we tried LADG for the treatment of AGCs without massive lymph node metastasis (n2) judged by prediagnostic examination using ultrasound and computed tomography (CT) and AGCs without serosal exposure (T2) diagnosed by laparoscopic examination before LADG.

Techniques of LADG with D1+β Lymph Node Dissection

Patient Positioning and Port Placement

After general anesthesia, the patient is placed supine in 10° reverse Trendelenburg position with the patient's legs abducted on the operating table (Fig. 10.2). The operator stands to the patient's right or left side according to the operative area, and the camera assistant stands between the patient's abducted legs.

After the Hasson trocar is placed in the subumbilical portion in an open manner, a CO_2 pneumoperitoneum at 10 mmHg is created. Under laparoscopic observation, four trocars are placed as follows. Two 10 mm trocars are placed above the umbilicus, one to the right and the other to the left of it, as shown in Fig. 10.3. Two 5 mm trocars are then inserted, into the left and right upper quadrants.

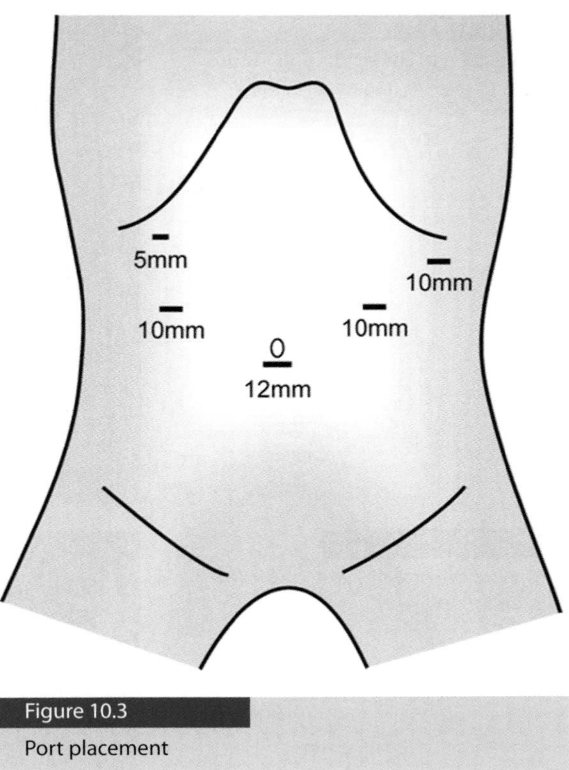

Figure 10.3
Port placement

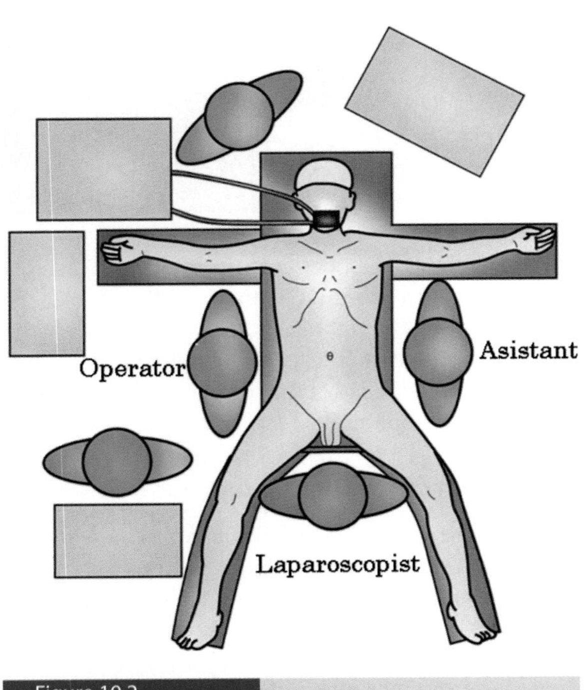

Figure 10.2
Patient positioning for LADG

Dissection of the Greater Omentum (No. 4d Ln Dissection) and the Left Gastroepiploic Vessels (No. 4sb Ln Dissection)

Using laparoscopic techniques, the greater omentum and gastrocolic ligament are opened with laparoscopic ultrasonic coagulation shears (LCS) from the area near the inferior pole of the spleen to the infrapyloric area (No.4d LN dissection) (Fig. 10.4). Near the inferior pole of the spleen, the left gastroepiploic vessels are gently divided by clipping and ultrasonic coagulation (No. 4sb LN dissection).

Dissection of the Right Gastroepiploic Vessels (No. 6 LN Dissection)

To dissect the right gastroepiploic vein, the surface of the pancreas head is exposed. For that purpose, in the infrapyloric area, the greater omentum and gastrocolic ligament are dissected layer by layer. After the right gastroepiploic vein is identified, it is clipped

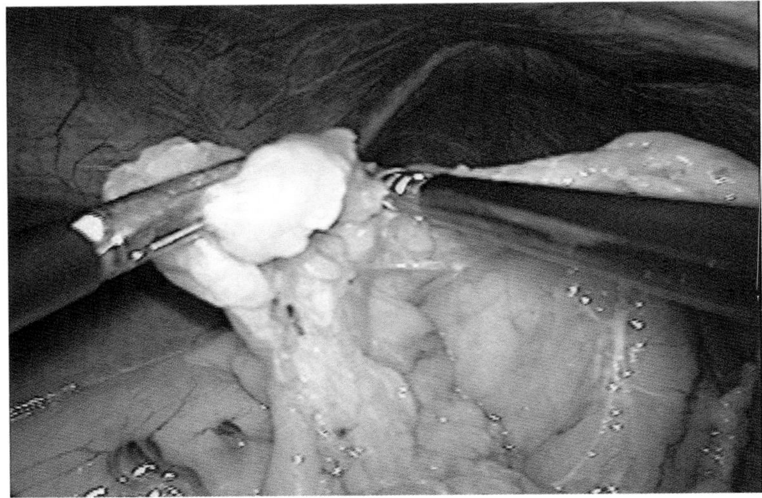

Figure 10.4
Dissection of the greater omentum

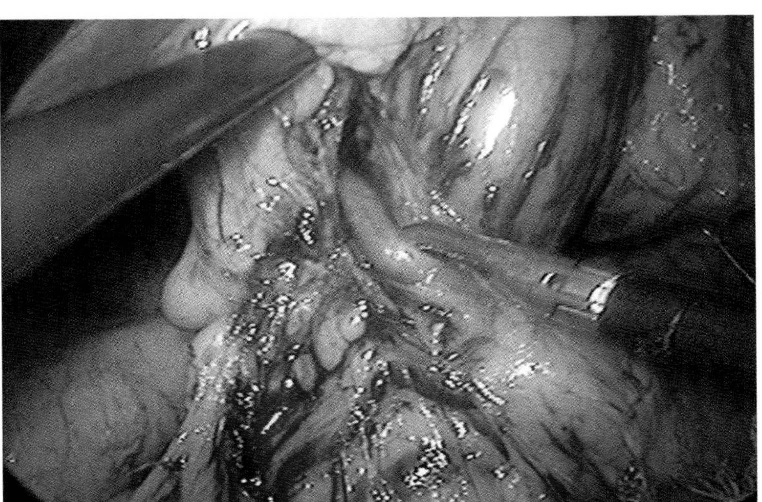

Figure 10.5
Dissection of the right gastroepiploic vessel

and divided to dissect the infrapyloric lymph nodes (No. 6) (Fig. 10.5). Next, when the gastroduodenal artery is recognized on the anterior surface of the pancreas, the root of the right gastroepiploic artery can be easily exposed. This artery is divided by clipping and ultrasonic coagulation.

Dissection of the Lesser Omentum (No. 3 LN Dissection) and Division of the Right Gastric Vessels (No. 5 LN Dissection)

After the liver is lifted with a retractor, the lesser omentum is dissected from the left side of the hepatoduodenal ligament to the right side of the esophagocardial junction (No. 3 LN dissection). When the assistant lifts the right gastric vessels, the nonvascular area above the bulbus of the duodenum can be seen. This area is opened and the connective tissue is dissected at the right side along the right gastric vessels to identify the root of the right gastric artery. The right gastric vessels are clipped and divided at the root for dissection of the suprapyloric lymph nodes (No. 5 LN dissection).

Transection of the Duodenum

Recently, the frequency of reconstruction with the Roux-en-Y method has gradually increased in Japan to prevent reflux gastritis and esophagitis. When using Roux-en-Y reconstruction, the duodenum is transected before dissection of the left gastric vessels. After the assistant lifts the antrum of the stomach, the duodenum is transected at the bulbus with a linear stapler (Fig. 10.6).

Figure 10.6
Transection of the duodenum

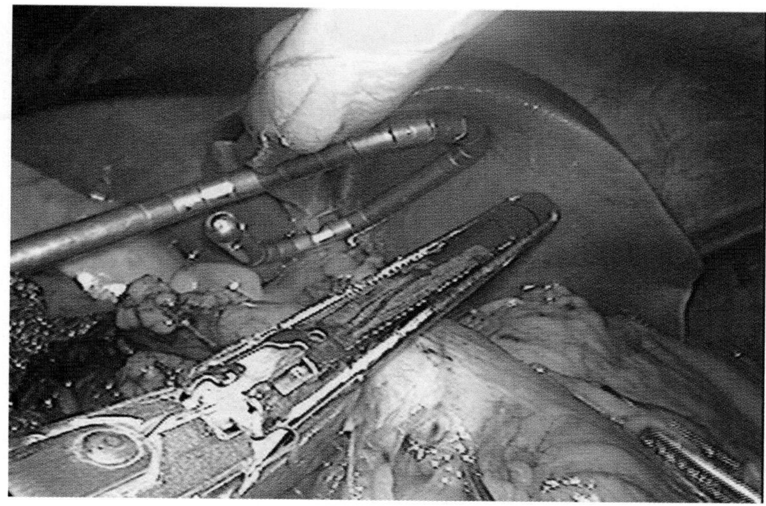

Dissection of Lymph Nodes Along the Common Hepatic Artery and Celiac Artery (Nos. 8, 9 LN Dissections)

The peritoneum is incised along the upper margin of the pancreas from the distal side of the common hepatic artery to the root of the celiac artery. The operator lifts the connective tissue containing lymph nodes (Nos. 8a, 9) and dissects the lymph nodes from the common hepatic artery and proximal splenic artery with LCS (Fig. 10.7).

Division of the Left Gastric Vessels (No. 7 LN Dissection)

During dissection of lymph nodes along the common hepatic artery, the left gastric vein is found. This vein is clipped and divided. The peritoneum is incised along the upper margin of the right crus and the root of the left gastric artery can then be recognized. After the connective tissue at the left side of the left artery is dissected, the left gastric artery is clipped and dissected, as shown in Fig. 10.8.

Dissection of the Left Cardiac and Superior Gastric Lymph Nodes (Nos. 1, 3 LN Dissection)

From both the anterior and the posterior sides of the stomach, the left cardiac and superior gastric lymph nodes are dissected by using LCS.

Mini-Laparotomy and Roux-en-Y Reconstruction

A 5 cm mini-laparotomy is made at the upper midline of the abdomen, and a wound protector is

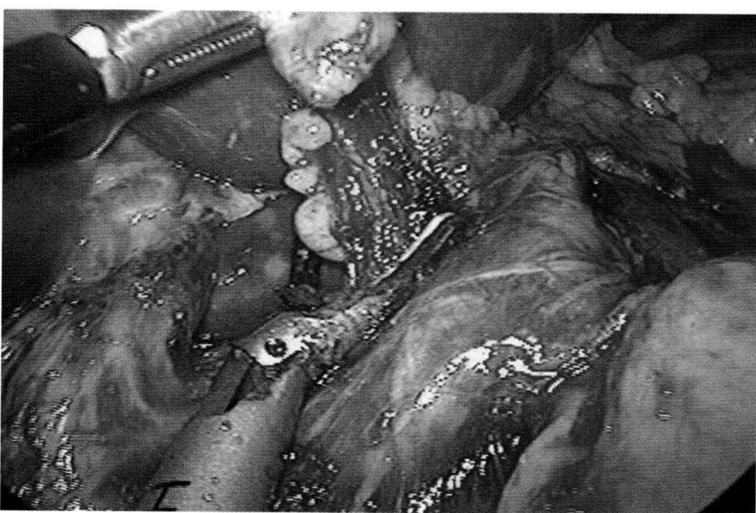

Figure 10.7
Dissection of LNs along the common hepatic artery

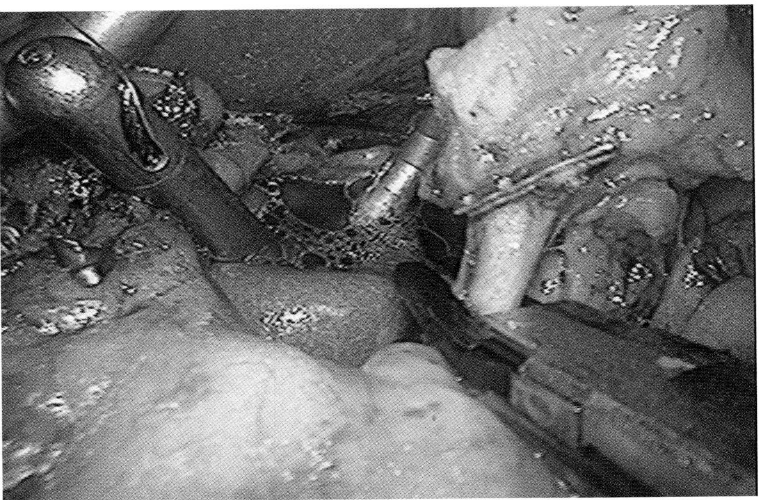

Figure 10.8
Division of the left gastric vessels

attached. Through this mini-laparotomy, the distal stomach is exteriorized and distal gastrectomy is performed. Under re-pneumoperitoneum, the jejunum at 20 cm from the ligament of Treitz is recognized, and this jejunum is pulled out through the mini-laparotomy. After the jejunum is transected with a linear cutter, jejuno-jejunostomy (Y-anastomosis) and gastro-jejunostomy are performed as a functional end-to-end anastomosis in the manner of open surgery (Fig. 10.9).

Irrigation and Drainage

After irrigation of the abdominal cavity, a closed-suction drain is placed near the stump of the duodenum and the operative wounds are closed.

Evaluations of LADG for Early Gastric Cancer (EGC)

To our knowledge, there are two meta-analyses of short-term outcomes after laparoscopic and open distal gastrectomy (ODG) for cancer: those of Hosono et al. and Memon et al. [16, 17]. In their meta-analysis, Hosono et al. analyzed the outcomes of 1,611 procedures (837 LADGs and 774 ODGs) from 4 randomized controlled trials (RCTs) and 12 retrospective studies were analyzed [18–33]. On the other hand, Memon et al. evaluated the outcomes of 162 operations (82 LADGs and 80 ODGs) from 4 RCTs [18–21]. In this chapter, technical safety, oncologic feasibility, and the advantages of LADG for EGC are evaluated based on the data from these meta-analyses.

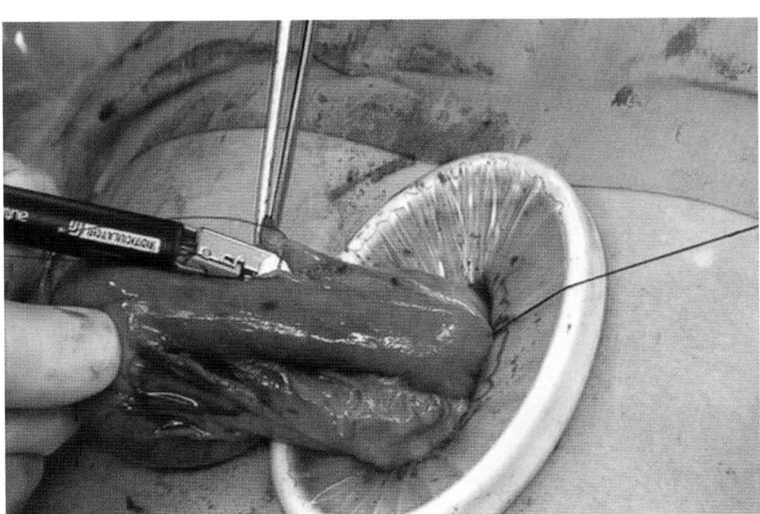

Figure 10.9
Reconstruction by Roux-en-Y method (gastro-jejunostomy)

Table 10.3. Operative findings of LADG with extended lymph node dissection (D2)

Study	Cases		Lymph node dissection	Operation time (min)		Blood loss		Number of disease node		Conversion to open (%)	Morbidity		Mortality of LADG
	LADG	ODG		LADG	ODG	LADG	ODG	LADG	ODG		LADG	ODG	
Case-controlled study													
Tanimura et al. [44]	235	200	D2	236>	184	134<	466[a]	31	30	–	–	–	0
Noshiro et al. [45]	37	31	D2	320>	277[a]	163	488	43	41	0	5.4	12.9	0
Ziqiang et al. [46]	44	58	D1, D2	282>	227	139<	331	30	33	2.3	13.6	20.7	0
Song et al. [47]	44	31	D2	264>	184[a]	158<	392[a]	37	42	0	11.3	19.1	0
Randomized controlled study													
Husher et al. [21]	30	29	D1, D2	196	168	229	391	–	–	0	23.3	27.6	3.3

LADG: laparoscopy-assisted distal gastrectomy, ODG: open distal gastrectomy.
[a]Significant difference.

Table 10.4. Postoperative course after LADG with extended lymph node dissection (D2)

Study	Cases		Time to first flatus (POD)		Time to diet (POD)		Time to first walking (POD)		Length of stay (days)		Other advantages
	LADG	ODG	LADG	ODG	LADG	ODG	LADG	ODG	LADG	ODG	
Case-controlled study											
Tanimura et al. [44]	235	200	2.6<	3.6[a]	3.3<	6.0	–	–	–	–	–
Noshiro et al. [45]	37	31	2.8<	3.4[a]	3.2<	4.2[a]	1.1	1.2	–	–	–
Ziqiang et al. [46]	44	58	4.1<	5.3[a]	–	–	3.2<	5.2[a]	–	–	Less pain
Song et al. [47]	44	31	3.3<	4.4[a]	5.8	6.4[a]	–	–	7.7<	9.4	Less pain

LADG: laparoscopy-assisted distal gastrectomy, ODG: open distal gastrectomy.
[a]Significant difference.

References

1. Kitano S, Iso Y, Moriyama M et al (1994) Laparoscopy-assisted Billroth I gastrectomy. Surg Laparosc Endosc 4: 146–148
2. Japan Society for Endoscopic Surgery (2008) Nationwide survey on endoscopic surgery in Japan. J Jpn Soc Endosc Surg 13(5):499–604
3. Swanstrom LL, Pennings JL (1995) Laparoscopic control of short gastric vessels. J Am Coll Surg 181:347–351
4. Japanese Gastric Cancer Association (2001) The guidelines for the treatment of gastric cancer. Kanahara Co, Tokyo
5. Kitano S, Shiraishi N, Uyama I et al (2006) A multicenter study on oncologic outcome of laparoscopic gastrectomy for early cancer in Japan. Ann Surg 245:68–72
6. Yasuda K, Inomata M, Shiraishi N et al (2004) Laparoscopy-assisted distal gastrectomy for early gastric cancer in obese and nonobese patients. Surg Endosc 18:1253–1256
7. Noshiro H, Shimizu S, Nagai E et al (2003) Laparoscopy-assisted distal gastrectomy for early gastric cancer. Is it beneficial for patients of heavier weight? Ann Surg 238: 680–685
8. Yasuda K, Sonoda H, Shiroshita H et al (2004) Laparoscopically assisted distal gastrectomy for early gastric cancer in the elderly. Br J Surg 91:1061–1065
9. Uyama I, Sugioka A, Fujita J et al (1999) Laparoscopic total gastrectomy with distal pancreatosplenectomy and D2 lymphadenectomy for advanced gastric cancer. Gastric Cancer 2:230–234
10. Kitano S, Adachi Y, Shiraishi N et al (1999) Laparoscopic-assisted proximal gastrectomy for early gastric carcinomas. Surg Today 29(4):389–391
11. Uyama I, Sugioka A, Matsui H et al (2001) Laparoscopic side-to-side esophagogastrostomy using a linear stapler after proximal gastrectomy. Gastric Cancer 4(2):98–102
12. Ikeda Y, Sasaki Y, Niimi M et al (2002) Hand-assisted laparoscopic proximal gastrectomy with jejunal interposition and lymphadenectomy. J Am Coll Surg 4:578–581
13. Mochiki E, Kamimura H, Haga N et al (2002) The technique of laparoscopically assisted total gastrectomy with jejunal interposition for early gastric cancer. Surg Endosc 16:540–544
14. Takaori K, Nonura E, Mabuchi H et al (2005) A secure technique of intracorporeal Roux-Y reconstruction after laparoscopic distal gastrectomy. Am J Surg 189: 178–183
15. Dulucq JL, Wintringer P, Perissat J et al (2005) Completely laparoscopic total and partial gastrectomy for benign and malignant disease: a single institute's prospective analysis. J Am Coll Surg 200:191–197
16. Hosono H, Arimoto Y, Ohtani H et al (2006) Meta-analysis of short-term outcomes after laparoscopy-assisted distal gastrectomy. World J Gastroenterol 12: 7676–7683
17. Melon MA, Khan S, Yunus RM et al (2008) Meta-analysis of laparoscopic and open distal gastrectomy for gastric carcinoma. Surg Endosc 22:1781–1789
18. Kitano S, Shiraishi N, Fujii K et al (2002) A randomized controlled trial comparing open vs laparoscopy-assisted distal gastrectomy for the treatment of early gastric cancer: an interim report. Surgery 131:S306–S311
19. Lee JH, Han HS, Lee JH et al (2005) A prospective randomized study comparing open vs laparoscopy-assisted distal gastrectomy in early gastric cancer: early results. Surg Endosc 19:168–173
20. Hayashi H, Ochiai T, Shimada H et al (2005) Prospective randomized study of open versus laparoscopy-assisted distal gastrectomy with extraperigastric lymph node dissection for early gastric cancer. Surg Endosc 19:1172–1176
21. Husher CGS, Mingoli A, Sgarzini G et al (2005) Laparoscopic versus open subtotal gastrectomy for distal gastric cancer. Five-year results of a randomized prospective trial. Ann Surg 241:232–237
22. Adachi Y, Shiraishi N, Shiromizu A et al (2000) Laparoscopy-assisted Billroth I gastrectomy compared with conventional open gastrectomy. Arch Surg 135: 806–810

23. Shimizu S, Uchiyama A, Mizumoto K et al (2000) Laparoscopically assisted distal gastrectomy for early gastric cancer: is it superior to open surgery? Surg Endosc 14:27–31
24. Yano H, Monden T, Kinuta M et al (2001) The usefulness of laparoscopy-assisted distal gastrectomy in comparison with that of open distal gastrectomy for early gastric cancer. Gastric Cancer 4:93–97
25. Migoh S, Hasuda K, Nakashima K et al (2003) The benefit of laparoscopy-assisted distal gastrectomy compared with conventional open distal gastrectomy: a case-matched control study. Hepato-Gastroenterol 50:2251–2254
26. Noshiro H, Nagai E, Shimizu A et al (2005) Laparoscopically assisted distal gastrectomy with standard radical lymph node dissection for gastric cancer. Surg Endosc 19:1592–1596
27. Tanimura S, Higashino M, Fukunaga Y et al (2005) Laparoscopic distal gastrectomy with regional lymph node dissection for gastric cancer. Surg Endosc 19:1177–1181
28. Mochiki E, Kamiyama Y, Aihara R et al (2005) Laparoscopic assisted distal gastrectomy for early gastric cancer: five years' experience. Surgery 137:317–322
29. Naka T, Ishikura T, Shibata S et al (2005) Laparoscopy-assisted and open distal gastrectomy for early gastric cancer at a general hospital in Japan. Hepato-Gastroenterol 52:293–297
30. Kim MC, Kim KH, Kim HH et al (2005) Comparison of laparoscopy-assisted by conventional open distal gastrectomy and extraperigastric lymph node dissection in early gastric cancer. J Surg Oncol 91:90–94
31. Kim YW, Bae JM, Lee KW et al (2005) The role of hand-assisted laparoscopic distal gastrectomy for distal gastric cancer. Surg Endosc 19:29–33
32. Ikenaga N, Nishihara K, Iwashita T et al (2006) Long-term quality of life after laparoscopically assisted distal gastrectomy for gastric cancer. J Laparoendosc Adv Surg Tech 16:119–123
33. Lee SI, Choi YS, Park DJ et al (2006) Comparative study of laparoscopy-assisted distal gastrectomy and open distal gastrectomy. J Am Coll Surg 202:874–880
34. Hyung WJ, Song C, Cheong JH et al (2007) Factors influencing operation time of laparoscopy-assisted distal subtotal gastrectomy: analysis of consecutive 100 initial cases. EJSO 33:314–319
35. Fujiwara M, Kodera Y, Miura S et al (2005) Laparoscopy-assisted distal gastrectomy with systemic lymph node dissection: a phase II study following the learning curve. J Surg Oncol 91:26–32
36. Kim MC, Jung GJ, Kim HH (2005) Learning curve of laparoscopy-assisted distal gastrectomy with systemic lymphadenectomy for early gastric cancer. World J Gastroenterol 11:7508–7511
37. Ryu KW, Kim YW, Lee JH et al (2008) Surgical complications and the risk factors of laparoscopy-assisted distal gastrectomy in early gastric cancer. Ann Surg Oncol 15:1625–1631
38. Bonenkamp JJ, Songun I, Hermans J et al (1995) Randomized comparison of morbidity after D1 and D2 dissection for gastric cancer in 996 Dutch patients. Lancet 345:745–748
39. Cuschieri A, Fayers P, Fielding J et al (1996) Postoperative morbidity and mortality after D1 and D2 resections for gastric cancer: preliminary results of the MRC randomized controlled surgical trial. The Surgical Cooperative Group. Lancet 347:995–999
40. Yasuda K, Shiraishi N, Etoh A et al (2007) Long-term quality of life after laparoscopy-assisted distal gastrectomy for gastric cancer. Surg Endosc 21:2150–2153
41. Kim KH, Kim MC, Jung GJ et al (2006) The impact of obesity on LADG for early gastric cancer. Gastric Cancer 9:303–307
42. Yamada H, Kojima K, Inokuchi M et al (2008) Effect of obesity on technical feasibility and postoperative outcomes of laparoscopy-assisted distal gastrectomy – Comparison with open distal gastrectomy. J Gastrointest Surg 12: 997–1004
43. Singh KK, Rohatgi A, Rybinkina I et al (2008) Laparoscopic gastrectomy for gastric cancer: early experience among the elderly. Surg Endosc 22:1002–1007
44. Tanimura S, Higashino M, Fukunaga Y et al (2005) Laparoscopic distal gastrectomy with regional lymph node dissection for gastric cancer. Surg Endosc 19: 1177–1181
45. Noshiro H, Nagai E, Shimizu A et al (2005) Laparoscopically assisted distal gastrectomy with standard radical lymph node dissection for gastric cancer. Surg Endosc 19:1592–1596
46. Ziqiang W, Feng Q, Zhimin C et al (2006) Comparison of laparoscopically assisted and open radical distal gastrectomy with extended lymphadenectomy for gastric cancer management. Surg Endosc 20:1738–1743
47. Song KY, Kim SN, Park CH (2008) Laparoscopy-assisted distal gastrectomy with D2 lymph node dissection for gastric cancer: technical and oncologic aspects. Surg Endosc 22:655–659
48. Topal B, Leys E, Ectors N et al (2008) Determinants of complications and adequacy of surgical resection in laparoscopic versus open total gastrectomy for adenocarcinoma. Surg Endosc 22:980–984
49. Pugliese R, Maggioni D, Sansonna F et al (2007) Total and subtotal laparoscopic gastrectomy for adenocarcinoma. Surg Endosc 21:21–27
50. Kim YW, Han HS, Fleischer GD (2003) Hand-assisted laparoscopic total gastrectomy. Surg Laparosc Endosc Percuta Tech 13:26–30
51. Tanaka K, Tonouchi H, Kobayashi M et al (2004) Laparoscopically assisted total gastrectomy with sentinel node biopsy for early gastric cancer: preliminary results. Am Surg 70:976–981
52. Takiguch S, Sekimoto M, Fujiwara Y et al (2005) A simple technique for performing laparoscopic purse-string suturing during circular stapling anastomosis. Surg Today 35:896–899
53. Omori T, Nakajima K, Endo T et al (2006) Laparoscopically assisted total gastrectomy with jejunal pouch interposition. Surg Endosc 20:1497–1500
54. Kitanno S, Adach Y, Shiraishi N et al (1999) Laparoscopic-assisted proximal gastrectomy for early gastric carcinoma. Surg Today 29:389–391
55. Song KY, Park CHP, Kang HC et al (2008) Is totally laparoscopic gastrectomy less invasive than laparoscopy-assisted gastrectomy? Prospective, multicenter study. J Gastrointest Surg 12:1015–1025

Part III

Management of Hepatopancreaticobiliary Cancer

Minimal Access Management of Pancreatic Cancer

Nicholas A. Hamilton, Brent D. Matthews

Contents

Pancreatic adenocarcinoma (PC) is the fourth leading cause of cancer-related death in the United States, accounting for over 33,000 deaths in 2008 [1]. The peak incidence occurs in the seventh and eighth decades [2]. Only approximately 15% of patients have resectable disease at the time of presentation [3] and nearly all patients die from the disease within 7 years of surgery [4, 5], with a median survival of only 6 months in patients with unresectable disease. Surgical resection remains the only hope for cure of this devastating disease.

Historically, laparoscopic management of PC has been limited to diagnostic staging and palliative procedures and is not universally accepted as the best surgical management for pancreatic malignancy. The retroperitoneal location of the pancreas and its relationship with major surrounding structures make operating on the pancreas technically demanding. Concerns over the need to palpate the gland to determine extent of disease, lack of a standardized methodology, concern over achieving a negative margin, and low frequency of patients requiring pancreatic resection have also contributed to a relatively slow development of laparoscopic pancreas resection. However, progress is being made in laparoscopic technologies, including laparoscopic ultrasonography, stapling devices, and parenchymal coagulators, all of which have advanced the laparoscopic treatment of the pancreas. Many surgeons have applied laparoscopic techniques initially used in benign pancreatic disease to distal pancreas tumors. Others have used minimally invasive techniques to perform ampullectomies. Some have even developed laparoscopic techniques to perform a pancreaticoduodenectomy.

F.L. Greene, B.T. Heniford (eds.), *Minimally Invasive Cancer Management*,
DOI 10.1007/978-1-4419-1238-1_11,

Laparoscopic Staging of Pancreatic Cancer

The application of diagnostic laparoscopy in patients with pancreatic cancer to detect metastatic disease has been in use since the early 1960s and, until recently, was one of the few areas in which minimally invasive surgery could be applied to the pancreas. Exploratory laparotomy alone has the potential for morbidity and mortality that carries with it significant socioeconomic implications [6, 7]. Ideally, only patients with resectable disease should undergo exploratory laparotomy for resection. Therefore, accurate preoperative staging is paramount. The aim of staging should be to determine the extent of disease, allowing for the appropriate therapy to be administered. Laparoscopy offers the benefit of sparing the patient with potentially unresectable disease a laparotomy while still allowing for a laparotomy for curative resection in those patients who are candidates.

Continued advances in radiographic technology have brought into question the routine use of laparoscopy for the staging of pancreatic malignancies. Contrast-enhanced computed tomography (CT) scan or specific "pancreatic protocol" CT scans are now the study of choice when evaluating suspected PC and have been shown to predict unresectability in 85–90% of patients. However, one of the shortcomings of CT imaging is its assessment of tumor extension into mesenteric vessels and small liver and peritoneal metastases [8, 9]. Several studies demonstrated that the use of laparoscopy is able to detect radiographically occult metastatic disease. Merchant and Conlon reviewed their patients from 1992 to 1996 and found a 9% false-negative rate in patients who did not have evidence of metastatic or locally advanced, unresectable PC on preoperative CT imaging [10].

Another diagnostic tool that has recently come into use is that of the endoscopic ultrasound. It is beneficial in that it can provide visualization of the lesion, surrounding lymph nodes and some vasculature as well as provide tissue diagnosis. However, it is very user dependent and is to be limited in its ability to predict resectability, with mixed results in comparison to CT [11, 12].

Some have criticized the yield of diagnostic laparoscopy in the face of improved radiographic imaging. White et al. recently reviewed their patients from 1995 to 2005 who had radiographically resectable disease. They found the yield of laparoscopy to be 12% in patients with PC [13]. This is comparable to the 21–24% yields found by groups at the University of Nebraska [14] and Washington University [15] and the historic 22–48% in older studies [9, 16–18]. Arguments have also been made against diagnostic laparoscopy in PC in terms of cost-effectiveness. To address this, one study found the prevalence of unresectable disease diagnosed at laparotomy or laparoscopy to be 14.1% and concluded that the mean charge per patient was not significantly different between patients undergoing laparotomy vs. laparoscopy [19]. Another group found a reduction in hospital charges by 25% in patients who underwent laparoscopic staging [20].

The selective use of laparoscopy has been suggested to improve the positive-predictive value of diagnostic laparoscopy. Shah et al. [21] proposed a staging algorithm based on tumor size, amount of weight loss, the presence of ascites, or markedly elevated serum CA 19–9 to define patients with radiographically resectable disease who received diagnostic laparoscopy. They found 53% of patients who met their staging criteria had unresectable disease on laparoscopy. One patient (5.8%) underwent a laparotomy and was found to have unresectable disease after laparoscopy. Of patients that did not meet the staging criteria, 10% of patients underwent laparotomy and were found to have unresectable disease [21].

The addition of laparoscopic ultrasound (LUS) further improves diagnostic certainty, proving to be more predictive of resectablity than CT [22]. Scheel-Hincke and colleagues evaluated the accuracy of LUS in assessing TNM staging. They found it was 80% accurate in determining the T category, 76% accurate for the N category, and 68% accurate for the M category [23]. John et al. found LUS to be much more accurate in predicting T (100% vs. 64%) and metastatic disease (94% vs. 33%) than CT [22]. Others have examined the role of LUS in detecting vascular invasion. One group found the accuracy for detecting vascular invasion by LUS to be 87%, compared to 69% for CT [24].

A number of centers have demonstrated that CT scanning in conjunction with extended staging laparoscopy and intraoperative ultrasound increases the resectablity rate close to 98% [9, 16, 22, 25–27] with a positive-predictive value of 100% and a negative-predictive value of 96–98% [16, 28], suggesting this may currently be the ideal combined diagnostic modality. Creating a staging algorithm to better differentiate patients who would most benefit from staging laparoscopy may be of benefit as CT imaging continues to improve, and the indications for diagnostic laparoscopy should continue to be evaluated as technology progresses.

Technique

The peritoneal cavity is entered via periumbilical vertical skin incision and either through open Hasson technique or through closed technique with a Veress needle, a 10-mm blunt port is placed into the umbilical area. The abdomen is insufflated and a 30° laparoscope is inserted through the port. Additional ports are then inserted under direct vision in the right upper quadrant and left upper quadrant. Any ascites present is aspirated and sent for cytology. Peritoneal washings for cytology are also collected after separately instilling 200 ml of saline into the right upper quadrant, left upper quadrant, and pelvis.

The peritoneum is systematically examined and any masses are biopsied. The patient is placed in 20° reverse Trendelenburg with a 10° left lateral tilt and the liver is systematically inspected on all surfaces. Visualization of the posterior and diaphragmatic surfaces may be improved by moving the camera to one of the other ports. Blunt instruments are used to palpate the liver for any irregularities.

The gastrohepatic omentum is then incised to visualize the caudate lobe of the liver, celiac axis, and vena cava. The hepatic artery in its course to the porta is visualized. Portal, perigastric, and celiac lymph nodes are biopsied if enlarged. The lesser sac is entered with the camera in the right upper quadrant port for evaluation of the primary tumor (see Fig. 11.1). The patient is then placed in 10° Trendelenburg and the omentum is placed in the left upper quadrant. The transverse colon is lifted to visualize the ligament of Treitz and transverse mesocolon. The middle colic vein is usually visible and nodes around this vein are noted.

Laparoscopic ultrasound is performed to evaluate small intraparenchymal hepatic lesions, vascular invasion into the portal vein, superior mesenteric artery or superior mesenteric vein, and peripancreatic extension of the tumor. The laparoscopic ultrasound probe is inserted via the 10-mm right upper quadrant port and the liver is examined using the articulated 6-MHz probe, using Couinaud's anatomy as a guide. Initially, segments 1, 2, and 3 are examined. The vena cava is then visualized in the back on the dome of the right lobe and followed to the porta anteriorly with identification of the hepatic veins along the way. The segments of the liver are examined sequentially by moving the probe slowly and rotating as necessary.

The hepatoduodenal ligament is evaluated by placing the probe transversely and the portal and superior mesenteric veins (SMV) are examined. The common bile duct, common hepatic duct, and hepatic artery are identified using the pulse and color flow Doppler.

The transducer is then placed transversely on the gastrocolic omentum and the superior mesenteric artery (SMA) is identified from its origin on the aorta and followed distally. It is also possible to visualize the confluence of the portal vein and SMV and inspect its relationship to the tumor.

Finally, the pancreas is examined by placing the transducer through the window in the gastrohepatic

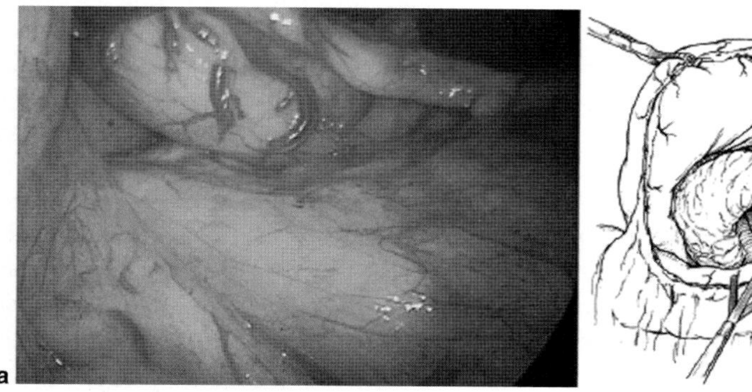

Figure 11.1

Exploration of the pancreas. A laparoscopic Babcock forceps grasps the greater curvature of the stomach, retracting it upward. The gastrocolic ligament is dissected below the gastroepiploic vessels, and the lesser sac is entered. (Reprinted with permission from Mori et al. [102])

omentum directly on the surface of the gland. The tumor and its relation to the pancreatic duct are noted. Rotation of the probe allows for evaluation of the celiac axis and the proximal hepatic artery.

Abnormal findings are photographed and video recording of ultrasound is performed. Frozen section examination of all biopsies is performed.

Any of the following findings removes the patient from being a candidate for surgery: histologically confirmed hepatic, serosal, peritoneal or omental metastasis, tumor extension outside the pancreas (i.e., mesocolic involvement), celiac or portal node involvement confirmed by frozen section, high portal vein involvement by tumor or invasion/encasement of the celiac axis, hepatic artery or superior mesenteric artery. Portal or superior mesenteric vein involvement is not a contraindication.

Laparoscopic Distal Pancreatectomy

While initially reported in the early twentieth century [29, 30], distal pancreatectomy remained a relatively rare procedure through much of the century because of the significant morbidity and mortality [31, 32]. Open distal pancreatectomy has only recently seen its associated morbidity and mortality decrease [31, 33]. Most of this improvement is due to increased experience with the procedure, with complication rates ranging from 20 to 31% in the two largest series [31, 33]. However, the anatomy of the distal pancreas presents itself as promising for minimally invasive intervention, as there is little to be done in the way of complex anastomosis and the laparoscope may actually aid in visualization of the pancreas. For these reasons, laparoscopic distal pancreatectomy is rapidly becoming the most common laparoscopic procedure performed involving resection of the pancreas. It has become the procedure of choice for removal of benign or low-grade malignant lesions at some high-volume, specialized centers. Initially attempted in benign pancreatic disease, comparisons to historical outcomes and internal open pancreatic resection controls revealed similar operative times, morbidity, and mortality [34, 35].

Distal pancreatectomy is slowly being applied to pancreatic malignancy, with initial studies showing the ability to attain negative surgical margins and attain adequate lymph node dissection [36]. Still, concern exists for the feasibility, safety, and long-term outcome of the laparoscopic approach in patients with malignant lesions of the pancreas. In an institutional review, Fernandez-Cruz et al. found in 13 patients with ductal adenocarcinoma undergoing laparoscopic distal pancreatectomy that they could safely complete the procedure in 10 of 13 patients and had positive margins in one patient completed laparoscopically. Perioperative morbidity included one pancreatic fistula, one case of delayed gastric emptying, and one post-operative pneumonia with no post-operative mortality. Median survival was 14 months, with three patients dying within 1 year due to local recurrence and liver metastases [37].

Of note, diagnostic laparoscopy should always be performed in patients with suspected or known PC of the pancreatic body or tail undergoing distal pancreatectomy, as radiographically negative intraabdominal spread is more common in tumors of the body and tail of the pancreas (44%) than in tumors of the pancreatic head (18%) [38].

Technique

Several methods have been described. The method here is the one used by the authors' institution [39]. The patient is positioned on the operating table either supine or, in select cases, on a bean-bag mattress with the legs abducted on spreader bars on a modified (30°) right lateral decubitus position. Sequential leg compression devices and a urinary bladder catheter are placed. The abdomen is entered under direct vision at the umbilicus using the Hasson (open) technique to establish the initial pneumoperitoneum. A total of four to five trocars are then placed under direct vision. The access configuration typically consists of two 5-mm and either two or three 10–12 mm trocars in a semicircular configuration (see Fig. 11.2). When a hand-assisted approach is chosen, a 7–8 cm incision is made in the midline to allow for the hand port insertion.

Once abdominal access is established, and a four-quadrant laparoscopy is performed, the gastrocolic omentum is divided, the lesser sac entered and the splenic flexure is mobilized. The short gastric vessels are then divided with either bipolar cautery or ultrasonic coagulating shears. The stomach is then elevated anteriorly with a flexible retractor and the pancreas is visualized (see Fig. 11.3).

A laparoscopic probe is then inserted and ultrasonography is performed to identify the lesion and any

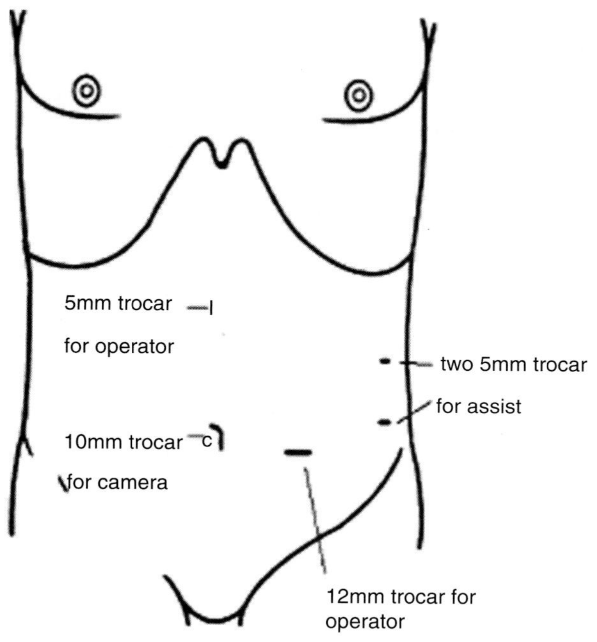

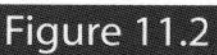

Figure 11.2
Trocar placement for laparoscopic distal pancreatic resection. (Reprinted with permission from Kim et al. [42])

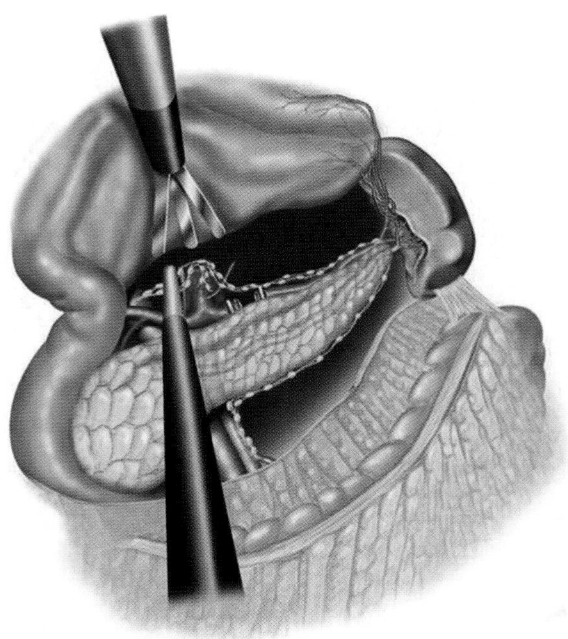

Figure 11.3
Visualization of the pancreas. Identification of the celiac trunk and its branches, lymphadenectomy in the area of the common hepatic artery, celiac artery and left gastric artery, and clipping of the splenic artery at its origin. (Reprinted with permission from Fernandez-Cruz et al. [37])

enlarged lymph nodes. The peritoneum along the inferior and superior borders of the pancreas is divided, taking caution to avoid damage to the splenic artery.

The pancreas is then mobilized along the posterior border, moving in a head-to-tail direction, using either the bipolar cautery device or ultrasonic coagulating shears to control any small vessels. After establishing the posterior plane, the body and tail of the pancreas are carefully dissected away from the splenic vein and artery, if necessary. If a splenectomy is to be performed, these vessels are generally transected at this time, either between vascular clips or via an endoscopic linear stapler loaded with a vascular cartridge.

Once this step is complete, or if a spleen-sparing procedure is to be performed, the pancreas is divided so as to leave a negative resection margin (see Fig. 11.4). This can be accomplished with the use of the bipolar cautery device, followed by identification and suture ligation of the pancreatic duct and then oversewing of the pancreatic stump or by using the endoscopic linear stapler device (see Fig. 11.5).

After the pancreas is transected, the specimen is placed in an entrapment bag and removed from the abdomen. If a splenectomy is also performed, the spleen is likewise placed in an entrapment bag and either removed through a hand port or mechanically fragmented and then extracted piecemeal through a trocar site. A closed suction drain is placed in the operative bed to monitor for pancreatic leakage.

Pancreatic Leak

Pancreatic leak remains the main complication in distal pancreatectomy, reported to occur in 15–20% of patients [40]. Leak rates are similar between laparoscopic and open distal pancreatectomies [41–43]. Many different approaches have been taken to attempt to reduce post-operative pancreatic leak. The authors' institution performed a non-randomized prospective study comparing absorbable mesh reinforcement (see Fig. 11.6) of the stapled transection line with a conventional, non-reinforced staple-line in both

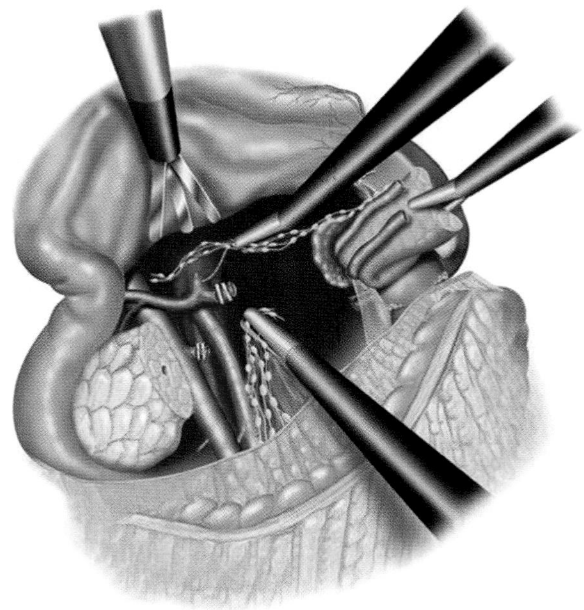

Figure 11.4

Division of the pancreas with lymphadenectomy on the superior border of the pancreas. (Reprinted with permission from Fernandez-Cruz et al. [37])

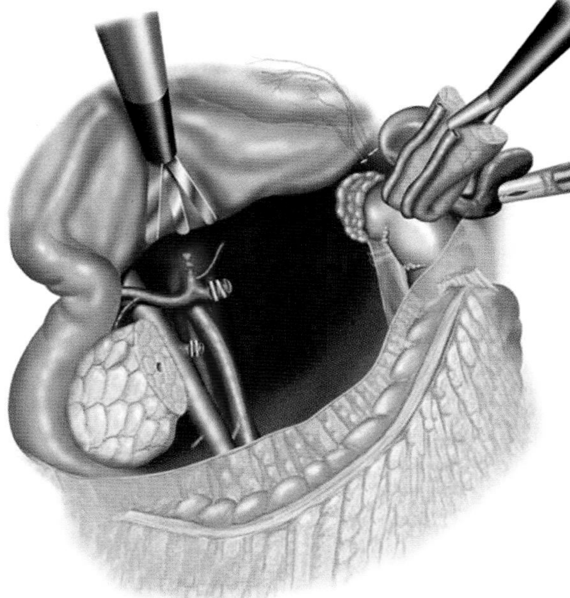

Figure 11.5

Completed distal pancreatectomy with splenectomy. (Reprinted with permission from Fernandez-Cruz et al. [37])

open and laparoscopic distal pancreatectomies for both benign and malignant diseases. We found the leak rate was reduced from 22 to 3.5% [44]. A randomized, controlled trial is currently ongoing. Other adjuvant therapies that have shown potential benefit in small studies include the use of tissue sealant on the cut edge of the pancreatic remnant [45]. Randomized trials do exist exploring the benefits of the use of somatostatin analogues [46–48] and fibrin glue sealants [49, 50] in open distal pancreatectomy for malignancy without demonstrating any conclusive advantage in using either. Further technology is needed to decrease leak rate for both open and minimally invasive approaches to distal pancreatectomy.

Splenectomy

Splenectomy is often performed at the same time as distal pancreatectomy, particularly in resection of PC, mostly to avoid compromising an oncologic resection. However, Warshaw described a splenic preservation technique that allows for resection of the splenic vasculature (thus allowing for an oncologically sound resection) but preserves short gastric vessels to the spleen [51]. In 1999, Schwarz et al. examined the

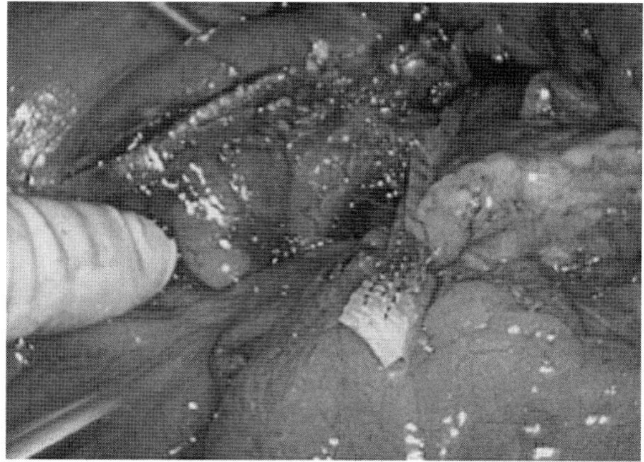

Figure 11.6

Transected staple-line with mesh reinforcement. (Reprinted with permission from Thaker et al. [44])

impact of splenectomy on the outcomes of patients undergoing resection of PC. They found that patients who had a splenectomy with resection of PC had increased operative blood loss increased blood transfusion, but no difference in immediate post-operative complications. They also found that splenectomy was an independent predictor of shortened survival. This was attributed by the authors to systemic disease progression that led to the need for splenectomy, but they also speculated that it could be based on an altered immune response to micrometastatic cancer or a result of different growth characteristics of lymphatic micrometastases [52]. Others also advocate for spleen preservation when possible during distal pancreatectomy for PC [53–56]. Vezakis et al. was the first to demonstrate Warshaw's spleen-preserving technique laparoscopically [57]. However, no studies exist comparing outcomes following laparoscopic distal pancreatectomy with or without splenectomy in patients with PC, so the outcomes using minimally invasive techniques are currently unknown and should be evaluated.

Laparoscopic distal pancreatectomy is still in its infancy, particularly for PC, but is becoming more common and shows promise as an oncologically and technically safe procedure. Overall, it has been demonstrated by non-randomized controlled trials that, in a carefully selected patient population, laparoscopic distal pancreatectomy is at least equal to open distal pancreatectomy [58] and may actually provide a faster return to normal activity and shorter hospital stays [34, 41]. Post-operative pancreatic leak is still unfortunately common and many technologies are being tried to prevent this troublesome complication. The debate over splenectomy or splenic preservation continues without any definitive answers in laparoscopic resection.

Laparoscopic Pancreaticoduodenectomy

The first laparoscopic Whipple procedure was reported in 1994 and was performed for a patient with chronic pancreatitis. This was expanded to include cystic masses, neuroendocrine tumors and, in select cases, ductal adenocarcinomas of the head and neck of the pancreas. Initially, it was performed with six trocars [59], but has been since modified to include a hand port for better tactile sensation [60]. Reviewing the literature, there are still very few reported laparoscopic pancreaticoduodenectomies (see Table 11.1), and even fewer for pancreatic adenocarcinoma.

Technique

After the decision to proceed with the procedure is made (negative diagnostic laparoscopy), five trocars are inserted and an 8-cm incision is made in the right subcostal area through which the non-dominant hand is introduced (see Fig. 11.7) [61]. This hand is used to assist in a Kocher maneuver by dissecting in the retroduodenal area while using endoscopic scissors for adhesiolysis. The peritoneal reflection is opened along the lateral curve of the duodenum from the hepatoduodenal ligament to the mesocolon. The small vessels

Table 11.1. Laparoscopic pancreaticoduodenectomy in the literature

Study	Year	Patients	Pancreas cancer	Mean operation time (min)	Operative complications
Sa Cunha et al. [103]	2008	2	n/a	450	Fistula [1]
Pugliese et al. [63]	2008	19	11	446	Fistula [1], Hemorrhage [1]
Dulucq et al. [104]	2006	11	4	268	Intraperitoneal bleeding [1], small bowel obstruction [1]
Staudacher et al. [105]	2004	4	1	416	None
Masson et al. [106]	2003	1	0	480	n/a
Gagner and Pomp [60]	1997	10	4	510	In converted patients
Uyama et al. [107]	1996	1	0	373	None
Cushieri [108]	1994	2	0	n/a	None

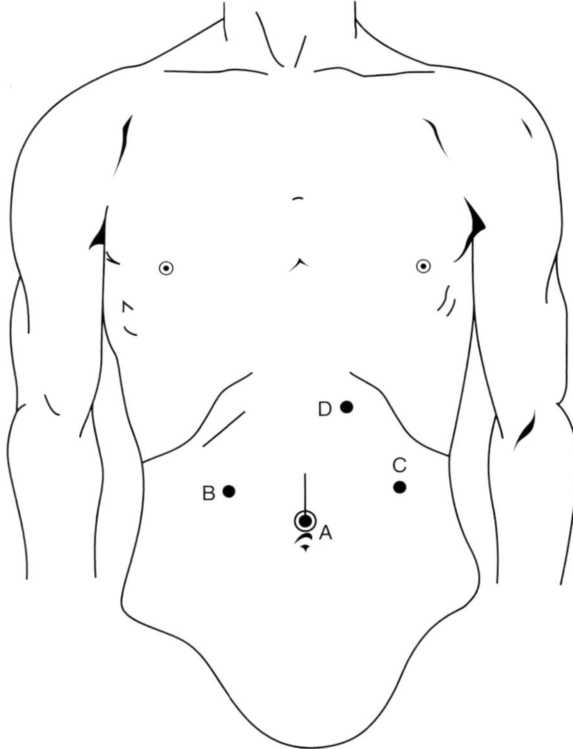

Figure 11.7

Trocar placement for laparoscopic pancreaticoduodenectomy. (Reprinted with permission from Staudacher et al. [105])

under the peritoneum are then cauterized, allowing for blunt dissection in an avascular plane behind the pancreas anterior to the vena cava.

The right colonic flexure is then mobilized and reflected downward using the hand port. The avascular peritoneum reflection covering the third portion of the duodenum is divided to the large vessels at the mesenteric root. Now, the second, third, and fourth portions of the duodenum are dissected and mobilized. The vena cava is exposed and the peritoneum covering the common bile duct is opened anteriorly and laterally.

The peritoneal sheet of the hepatoduodenal ligament and the lesser omentum is divided close to the hepatic hilum, thus exposing the structures within the ligament. A laparoscopic right-angled dissector is used to isolate the bile duct, portal vein, and right hepatic artery. A cholecystectomy with cholangiogram is then performed. The gastrocolic ligament is then opened with the harmonic scalpel laterally to the gastroepiploic artery, which is preserved. All transverse branches are divided.

The dissection then continues toward the pylorus, with transection of the first portion of the duodenum at 1 cm from the pylorus using an Endo-GIA stapler. The bile duct is suspended with an umbilical tape and transected with a 30-mm Endo GIA stapler approximately 3 cm above the superior border of the pancreas. The gastroduodenal artery is then exposed and transected with an endoscopic stapler, vascular load.

The superior mesenteric vein and the portal vein are dissected from the head of the pancreas using a suction/irrigation probe in a blunt fashion. With this maneuver, the neck of the pancreas is carefully cleared from the portal vein by gentle blunt dissection and hand assistance (see Fig. 11.8). The pancreas is then transected, starting inferiorly and moving toward the superior border anterior to the portal vein and the mesenteric vessels. The harmonic scalpel aids in limiting blood loss (see Fig. 11.9).

The fourth portion of the duodenum, medial to the mesenteric vessels, is transected with a stapler. The harmonic scalpel is used to mobilize the uncinate process from the mesenteric artery and vein. The specimen is placed in a specimen bag and extracted through the hand port.

The three anastomoses are created by intracorporeal suturing techniques. The proximal jejunal loop is pulled behind the mesenteric vessels and its antimesenteric side is approximated to the pancreatic duct in 2 layers, using a 5 cm long 5-F pediatric tube as a stent, inserting one half into the pancreatic duct and then sutured to the duct and jejunal opening with a running 4-0 monofilament absorbable suture. A layer of silk interrupted sutures is then applied between the anterior capsule of the pancreas and the serosal side of the jejunal loop.

The hepaticojejunostomy is then performed with a running posterior and anterior 3-0 monofilament absorbable suture. Finally, the third anastomosis is carried out with the same suture between the pylorus and the jejunum end to end. A feeding jejunostomy tube (T-tube, 14-F) is inserted through one of the trocar sites and two large Jackson–Pratt drains are left anterior and posterior to the anastomoses.

Some criticize the laparoscopic pancreaticoduodenectomy as a compromised cancer operation because a remnant of the pancreas is attached to the

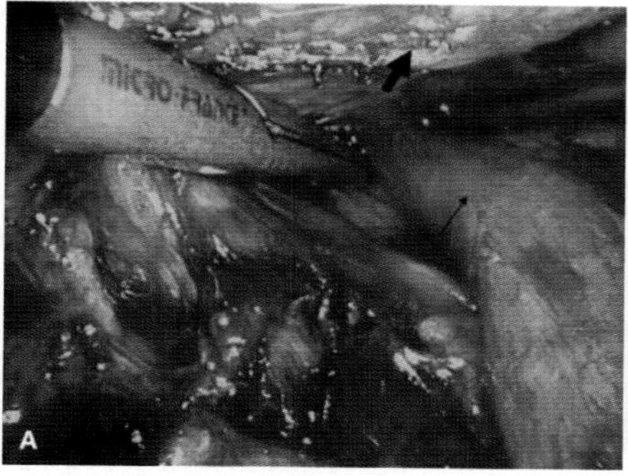

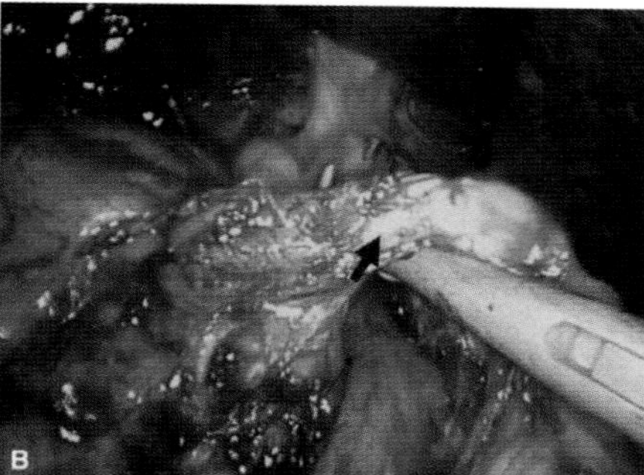

Figure 11.8

Dissection of the posterior pancreas from the portal vein using a 5-mm irrigation suction probe under direct laparoscopic vision. (**a**) Beginning of dissection. (**b**) The pancreas is separated from the portal vein and ready for transaction. The *thick arrow* shows the pancreas and the *thin arrow* shows the portal vein. (Reprinted with permission from Dulucq et al. [36])

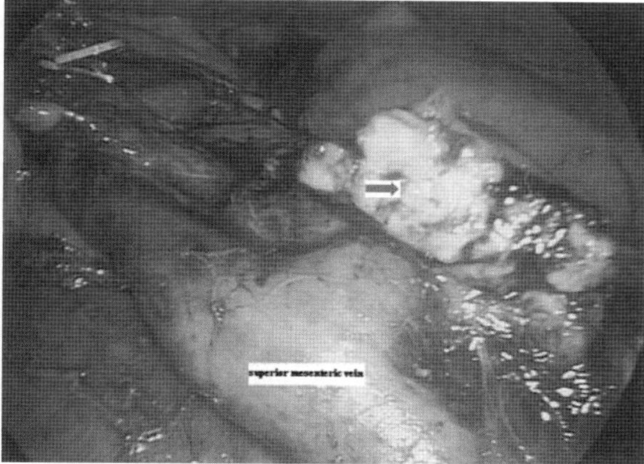

Figure 11.9

Laparoscopic view of the transected pancreas. *Arrow* shows the stump of the pancreatic duct. (Reprinted with permission from Staudacher et al. [105])

superior mesenteric vein while dissecting the uncinate process with a linear stapler [62]. This can be solved by using an ultrasonic dissector in the dissection of the superior mesenteric vessels from the uncinate process [36]. Other concerns arise over the blind passage of the laparoscopic instrument along the superior mesenteric vein behind the neck of the pancreas [62]. This can be avoided by using a 5-mm irrigation suction probe under direct laparoscopic vision for dissection of the pancreas from the large vessels [36].

Concerns over adequate extended lymphadenectomy as well as the steep learning curve and no proven decrease in the length of hospital stay or post-operative complications [63] continue to keep this procedure limited to only the most experienced laparoscopic surgeons.

Laparoscopic Palliation of Pancreatic Adenocarcinoma

Despite the advances in diagnostic technology, only 15–20% of all patients with PC are respectable for cure at the time of initial presentation [3]. Thus, it is necessary to include palliative options when discussing minimally invasive treatment for PC, as 70–80% of patients will develop common bile duct obstruction and digestive tract obstruction will occur in 5–10% [64]. MIS for palliation in patients with advanced PC is appealing because of the limited survival in these patients.

Palliation is directed at three main problems: biliary obstruction, duodenal obstruction, and pain. The aim of treatment is to provide symptomatic relief with minimal morbidity and rapid return of function. This can be done surgically by either with biliary bypass or without gastric bypass. Non-surgical options include endoscopic biliary and duodenal stenting.

Many controversies exist in the realm of the palliation of PC. Among them, the effectiveness of stenting vs. surgical bypass, the feasibility of performing a biliary bypass via a minimally invasive technique and the prophylactic surgical bypass when metastatic or locally advanced disease are found at the time of diagnostic laparoscopy or laparotomy.

Endoscopic Biliary and Duodenal Stenting

Endoscopic stenting of the common bile duct for palliation of malignant obstruction has proven to be effective. Approximately 90% of patients with unresectable PC have resolution of symptoms and jaundice following endoscopic stenting [65].

The major complication associated with stenting is obstruction, a complication frequently seen in plastic stents and one that predisposes patients to recurrent jaundice and cholangitis. This occlusion is secondary to a bacterial biofilm that coats the stent. This film then adheres to the bile proteins adsorbed to the stent surface. Bacterial enzymes then deconjugate bilirubin, promoting sludging and occlusion [66]. Stent size and material of construction appear to affect occlusion rates. A 10-French (Fr) stent is believed to be the optimal size for an obstructed common bile duct and Teflon construction may reduce protein adsorption [67].

Self-expanding metal stents have been found superior to plastic stents in terms of occlusion.

Several randomized trials exist (see Table 11.2) that demonstrate decreased rates of occlusion and reintervention, although they cannot prevent tumor ingrowth, which is the primary cause of occlusion [68]. They were also found to be cost-effective in patients surviving longer than 6 months [69]. Metal stents are not without their own issues. A higher cost and difficulty positioning and removing the stent were initial problems faced with the use of metal stents. However, a recent cost analysis found that metal stents are cost effective if the unit cost of additional endoscopic retrograde cholangiopancreatographies exceeds $1,820 [70]. A recent Cochrane meta-analysis found that metal stents are the intervention of choice in patients with unresectable PC experiencing distal obstructive jaundice [71].

Gastric outlet obstruction is a well-known complication of PC and occurs in as many as 33% of patients with unresectable PC [72]. There are many philosophies held by surgeons regarding the treatment of gastric outlet obstruction that lead to the various approaches taken in the management of these patients.

Endoscopic duodenal stenting is a minimally invasive option for management of gastric outlet obstruction. There is a high technical success rate, a low intervention-related mortality, a short procedure-related hospital stay, and rapid return of toleration of oral intake [73, 74]. Complications range from stent migration, pain, re-obstruction or biliary obstruction to bleeding or perforation. A recent retrospective multicenter study found an 85% clinical success rate and a 17% 30-day complication rate, including a 3% perforation rate, with a mean hospital stay of 6 days [75]. Long-term stent patency was found to be 78%, with a median stent patency time of 5.5 weeks in a patient population with a median survival of 7 weeks [76].

Endoscopic Biliary Stents Versus Surgical Bypass

Endoscopic biliary stenting has been compared to open biliary bypass in numerous studies. Three prospective, randomized trials compared these two approaches

Table 11.2. Randomized trials of metal vs. plastic stents for palliation in malignant biliary obstruction

Authors	Patients	Pancreatic carcinoma (%)	Metallic stent dysfunction (%)	Plastic stent dysfunction (%)
Davids et al. [109]	105	89	33	54
Carr-Locke et al. [68]	163	52	13	13
Knyrim et al. [110]	55	78	22	43
Prat et al. [69]	101	64	18	73
Rosch and Schinner [111]	75	N/A	8	25
Kaassis et al. [112]	118	75	19	37
Soderlund and Linder [113]	100	78	18	43

tumors are now detected earlier with increased use of high-definition CT scanners.

The majority of PETs are sporadic and have no identifiable risk factors [28], but PET is, however, more frequent in certain genetic syndromes. Multiple endocrine neoplasia type one (MEN 1) is an autosomal dominant syndrome associated with endocrine lesions of the parathyroid, pancreas, pituitary, and upper gastrointestinal tract [29]. Over 60% of patients with MEN 1 will develop PETs, which are usually multiple. These tumors may remain clinically insignificant for a long time interval [30]. Inversely, the most common PET in this population is gastrinoma, and 20–30% of patients with Zollinger–Ellison syndrome have MEN 1 [31]. Pancreatic endocrine tumors are found in 5–10% of patients with Von Hippel–Lindau syndrome [32], and these are usually small, multiple, and nonfunctional [33]. Associations between PETs and neurofibromatosis type 1 as well as tuberous sclerosis have also been described [20].

Overall survival in patients with PETs is significantly better than that for patients with pancreatic adenocarcinoma. A 2005 study using the Surveillance, Epidemiology, and End Results (SEER) data for 35,276 patients demonstrated overall survival of 27 months for PET cases vs. 4 months for adenocarcinoma [34]. Patients with functioning tumors have a better overall survival than those with nonfunctioning tumors [18, 35]. For patients with functioning tumors, the 5-year survival for insulinoma and gastrinoma is higher than that for other types such as glucagonoma [35]. The mixed cell variety is, however, much more aggressive and resembles that of adenocarcinoma, warranting an aggressive surgical approach.

Medical therapy for cure or palliation of PETs has been disappointing, although some response has been shown with streptozocin and tozolomide combination regimens [36, 37]. A recent study indicates sunitinib, a tyrosine kinase inhibitor, may offer some benefit [38]. Therefore, surgery is considered by most to offer the best chance for long-term survival or cure. A review of SEER data from 1998 to 2000 showed that resection, of any type, improved outcome to a median overall survival of 58 months compared with 15 months in patients not undergoing resection [18]. However, due to controversy in classification schemes for both grading and staging, prognosis has been difficult to determine. The 2000 WHO Classification [5] is the most widely accepted standard for grading of PETs. In this classification, tumors <2 cm, confined to the pancreas, nonangioinvasive, ≤2 mitosis/HPF, and ≤ 2% Ki-67-positive cells are considered benign. The majority of these tumors are either insulinomas or small nonfunctional tumors, and resection is usually curative. Uncertain malignant potential is differentiated from low-grade malignant based on invasion and/or metastases.

A widely accepted TNM staging classification for PETs has not previously existed. Proposed classifications have been based on endocrine tumors found in specific regions of the gut [39] and based on exocrine tumors of the pancreas [40]. The American Joint Committee on Cancer (AJCC) *Cancer Staging Manual*, 6th edition, published in 2002 specifically excluded PETs [41], although there have been attempts to validate this system to PETs, with some success. The 7th edition (in press), will contain a chapter specific to PETs.

Patients with a functioning PET usually present with the associated paraneoplastic syndrome, while those with nonfunctioning PETs are either asymptomatic or have nonspecific symptoms such as abdominal pain or nausea. These nonspecific symptoms may be due to localized invasion, obstruction of the pancreatic duct, or metastatic lesions to the liver [9]. Many, and perhaps the growing majority, of the nonfunctioning PETs are found incidentally. Nearly half (48%) of all PETs occur in the tail of the pancreas, 31% in the head, and 16% in the body [28]. With the exception of insulinoma, the majority of patients (50–60%) with either functioning or nonfunctioning PETs have metastases at the time of presentation [40, 42, 43]. Metastasis to the liver is described as the cause of death in up to 80% of patients [11, 43].

Diagnosis and Treatment

The evaluation of a patient suspected of having a PET usually begins with noninvasive imaging such as CT, MRI, or transabdominal ultrasound. However, as noted previously, a growing number of PETs are discovered incidentally. PETs typically have increased vascularity and are best seen on the arterial phase images of a contrasted CT or the T2 phase images of an MRI. On transabdominal ultrasound, they are usually solid and hypoechoic, but are often not well visualized due to bowel gas interference or patient's body habitus. Transabdominal ultrasound may detect larger lesions in the pancreas or metastasis within the liver, but should not be relied upon for definitive imaging of PETs. Detection with all of these modalities decreases significantly with smaller tumor size [44], requiring additional modalities for aid in detection. CT and MRI are both significantly more sensitive than transabdominal ultrasound for detecting most pancreatic masses, but still lack the specificity required to consistently differentiate PETs from other pancreatic neoplasms. Newer imaging modalities are selectively employed to aid in the differentiation, include positron emission tomography, indium octreotide scintigraphy, and endoscopic ultrasound (EUS). Of the three, EUS has become increasingly effective in both imaging and diagnosis of PETs via fine needle aspiration. Operator expertise is an important factor in the sensitivity of EUS [45], but lesions as small as 0.5 cm can be detected [46].

Our initial enthusiasm for EUS has been recently tempered by the occurrence of complications as a result of the biopsy performed during the procedure. Bleeding, focal acute necrotizing pancreatitis, as well as adhesion formation in the lesser sac have all been seen after EUS-FNA. We therefore no longer routinely attempt to obtain definitive histological diagnosis unless it will play a significant factor in determining the individual patient management. This practice is consistent with the time-honored medical dictum of "do not order a test unless the result will change what you will do for the patient." In a corollary to this, increased detection of pancreatic lesions on imaging for vague abdominal symptoms can result in aggressive therapy for indolent lesions that may otherwise have been left untreated.

Selection of patients for surgical resection depends on their overall medical status, Eastern Cooperative Oncology Group (ECOG) performance, as well as the tumor size, number, and localization. The patient's age and their desire for surgical resection also play an important role in determining management and should not be underestimated. For example, a 75-year-old man with a small, 1.2 cm, well-circumscribed, hypervascular solid lesion in the tail of the pancreas likely has a benign PET. It may certainly be a better decision to observe this patient, since the disease-specific mortality for him is extremely low. Conversely, a 34-year-old woman with the same tumor may be facing years and years of surveillance scans and anxiety and may actually do better with a pancreatic resection. Aside from these two extremes, most patients with solid pancreatic neoplasms suspected of being a PET should be offered surgical resection unless there are absolute contraindications for surgery. For patients with metastases isolated to the liver, the most recent recommendation by the European Neuroendocrine Tumour Society (ENETS) is to attempt a curative resection that includes the pancreatic primary and the lesions in the liver [30]. Patients with widespread metastases or invasion of other organs should be treated medically. Surgical treatment for pancreatic lesions is to a large extent dictated by the location of the tumor in the pancreas, as will be discussed later.

Lesions Located in the Head and Uncinate Process

For lesions located in the head and uncinate process, the decision as to which type of resection to perform is determined in part by size, depth, and location of the tumor. A small tumor located superficially on the anterior or posterior (uncinate) surface may be safely removed by enucleation (Fig. 12.1), and this can often be performed laparoscopically. Enucleation is usually considered adequate for small tumors (<2 cm), since the majority of these are benign with a low risk of nodal metastasis. However, enucleation of tumors located in the pancreatic head or uncinate is often difficult due to the convergence of mesenteric venous and arterial arcades of the transverse mesocolon, duodenum, gastric antrum, and pancreatic head, making this a treacherous area for laparoscopic dissection. Additionally, proximity to one or more of the major pancreatic ducts also increases the risk of pancreatic leaks and fistulae. Indeed, the biggest concern after enucleation is pancreatic fistula, with the incidence ranging between 5 and 25% [47–49]. For large tumors in this location or for lesions seated deep within the parenchyma, a more conservative and probably a safer approach is to perform a formal en bloc resection in the form of a pancreaticoduodenectomy, or Whipple procedure. This resection also allows for the removal of the primary lymph nodes draining the head and uncinate, facilitating a more thorough staging and reducing the risk of an inadequate (R1) resection. While the more conservative surgical approach to tumors in the pancreatic head and uncinate would be to perform a pancreaticoduodenectomy, enucleation remains a reasonable alternative if technically feasible [30], especially for insulinoma or small nonfunctional PETs.

Laparoscopic pancreaticoduodenectomy or Whipple procedure is, arguably, the last frontier in minimally

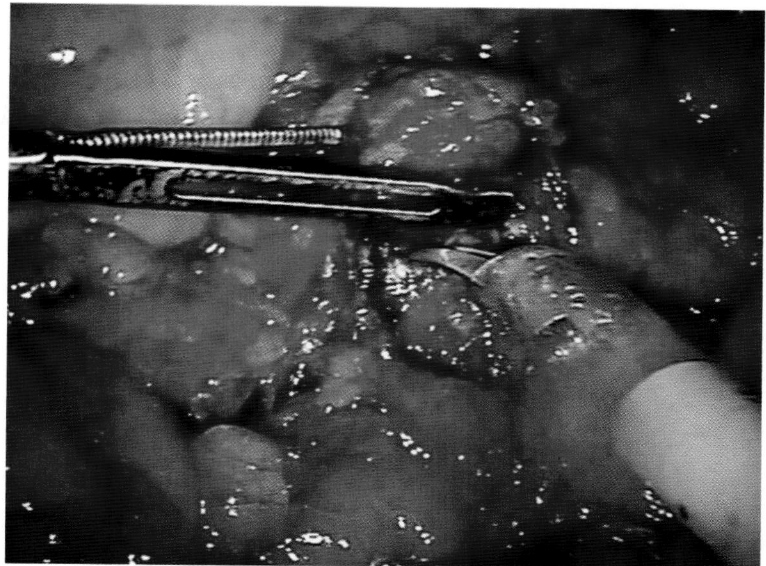

Figure 12.1

Enucleation of PET with monopolar electrocautery and shears

invasive surgery. Since Gagner's [50] initial description of this tremendous laparoscopic feat, there have been several reports validating the safety of the procedure, albeit in highly selected patients [51, 52, 53]. In a thin, healthy patient with a localized solid or cystic neoplasm in the head of the pancreas, laparoscopic Whipple could be contemplated if an adequate oncological resection and lymphadenectomy can be ensured. Yet most surgeons, regardless of their backgrounds, are wary of considering such a daunting task even under the most ideal circumstances. Perhaps this is due to the widely held belief that the morbidity of a pancreaticoduodenectomy is not so much derived from the length of the incision, but rather from the physiological impact of the resection and reconstruction. It is feared that the potentially lethal complication of an anastomotic leak may be higher when a laparoscopic reconstruction is performed. This, however, has not been demonstrated in the small number of publications of the technique [51]. The average length of hospital stay and time to return of normal GI function does not appear to be improved when laparoscopic techniques are employed [54]. Therefore, it is the author's (JBM) belief that a laparoscopic Whipple should only be performed at high volume centers with extensive experience in pancreatic and minimally invasive techniques, in highly selected patients, and with the oversight of an IRB study protocol. It may take several more years to demonstrate outcome equivalence for laparoscopic pancreaticoduodenectomy.

Lesions in the Neck, Body, and Tail

The majority of PETs are located in the body and tail of the pancreas, extending from the superior mesenteric vein–portal vein confluence to the spleen. This portion of the pancreas has a more predictable blood supply and ductal anatomy and lends itself to laparoscopic resection techniques better than tumors in the head and uncinate. Once the lesser sac is entered through the gastrocolic omentum, the body and tail of the pancreas are easily visualized and accessible to a variety of resection techniques. Laparoscopic ultrasound can aid in the localization of small tumors which are not plainly visible and should be employed routinely. Occasionally the lesser sac is difficult to enter due to inflammatory adhesions which may be the result from prior episodes of pancreatitis or from attempts to biopsy the tumor.

For lesions in the body and tail of the pancreas, the decision on the type of resection to perform again depends on the size and location of the tumor as well as the amount of normal pancreas which requires resection. For small lesions near the neck or proximal body of the pancreas, it may be reasonable to try to preserve the tail of the pancreas by performing either an enucleation or a central pancreatectomy. The latter procedure has been described for open techniques by Roggin et al. [55] and is a useful technique for preserving pancreatic parenchyma when a formal oncological resection and lymphadenectomy are not indicated. Laparoscopic central pancreatectomy has also been described

[56, 57], but probably remains outside the arsenal of most pancreatic surgeons who perform LPS, due to the difficulty in performing the pancreaticojejunostomy laparoscopically.

The majority of tumors over 2 cm, in close proximity to the pancreatic duct, or located in the body or tail of the gland are best managed by performing a laparoscopic distal pancreatectomy. There are several variations on the technique of this procedure, which essentially differ in preserving or sacrificing the spleen and its vessels.

Techniques

Since 1994, when Cuschieri first described the laparoscopic distal pancreatectomy, a growing body of literature supporting a variety of minimally invasive approaches to pancreatic surgery has been established. Laparoscopic distal pancreatectomy with splenectomy, with splenic preservation (with and without vessel preservation), enucleation, and even Whipple's operation have successfully been performed [50,51,58,59]. In a nice review, Fernandez-Cruz et al. [60] recently summarized the literature analyzing the role of LPS for PETs.

The specific techniques employed for LPS for any particular patient depend on several factors. Individual characteristics of the tumor, such as size, location within the pancreas, proximity to a major pancreatic duct, histological identity, and risk of nodal involvement dictate the choice for a particular surgical approach. Additionally, characteristics of the patient, such as age, body mass index, previous surgeries, physiological condition, as well as the training and experience of the surgeon, guide the decision making.

Patient Positioning and Setup

The positioning of patients for LPS obviously depends again on several factors, including the surgeon's preference and dexterity, as well as body habitus of the patient, and positioning of assistants. It is critically important to utilize an operating table that allows for maximum versatility and positioning. We currently use one that allows for split-leg positioning without the need for stirrups (Maquet, Inc., Bridgewater, NJ) and lateral rotation and goes extremely low to the floor, which is beneficial for operating on obese patients. We often have the operative surgeon stand between the patients' legs, in the so-called French position, although for thin patients it is probably not necessary (Fig. 12.2). The patient's arms need not be tucked since both the surgeon and the assistant will typically be in positions below the level of the umbilicus, looking up toward the patient's head. The patient is placed supine in the OR table, although it is often beneficial to have a roll under the left side to achieve a

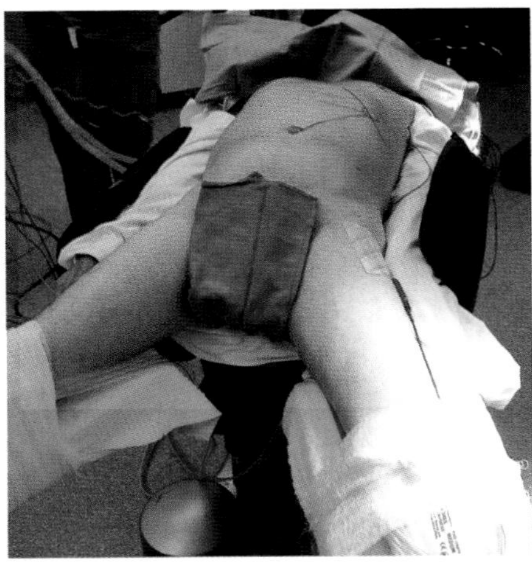

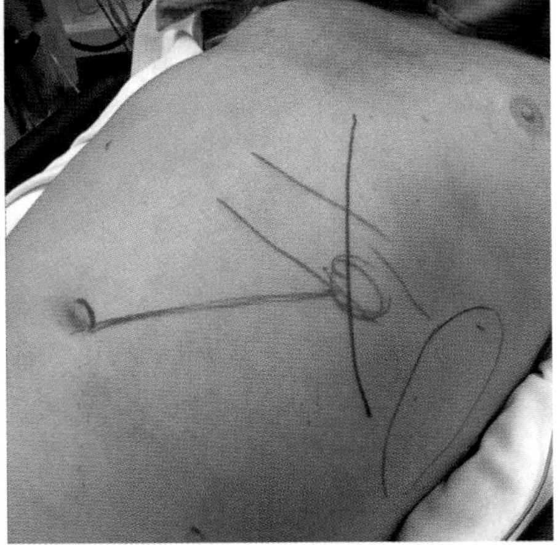

Figure 12.2

Patient positioning for laparoscopic distal pancreatectomy

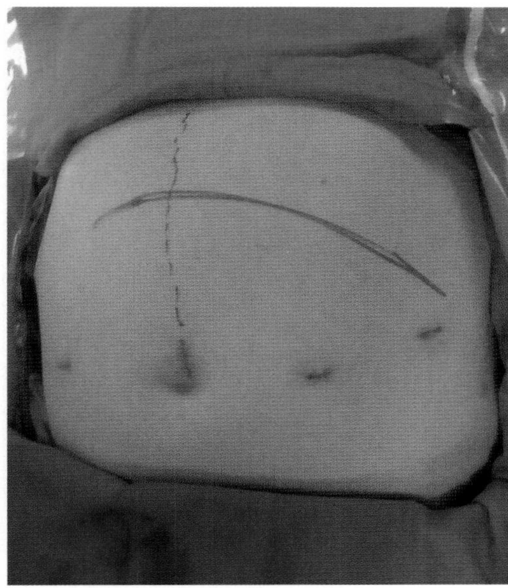

Figure 12.3

Post-operative view of trochars for laparoscopic distal pancreatectomy

semi-lateral position. We do not routinely do this, as the table we employ allows for 45° lateral roll, which essentially achieves the same result. We typically begin the procedure by placing the camera port near the umbilicus, then place three or four accessory operative ports in a semi-circular array, and use a variety of 5 and 12 mm ports to allow for maximum flexibility (Fig. 12.3). If a hand port is to be placed, we do so at the beginning of the case, and it is usually placed in the upper midline position. Finally, the importance of having high-quality video monitors arranged in positions which are ergonomically optimal cannot be emphasized strongly enough. We prefer to have a flat-panel screen directly over the patient's head so that the operative surgeon stands between the patient's legs and looks directly in the direction of the pancreas, in a so-called mono-axial position.

Hand-Assisted Laparoscopic Techniques

Laparoscopic pancreatic surgery requires the combination of advanced technical skills and comprehensive surgical knowledge which were taught, until recently, in two largely divergent surgical subspecialties. Because many experienced pancreatic surgeons had little or no initial laparoscopic training or were not comfortable with advanced laparoscopy, many were slow to adopt LPS. In addition, until recently, most fellowships in hepatopancreatobiliary surgery and surgical oncology offered limited training and experience in minimally invasive procedures. The technique of hand-assissted laparoscopy (HALS) offers many distinct advantages over conventional laparoscopy and has served as a bridge from open to complete laparoscopic techniques for many pancreatic surgeons. Having a hand in the abdomen to assist with retraction, dissection, and proprioception adds a significant level of comfort to the surgeon who is learning LPS. It is also particularly useful in the training environment and allows the teaching surgeon to retain some level of control over the procedure when the laparoscopic dissection is being done by a fellow or resident. The added advantage of having an 8 cm hand-port incision allows for rapid conversion to an open procedure if necessary. In the event of sudden, unexpected, or difficult to control hemorrhage, the surgeon can often tamponade the bleeding with manual finger compression until a full open incision and conversion to an open approach is made. Finally, many surgeons justify the placement of a hand-port incision due to the fact that the pancreas and possibly the spleen will require some sort of incision for retrieval at the end of the case. We utilize a hand port (GelPort® Applied Medical, Rancho Santa Margarita, CA), which allows for either hand or multiple trocar access. This device also serves as a wound protector and retractor during specimen retrieval. We frequently employ a hand-assist approach when teaching LPS to residents and employ it in cases when we anticipate difficulty with the dissection or specimen retrieval (Fig. 12.4).

Laparoscopic Distal Pancreatectomy and Splenectomy

In 2003, Strasberg [61] described the technique known as radical antegrade modular pancreatosplenectomy (RAMPS) for open procedures. Most open and laparoscopic procedures today are modifications of this technique, and the majority of surgeons today perform a laparoscopic distal pancreatectomy and splenectomy. Certainly for known malignancies, splenectomy allows for more thorough lymphadenectomy and oncological staging. For PETs, or other pancreatic neoplasms of undefined malignant potential, the necessity of

Figure 12.4

Hand-assisted stapling of pancreas

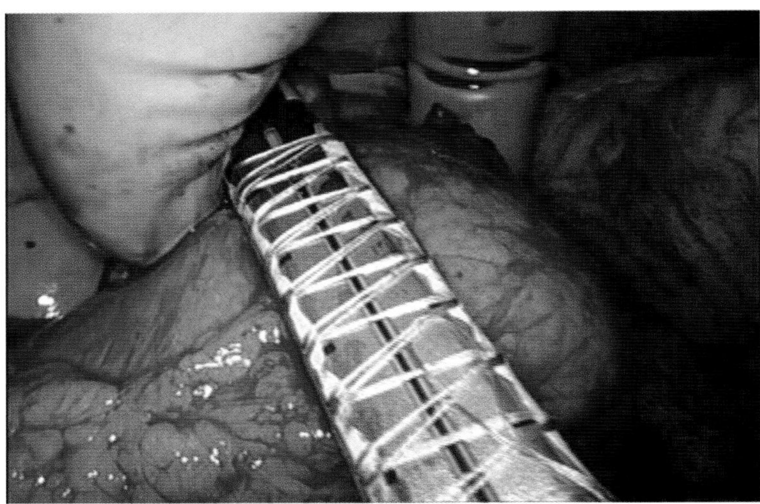

splenectomy remains controversial. For PETs over 2 cm or involving the splenic vessels or hilum, we perform en bloc splenectomy routinely.

After establishing pneumoperitoneum and port placement, we begin by performing thorough inspection of the peritoneal cavity to look for unexpected metastatic disease or local advancement. The gastrocolic omentum is widely opened using ultrasonic shears, monopolar or bipolar sealing/cutting devices, to enter the lesser sac (Fig. 12.5). The anterior surface of the pancreas should now be visualized, and we make attempts to confirm the location of the tumor, as well as vascular anatomy, using intraoperative ultrasound (Fig. 12.6). The dissection is continued toward the spleen, taking care to avoid either the gastroepiploic vessels or the colon. The splenocolic ligament is divided and the splenic flexure mobilized caudally. From here, the surgeon must decide to work either medial to lateral, or the opposite, taking the splenic attachments first. We usually choose to work in the former direction, and dissection progresses medial to lateral. The celiac axis is identified and adjacent lymph nodes resected if feasible. Progressing laterally, a complete dissection is made of the anterior pancreas with care to identify the left gastric and splenic artery. After the splenic artery is identified, attempts are made to dissect and divide the artery outside of the pancreatic capsule. If it is not possible to divide the artery in such a manner, it is usually stapled along with the pancreatic parenchyma at the appropriate

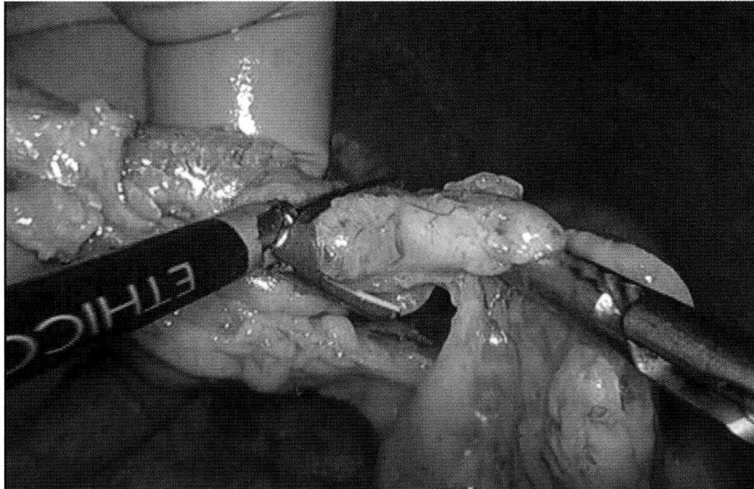

Figure 12.5

Opening of gastrocolic omentum with ultrasonic shears

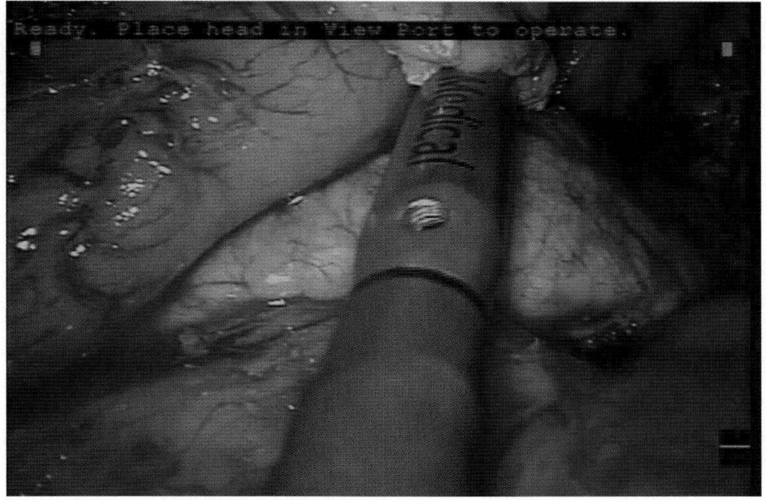

Figure 12.6

Intraoperative ultrasound of pancreas

stage. Careful dissection of the inferior border of the pancreas allows for mobilization of the body and tail away from the retroperitoneum, and the splenic vein is brought up along with the pancreas. A Penrose drain or umbilical tape can be passed posterior to the pancreatic gland to aid in traction and elevation of the gland during the dissection (Fig. 12.7.), the so-called lasso technique [62]. The splenic vein is identified on the posterior portion of the gland and then either clipped or stapled independent of the pancreas or stapled together with the pancreatic parenchyma. The pancreas is lifted and transected through its narrowest region, typically at the neck, with a laparoscopic linear stapler (Endo-GIA, ValleyLab, Boulder, CO) or similar device with 3.5 mm staples. There has yet to be developed a fail-proof method of pancreatic parenchymal transection, as demonstrated by the persistently high rates of pancreatic fistulae, this, despite the use of a variety of devices and so-called vascular staplers with a 1.8–2.0 mm staple length. There has been recent evidence to support the use of a combination of a linear stapling device with a bioabsorbable staple line reinforcement (SeamGuard®, W.L. Gore and Associateds, Inc., Flagstaff, AZ) to reduce the rate of post-op leaks [63]. We now routinely use a laparoscopic stapler with an even longer, 4.8 mm staple height than we had in the past, in combination with the bioabsorbable staple line reinforcement (Fig. 12.8). This technique seems

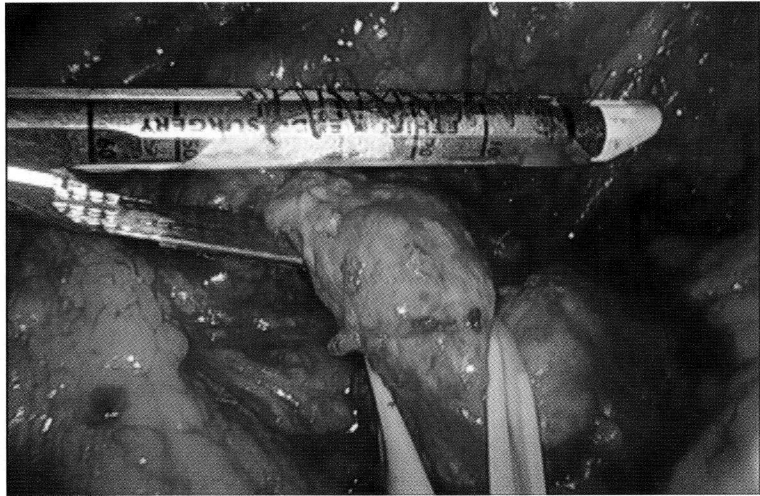

Figure 12.7

Lasso technique for transecting the pancreatic neck

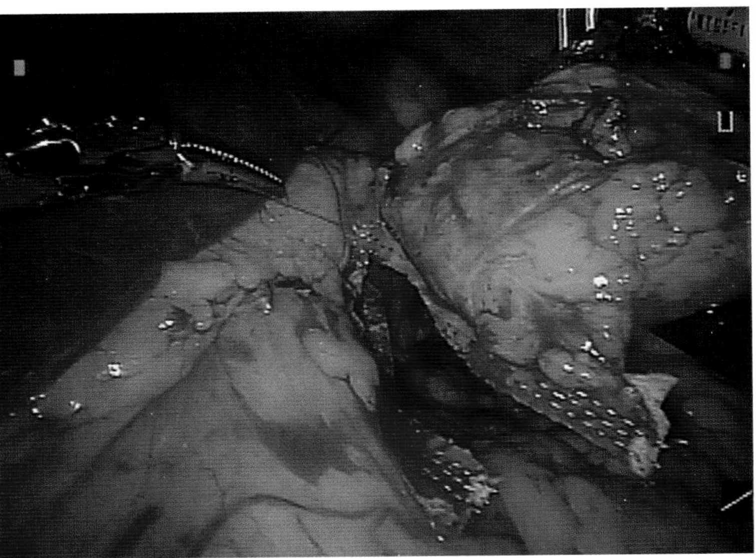

Figure 12.8
Bioabsorbable staple line reinforcement

to prevent the staples from simply tearing through or "crumbling" the pancreatic parenchyma, and the staple line reinforcement produces the effect of pledgets, compressing the tissue without disrupting its integrity. Once the pancreas has been divided, the splenic artery is appropriately divided if not done so previously. Attention is now turned to completing the mobilization of the body and tail. The posterior dissection is in a relatively avascular plane, and much of this can be done with either electrocautery or ultrasonic shears. Lymphadenectomy is performed from the superior border to the anterior superior mesenteric artery, simply by including the splenic artery and vein with the resection. Posterior lymph nodes are also removed while mobilizing the body and tail from the retroperitoneum over the left kidney. Dissection continues up the superior border of the pancreas toward the apex of the spleen and the short gastric vessels are controlled with the ultrasonic shears. Finally, the avascular attachments of the spleen are divided, and the entire specimen should be ready for retrieval. In order to reduce the size of the specimen and length of incision needed for its removal, we often will staple the distal tip of the pancreas to allow the spleen to be removed separately. This allows for a specimen to be removed from an incision about half as long as a typical hand-port incision and may be placed in a more cosmetically pleasing location. The pancreatic staple line is inspected and fibrin sealant (TISSEEL®, Baxter Healthcare, Westlake Village, CA) is applied to the staple line routinely. A drain is selectively placed in the resection bed if extensive dissection has taken place to drain seroma and not left in place in anticipation of leaks.

Laparoscopic Distal Pancreatectomy with Spleen Preservation

For body and tail lesions that are of benign or indeterminate nature, many surgeons recommend a spleen-preserving distal pancreatectomy [28], as the splenectomy certainly adds little if any to the oncological outcome and may increase morbidity. This resection can be accomplished either with or without splenic vessel sparing. The choice of procedure depends on the status of the splenic artery and vein as well as surgeon preference. Vessel sparing requires meticulous and time-consuming dissection, often resulting in sacrificing the spleen due to either bleeding or thrombosis of the splenic vessels. There is no significant literature supporting one method over the other, although proponents of vessel preservation cite the increased risk of splenic infarction or decreased immunological function. Our preference is the nonvessel sparing method, first described for open procedures by Warshaw in 1988 [64] and frequently referred to as the "Warshaw technique." The splenic artery and vein are initially divided at the proximal pancreatic transection point, and again as distal as possible, trying to stay as far out of the splenic hilum as possible. It is critically important to preserve the entering short gastric and left gastroepiploic vessel, as well as any of the branching collaterals in the splenic hilum, as the spleen will remain vascularized solely from these vessels.

For a spleen-preserving, vessel-sparing distal pancreatectomy, the inferior border of the pancreas body and tail are carefully dissected away from the vein while taking any feeders. Sealing compounds may need to be used liberally. After the splenic hilum is reached and the body and tail are completely mobilized from the retroperitoneum, the pancreas can be transected.

Robotics

Recently there has been exponential growth in the application of surgical robotic devices to a variety of surgical disciplines, most notably in urology and gynecology. Yet there has been slow acceptance and limited application of robotics to general surgical procedures, and minimally invasive pancreatic surgery in particular. There have been only a handful of publications discussing the use of robotics for pancreatic resections, most of which are small, limited case series, and certainly there is no literature which might suggest a benefit from utilizing the robot. Yet there is a growing body of clinical experience with the use of robotics to perform a variety of pancreatic resections, and it is estimated that there have been over 500 procedures performed worldwide to date (unpublished data, personal communications).

The most widely used robotic system is currently the daVinci surgical system (Intuitive Surgical, Sunnyvale, CA), which has two platforms available. We have been utilizing the daVinci robot since 2006 for selected cases and exploring the benefits and limitations for complex hepatobiliary and pancreatic cases. Certainly, it will be hard to demonstrate a clear advantage over standard laparoscopic techniques, especially to expert surgeons who have already mastered LPS techniques. The greatest advantages of the system include improved optics, magnification and lighting, depth perception, and increased range of motion and dexterity of the instrumentation. There is the ability to perform complex, difficult tasks with relative ease (Fig. 12.9). There is perhaps no better example of this than the performance of creating a hand-sewn biliary or pancreatic anastomosis. Its limitations include having to re-learn many aspects of the laparoscopic procedures that may have taken years to master. The initial learning curve of patient positioning, trocar placement, and docking of the robot to the patient is overcome with a handful of cases. The actual operative times of the dissection appear comparable to laparoscopic pancreas tail resection in our experience, although cases in which suturing was required were completed with much less effort. Early experience with the robotic-assisted laparoscopic techniques suggests these techniques to be equivalent with respect to blood

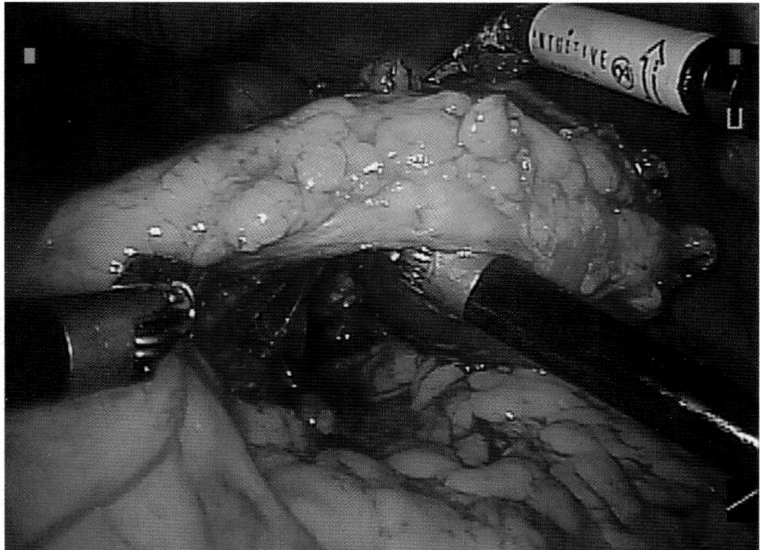

Figure 12.9

Robotic retroperitoneal dissection

loss, OR time, and convalescence, but further investigations are required.

Conclusion

Minimally invasive surgery has grown exponentially since its early days and there are now very few procedures to which these techniques have not been applied. Laparoscopic pancreatic surgery was until recently beyond the reach of most surgeons for a variety of reasons, including inexperience, lack of adequate training programs, and complexity of the anatomy and diseases. Advances in tumor localization and imaging, as well as instrumentation and robotics will hopefully aid in the utilization of LPS techniques by a larger number of surgeons who treat pancreatic neoplasms. Certainly it must have been difficult, if not impossible, for surgeons of prior generations to foresee the current widespread use of minimally invasive techniques to complicated pancreatic surgery. It is with that in mind that one must look to the future with cautious optimism and realize that many of the procedures we perform today will long be replaced by less invasive treatments.

References

1. Frankel WL (2006) Update on pancreatic endocrine tumors. Arch Pathol Lab Med 130:963–966
2. Stephen AE, Hodin RA (2006) Neuroendocrine tumors of the pancreas, excluding gastrinoma. Surg Oncol Clin N Am 15:497–510
3. Nicholls A (1902) Simple adenoma of the pancreas arising from an island of Langerhans. J Med Res 8:358–395
4. Oberndorfer S (1907) Karzinoide Tumoren des Dunndarms. Frankf Z Pathol 1:426–432
5. Kloppel G, Perren A, Heitz PU (2004) The gastroenteropancreatic neuroendocrine cell system and its tumors: the WHO classification. Ann NY Acad Sci 1014:13–27
6. Wilder R (1927) Carcinoma of the island of the pancreas, hyperinsulinism and hypoglycemia. JAMA 89:348–355
7. Hochwald SN, Zee S, Conlon KC et al (2002) Prognostic factors in pancreatic endocrine neoplasms: an analysis of 136 cases with a proposal for low-grade and intermediate-grade groups. J Clin Oncol 20:2633–2642
8. Kloppel G, Heitz PU (1988) Pancreatic endocrine tumors. Pathol Res Pract 183:155–168
9. Kent RB 3rd, van Heerden JA, Weiland LH (1981) Nonfunctioning islet cell tumors. Ann Surg 193:185–190
10. Bettini R, Boninsegna L, Mantovani W et al (2008) Prognostic factors at diagnosis and value of WHO classification in a mono-institutional series of 180 non-functioning pancreatic endocrine tumours. Ann Oncol 19:903–908
11. Chu QD, Hill HC, Douglass HO Jr. et al (2002) Predictive factors associated with long-term survival in patients with neuroendocrine tumors of the pancreas. Ann Surg Oncol 9:855–862
12. Vagefi PA, Razo O, Deshpande V et al (2007) Evolving patterns in the detection and outcomes of pancreatic neuroendocrine neoplasms: the Massachusetts General Hospital experience from 1977 to 2005. Arch Surg 142:347–354
13. Lloyd RV, Mervak T, Schmidt K, Warner TF, Wilson BS (1984) Immunohistochemical detection of chromogranin and neuron-specific enolase in pancreatic endocrine neoplasms. Am J Surg Pathol 8:607–614
14. Chang F, Chandra A, Culora G, Mahadeva U, Meenan J, Herbert A (2006) Cytologic diagnosis of pancreatic endocrine tumors by endoscopic ultrasound-guided fine-needle aspiration: a review. Diagn Cytopathol 34:649–658
15. Chetty R, Clark SP, Pitson GA (1993) Primary small cell carcinoma of the pancreas. Pathology 25:240–242
16. Ballas KD, Rafailidis SF, Demertzidis C, Alatsakis MB, Pantzaki A, Sakadamis AK (2005) Mixed exocrine-endocrine tumor of the pancreas. JOP 6:449–454
17. Carriaga MT, Henson DE (1995) Liver, gallbladder, extrahepatic bile ducts, and pancreas. Cancer 75:171–190
18. Halfdanarson TR, Rabe KG, Rubin J, Petersen GM (2008) Pancreatic neuroendocrine tumors (PNETs): incidence, prognosis and recent trend toward improved survival. Ann Oncol 19:1727–1733
19. Vortmeyer AO, Huang S, Lubensky I, Zhuang Z (2004) Non-islet origin of pancreatic islet cell tumors. J Clin Endocrinol Metab 89:1934–1938
20. Alexakis N, Connor S, Ghaneh P et al (2004) Hereditary pancreatic endocrine tumours. Pancreatology 4:417–433, discussion 34–5
21. Lepage C, Bouvier AM, Phelip JM, Hatem C, Vernet C, Faivre J (2004) Incidence and management of malignant digestive endocrine tumours in a well defined French population. Gut 53:549–553
22. Panzuto F, Nasoni S, Falconi M et al (2005) Prognostic factors and survival in endocrine tumor patients: comparison between gastrointestinal and pancreatic localization. Endocr Relat Cancer 12:1083–1092
23. Heitz PU, Kasper M, Polak JM, Kloppel G (1982) Pancreatic endocrine tumors. Hum Pathol 13:263–271
24. Soga J, Yakuwa Y (1999) Somatostatinoma/inhibitory syndrome: a statistical evaluation of 173 reported cases as compared to other pancreatic endocrinomas. J Exp Clin Cancer Res 18:13–22
25. Vinik AI, Strodel WE, Eckhauser FE, Moattari AR, Lloyd R (1987) Somatostatinomas, PPomas, neurotensinomas. Semin Oncol 14:263–281
26. Grosfeld JL, Vane DW, Rescorla FJ, McGuire W, West KW (1990) Pancreatic tumors in childhood: analysis of 13 cases. J Pediatr Surg 25:1057–1062
27. Jaksic T, Yaman M, Thorner P, Wesson DK, Filler RM, Shandling BA (1992) 20-year review of pediatric pancreatic tumors. J Pediatr Surg 27:1315–1317
28. Alexakis N, Neoptolemos JP (2008) Pancreatic neuroendocrine tumours. Best Pract Res Clin Gastroenterol 22: 183–205
29. Lewis CE, Yeh MW (2008) Inherited endocrinopathies: an update. Mol Genet Metab 94:271–282

30. Plockinger U, Rindi G, Arnold R et al (2004) Guidelines for the diagnosis and treatment of neuroendocrine gastrointestinal tumours. A consensus statement on behalf of the European Neuroendocrine Tumour Society (ENETS). Neuroendocrinology 80:394–424
31. Roy PK, Venzon DJ, Shojamanesh H et al (2000) Zollinger-Ellison syndrome. Clinical presentation in 261 patients. Medicine (Baltimore) 79:379–411
32. Corcos O, Couvelard A, Giraud S et al (2008) Endocrine pancreatic tumors in von Hippel-Lindau disease: clinical, histological, and genetic features. Pancreas 37: 85–93
33. Libutti SK, Choyke PL, Bartlett DL et al (1998) Pancreatic neuroendocrine tumors associated with von Hippel Lindau disease: diagnostic and management recommendations. Surgery 124:1153–1159
34. Fesinmeyer MD, Austin MA, Li CI, De Roos AJ, Bowen DJ (2005) Differences in survival by histologic type of pancreatic cancer. Cancer Epidemiol Biomarkers Prev 14: 1766–1773
35. Lepage C, Rachet B, Coleman MP (2007) Survival from malignant digestive endocrine tumors in England and Wales: a population-based study. Gastroenterology 132:899–904
36. Delaunoit T, Neczyporenko F, Rubin J, Erlichman C, Hobday TJ (2008) Medical management of pancreatic neuroendocrine tumors. Am J Gastroenterol 103:475-483, quiz 84
37. Kouvaraki MA, Ajani JA, Hoff P et al (2004) Fluorouracil, doxorubicin, and streptozocin in the treatment of patients with locally advanced and metastatic pancreatic endocrine carcinomas. J Clin Oncol 22:4762–4771
38. Kulke MH, Lenz HJ, Meropol NJ et al (2008) Activity of sunitinib in patients with advanced neuroendocrine tumors. J Clin Oncol 26:3403–3410
39. Williams ED, Sandler M (1963) The classification of carcinoid tum ours. Lancet 1:238–239
40. Bilimoria KY, Bentrem DJ, Merkow RP et al (2007) Application of the pancreatic adenocarcinoma staging system to pancreatic neuroendocrine tumors. J Am Coll Surg 205:558–563
41. Greene FL, Page DL, Fleming ID et al (eds) (2002) AJCC cancer staging manual, 6th edn. Springer, New York, NY
42. La Rosa S, Sessa F, Capella C et al (1996) Prognostic criteria in nonfunctioning pancreatic endocrine tumours. Virchows Arch 429:323–333
43. Weber HC, Venzon DJ, Lin JT et al (1995) Determinants of metastatic rate and survival in patients with Zollinger-Ellison syndrome: a prospective long-term study. Gastroenterology 108:1637–1649
44. Boukhman MP, Karam JM, Shaver J, Siperstein AE, DeLorimier AA, Clark OH (1999) Localization of insulinomas. Arch Surg 134:818–822, discussion 22–3
45. Mertz H, Gautam S (2004) The learning curve for EUS-guided FNA of pancreatic cancer. Gastrointest Endosc 59:33–37
46. Vilmann P, Hancke S, Henriksen FW, Jacobsen GK (1993) Endosonographically guided fine needle aspiration biopsy of malignant lesions in the upper gastrointestinal tract. Endoscopy 25:523–527
47. Assalia A, Gagner M (2004) Laparoscopic pancreatic surgery for islet cell tumors of the pancreas. World J Surg 28:1239–1247
48. Ayav A, Bresler L, Brunaud L, Boissel P (2005) Laparoscopic approach for solitary insulinoma: a multicentre study. Langenbecks Arch Surg 390:134–140
49. Pierce RA, Spitler JA, Hawkins WG et al (2007) Outcomes analysis of laparoscopic resection of pancreatic neoplasms. Surg Endosc 21:579–586
50. Gagner M, Pomp A (1994) Laparoscopic pylorus-preserving pancreatoduodenectomy. Surg Endosc 8:408–410
51. Pugliese R, Scandroglio I, Sansonna F et al (2008) Laparoscopic pancreaticoduodenectomy: a retrospective review of 19 cases. Surg Laparosc Endosc Percutan Tech 18:13–18
52. Cai X, Wang Y, Yu H, Liang X, Xu B, Peng S (2008) Completed laparoscopic pancreaticoduodenectomy. Surg Laparosc Endosc Percutan Tech 18:404–406
53. Menon KV, Hayden JD, Prasad KR, Verbeke CS (2007) Total laparoscopic pancreaticoduodenectomy and reconstruction for a cholangiocarcinoma of the bile duct. J Laparoendosc Adv Surg Tech A 17:775–780
54. Gagner M, Pomp A (1997) Laparoscopic pancreatic resection: is it worthwhile? J Gastrointest Surg 1:20–25, discussion 5–6
55. Roggin KK, Rudloff U, Blumgart LH, Brennan MF (2006) Central pancreatectomy revisited. J Gastrointest Surg 10:804–812
56. Orsenigo E, Baccari P, Bissolotti G, Staudacher C (2006) Laparoscopic central pancreatectomy. Am J Surg 191: 549–552
57. Sa Cunha A, Rault A, Beau C, Collet D, Masson B (2007) Laparoscopic central pancreatectomy: single institution experience of 6 patients. Surgery 142:405–409
58. Cuschieri A, Jakimowicz JJ, van Spreeuwel J (1996) Laparoscopic distal 70% pancreatectomy and splenectomy for chronic pancreatitis. Ann Surg 223:280–285
59. Cuschieri SA, Jakimowicz JJ (1998) Laparoscopic pancreatic resections. Semin Laparosc Surg 5:168–179
60. Fernandez-Cruz L, Cosa R, Blanco L, Levi S, Lopez-Boado MA, Navarro S (2007) Curative laparoscopic resection for pancreatic neoplasms: a critical analysis from a single institution. J Gastrointest Surg 11:1607–1621, discussion 21–2
61. Strasberg SM, Drebin JA, Linehan D (2003) Radical antegrade modular pancreatosplenectomy. Surgery 133: 521–527
62. Velanovich V (2006) The lasso technique for laparoscopic distal pancreatectomy. Surg Endosc 20:1766–1771
63. Thaker RI, Matthews BD, Linehan DC, Strasburg SM, Eagon JC, Hawkins WG (2007) Absorbable mesh reinforcement of a stapled pancreatic transection line reduces the leak rate with distal pancreatectomy. J Gastrointest Surg 11(1):59–65
64. Warshaw AL (1988) Conservation of the spleen with distal pancreatectomy. Arch Surg 123:550–553

Laparoscopic Approaches to Hepatobiliary Cancer

Michael B. Ujiki, Lee L. Swanstrom, Paul D. Hansen

Contents

Primary cancers of the liver and extrahepatic biliary tree are uncommon malignancies in North America, annually affecting approximately 30,000 people and resulting in 21,000 deaths [1]. Metastatic liver tumors, mostly from nonhepatobiliary primaries, are 15–20 times more common than primary cancers and more than 40% of people dying with cancer will have liver involvement [2, 3]. Primary and secondary liver tumors include a wide variety of cell types, as essentially any cancer can involve the liver (Table 13.1) [4]. Patients with primary or metastatic hepatic malignancies generally have a poor prognosis due to the aggressive nature of the tumors, the late onset of symptoms, and the rarity of isolated liver disease. In the past, depending on tumor type, the majority of patients died within 12 months of diagnosis [5, 6]. Recently, dramatic improvements have been made in the medical and surgical management of metastatic hepatic tumors in particular, so that studies are now more commonly reporting 5 and 10 year survival rates [7–9]. Modern chemotherapeutics are more effective and have expanded the number of patients suitable for potential curative resection which has led to an increase in survival for many cancers after resection [10–12].

Multimodality approaches play a large role in the curative treatment for hepatobiliary and secondary malignancies and include chemotherapy, ablative therapies, and surgical resection [13–15]. Adjuvant chemotherapy, chemoembolization, ablation, and, rarely, radiotherapy play a role in palliative treatment [16]. In those with hepatobiliary cancer that are incurable, treatment outcomes must be expressed not only in terms of survival rates but also in terms of quality of life. Therapeutic goals may be best achieved by avoiding aggressive interventions in futile cases and successful palliation when possible. Based on this assumption, the current therapy for treatment of hepatobiliary cancer can be summarized by the precepts of:

F.L. Greene, B.T. Heniford (eds.), *Minimally Invasive Cancer Management*,
DOI 10.1007/978-1-4419-1238-1_13,

Table 13.1. Primary and metastatic tumors of the liver

Primary hepatobiliary cancers
Hepatocellular
Fibrolamellar
Cholangiocarcinoma
Gallbladder cancer
Angiosarcoma
Leiomyosarcoma
Rhabdomyosarcoma
Fibrosarcoma
Mesenchymal sarcoma
Metastatic liver tumors
Bronchogenic
Colon
Pancreas
Breast
Stomach
Unknown primary
Ovary
Prostate
Gallbladder
Cervix
Kidney
Melanoma
Bladder/ureter
Esophagus
Testis
Endometrial
Thyroid

Metastatic liver tumors are listed in order of number of autopsies with hepatic metastasis. Data are obtained from Los Angeles County University of Southern California Medical Center [1970–1979] and John Wesley County Hospital [1960–1976].

- accurate diagnosis
- careful selection of patients and surgery
- aggressive treatment when appropriate

Because of inherent difficulties in studying surgical outcomes in patients with metastatic disease, the effectiveness of many therapeutic interventions for these patients has been difficult to assess. The rarity of isolated hepatic tumors and the perceived hopeless prognosis disincline many treating physicians from further referral of these patients for inclusion in outcome trials. This is compounded by a reluctance to subject patients with advanced disease to extensive surgical morbidity with dubious survival benefit [17, 18]. The introduction of minimally invasive surgical (MIS) techniques for accurate diagnosis and staging and less morbid treatment should generate a wider acceptance of surgical intervention. This in turn may help generate the outcome data needed to accurately inform patients of the benefits of palliative therapy and the likelihood of success from curative therapy.

Nonsurgical, minimally invasive therapy has long played a major role in the treatment of patients with hepatobiliary cancer. Advanced radiologic techniques, both diagnostic and interventional, have been crucial in staging, determining resectability, treatment, and palliation [19–21]. Flexible endoscopy, particularly endoscopic retrograde cholangiopancreatography (ERCP) and, more recently, endoscopic ultrasound (EUS), has also had a large and growing role in the diagnosis, staging, and palliation of cancer patients [22]. Minimally invasive surgical treatments primarily rely on laparoscopic techniques. Laparoscopy, much like advanced radiologic imaging and flexible endoscopy, has demonstrated a vital role in the staging and palliation [23–28], as well as presenting a potential role in curing these cancer patients [29].

The use of the laparoscope as a diagnostic and staging tool goes back 90 years. Jacobaeus [30] described in 1911 its use in 187 patients, and innumerable others have supported its accuracy and utility since that time [23, 27, 29]. Improved video technology, better instrumentation, broader recognition of the possibilities of MIS techniques, and an increasing awareness of the benefits associated with MIS techniques (Table 13.2) have led to a paradigm shift in general surgery. There is tremendous potential for laparoscopy, even in the technically demanding field of hepatobiliary surgery. The addition of laparoscopic ultrasound, in particular, has improved the ability of the surgeon to stage patients with hepatobiliary cancers by allowing the identification of involved lymph nodes, invasion of vital structures, and dissemination of intrahepatic tumors [23–25]. Other technologies, such as radiofrequency ablation (RFA) and cryotherapy, are uniquely applicable to laparoscopic access and have shown promise as palliative and possibly curative approaches to hepatic tumors [29, 31]. Finally, laparoscopic surgical skills in some institutions have progressed enough to allow the performance of safe hepatic resections that can reproduce standard curative techniques [32–36]. Much work

Table 13.2. Potential and proven benefits of laparoscopic surgery

Operative
Improved visualization
Visual magnification
Reduced blood loss
Reduced fluid shifts
Less adhesion formation
Recovery
Less postoperative pain
Reduced postoperative narcotic requirement
Earlier ambulation
Improved perioperative pulmonary function
Fewer wound complications
Reduced perioperative immune suppression
Shorter postoperative recovery time

still remains to be done in the development, validation, and teaching of these techniques before widespread utilization can occur.

General Considerations

The ability to overcome purely technical obstacles in the application of MIS techniques has been widely demonstrated throughout all of general surgery. Problems inherent in the laparoscopic approach to cancer surgery were suggested by early reports describing missed cancers, inadequate tumor margins, and the development of port-site metastasis [37, 38]. Subsequent trials involving well-trained laparoscopic surgeons comparing laparoscopic vs. open colectomies for colon cancer have shown that these early concerns were related to technical errors that disappear when classic oncologic surgical principles were applied [39–41]. Similarly, as experience with hepatobiliary surgery has increased, the ability to perform safe hilar dissections, to isolate and control large vascular structures, to safely transect the hepatic parenchyma, and to ensure adequate tumor margins has and will continue to improve [42–46].

The equipment and skills required to perform laparoscopic hepatobiliary surgery vary widely depending on the procedure being performed. Basic staging laparoscopy can be accomplished, using fairly simple instrumentation, by any surgeon with a sound foundation in the basics of laparoscopic surgery. More advanced procedures require additional skills, including the ability to perform laparoscopic ultrasound, retroperitoneal dissections, advanced bowel manipulation, solid organ resection, and laparoscopic suturing. In addition, hybrid techniques, such as hand-assisted laparoscopy, may play a transitional role in some procedures. Several of the instruments found to be helpful in performing hepatobiliary procedures are listed in Table 13.3. Adequate training should be obtained by the surgeon before attempting even the

Table 13.3. Instrumentation used in advanced laparoscopic hepatobiliary procedures

	Comment
Scopes	
Three-chip camera	For highest quality image
Large-format monitors	
Xenon light source	
5 mm or 10 mm, 30°–45° angled laparoscope	Provides control of visual perspective
1.7–3.0 mm "mini" laparoscope	For diagnostic laparoscopy only
Instruments	
Liver retractor	
Atraumatic grasper	Allows manipulation of bowel for staging
Fine-tipped dissector	Allows dissection of vascular structures
Right-angle dissector	
Bipolar scissors	
Harmonic shears	
Retractable scalpel	
Suction – Irrigation	
Monopolar cautery	
Needle drivers	
Parenchymal division	
Harmonic shears	Slow, but generally reliable hemostasis
CUSA	Very slow, requires the use of numerous clips
Clip appliers	Single or multifire
GIA staplers	Triple rows of staples for vascular control

Table 13.3. (continued)

	Comment
Additional equipment	
Ultrasound	5–7.5 MHz, flexible tip, color flow
Argon beam coagulation	Must vent peritoneum during use
Biopsy needles	8 in. or longer
Radiofrequency ablation	
Cryotherapy	
Thrombogenic agents	

most basic laparoscopic procedures on patients with liver and bile duct cancers. Inexperience can lead to misdiagnosis, perioperative complications, inadequate margins, tumor spillage, or inadequate staging. Early in surgeons' learning curve, they should seek assistance from an experienced proctor to safely develop the necessary skills.

Laparoscopy and Immune Function

Early in the laparoscopic experience with oncologic disease, a small number of animal studies suggested that CO_2 pneumoperitoneum might cause an increase in tumor dissemination and/or growth rate [47, 48]. Only limited data have supported this and conversely, more recent long-term data have shown similar if not improved oncologic outcomes associated with laparoscopy [41, 49].

Immune function is known to be suppressed by surgical trauma, and the degree of immune suppression correlates with the severity of the surgical trauma [50–53]. Since laparoscopic surgery is associated with less trauma than open surgery, it can be assumed that laparoscopic surgery also causes less trauma-related immune suppression. Cortisol, catecholamines, and cytokines are markers of physiologic stress and immune response and are altered by surgical trauma [54–58]. Changes in serum levels of these markers are significantly reduced following laparoscopic surgery when compared to a corresponding open surgery (Table 13.4). Delayed type II hypersensitivity, another marker of humoral immune response, has been demonstrated to be more suppressed by laparotomy than laparoscopy in both animal models and human trials [50, 52, 53, 59]. Further, there is

Table 13.4. Markers of immune function that may be altered in laparoscopic or open surgery

	Change in open versus laparoscopic surgery
Cytokines	
TNF alpha	Unchanged
IL-1	Increased
IL-6	Increased
IL-8	Increased
Neuroendocrine	
Cortisol	Unchanged
Catecholamines	Increased
DTH[a]	Suppressed

[a] DTH = delayed type hypersensitivity response.

evidence from animal experiments demonstrating a reduced rate of tumor implantation, tumor spread, and tumor growth in laparoscopic vs. open surgical procedures [47, 50, 60]. All of these data are preliminary, but draw attention to the limited understanding we have regarding the possible long-term effects of laparoscopic surgery for cancer.

Laparoscopic Staging and Determination of Resectability

Staging for hepatobiliary malignancies depends on the size of the primary tumor, on the depth of invasion, the presence of vascular invasion, the involvement of adjacent organs, and the presence of nodal involvement and metastasis (Table 13.5). The tumor, node, metastasis (TNM) staging criteria of the American Joint Committee on Cancer are the most frequently used staging system for both liver and extrahepatic biliary malignancies. Accurate staging is critical to optimize the care of hepatobiliary cancer patients. Since cure depends in almost all cases on the total eradication of the cancer and the absence of nodal or extrahepatic disease, the determination of resectability is crucial [14, 61, 62]. This determination should be accomplished in the least invasive way.

Preoperative evaluation of hepatobiliary cancers always includes diagnostic imaging. The value of diagnostic imaging to accurately stage most hepatobiliary cancers cannot be understated [25, 63]. Modalities of diagnostic imaging, such as contrast-enhanced

Table 13.5. Tumor, node, metastasis staging of hepatobiliary cancers

	Primary tumor	Regional lymph nodes	Distant metastasis
Liver (including intrahepatic bile ducts)	**TX** Primary tumor cannot be assessed	**NX** Regional lymph nodes cannot be assessed	**MX** Distant metastasis cannot be assessed
	T0 No evidence of primary tumor	**N0** No regional lymph node metastasis	**M0** No distant metastasis
	T1 Solitary tumor without vascular invasion	**N1** Regional lymph node metastasis	**M1** Distant metastasis
	T2 Solitary tumor with vascular invasion or multiple tumors none more than 5 cm		
	T3 Multiple tumors more than 5 cm or tumor involving a major branch of the portal or hepatic vein(s)		
	T4 Tumor(s) with direct invasion of adjacent organs other than the gallbladder or with perforation of visceral peritoneum		
Gall bladder	**TX** Primary tumor cannot be assessed	**NX** Regional lymph nodes cannot be assessed	**MX** Distant metastasis cannot be assessed
	T0 No evidence of primary tumor	**N0** No regional lymph node metastasis	**M0** No distant metastasis
	Tis Carcinoma in situ		
	T1 Tumor invades lamina propria or muscle layer	**N1** Regional lymph node metastasis	**M1** Distant metastasis
	T1a Tumor invades lamina própria		
	T1b Tumor invades muscle layer		
	T2 Tumor invades perimuscular connective tissue; no extension beyond serosa or into liver		
	T3 Tumor perforates the serosa (visceral peritoneum) and/or directly invades the liver and/or one other adjacent organ or structure, such as the stomach, duodenum, colon, pancreas, omentum, or extrahepatic bile duct		
	T4 Tumor invades the main portal vein or hepatic artery or invades multiple extrahepatic organs or structures		
Extrahepatic Bile Ducts	**TX** Primary tumor cannot be assessed	**NX** Regional lymph nodes cannot be assessed	**MX** Distant metastasis cannot be assessed
	T0 No evidence of primary tumor	**N0** No regional lymph node metastasis	**M0** No distant metastasis
	Tis Carcinoma in situ		

Table 13.5. (continued)

	Primary tumor	Regional lymph nodes	Distant metastasis
	T1 Tumor confined to the bile duct	**N1** Regional lymph node metastasis	**M1** Distant metastasis
	T2 Tumor invades beyond the wall of the bile duct		
	T3 Tumor invades the liver, gall bladder, pancreas, and/or unilateral branches of the portal vein (right or left) or hepatic artery (right or left)		
	T4 Tumor invades any of the following: main portal vein or its branches bilaterally, common hepatic artery, or other adjacent structures, such as the colon, stomach, duodenum, or abdominal wall		

Used with permission of the American Joint Committee on Cancer (AJCC®), Chicago, Illinois. The original source for this material is the AJCC Cancer Staging Manual, Sixth Edition (2002) published by Springer Science and Business Media LLC, www.springerlink.com

spiral computed tomography (CT), magnetic resonance imaging (MRI), visceral angiography, EUS, and positron emission tomography (PET) scans, can determine the size and anatomic relationships of the primary tumor, detect invasion of vasculature or adjacent organs, and identify distant metastases (Figs. 13.1 and 13.2) [20, 64, 65]. Most imaging studies are less accurate at determining the status of lymph node metastases, detecting the presence of carcinomatosis, or identifying small satellite lesions [63]. Put another way, radiologic imaging is least accurate in differentiating the subtleties of stages II, III and early stage IV disease. Radiologically guided percutaneous biopsy is an excellent method of obtaining tissue to confirm staging and diagnosis (Fig. 13.3) [19]. When percutaneous biopsies cannot be obtained due to anatomic considerations or technical constraints, laparoscopy can play an important role.

Indications for laparoscopic staging procedures include as follows:

- Obtaining tissue samples

  When percutaneous needle biopsy is contraindicated
  When percutaneous biopsy fails to access lesion or obtain sufficient tissue to make a diagnosis
  When large amounts of tissue are needed for an accurate pathologic diagnosis

- When standard imaging techniques are inconclusive or require confirmation

  Radiologist's report is noncommittal
  Borderline staging would change treatment discussions
  Imaging studies conflict

- Determining the resectability of a primary or secondary hepatobiliary cancer

  Evaluating ascites
  Examining for carcinomatosis

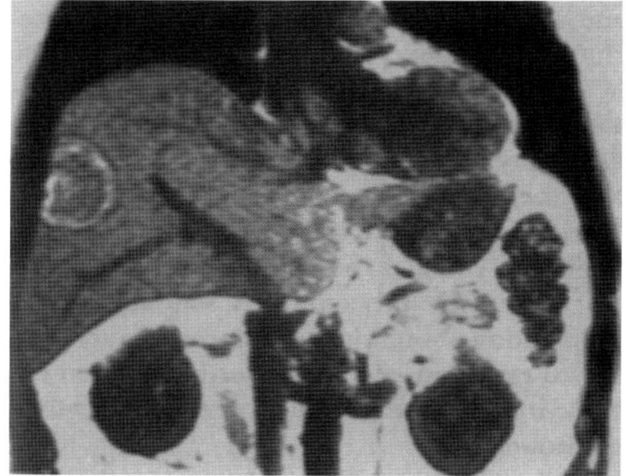

Figure 13.1
Magnetic Resonance Imaging (MRI) showing metastatic colorectal carcinoma

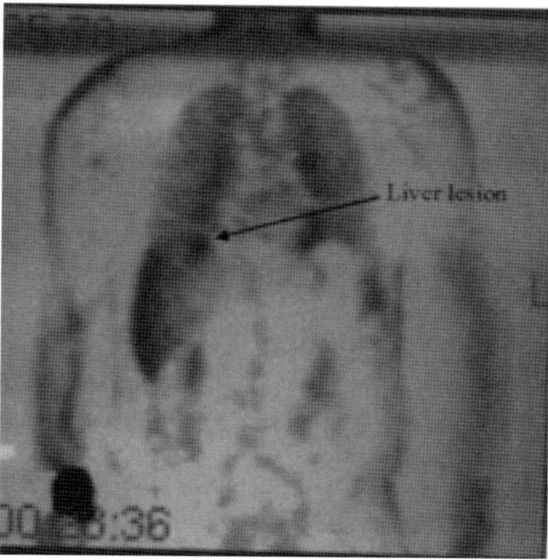

Figure 13.2

Positron Emission Tomography (PET) scans provide sensitive detection of hepatic metastasis

Identifying satellite lesions or bilobar hepatic metastasis
Identifying vascular invasion (with laparoscopic ultrasound)
Identifying retroperitoneal adenopathy (with ultrasound and/or biopsy)
Identifying invasion of adjacent structures

- When laparoscopic surgery for another reason is indicated.

Laparoscopic Staging Techniques for Hepatobiliary Cancer

Laparoscopic staging may be done as a one- or two-stage procedure [27, 28]. In a one-stage procedure, the definitive procedure is undertaken immediately in the absence of contraindications to curative or palliative treatment. A two-stage method allows a thoughtful analysis of the laparoscopic findings, thorough histologic review of biopsies, and full consultation and informed consent with the patient and cancer care team. Table 13.6 lists the surgical findings that would traditionally make a hepatobiliary cancer patient inoperable. The downside to performing laparoscopic staging as a separate procedure is the added risk, inconvenience, and cost of a separate surgical procedure, as well as the possibility that it may result in some delay in the patient's definitive treatment.

Patient preparation should begin with adequate informed consent regarding the procedure and why it is being performed. This will preclude a patient's confusion following a surgery in which "nothing was done." Nasogastric tubes are rarely needed, but the anesthetist should decompress the stomach with an orogastric tube before laparoscopic access is obtained. The patient should void before entering the operating room or be catheterized at the beginning of the procedure. A standard bowel preparation should be

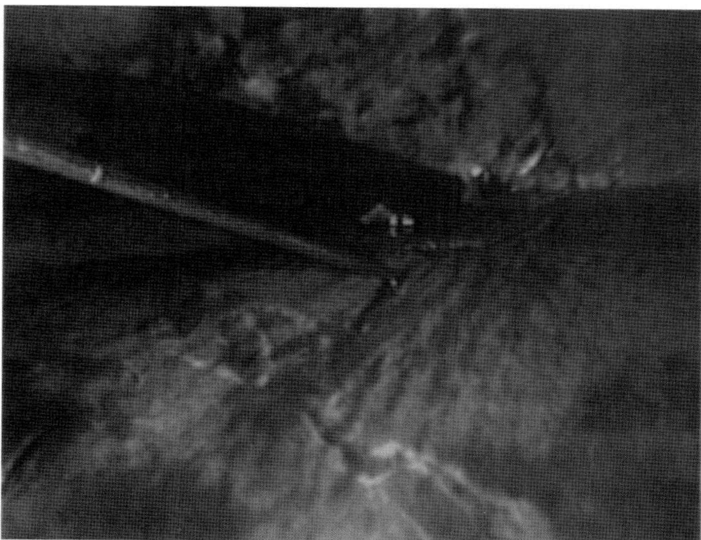

Figure 13.3

Laparoscopic image directed biopsy is a useful and accurate method of obtaining a tissue diagnosis

Table 13.6. Local and distant factors that make hepatobiliary tumors unresectable

Local
Bilobar or diffuse disease
Inadequate residual hepatic parenchyma
Incorporation of vital vascular structures
Incorporation of vital biliary structures
Invasion of adjacent viscera
Unsuspected cirrhosis
Portal vein thrombosis
Distant
Carcinomatosis
Extrahepatic metastasis
Involved portal, para-celiac, or periaortic lymph nodes

considered if retroperitoneal exploration is to be performed and because it makes it easier and safer to manipulate the bowel.

Patients are positioned supine with both arms padded and tucked to allow the surgeon full access to all quadrants of the abdomen. Initial access is typically obtained via the umbilicus with a 5- or 10-mm trocar and laparoscope. Additional trocars are placed under direct vision and can be 5 mm or smaller unless laparoscopic ultrasound is being used. In today's operating room, laparoscopic ultrasound should be considered a routine part of a staging procedure. All current commercially available laparoscopic ultrasound probes require 10 mm trocar access. For hepatobiliary work, the ultrasound probe port should be placed within reach of the porta hepatis and the right and left domes of the liver.

Staging laparoscopic examinations should proceed in a systematic fashion and include all areas of the abdominal cavity (see Chapter 3). This will minimize the chance of missing a critical finding. Initial exam includes the omentum and root of the mesentery, deep pelvis, anterior abdominal wall, right and left paracolic gutters, left hemidiaphragm and spleen, and right hemidiaphragm. Close attention should be paid to the liver, porta hepatis, gallbladder, and peripancreatic areas. Inspection is made of the serosal surface of the liver and perihepatic peritoneal surfaces using an angled laparoscope as well as an atraumatic grasper to help provide exposure to deeper areas of interest such as Morrison's pouch, the anterior stomach wall, and the right hemidiaphragm.

The goal of inspection is to detect unresectable disease and to assess the primary tumor, its size, and its relationship to critical adjacent structures. In addition, laparoscopy allows the assessment of any non-cancer-related anatomic abnormalities, such as adhesions, evidence of portal hypertension, or organomegaly, which may affect the possibility of definitive surgery or future therapies. It is helpful to record all abnormal findings with photographs or on videotape for later review and pathologic correlation (Fig. 13.4). The magnification offered by laparoscopy allows the surgeon to detect even small, subtle peritoneal or serosal abnormalities, which should always be biopsied. Suspected deep masses should have a needle biopsy with frozen section. Such biopsies should be done only under laparoscopic ultrasound guidance to avoid injury to deeper structures. The key element of the staging laparoscopy is visual inspection; palpation, the key to open staging exams, is less important in laparoscopy but can still play a role. Careful palpation with a blunt laparoscopic tool can provide some feedback, particularly about larger, deep lesions in the retroperitoneum or liver, which can then be biopsied under ultrasound guidance.

Minilaparoscopy

As the result of improvements in technology, laparoscopes, laparoscopic cameras, and laparoscopic instrumentation have become progressively smaller and of higher quality [66]. Current laparoscopes measuring 3 mm in diameter offer the same resolution and illumination as 10 mm scopes of the past. Likewise, laparoscopic instruments have adopted new alloys and construction techniques to allow very small yet functional instruments to be designed (Fig. 13.5). The field of minilaparoscopy has generated enormous interest from surgeons. Aside from improved cosmesis and decreased pain, there are hopes that minilaparoscopy will eventually facilitate outpatient procedures such as staging laparoscopy to be performed under local anesthesia and perhaps in an office setting [67]. This would contribute to the acceptance and cost-effectiveness of preoperative staging laparoscopy.

Laparoscopic Ultrasound

Laparoscopic ultrasound probes have dramatically increased the ability of laparoscopic surgeons to stage

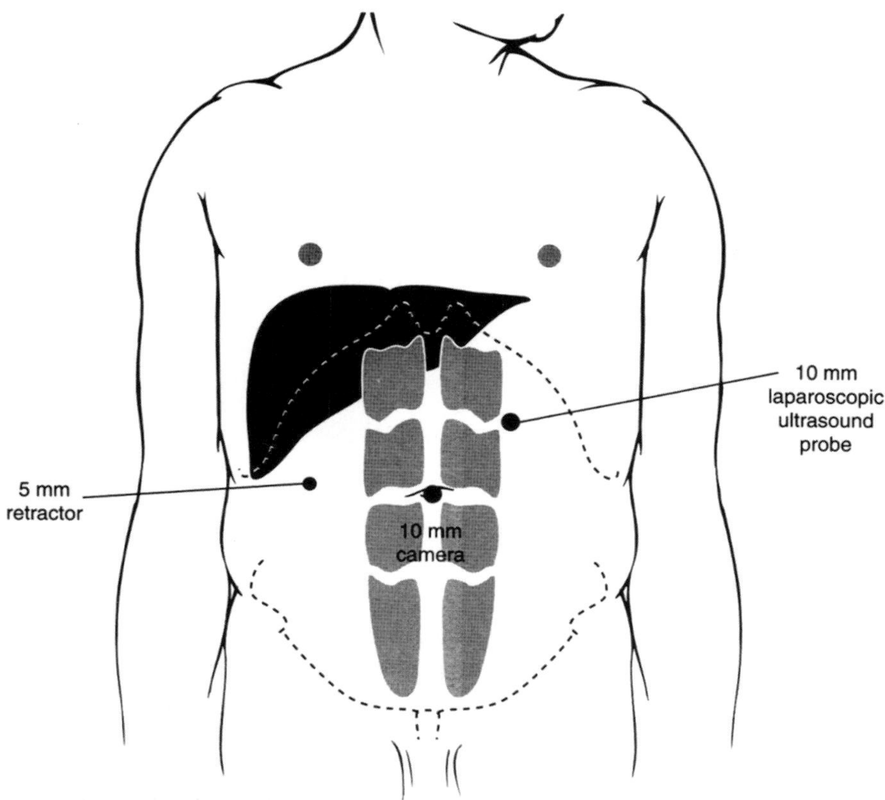

Figure 13.4
Typical port placement for laparoscopic ultrasound

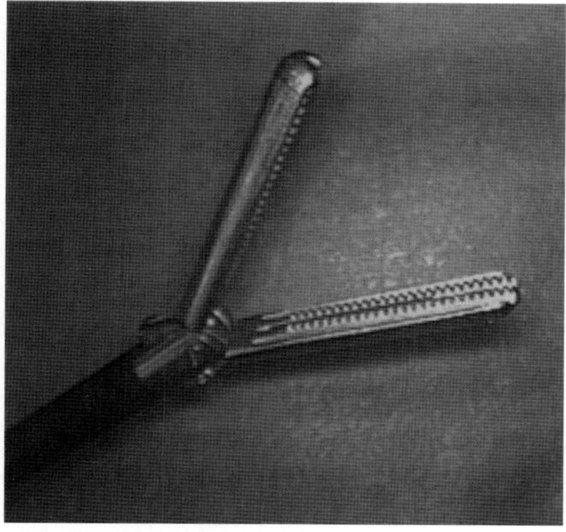

Figure 13.5
3 mm and smaller laparoscopic instruments allow even less invasive staging procedures

hepatobiliary cancers with a high degree of accuracy [23, 25]. They have become mandatory equipment in centers performing even a moderate amount of staging laparoscopy. Several companies have produced ultrasound handpieces that fit through a 10-mm port (Fig. 13.6). These handpieces have several configurations, including articulating and non-articulating tips with 5–7.5 MHz linear or curvilinear arrays. Most recently, prototype handpieces with guides for needle biopsy have been developed. For most hepatobiliary staging procedures, the flexible-tip, curvilinear-array handpieces offer the widest applicability. Successful use of laparoscopic ultrasound requires a fair degree of experience and familiarity both with standard open intraoperative ultrasonography and with manipulating the probe through a laparoscopic port. The fixed entry point in laparoscopy is initially disorienting and requires thoughtful placement of the ultrasound port.

It is helpful to establish a routine scanning pattern to use in all cases of hepatobiliary staging. We recommend

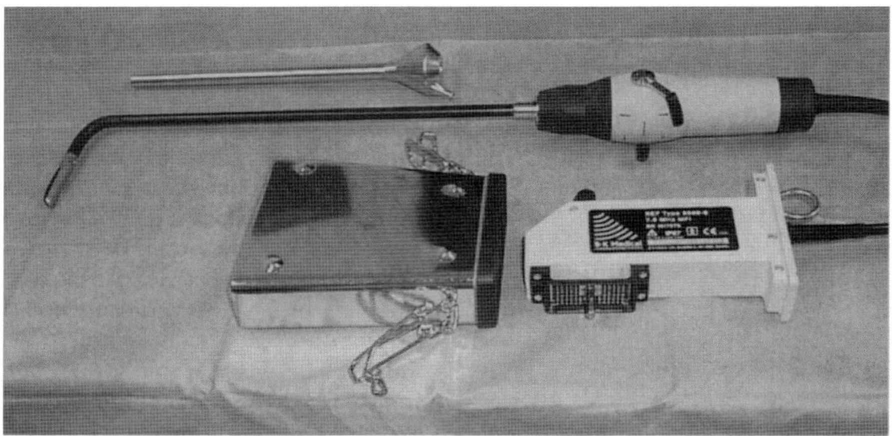

Figure 13.6

Laparoscopic ultrasound probe

placement of the ultrasound access port at or above the umbilicus. Scanning should start with the lateral right lobe of the liver and move medially. Transhepatic views of the retroperitoneum, gallbladder, vena cava, and porta hepatis should be obtained as the probe is progressively moved toward the falciform ligament. The left lateral segments of the liver should next be scanned starting from the left side of the falciform ligament and moving laterally. During the left-sided sweep, transhepatic views of the celiac plexus, periaortic nodes, and portal vein are visible. Direct views of the porta hepatis, paraceliac, and periaortic areas are also required (Figs. 13.7, 13.8, 13.9). Biopsies of suspicious masses should be obtained either by excising them laparoscopically or, for deep lesions, with core needle biopsy. If a biopsy needle guide is not available for the handpiece being used, the biopsy must be performed freehand, which requires more laparoscopic skill and experience. Again, any findings that would render the patient unresectable should be noted and clearly described. Photodocumentation (which is available as a feature on most ultrasound machines) can be helpful later in determining the patient's therapy.

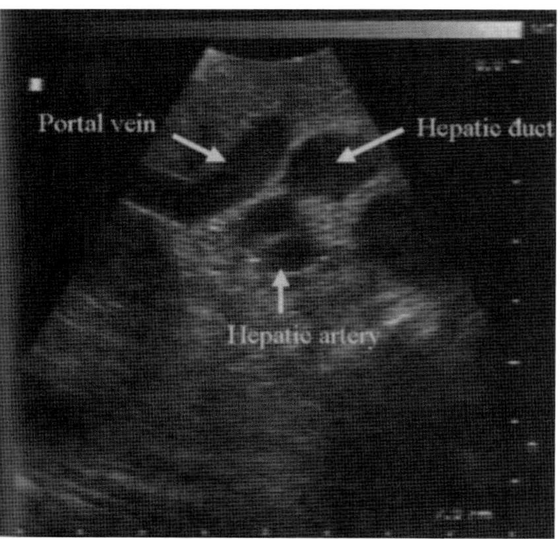

Figure 13.7

Ultrasound of the liver should always include views of the porta hepatis

Biopsy Techniques

It is often important to obtain tissue samples either of unsuspected findings or of the primary tumor in order to determine stage or tissue type. There are several methods for obtaining such biopsies, ranging from peritoneal washings to total excision. Peritoneal washings are easily done laparoscopically, requiring little more than a laparoscopic suction/irrigator and the ability to capture 300 cc of irrigation fluid. The utility of peritoneal washings is limited, as most patients with positive washings have otherwise identifiable evidence

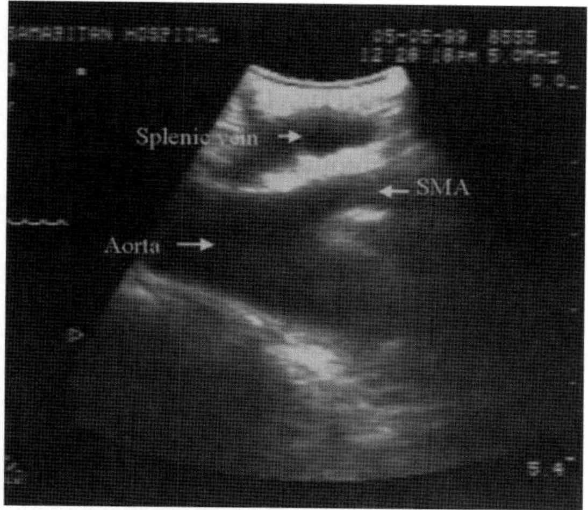

Figure 13.8
The celiac plexus, periaortic, and periportal areas should be carefully scanned

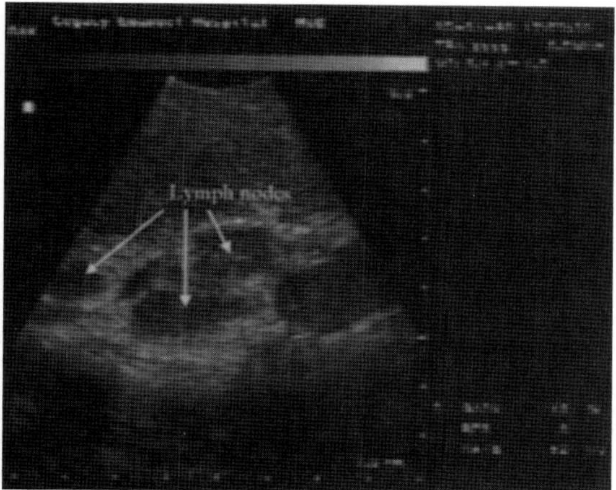

Figure 13.9
Laparoscopic ultrasound is accurate at determining unresectability due to vascular inversion, extrahepatic spread, or positive lymph nodes

of advanced disease [27, 68]. Needle biopsy is done either using a fine needle histologic technique or, more commonly, using a core needle biopsy. Core biopsies have a better diagnostic yield because they provide more information on tissue architecture. Any needle biopsy device should be at least 8 in. long to allow it to traverse the abdominal wall and the pneumoperitoneum to reach the target tissue. Incisional biopsy can be performed with a laparoscopic scissors or ultrasonic shears or by using endoscopic stapling devices to perform a true wedge biopsy (Fig. 13.10). The choice of technique depends on the position of the tumor and on the amount of tissue required. Any tissue specimen removed should be protected from contact with the abdominal wall tract either by making sure it is within the cannula of a needle, or by placing it into an intracorporeal tissue sack (e.g., cut-off thumb from a surgical glove) for retrieval.

Procedure Completion

At the completion of the staging laparoscopy, several procedures should be routinely followed. A final survey of the abdomen should be performed to ensure adequate hemostasis and the absence of injury to any viscera. Access ports should be withdrawn under direct vision to ensure that the port site is not bleeding. An effort should be made to completely evacuate the pneumoperitoneum to minimize postoperative referred pain. All port sites larger than 10 mm should undergo fascial closure. There are many techniques for this, but all should include the closure of the posterior fascia to minimize the chance of a postoperative Richter's-type hernia. Patients can often be discharged the same day following a brief recovery period. Two to 4 days of oral narcotics may be needed after discharge.

Results

Staging laparoscopy has been available for many years, and the usefulness and accuracy of laparoscopy with ultrasound as a staging tool has been evaluated by many authors and for many malignancies. Hepatobiliary malignancies, in particular, are well suited to staging laparoscopy with ultrasound. Despite the tremendous advances in imaging of the hepatobiliary system, modern series still report 20–30% unresectability rates at laparotomy [69]. The rate is even higher (50–75%) for extrahepatic biliary tumors such as gallbladder cancer and common bile duct tumors [70]. Given these high rates and the fact that unresectable disease found through laparoscopy may save days in the hospital as well as cost (especially

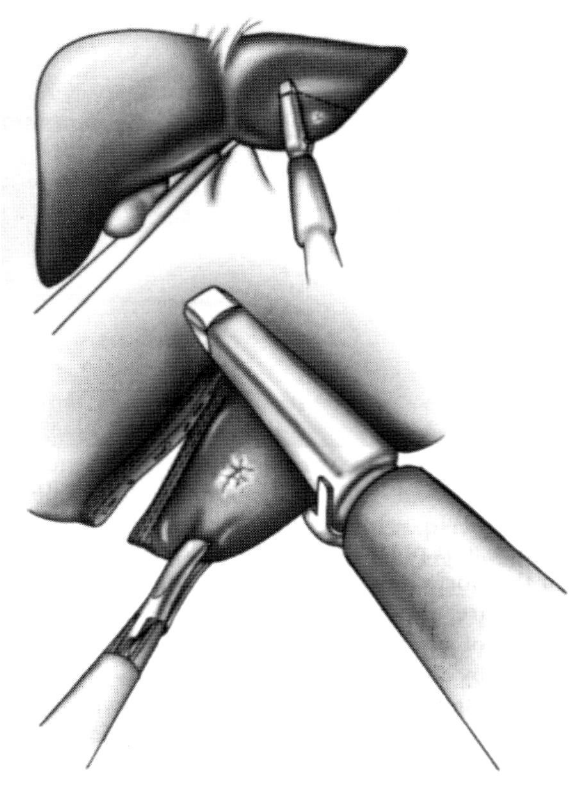

Figure 13.10

Large wedge biopsies can be obtained with the ultrasonic scissors or by use of the endoscopic GIA

important in the current economic climate), few can argue against the utility of staging laparoscopy for hepatobiliary tumors. Thaler et al. and Pomel et al. each reported that when patients were taken to the operating room for surgical management of colorectal liver metastases, 50% of procedures were altered by findings at staging laparoscopy with intraoperative ultrasound [71, 72]. The principle findings were extrahepatic disease, unexpected nodal and peritoneal disease, and the identification of additional intrahepatic tumors.

D'Angelica et al., recently reported the results of 401 patients followed prospectively after staging laparoscopy for hepatobiliary tumors [73]. The authors found that 21% of patients were unresectable and nearly all were spared laparotomy. Resectability increased from 62 to 78% with only a 22% false-negative rate. Vascular invasion and lymph node metastases were the most difficult to identify laparoscopically. If patients went on to laparotomy, staging laparoscopy added 30 min to the procedure time, but overall significantly decreased hospital length of stay and cost if laparotomy was not performed. As preoperative staging techniques improve, staging laparoscopy may become more of a selective tool, but for now it appears to continue to have advantages both for the patient and for surgeon.

Indications for Laparoscopic Surgery in Patients with Hepatobiliary Cancers

The morbidity associated with open surgical palliation is well described. Laparotomy for biliary or duodenal bypass in patients with unresectable pancreatic head tumors has a morbidity of 29–40% and a 30-day mortality of 14–31% [22, 74]. Following exploratory laparotomy, patients generally spend 5–10 days in the hospital and another 6–8 weeks recovering at home. With a limited life expectancy and little chance of cure for these patients, many physicians believe it is useless to expose patients with poor prognosis to any surgical intervention. More recent advances in endoscopic stenting of the biliary and intestinal tract have resulted in less need for surgical palliative procedures. There are still some situations in which endoscopic approaches are not possible and for these,

be used for mobilization and even parenchymal transection. Saline-linked cautery (Tissue Link EndoSH2.0 Sealing Hook) is another device preferred by some due to a near bloodless transection through precoagulation [46]. Some have suggested and reported the use of radiofrequency energy during transection [44].

Hand-Assisted Laparoscopic Resection

Hand-assisted techniques may be useful to control blood loss, and the additional incision may facilitate specimen extraction. These techniques are particularly useful in surgeries where inflow control is not performed, such as sectional or segmental resections. In these cases, the hand can be used for assistance in mobilization, parenchymal transection, and digital control of hemorrhage. A number of different hand-port devices are currently marketed. Hand assistance requires an incision length, in centimeters, that is equivalent to the glove size of the surgeon. The incision is made away from the operative field to keep the assisting hand from obstructing the camera's view (Fig. 13.13). Typically, operating surgeons use their nondominant hand to retract, expose, and compress the cut surface of the liver.

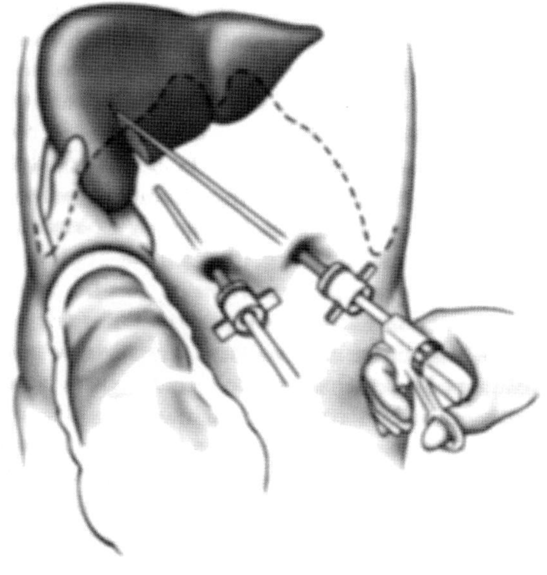

Figure 13.13

Hand-assisted laparoscopy is a useful tool, particularly for extensive, formal liver resection

Laparoscopy-Assisted Open Resection

Similar to the hand-assisted technique described earlier, a vertical incision just below the xiphoid is created for a hand port, but through it, open hilar dissections and even portions of the parenchymal transection can be performed under direct vision. Mobilization of the target lobe is carried out in a hand-assisted fashion. This technique is ideal for hepatobiliary surgeons early in their laparoscopic experience.

Following excision, the specimen may be placed in a nonpermeable specimen bag and extracted through the hand-port site. In the absence of a hand port for specimen retrieval, one of the lower and midline port sites is enlarged to a size adequate for extraction. If pathologic evaluation of tumor margin is not required, the specimen may be placed in a nonpermeable specimen bag, morcellated, and extracted piecemeal. It may be helpful to place ink in the specimen bag prior to morcellization to mark the exterior of the specimen. The excess ink is aspirated and the specimen fractured and removed. As the tumor is extracted, inked tissue can give helpful information regarding the proximity of the margin to the tumor.

Although CO_2 embolization has not been described during laparoscopic liver resection, careful measures should nevertheless be routinely applied to minimize the risk. Pneumoperitoneum pressures should be kept as low as possible while allowing adequate visualization (8–12 mmHg). The CVP should be kept at 12 mmHg and the patient should be maintained in a slight Trendelenburg position during parenchymal division. Major hepatic veins should be identified with ultrasound and controlled at the earliest reasonable stage of the resection. Medium-sized hepatic veins (3–5 mm) should be controlled with clips or sutures, but primary hepatic veins may need to be controlled with a vascular stapler.

For a left lateral segmentectomy, the patient is placed supine in a split leg position. Four or five ports are placed in a subcostal array extending as far left as possible. The falciform ligament is divided from the round ligament to the suprahepatic vena cava. The left triangular ligament is divided to the left side of the vena cava. This will allow identification of the left hepatic vein, although bulky tumors can sometimes make this exposure difficult. The gastrohepatic ligament is divided from the hepatoduodenal ligament to the right crus. An ultrasound evaluation of the liver will demonstrate the location of the tumor to be resected and identify the left portal vein, left hepatic artery, left hepatic duct, and left hepatic vein. The capsule of the liver is scored along the planned line of dissection. The falciform ligament is grasped and retracted anteriorly. The bridge of liver tissue overlying the hilum of the left lateral segment is divided with the harmonic shears. This dissection is continued starting on the free lower anterior edge of the liver following the previously scored line. The portal structures entering segments two and three are identified and divided with a firing of an endoscopic linear cutting stapler. Progressive parenchymal division is continued with slow, steady use of the harmonic shears. The left hepatic vein is ultimately encountered and divided with a vascular stapler. At the completion of the resection the cut surface is inspected for hemorrhage or bile leak. These are controlled by ABC or suture ligation as appropriate. The specimen is placed in a nonpermeable specimen bag and retrieved through an extended incision or by morcellation.

Technique for Ablation

There are several modalities available for hepatic tumor ablation. The most commonly used methods are RFA and ethanol injection. These techniques can be applied percutaneously, laparoscopically, or at open laparotomy. There are advantages and disadvantages to each.

The percutaneous approach is the least invasive approach, but also the one with the least control. A percutaneous approach may be used to ablate lesions that are small, not peripherally located, and accessible by CT or ultrasound-guided needle placement. Occasionally a patient is felt to be too high risk for general anesthesia and may be approached percutaneously regardless of staging. One must be careful with this indication, however, as many patients have substantial discomfort associated with RFA under sedation and may require general anesthesia to complete the procedure.

Heating tumors may also injure adjacent viscera. In the laboratory we have induced full-thickness injuries to adjacent viscera when RFA was performed near the surface of the liver [93]. Scudamore et al. [94] have demonstrated similar injuries to the diaphragm, although these are clinically less concerning. Finally, it is probably mandatory to fully stage a patient prior to undertaking potentially complicated ablative procedures, and this is best done by an operative approach.

Our preferred approach for tumor ablation is laparoscopic. The patient is placed supine. If RFA or ethanol is being used, no specific preparative measures are taken. A complete staging laparoscopy is undertaken as described above. The presence of extrahepatic tumor is a contraindication for local treatment. Tumor biopsies are obtained for any suspicious findings. Surrounding viscera must be separated from the surface of the liver adjacent to the tumor and protected with packs or laparoscopic retractors.

Needle or probe placement is guided by real-time ultrasound (Fig. 13.14). To assure perfect placement, it is vital to obtain biplanar views demonstrating the probe tip centrally located within the target. When placement is confirmed, the ablation is performed. Ethanol injection is the simplest technique. The tumor is injected with 95% alcohol using a volume equal to the estimated volume of the tumor. Ethanol works best on small, soft tumors, and is generally not recommended for colorectal adenocarcinoma. It is particularly difficult to evenly diffuse the alcohol into hard colorectal tumors, and frequently colorectal

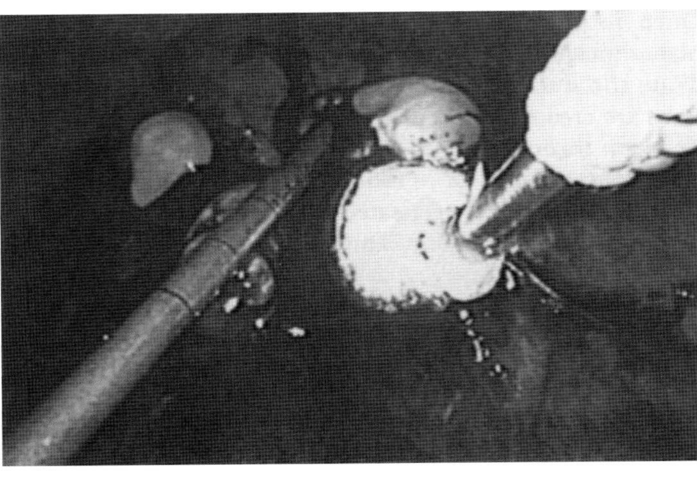

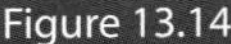

Figure 13.14

Ultrasound is needed to ensure placement of ablation probes into the center of the tumor and to follow the size of the ablation lesion

metastasis may fracture, spilling alcohol into the surrounding liver. Care must also be taken when injecting large-volume tumors, as the alcohol will enter the systemic circulation and volumes larger than 40 cc may be associated with significant hypotension.

RFA is performed by heating the tumor and a surrounding 1 cm margin to the point of protein denaturation and cell wall degradation. Different RFA devices measure different characteristics to monitor tissue destruction. They may monitor temperature, tissue impedance, or time, to determine when destruction is complete. Most of the current systems can reliably generate 3 cm ablation lesions, and recent improvements in technology have allowed devices that occasionally generate tissue ablation 4–5 cm in diameter. It is necessary to completely ablate the area of these lesions, and multiple applications are frequently necessary. Failure to completely destroy the surface of the target tumor will result in treatment failure. Ultrasound is used as a guide to RFA probe positioning, but is generally less helpful in the assessment of the completeness of ablation. Ultrasound has been shown to overestimate the size of the ablation [93]. In addition to failures due to misplaced probes or inadequate volume of ablation, treatment failures can occur along major vasculature. Blood vessels act as heat sinks or heat shields [70]. It can therefore be difficult to obtain complete destruction of tumors lying adjacent to, or invading, vascular structures. It is therefore necessary to perform treatments on multiple sides of an involved vessel to assure ablation. Techniques of vascular inflow occlusion reduce blood flow to the involved tissue and may facilitate complete ablations. This technique, however, may lead to dangerous thrombosis of adjacent major vessels. Major biliary structures are frequently protected from heat damage secondary to their proximity to major blood vessels. Temperatures in the portal triads are therefore relatively reduced. One of the principal advantages to RFA is the relative lack of associated complications [31]. Although patients frequently experience fevers, rigors, and pain post-ablation, serious complications, notably bleeding, seldom occur.

Hepatic Artery Infusion Pumps

High-dose chemotherapy delivered by direct organ perfusion has theoretical appeal for the treatment of unresectable liver cancers. By directly infusing the hepatic artery, high tissue dosing can be achieved with fewer systemic side effects. Regional chemotherapy may be administered via either the hepatic artery or the portal vein. The majority of experience in Western countries regarding hepatic artery infusion has been the treatment of isolated hepatic metastasis from colorectal primaries.

For patients with unresectable colorectal liver metastasis confined to the liver, hepatic artery perfusion can be accomplished by several minimally invasive techniques. Hepatic artery catheters can be placed angiographically via a femoral vessel for temporary perfusion. This technique is limited to short infusion periods (3–5 days) and requires anticoagulation to prevent hepatic artery thrombosis. Additionally, perfusion of the gallbladder, stomach, and duodenum is uncontrolled and may result in chemotherapy-induced cholecystitis, gastritis, or duodenitis. Both the chemotherapy and non -chemotherapy-related complication rates for this approach are higher than those seen when implantable pumps are used [95].

The preferable mode of perfusion is via subcutaneously implanted continuous perfusion hepatic artery pumps that can be placed by open or laparoscopic approaches. Laparoscopic pump placement follows the tenets developed for open surgical pump placements. Abdominal and pelvic CT scans, chest x-rays, and whole body fluorodeoxyglucose (FDG) PET scans are obtained to reduce the risk of performing a surgical procedure in a patient with extrahepatic disease. Patients found to have extrahepatic disease are not candidates for this procedure and should be referred for systemic chemotherapy instead. Preoperative visceral angiography is required to demonstrate hepatic arterial and venous anatomy. Accessory or replaced hepatic arteries may need to be embolized preoperatively or ligated intraoperatively.

A thorough exploratory laparoscopy is performed, including intraoperative ultrasound, to identify unsuspected extrahepatic disease. A cholecystectomy should be performed to prevent chemotherapy-induced cholecystitis. The hepatic and gastroduodenal arteries are dissected and the antral and pancreaticoduodenal branches are divided to prevent chemoperfusion of these structures. The pump is placed in a subcutaneous pocket on the anterior abdominal wall and the catheter is passed into the abdomen. After obtaining vascular control, the catheter is passed through an arteriotomy in the gastroduodenal artery and secured with its tip at the orifice of the hepatic artery.

The disadvantages of a laparoscopic approach for pump placement are the inability to manually palpate intraabdominal vascular structures and the technical difficulty in safely placing the pump. The loss of palpation, however, can be partially replaced by laparoscopic ultrasound. Increased familiarity and facility with advanced laparoscopic techniques are likely to make application of this technique easier and therefore more widely applicable.

No long-term study has evaluated the results of laparoscopic HAI pump placement compared to open arterial perfusion. It is hoped that patients will receive the benefits observed in other laparoscopic procedures, such as decreased perioperative pain, less perioperative morbidity, and, most importantly, a shortened recovery time. Reduced perioperative immune suppression may, in fact, contribute to improved long-term survival for patients receiving the pump laparoscopically.

Biliary Bypass

As mentioned earlier, biliary bypass for malignant obstruction is generally performed either percutaneously or by ERCP placed stents. Placement of large, covered, expandable stents will yield good short-term patency rates [96, 97]. Both the percutaneous and the endoscopic techniques require fluoroscopically guided passage of a wire across the biliary stenosis. Using over-wire technology, a balloon dilator is passed into the stenosis and inflated. A stent/balloon delivery system is next introduced into the stenosis and the stent is deployed by dilation of a second balloon. Uncovered stents allow tumor ingrowth, reducing long-term patency rates. The recent development of covered stents has provided a more effective long-term solution.

Cholecystojejunostomy

In cases of complete biliary obstruction where a channel cannot be established to place a stent, surgical bypass of the distal common bile duct obstruction may be indicated. Cholecystojejunostomy may be useful in cases where the patient has a normal gallbladder and the common bile duct is not involved near the junction with the cystic duct. Problems have arisen with cholecystojejunostomy because the cystic duct can be an inadequate or diseased conduit, making it inappropriate for a primary route of bile drainage. Tarnasky et al. [98] showed that only 50% of biliary cancer patients have ducts that will support such a drainage procedure and that 50% of bypassable patients ultimately fail due to tumor progression into the junction of cystic and common bile ducts.

The laparoscopic bypass technique begins with the patient being placed in a supine position. Four trocars are placed in a diamond fashion over the presumed sight of anastomosis. A loop of jejunum is selected by retracting the transverse colon cephalad and identifying the ligament of Treitz. The loop is selected 30 cm distal to the ligament and tested to assure that it will reach antecolic to the gallbladder without undue tension. This loop is then sewn to the gallbladder at two sites. A jejunostomy and cholecystostomy are created, and an endoscopic linear stapler is introduced to create a 3-cm anastomosis (Fig. 13.15). The remaining enterocystostomy, through which the stapler had been passed, is closed with a single-layer running suture. A loop jejunostomy is selected in this case because it is unlikely that significant small bowel content will enter the biliary tree through the cystic duct.

Choledochojejunostomy

In highly selected cases, laparoscopic choledochojejunostomy may be indicated. An unresectable distal common bile duct obstruction with a largely dilated and uninvolved proximal duct and an unusable or absent gallbladder is an indication for a choledochojejunostomy. A Roux-en-Y reconstruction using the same principles observed in open procedures is the indicated procedure.

The patient is placed in a 45° left lateral decubitus position on the operating table with both the feet and head down and kidney rest in place to open the space between the costal margin and iliac crest. Four or five ports may be necessary. These should include an array of right subcostal ports as well as an abdominal port to facilitate bowel and liver retraction.

A loop of jejunum is selected by elevating the transverse colon cephalad and identifying the ligament of Treitz at the base of the mesocolon. Approximately 30 cm distal to the ligament, the jejunum is divided by a single firing of an endoscopic intestinal stapler. The small bowel mesentery is elongated using

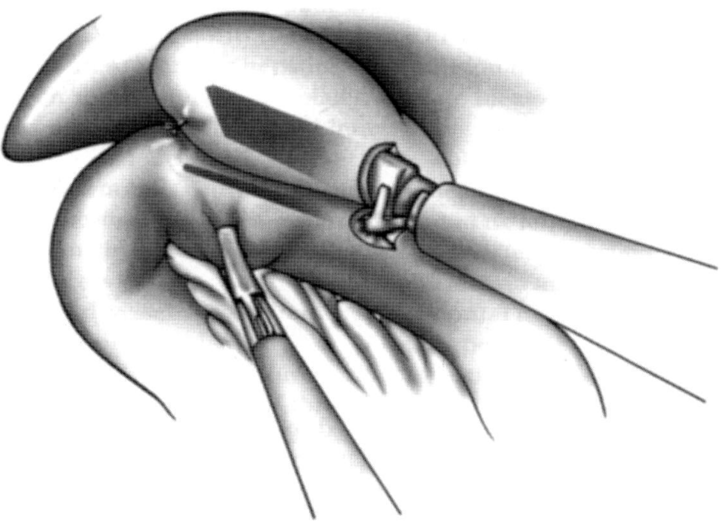

Figure 13.15
An endoscopic stapler is used to create cholecystojejunal anastomosis

ultrasonic coagulating shears or firings of endoscopic vascular stapler loads as necessary. An antecolic or retrocolic anastomosis can be performed as indicated. The common bile duct is carefully dissected and encircled. It is divided, and a distal specimen is sent for frozen section to ensure that the anastomosis will not be performed to malignant tissue. The distal duct is oversewn, and a one-layer choledochojejunostomy is performed using absorbable monofilament suture with the posterior row run in continuity and the anterior row sewn with carefully placed interrupted simple sutures. Alternatively, a side-to-side anastomosis could be constructed with interrupted or continuous suture (Fig. 13.15). This procedure obviously requires quite advanced laparoscopic skills and would primarily be performed at high-volume centers.

Segment Three Bypass

Gagner's group [99] has described a combination percutaneous and endoscopic method of biliary bypass using the segment three hepatic duct. The method involves obtaining percutaneous access to the left ductal system and passing a stiff guidewire and, subsequently, a stent out through the wall of the segment three duct and through the lesser curvature of the stomach (Fig. 13.16). Though his early reports were positive, it is unclear if this is truly a useful technique for those patients who cannot be drained via other methods.

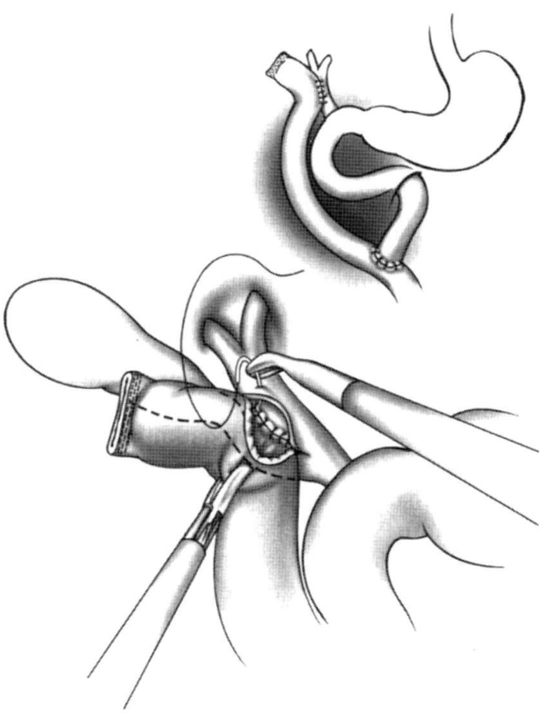

Figure 13.16
A formal choledochojejunostomy is occasionally indicated and can be performed laparoscopically if the surgeon has advanced skills

Enteric Bypass

Enteric bypass is seldom required, even when advanced distal common bile duct tumors are present. Large tumor masses that obstruct gastroduodenal continuity can occasionally develop. In most of these cases, curative resection is not indicated due to local invasion or metastatic spread, and a gastroduodenal bypass via a laparoscopic gastrojejunostomy is preferred for palliation. Again, the basic principles developed in open surgery should be applied when feasible. The anastomosis should be low and, if possible, on the posterior wall of the body or antrum. We prefer a Roux-en-Y, but many surgeons perform a loop jejunostomy. Regardless, the anastomosis must be widely patent and 5–6 cm is preferable.

The technique is performed with the patient supine. The operating surgeon may be on either the patient's right or left. Four ports are arranged in a diamond configuration over the assumed site of the anastomosis. The camera port is initially the midline port closest to the surgeon, and the surgeon's operating ports are on the right and left. The port furthest away from the surgeon will be an assistant's port.

A loop of jejunum is selected as described above (biliary bypass). We prefer an antecolic anastomosis to minimize the chance of late obstruction due to tumor invasion of the mesentery. A retrocolic approach is another acceptable alternative, although somewhat more technically challenging. The gastrocolic ligament is divided with a harmonic shears opening the lesser sac. The proximal Roux loop is attached at two sites, 6 cm apart, to the lower posterior body of the stomach. A small adjacent enterotomy and gastrotomy are created, and two firings of an endoscopic intestinal stapler are used to create a 6 cm anastomosis. The residual enterotomy is closed with a running inner layer of Vicryl and an interrupted outer layer of silk. A jejunojejunostomy is created in a similar fashion 30 cm down the Roux loop to restore intestinal continuity. Care must be taken to avoid narrowing the intestinal lumen when oversewing the enterotomy through which the stapler had been fired.

One must be cautioned when presented with a patient who has a hepatobiliary malignancy and complains of persistent nausea and vomiting. It is critical that mechanical duodenal obstruction be documented before committing such patients to a bypass procedure as nausea and vomiting are frequent symptoms of hepatobiliary tumors and, outside of true obstruction, are not improved by duodenal bypass.

Conclusion

The application of minimally invasive surgical techniques to all of general surgical practice has proliferated tremendously in recent years. It has been well demonstrated that thoughtful procedure design, development of appropriate instrumentation, and adequate surgical training and experience can overcome most technical obstacles. Even laparoscopic dissection of the porta hepatis, complete vascular control, and complex anastomosis may be performed safely and efficiently.

There are a number of frequently cited and documented advantages of using minimally invasive surgical approaches in hepatobiliary patients requiring surgical intervention. These include lower rates of perioperative morbidity, decreased blood loss, less pain, shorter hospital stays, and shorter posthospital recovery. Although these are important issues for all surgical patients, a shorter recovery may be especially important when we intervene in patients with a limited life expectancy. Shorter recovery time may also allow adjuvant therapies to be initiated sooner. Lastly, hepatobiliary malignancies are generally a disease of the elderly, the fastest growing segment of the population. There is little doubt that minimally invasive surgery will benefit this population more than any other.

An important potential advantage obtained by using a minimally invasive approach for the treatment of patients with hepatobiliary cancers is the reduction in surgery-induced immune suppression. Immune suppression has been associated with worsened overall survival in patients with malignancy. Measures of cellular and humoral immune function are less suppressed following minimally invasive procedures when compared to an open surgical procedure. The true impact of this phenomenon on patient outcomes and survival has not been demonstrated, but the theoretical implications are obvious.

The most obvious limitations of laparoscopic techniques are the technical challenges they present to surgeons. Universality is an important aspect of any new technique developed to be an important factor in patient care and is necessary for the uniform utilization of the procedure. Technology-intensive procedures are also generally more costly to perform, which may impede their adoption. While these costs may be recovered by shorter hospitalization and recovery times, they still present payer issues on the front end. From a technical perspective, minimally invasive techniques may provide a magnified and well-illuminated view of the selected operative field but typically provide less access to the remainder of the abdominal cavity as well as a loss of tactile feedback. This deficit can be partially replaced by laparoscopic ultrasound, but there is currently no surgical instrument designed that can totally replace the human hand.

There is little doubt that minimally invasive therapies, whether endoscopic, interventional radiologic techniques, or laparoscopic, currently play a major role in the treatment of all hepatobiliary cancers. Laparoscopy, in particular, brings the option of a fairly aggressive and accurate diagnosis and staging modality into the pretreatment algorithm of these patients. The addition of laparoscopic ultrasound and improved techniques of excisional biopsy and retroperitoneal dissection not only have increased the accuracy of staging patients but also help to identify patients who would not benefit from attempts at resection. Therapeutic laparoscopy may also offer the skilled laparoscopic surgeon the opportunity to provide palliation to many patients who are incurable. The performance of biliary-enteric bypass or placement of a hepatic artery chemotherapy pump, both relatively simple surgical procedures, is sometimes denied to patients simply because of the morbidity of the traditional open surgical approach. Laparoscopic access has demonstrated equal success palliating these patients with minimal morbidity and less pain. The benefit this provides to these unfortunate cancer sufferers can scarcely be measured.

Most recently, laparoscopic methods have been developed for performing curative hepatic resections. Surgeons have approached this concept with caution both because of the technical difficulties involved in open biliary surgery and because of concerns about the long-term cure rates and the unknown effects of pneumoperitoneum and laparoscopy on the host/cancer response. Ultimately the acceptance of laparoscopic surgery to cure hepatobiliary cancers depends on the use of meticulous technique to achieve operative results comparable to open procedures and by confirmation that long-term outcomes are acceptable.

In the future, there may be an increased emphasis on more directed or limited ablations as opposed to major resections, possibly with directed chemotherapy or other catheter, endoscopic, or laparoscopic delivered therapies. These truly minimally invasive approaches offer the potential for tremendous patient benefits if they are proven to be effective.

References

1. Jemal A, Siegel R, Ward E et al (2008) Cancer statistics, 2008. CA Cancer J Clin 58:79–96
2. Pickren J, Tsukada Y, Lane W (1982) Liver metastasis: analysis of autopsy data. In: Gilbert H, Weiss L (eds). Liver metastasis. Hall, Boston, MA, 2–18
3. Way L (1995) Liver. In: Way L (ed). Current surgical diagnosis and treatment. Appleton & Lange, Norwalk, CT, 505–519
4. Edmondson H, Craig J (1987) Neoplasms of the liver. In: Schiff L, Schiff E (eds). Diseases of the liver. IB Lippincott, Philadelphia, PA, 1109–1158
5. Nagasue N, Yukaya H, Hamada T, Hirose S, Kanashima R, Inokuchi K (1984) The natural history of hepatocellular carcinoma. A study of 100 untreated cases. Cancer 54:1461–1465
6. Wagner JS, Adson MA, Van Heerden JA, Adson MH, Ilstrup DM (1984) The natural history of hepatic metastases from colorectal cancer. A comparison with resective treatment. Ann Surg 199:502–508
7. Fong Y, Fortner J, Sun R et al (1999) Clinical score for predicting recurrence after hepatic resection for metastatic colorectal cancer. Ann Surg 230(3):309–321
8. Choti MA, Sitzman JV, Tiburi MF et al (2002) Trends in long-term survival following liver resection for hepatic colorectal metastases. Ann Surg 235(6):759–766
9. Abdalla EK, Vauthey J, Ellis LM et al (2004) Recurrence and outcomes following hepatic resection, radiofrequency ablation, and combined resection/ablation for colorectal liver metastases. Ann Surg 239:818–827
10. Khatri VP, Chee KG, Petrelli NJ (2007) Modern multimodality approach to hepatic colorectal metastases: solutions and controversies. Surg Oncol 16:71–83
11. Kemeny N (2007) Presurgical chemotherapy in patients being considered for liver resection. Oncologist 12: 825–839
12. De Jong KP (2007) Review article: multimodality treatment of liver metastases increases suitability for surgical treatment. Aliment Pharmacol Ther 26(Suppl 2): 161–169
13. Scheele JM, Stangl R, Altendorf-Hofmann A (1990) Hepatic metastases from colorectal carcinoma: impact of surgical resection on the natural history. Br J Surg 77:1241–1246
14. Geoghegan JG, Scheele J (1999) Treatment of colorectal liver metastases. Br J Surg 86:158–169
15. Fuhrman GM, Curley SM, Hohn DM, Roh MM (2000) Improved survival after resection of colorectal liver metastasis. Ann Surg Oncol 2:537–541
16. Fong YM, Kemeny NM, Paty PM, Blumgart LHM, Cohen AMM (2000) Treatment of colorectal cancer: hepatic metastasis. Semin Surg Oncol 12:219–252
17. Silen W (1989) Hepatic resection for metastases from colorectal carcinoma is of dubious value. Arch Surg 124:1021–1022
18. Scheele J, Stangl R, Altendorf-Hofmann A (1990) Hepatic metastases from colorectal carcinoma: impact of surgical resection on the natural history. Br J Surg 77: 1241–1246

19. van Leeuwen DJ, Wilson L, Crowe R (1995) Liver biopsy in the mid-1990s: questions and answers. Semin Liver Dis 15:340–358
20. Sheiner PA, Bower ST (1994) Treatment of metastatic cancer to the liver. Semin Liver Dis 14:170–177
21. Bhattacharya S, Novell JR, Winslet M, Hobbs KEF (1994) Iodized oil in the treatment of hepatocellular carcinoma. Br J Surg 11:1563–1571
22. Anderson JR, Sorensen SM, Kruse A et al (1989) Randomized trial of endoscopic endoprosthesis versus operative bypass in malignant obstructive jaundice. Gut 30:1132–1135
23. Gallery M, Strasbert S, Doherty G, Soper N, Norton J (1997) Staging laparoscopy with laparoscopic ultrasonography: optimizing resectability in hepatobiliary and pancreatic malignancy. Am Coll Surg 185:33–39
24. Lo C-M, Lai EC, Liu C-L, Fan EE-TF, Wong J (1998) Laparoscopy and laparoscopic ultrasonography avoid exploratory laparotomy in patients with hepatocellular carcinoma. Ann Surg 227:527–532
25. John T, Greig D, Crosbie J, Miles WA, Garden OJ (1994) Superior staging of liver tumors with laparoscopy and laparoscopic ultrasound. Ann Surg 220: 711–719
26. Velanovich V (1998) Staging laparoscopy in the management of intra-abdominal malignancies. Surgery 124: 773–781
27. Castillo CF, Rattner DW, Warshaw AL (1995) Further experience with laparoscopy and peritoneal cytology in the staging of pancreatic cancer. Br J Surg 82: 1127–1129
28. Warshaw AL, Gu Z, Wittenberg J, Waltman A (1990) Perioperative staging and assessment of resectability of pancreatic cancer. Arch Surg 125:230–233
29. Siperstein AM, Rogers SM, Hansen PM, Gitomirsky AM (2000) Laparoscopic thermal ablation of hepatic neuroendocrine tumor metastasis. Surgery 122: 1147–1155
30. Jacobaeus HG (1911) Kurze Ubersicht uber meine Erfahrungen mit der Laparothorakoskipie. Munch Med Wochenschr 58:2017
31. Curley SA, Izzo F, Delrio P et al (1999) Radiofrequency ablation of unresectable primary and metastatic hepatic malignancies: results in 123 patients [see comments]. Ann Surg 230:1–8
32. Huscher CG, Lirici MM, Chiodini S, Recher A (1997) Current position of advanced laparoscopic surgery of the liver. J R Coll Surg Edinb 42:219–225
33. Koffron AJ, Auffenberg G, Kung R et al (2007) Evaluation of 300 minimally invasive liver resections at a single institution. Ann Surg 246:385–394
34. Mala T, Edwin B, Gladhaug I et al (2002) A comparative study of the short-term outcome following open and laparoscopic liver resection of colorectal metastases. Surg Endosc 16:1059–1063
35. Gigot JF, Gilneur D, Azagra JS et al (2002) Laparosocpic liver resection for malignant liver tumors. Ann Surg 1: 90–97
36. Dagher I, Proske JM, Carloni A et al (2007) Laparoscopic liver resection: results for 70 patients. Surg Endosc 21: 619–624
37. Fusco MM, Paluzzi MM (2000) Abdominal wall recurrence after laparoscopic-assisted colectomy for adenocarcinoma of the colon. A case report. Dis Colon Rectum 36:858–861
38. Ortega AM, Beart R (2000) Laparoscopic bowel surgery registry. Preliminary results. Dis Colon Rectum 38: 681–686
39. Hoffman GM, Backer JM, Fitchett CM (2000) Laparoscopic-assisted colectomy: initial experience. Ann Surg 219:732–743
40. Nduka CM, Monson JM, Menzies-Gow NM (2000) Abdominal wall metastasis following laparoscopy. Br J Surg 81:648–652
41. Fleshman J, Sargent DJ, Green E et al (2007) Laparoscopic colectomy for cancer is not inferior to open surgery based on 5-year data from the COST study group trial. Ann Surg 246:655–664
42. Huscher CG, Napolitano C, Chiodini S, Recher A, Buffa PF, Lirici MM (1997) Hepatic resections through the laparoscopic approach. Ann Ital Chir 68: 791–797
43. Azagra JM, Goergen MM, Gilbart EM, Jacobs DM (2000) Laparoscopic anatomical (hepatic) left lateral segmentectomy—technical aspects. Surg Endosc 10: 758–761
44. Hompes D, Aerts R, Penninckx F et al (2007) Laparoscopic liver resection using radiofrequency coagulation. Surg Endosc 21:175–180
45. Gumbs A, Gayet B, Gagner M (2008) Laparoscopic liver resection: when to use the laparoscopic stapler device. HPB 10:296–303
46. Koffron AJ, Stein JA (2008) Laparoscopic liver surgery: parenchymal transection using saline-enhanced electrosurgery. HPB 10:225–228
47. Whelan R, Allendorf J, Gutt C et al (1998) General oncologic effects of the laparoscopic surgical approach. Surg Endosc 12:1092–1103
48. Jacobi C, Wenger F, Sabat R, Volk T, Ordemann J, Muller J (1998) The impact of laparoscopy with carbon dioxide versus helium on immunologic function and tumor growth in a rat model. Dig Surg 15:110–116
49. Lacy AM, Garcia-Valdecasas JC, Delgado S et al (2002) Laparoscopy-assisted colectomy versus open colectomy for treatment of non-metastatic colon cancer: a randomized trial. Lancet 359:2224–2229
50. Allendorf J, Bessler M, Trokel WBL, Reat M (1997) Postoperative immune function varies inversely with the degree of surgical trauma in a murine model. Surg Endosc 11:427–430
51. **Park** SK, Brody JI, Wallace HA, Blakemore WS (1971) Immunosuppressive effects of surgery. Lancet 1: 53–55
52. Slade M, Simmons R, Greenberg Y (1975) Immune depression after major surgery in normal patients. Surgery 78:363–372
53. Little DM, Regan M, Keane R, Bouchier-Hayes D (2000) Perioperative immune modulation. Surgery 114: 87–91
54. Glaser F, Sannwald GA, Buhr HJ et al (1995) General stress response to conventional and laparoscopic cholecystectomy. Ann Surg 221:372–380

55. Bellon JM, Manazano L, Bernardos L et al (1997) Cytokine levels after open and laparoscopic cholecystectomy. Eur Surg Res 29:27–34
56. Baigrie RJ, Lamont PM, Whiting S, Morris PJ (1993) Portal endotoxin and cytokine responses during abdominal aortic surgery. Am J Surg 166:248–251
57. Hensler T, Hecker H, Heeg K et al (1997) Distinct mechanisms of immunosuppression as a consequence of major surgery. Infect Immun 65(6):2283–2291
58. Redmond HP, Watson WG, Houghton T, Condron C, Watson RGK, Bouchier-Hayes D (1994) Immune function in patients undergoing open vs. laparoscopic cholecystectomy. Arch Surg 129:1240–1246
59. Waymack J, Rapien J, Garnett D et al (1986) Effect of transfusion on immune function in a traumatized animal model. Arch Surg 121:505–555
60. Chen WS, Lin W, Kou YR et al (1997) Possible effect of pneumoperitoneum on the spreading of colon cancer tumor cells. Dis Colon Rectum 40:791–797
61. Hughes KM, Scheele JM, Sugarbaker PM (1989) Surgery for colorectal cancer metastatic to the liver. Liver Surg 69:339–359
62. Vauthey JN, Marsh RD, Cendan JC, Chu NM, Copeland EM (1996) Arterial therapy of hepatic colorectal metastases [review]. Br J Surg 83:447–455
63. Feld RI, Liu JB, Nazarian L et al (1996) Laparoscopic liver sonography: preliminary experience in liver metastases compared with CT portography. J Ultrasound Med 15:288–295
64. Flamen P, Stroobants S, Cutsem E et al (1999) Additional value of whole-body positron emission tomography with fluorine-18-2-fluoro-2-deoxy-D-glucose in recurrent colorectal cancer. J Clin Oncol 17:894–901
65. Fong Y, Saldinger PF, Akhurst T et al (2000) Utility of 18F-FDG positron emission tomography scanning on selection of patients for resection of hepatic colorectal metastasis. Am J Surg 178(4):282–287
66. Jobe BA, Kenyon T, Hansen PD, Swanstrom LL (1998) Minilaparoscopy: current status, technology, and future applications. Minim Invasive Ther Allied Tech 7(3): 201–208
67. Cranstock LRF, Dillon JF, Hayes PC (1994) Diagnostic laparoscopy and liver disease: experience of 200 cases. Aust NZ J Med 24:258–262
68. Nieveen van Dijkum EJ, Sturm PD, de Wit LT, Offerhaus J, Obertop H, Gouma D (1998) Cytology of peritoneal lavage performed during staging laparoscopy for gastrointestinal malignancies: is it useful? Ann Surg 228(6): 728–739
69. Jarnagin WR, Conlon K, Bodniewicz J et al (2001) A clinical scoring system predicts the yield of diagnostic laparoscopy in patients with potentially resectable hepatic colorectal metastases. Cancer 91:1121–1128
70. Weber SM, DeMatteo RP, Fong Y et al (2002) Staging laparoscopy in patients with extrahepatic biliary carcinoma. Analysis of 100 patients. Ann Surg 235: 392–399
71. Thaler K, Kanneganti S, Khajanchee Y et al (2005) The evolving role of staging laparoscopy in the treatment of colorectal hepatic metastasis. Arch Surg 140(8): 727–734
72. Pomel C, Appleyard TL, Gouy S et al (2005) The role of laparoscopy to evaluate candidates for complete cytoreduction of peritoneal carcinomatosis and hyperthermic intraperitoneal chemotherapy. Eur J Surg Oncol 31(5):540–543
73. D'Angelica M, Fong Y, Weber S et al (2003) The role of staging laparoscopy in hepatobiliary malignancy: prospective analysis of 401 cases. Ann Surg Onc 10(2): 183–189
74. Smith AC, Dowsett JF, Russel RCG et al (1994) Randomised trial of endoscopic stenting versus surgical bypass in malignant low bile duct obstruction. Lancet 344:1655–1660
75. Meta-Analysis Group in Cancer (1996) Reappraisal of hepatic artery infusion in the treatment of nonresectable liver metastasis from colorectal cancer. J Nat Cancer Inst 88(5):252–258
76. Kemeny NE, Huang Y, Cohen AM et al (1999) Hepatic arterial infusion of chemotherapy after resection of hepatic metastasis from colorectal cancer. N Engl J Med 341(27):2039–2048
77. Kemeny N, Adak S, Gray B et al (2002) Combined-modality treatment for resectable metastatic colorectal carcinoma to the liver: surgical resection of hepatic metastases in combination with continuous infusion of chemotherapy – an Intergroup study. J Clin Oncol 20:1499–1505
78. Lorenz M, Muller H, Schramm H et al (1998) Randomized trial of surgery versus surgery followed by adjuvant hepatic arterial infusion with 5-fluorouracil and folinic acid for liver metastases of colorectal cancer. Ann Surg 228: 756–764
79. Board RE, Valle JW (2007) Metastatic colorectal cancer: current systemic treatment options. Drugs 67(13): 1851–1867
80. McEntee GP, Nagorney DM, Kvolls LK (1990) Cytoreductive hepatic surgery for neuroendocrine tumors. Surgery 108:1091–1096
81. Seifert JK, Cozzi PJ, Morris DL (1998) Cryotherapy for neuroendocrine liver metastasis. Semin Surg Oncol 14:175–183
82. Pitchumoni CS (1998) Chronic pancreatitis: pathogenesis and management of pain [review published erratum appears in J Clin Gastroenterol 1999;28(2):109]. J Clin Gastroenterol 27:101–107
83. Takahashi T, Kakita A, Izumika H et al (1996) Thoracoscopic splanchnicectomy for the relief of intractable abdominal pain. Surg Endosc 10:65–68
84. Buell JF, Thomas MT, Rudich S et al (2008) Experience with more than 500 minimally invasive hepatic procedures. Ann Surg 248(3):475–486
85. Cherqui D, Laurent A, Tayar C et al (2006) Laparoscopic liver resection for peripheral hepatocellular carcinoma in patients with chronic liver disease. Ann Surg 243:499–506
86. Shima Y, Horimi T, Ichikawa J et al (2003) Aggressive surgery for liver metastases from gastrointestinal stromal tumors. J Hepatobiliary Pancreat Surg 10: 77–80
87. Alves A, Adam R, Majno P et al (2003) Hepatic resection for metastatic renal tumors: is it worthwhile? Ann Surg Onc 10(6):705–710

88. Sakamoto Y, Ohyama S, Yamamoto J et al (2003) Surgical resection of liver metastases of gastric cancer: an analysis of a 17-year experience with 22 patients. Surgery 133(5): 507–511
89. Vlastos G, Smith DL, Singletary E et al (2004) Long-term survival after an aggressive surgical approach in patients with breast cancer hepatic metastases. Ann Surg Onc 11(9):869–874
90. Sandor J, Ihasz M, Fazekas T, Regoly-Merei J, Batorfi J (1995) Unexpected gallbladder cancer and laparoscopic surgery. Surg Endosc 9:1207–1210
91. Wibbenmeyer IA, Wade TP, Chen RC, Meyer RC, Turgeon RP, Andrus CH (1995) Laparoscopic cholecystectomy can disseminate in situ carcinoma of the gallbladder [see comments]. J Am Coll Surg 181:504–510
92. Anonymous (1994) Fatal gas embolism caused by overpressurization during laparoscopic use of argon enhanced coagulation. Health Devices 23:257–259
93. Hansen PD, Rogers SJ, Corless CL, Swanstrom LL, Siperstein AE (1999) Radiofrequency ablation lesions in a pig liver model. J Surg Res 87:114–121
94. Scudamore CH, Lee SI, Patterson EJ et al (1999) Radiofrequency ablation followed by resection of malignant liver tumors. Am J Surg 177:411–417
95. Curley SA, Hohn DC, Roh MS (1990) Hepatic artery infusion pumps: cannulation techniques and other surgical considerations. Langenbecks Arch Chir 375:119–124
96. Vitale GC, Larson GM, George M, Tatum C (1996) Management of malignant biliary stricture with self-expanding metallic stent. Surg Endosc 10:970–973
97. van Berkel AM, Boland C, Redekop WK et al (1998) A prospective randomized trial of Teflon versus polyethylene stents for distal malignant biliary obstruction [see comments]. Endoscopy 30:681–686
98. Tarnasky PR, England RE, Lail LM, Pappas TN, Cotton PB (1995) Cystic duct patency in malignant obstructive jaundice. An ERCP-based study relevant to the role of laparoscopic cholecystojejunostomy [Review]. Ann Surg 221:265–271
99. Soulez G, Therasse E, Oliva VL et al (1997) Left hepaticogastrostomy for biliary obstruction: long-term results. Radiology 204:780–786

Laparoscopic Approaches to Colonic Malignancy

Juliane Bingener, Heidi Nelson

Contents

The last two decades have witnessed the surge and success of laparoscopic approaches in several surgical arenas. Laparoscopic cholecystectomy, laparoscopic solid organ surgery, and laparoscopic gastric bypass have become the standard of care. Adoption of laparoscopic colectomy has remained low until the middle of this decade and is approaching 10% for benign disease [1].

Concerns over the appropriateness of laparoscopic colectomy for colon cancer had been raised with regard to possible limitations in tumor staging, patterns of tumor recurrences related to the use of the pneumoperitoneum, and effective cost containment. Well-designed prospective randomized trials have now reported data necessary to support laparoscopic colectomy as an alternative technique for colon cancer. This chapter analyzes the technical aspects of laparoscopic colectomy (LAC) as a cancer operation, discusses the results experienced with LAC, addresses cancer staging and unusual patterns of tumor recurrence, describes the results of prospective randomized trials and meta-analyses, and gives an outlook on possible future developments.

Techniques

Laparoscopic colon surgery is technically challenging and requires a thorough and systematic approach. Specific key principles dictate the general requirements for laparoscopic techniques; they should be simple, reproducible, easy to teach, easy to learn, and of reasonable cost. One manner of adhering to these principles is to design and implement laparoscopic techniques modeled after the same approach as performed open. For example, for both right and left colectomy, colon mobilization can be performed in the same fashion as in the open technique and the anastomosis is fashioned extracorporeally. When a lower anastomosis

F.L. Greene, B.T. Heniford (eds.), *Minimally Invasive Cancer Management*,
DOI 10.1007/978-1-4419-1238-1_14,

is anticipated such as for sigmoid colectomy, a circular stapler anvil is inserted in the proximal bowel segment. The use of a totally intracorporeal technique is technically more demanding and time consuming. It may be of benefit if a natural orifice can be used for specimen extraction, but currently data to support this are sparse. Rendering the procedure reproducible allows for maximizing proficiencies as the team gains experience; this keeps operating room costs to a minimum. Further reductions in costs can be accomplished by the application of reusable instruments.

Laparoscopic surgery for colorectal cancer mandates additional requirements. Liver and peritoneal surfaces should be routinely explored prior to any procedure. Bulky or T4 disease involving adjacent structures is likely an indication for conversion to open surgery. The initial assessment of the abdominal cavity should also be directed to check for massive adhesions, pelvic fixation of the small bowel, or extensive scarring in the right upper quadrant, which might prompt expeditious conversion to open surgery. Also, a number of critical steps should be adopted in each case to reduce the likelihood of port-site recurrences to a minimum, including minimal bowel handling, absolute avoidance of direct tumor handling, fixation of trocars to avoid leakage of pneumoperitoneum, irrigation of the peritoneum, irrigation of the wound, and the use of a wound protector at the extraction site. It is likely that attention to these details has allowed the drastic reduction of trocar-wound tumor recurrences witnessed over the last few years.

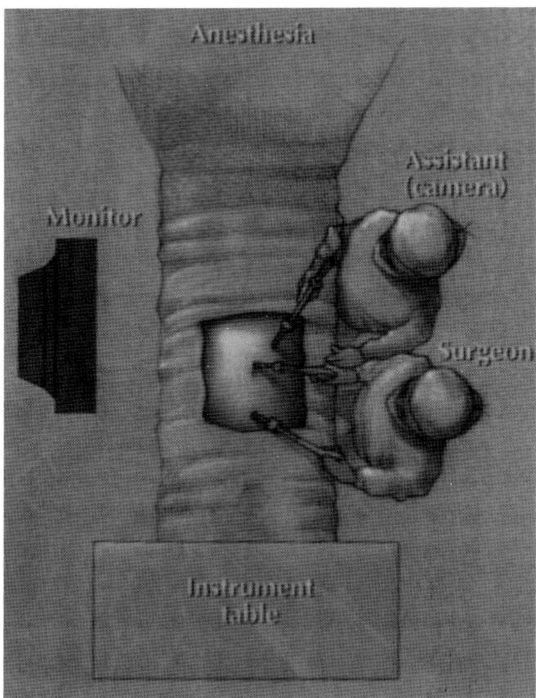

Figure 14.1

Positioning of the personnel and equipment in the operating room (Reproduced with permission from Young-Fadok and Nelson [58])

Resection of the Right Colon

Three cannulas (one or two 10–12 mm, one or two 5 mm) are inserted supraumbilically in the lower midline and in the left upper quadrant. The supraumbilical cannula is usually inserted first, using a direct cut-down technique. As an alternative, the left upper quadrant can be used as the first portal of entry to avoid midline scars and adhesions. It is extremely rare to find left upper quadrant scars. Pneumoperitoneum (not exceeding 14 mmHg) is established more readily using the cut-down approach. The operator stands on the left side of the patient opposite the monitor and the pathology. The video camera is controlled by an assistant standing by the left upper quadrant (Fig. 14.1). With the patient in the Trendelenburg position, with the right side up and the small bowel out of the field, dissection of the lateral attachments of the right colon is commenced from the cecum and terminal ileum cephalad with early identification of the right ureter. Typically, the ureter is first seen crossing the iliac vessels under the peritoneum. With the cecum retracted toward the left upper quadrant, the initial peritoneal incision is made near the base of cecum and mesoappendix. Now the ureter can be directly visualized and the mesentery swept cephalad off the critical retroperitoneal structures.

Care is taken to grasp only the tissue immediately adjacent to the bowel, but not the bowel itself, to prevent injuries (Fig. 14.2). When the mobilization of the ascending colon is completed, the patient is placed in reverse Trendelenburg and the hepatic flexure is mobilized with identification of the duodenum (Fig. 14.3). Once the bowel is fully freed up from its peritoneal attachments from the ileocecal valve to the midtransverse colon, the bowel is exteriorized through a 4- to

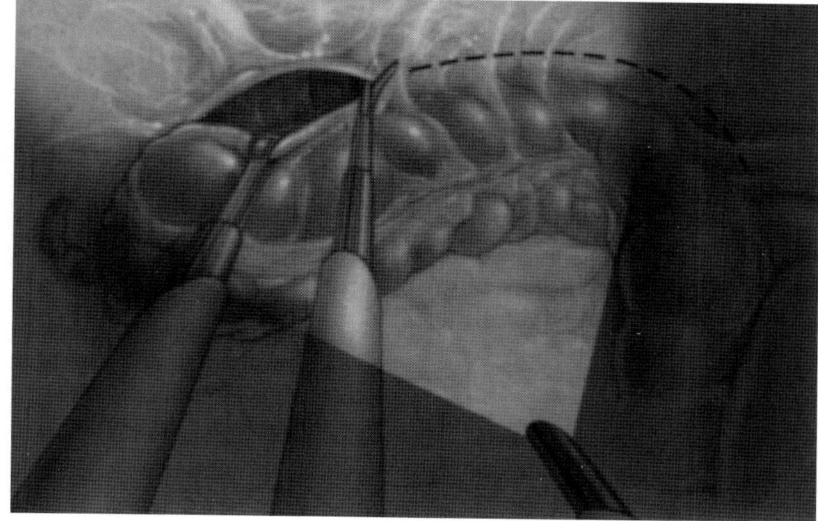

Figure 14.2

Mobilization of the ascending colon (Reproduced with permission from Young-Fadok and Nelson [58])

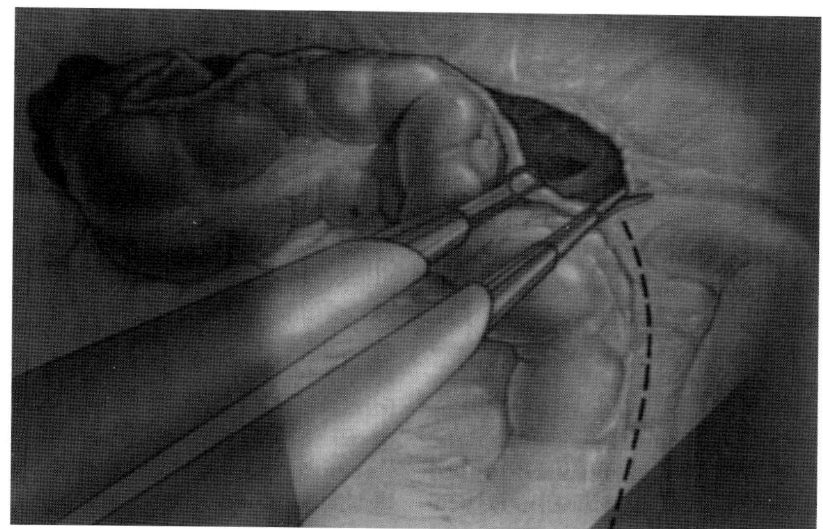

Figure 14.3

Mobilization of the hepatic flexure (Reproduced with permission from Young-Fadok and Nelson [58])

6-cm laparotomy (Fig. 14.4). Resection and anastomosis are then performed, and the bowel is replaced into the abdominal cavity and the minilaparotomy closed. Pneumoperitoneum is reestablished, and a further inspection of the peritoneal cavity is carried out before all the cannulas are removed and fascial defects closed. In some cases, it is possible to inspect the cannula sites for bleeding and to close them under direct visualization through the midline wound, thus avoiding the need to reestablish the pneumoperitoneum. This is only advised when there is no suspicion of residual bleeding at the operative site.

Resection of the Left Colon

This resection is essentially performed as the symmetrical opposite of the right colectomy. The left ureter should be identified when the sigmoid and left colon are freed from their lateral peritoneal attachments. Unlike the right colon where the ileocolic and right colic can be ligated extracorporeally, the left colic vessels should be ligated intracorporeally for cancer cases. This ensures proximal pedicle ligation and allows for ease of exteriorization. After mobilization of the splenic flexure, the omentum can be freed off the bowel

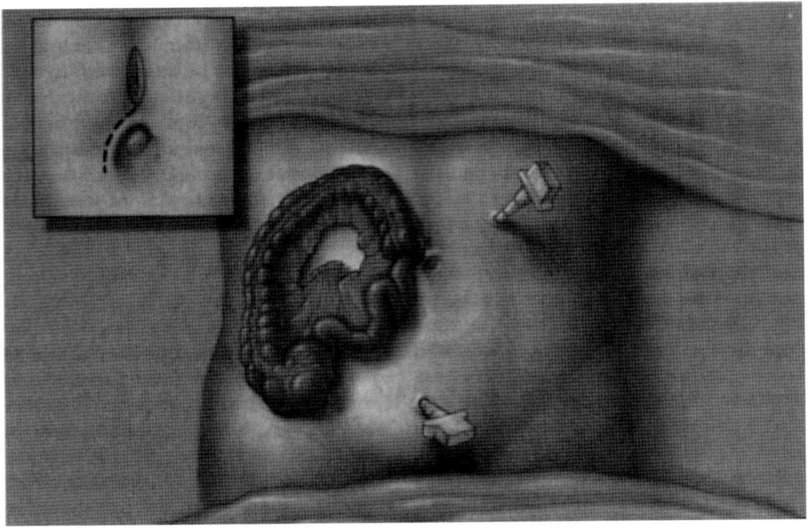

Figure 14.4
Minilaparotomy and exteriorization of the bowel (Reproduced with permission from Young-Fadok and Nelson [58])

and exteriorization with resection and anastomosis carried out in the same fashion as above.

Resection of the Sigmoid Colon

For this resection, the patient is placed in the combined legs-up position. Once the left colon is mobilized, the monitor is moved between the legs of the patient and the surgeon stands on the left side. The presacral space is entered on the left with the sigmoid colon retracted cephalad and to the right, and the same maneuver is then repeated on the opposite side. Vascular ligation of the superior hemorrhoidal vessels is performed with a vascular endostapler, clips, or endoloops according to the surgeon's preference. Following that, the proximal rectum is divided using a 60-mm linear stapler introduced through a 12-mm cannula (lower port). The proximal bowel is then exteriorized and resected. At this point, a circular stapler anvil is placed in the proximal bowel, secured with a purse-string suture, and replaced into the abdominal cavity where a pneumoperitoneum is then reestablished. The anvil is grasped and laparoscopically inserted into the shaft of the instrument introduced per anus as in the open-stapled technique. Anastomotic rings are checked for completeness and the anastomosis visualized with a proctoscope after the instrument is fired.

Above methods approach the colon resection in a manner similar to open surgical approaches (lateral to medial). Alternatively, approaches commencing with vascular pedicle ligation and then colon dissection from the peritoneal attachments (medial to lateral) can be performed.

Results

Following the LAC, patients resume oral intake as soon after surgery as they are ready, that is, when they are hungry. Typically, patients resume liquids within 24 h and solids within 48 h after surgery and have passage of flatus within 2–4 days and bowel movements within 4–5 days. This allows them to be ready for hospital dismissal within 3.6–7.8 days when considering right, left, and sigmoid colectomy combined [2–16],typically 4 days for right colectomy and 5 days for sigmoid resection. Different postoperative feeding policies can affect postoperative recovery times. In fact, while many surgeons follow the postoperative treatment described above, some have reported starting patients on food only after passage of flatus [12, 17]. European countries tend to have a longer length of stay (LOS), which is probably due more to patient expectation and societal practices than to variations specifically related to LAC [18, 19].

For patients over 75 years of age, we found a higher proportion of patients with comorbidities [American Society of Anesthesiology (ASA) classification III = 55%] and accordingly found that a longer time is required for return of bowel function (3.9 days) and time to discharge (6.5 days). These results still compare favorably to open surgery, that is, reduction of recovery parameters is in the range of 4 days. A further interesting finding from this study pertains to preservation of functional independence in the elderly using laparoscopic approaches. In a case-matched series of elderly patients, 95% of those who were independent at admission were also independent at discharge in the laparoscopic group; in contrast only 76% were independent at discharge in the open group [20].

Contraindications

Although increasing experience has resulted in a decreased incidence of contraindications to LAC, which is often relative more than absolute, there are still a number of conditions where the status of the patient does not allow a sufficiently safe laparoscopic approach. For example, active bleeding or a coagulopathy not correctable before surgery would increase the risk of severe intraoperative bleeding, which cannot be controlled using laparoscopic techniques. Although LAC has shown benefits in high-risk patients, when cardiovascular or respiratory functions are so compromised as to render the patient unstable, a laparoscopic procedure should not be attempted. In this setting, we prefer open surgery to avoid cardiovascular or respiratory labilities that can be associated with pneumoperitoneum. Significant dilatation of the bowel or complex enteroenteric or enterovesical fistulas would warrant consideration of an open approach for technical safety.

Complications

In general, medical complications such as cardiac and respiratory are qualitatively similar to what can generally occur after any type of surgery. Although most of the complications are qualitatively the same as for open surgery, a number of laparoscopic-specific complications have been described. Trocar-related complications have been reported but theoretically at least are diminished when the laparoscopic technique can be effectively mastered. In addition, it appears that potential damages deriving from the use of the Veress needle to induce pneumoperitoneum can be reduced by the adoption of the cut-down technique (Hasson technique), which allows for direct visualization of the planes of dissection. Inadvertent enterotomies can be attributed to the laparoscopic manipulation of the small intestine. In this regard, grasping of the bowel should always be gentle, and forceps should be preferentially applied to the pericolic or peritoneal tissues and not directly to the bowel. Cauterization should also be used with caution to prevent the risk of inadvertent burns that could result in a subsequent small bowel perforation. Inadvertent burn injuries are best avoided by having the entire length of the non-insulated portion of the cauterizing instrument in the viewing field.

A Cochrane review concerning the short-term benefits for laparoscopic colorectal resection reported on 25 randomized controlled trials with a total of 3,526 patients. Under traditional perioperative treatment, laparoscopic colonic resections showed clinically relevant advantages regarding intraoperative blood loss, postoperative pain, ileus, pulmonary function, and quality of life [21]. This systematic review of randomized controlled trials comparing laparoscopic and conventional colorectal resection for benign or malignant colorectal disease detailed the results for total complications as well as for several subgroups.

(1) Total morbidity: In 20 trials assessing morbidity, 2,879 participants were included. The overall morbidity was 20.6%. The incidence of postoperative complications was lower in the laparoscopic group (18.2%) compared to the conventional group (23.0%). The overall relative risk (RR) was 0.72 (95% CI 0.55–0.95; $p = 0.02$).
(2) General medical morbidity: The general medical morbidity was quite low with 129 events in 1,771 patients from 17 trials (7.3%). There was no significant difference in the medical morbidity between the laparoscopic groups (58 of 895; 6.5%) and the conventional groups (71 of 884; 8.0%) (RR 0.82 [95% CI 0.57–1.19; $p = 0.30$]). Pulmonary complications were observed in 35 patients (2%). Overall, there was no difference in the incidence of pulmonary complications between both groups (laparoscopic: 13 of 887 or 1.5%; conventional: 22 of 884 or 2.5%; RR: 0.69 [95% CI 0.35–1.35; $p = 0.27$]). Cardiac complications were reported in 25 of 1,688 patients (1.5%) during 16 trials. Again, there was no difference in cardiac morbidity between the laparoscopic and the conventional groups (RR 0.81 [95% CI 0.37–1.78; $p = 0.60$]) [21].

Thrombosis of the deep venous system in the lower extremities was a rare event, diagnosed in 9 of 1,688 patients from 16 trials (0.5%). The incidence of DVT was 0.35% (3/850) in the laparoscopic and 0.72% (6/838) in the conventional groups. This difference between both groups was not significant (RR 0.76 [95% CI 0.21–2.78; $p = 0.68$]) [21]).

(3) Surgical morbidity: Specific surgical morbidity was reported in 16 trials with a total of 1,688 participants. The overall surgical morbidity was 12.7% (215 out of 1,688 participants). Surgical complications were observed more often after conventional than after laparoscopic surgery (141 of 838 vs. 74 of 850 events: RR 0.55 [95% CI 0.39–0.77; $p = 0.0005$]).

Despite the shorter surgical incisions and limited communication between the skin, peritoneum, bowel, and wound infections do occur. The data on wound infections from 17 trials including 1,771 patients revealed that wound infections were less common in laparoscopic patients (41 out of 887 or 4.6%) than in conventional patients (77 out of 884 or 8.7%). The RR was 0.56 (95% CI 0.39–0.81; $p = 0.002$). Intraabdominal infections or abscesses were observed only in 5 of the 16 trials. The total number of patients included in the trials was 1,688. The reported incidence of intraabdominal abscess was not different between the laparoscopic groups (8 out of 850; 0.9%) and the conventional groups (11 out 838; 1.3%) (RR 0.71 [95% CI 0.28–1.80; $p = 0.47$]). In addition to the intraabdominal abscesses, 17 trials gave data concerning anastomotic leaks. The overall leak rate was 2.0%, and there was no difference in the leak rate between the laparoscopic and the conventional groups [21, 22]. Vascular and ureteral injuries are also comparable in frequency and presentation [21, 22].

Partial small bowel obstruction and postoperative ileus also have to be expected after laparoscopic colon resection. However, it appears less frequent in the laparoscopic groups and only was reported in 15 out of 887 patients or 1.7% compared to the conventional group which revealed 41 out of 887 patients or 4.6% with postoperative ileus in this report of 17 trials. The RR for the development of a postoperative ileus was 0.40 (95% CI 0.22–0.73; $p = 0.003$) in favor of the laparoscopic technique [23].

We have not found it imperative to close the mesenteric defect at completion of a laparoscopic colonic anastomosis. Although this could theoretically be associated with an increased risk of internal hernias, no report to date has been able to substantiate an increased incidence of this complication that would dictate a different technical approach. Retrieval of the wrong segment of bowel, i.e., the segment not bearing the tumor, or the inability to identify a synchronous colonic carcinoma has been reported [8], but is unlikely to occur when adequate caution is taken to ensure the site of the tumor. Should any doubts persist, intraoperative colonoscopy can be a valuable adjunct to help localize the lesion and plan the most appropriate management.

There is some evidence that LAC can actually be beneficial for preservation of cardiac and respiratory function in high-risk groups. In a matched-control study on patients older than 75, a significant decrease in morbidity after LAC has been found, where the specific complications were mainly medical, 12% in the LAC group vs. 26% after open colectomy [20]. It is of note that 55% of the patient population had an ASA classification of III or IV.

Laparoscopic procedures should also be an attractive option due to the possible advantages in reduction of certain long-term complications. Theoretically, a minimal abdominal incision should allow for lower incidence of incisional hernias. Most series do not report long-term follow-up; however, in an early study on 100 patients treated laparoscopically for diverticulitis with a median follow-up of 37 months, no incisional hernias were encountered [24]. Since then, two systematic reviews of the long-term outcome of laparoscopic surgery for colorectal cancer have not been able to demonstrate a decrease in hernia occurrence compared to open surgery [22, 25]. In addition, the use of the laparoscopic technique should allow for the reduction in postoperative adhesions, which would result in a major impact for cost containment. Data to support this potential advantage are insufficient. In a prospective cohort study analyzing the presence of postoperative adhesions to the anterior abdominal wall following laparoscopy, none of the 45 patients evaluated was shown to have postoperative adhesions at subsequent surgery [26]. Braga et al. reported on a randomized trial concerning 391 patients with long-term follow-up including re-operations for adhesions and did not observe a significant difference between open and laparoscopic procedures 1.1% vs. 2.5% with an odds ratio of 0.42 [27].

A further fascinating benefit associated with LAC, which is still being investigated, is the improved preservation of the immune system postoperatively. It is theorized that enhanced preservation of the immune response might result in reduced recurrence rates and improved survival. A number of substances have been considered as markers of a complex phenomenon, which most likely involves various systems.

Delayed-type hypersensitivity (DTH) has been studied as a marker of cell-mediated immune response and has been shown to be better preserved after laparoscopic cholecystectomy [28] and after LAC in an experimental model [29]. Interleukin-6 (IL-6) has been considered as a marker of inflammatory response and has been found to be significantly less responsive to surgical stress following LAC compared to open colectomy [30]. A randomized trial by the Barcelona group revealed significantly higher IL-6 and C-reactive protein (CRP) levels in patients undergoing open vs. laparoscopic colectomy [31]. Similar findings were reported in a randomized trial from Hong Kong with significantly attenuated responses in IL-1β, IL-6, and CRP [32].

Learning Curve

Several aspects of LAC contribute to its complexity. A laparoscopic colonic resection requires working in several different surgical fields, which requires a three-dimensional view including other organs contiguous with the colon that needs to be visualized during the procedure. To compound the difficulties, vascular ligation and an anastomosis are performed. It is therefore not surprising that technical proficiency is not immediate with this procedure. While several series have confirmed that LAC is safe and feasible, the amount of experience required to achieve proficiency in laparoscopic colon techniques is not yet established. Previous experience in laparoscopic surgery is no doubt helpful to develop confidence with LAC. Patient characteristics also affect the outcome of laparoscopic procedures early on, since it has been shown that obese patients or patients with multiple previous abdominal procedures are more prone to conversion to open surgery in one early report [33]. Surgeons approaching LAC for the first time should probably select a suitable candidate to insure a successfully completed laparoscopic procedure.

Since it is difficult to exactly predict how much experience is necessary before approaching a colon cancer operation, emphasis has been placed on standardizing the teaching of LAC. It is generally recommended that at least 20 cases of colonic resection for benign disease should be completed before proceeding to an LAC for malignancy. On the other end of the spectrum of laparoscopic colonic procedures, the creation of a palliative diverting colostomy or ileostomy is probably more reasonable as a starting point. Less experienced surgeons could therefore have the option to increase their experience in this novel approach and confer benefits to patients at the same time. In fact, stoma creation using a laparoscopic approach has been shown to be associated with the traditional advantages attributed to laparoscopy in a matched-control study when compared to open technique [34].

The learning curve has been estimated by looking at operative times, complications, and conversion rates; and the neophyte laparoscopic colorectal surgeon may expect improvements in all these areas. However, different series have shown a decrease in operative times, which can be variable according to the individual surgeon. Accordingly, different cutoff points where surgery becomes more expeditious have been detailed (Table 14.1).

With regard to learning the technique, the objection has been made that satisfactory results can be achieved only in selected centers with a wide experience in laparoscopic colon surgery. However, LAC is teachable and potentially applicable on a large basis. Kockerling and colleagues [35] have conducted a multicenter retrospective study on 231 laparoscopic procedures for colorectal cancer performed in 45 different institutions and analyzed the outcome for tumor perforation rate, distal resection margin, and number of harvested lymph nodes. No case of removal of incorrect colonic segment was reported, and the overall tumor perforation rate was 1.8%, which is comparable to open surgery. The number of harvested lymph nodes was significantly different among different institutions, although the number of positive nodes was not. This study suggests, therefore, that the quality of laparoscopic colon surgery appears acceptable, although it is variable among different surgeons, and feasible on a general basis and not only in few specialized centers. In addition, studies on the evaluation of laparoscopic surgical skill programs suggest that advanced laparoscopic procedures are not prohibitive, especially for those surgeons who have already been trained in laparoscopic surgery. In fact, there is evidence that residents can perform as well as trained open surgeons in a course on basic laparoscopic skills. In a survey comparing 291 trained surgeons and 99 residents, the two groups were equivalent for suturing exercises in a standardized training program [36]. Although it is not strictly appropriate to extrapolate these results to the complexity of a real laparoscopic procedure, it appears that current studies on learning curves are limited to analyzing the performance of surgeons who have become apprentices in laparoscopic surgery when

Table 14.1. The effect of the learning curve on operative times for laparoscopic colorectal procedures[a]

Authors	Year	No. of patients	Type of operation	Early[b]	Late[b]	Time reduction (%)	Breakpoint (cases)
Hoffman et al. [6]	1994	80	Colon and rectal	258	185	28	40
Jansen [60]	1994	19	Rectosigmoidectomy	294	186	37	5
Simons et al. [61][c]	1995	144	Right, left, and sigmoid colectomy	160	130	19	11–15
Wishner et al. [62]	1995	150	Colon and rectal	250	140	44	35–50
Stitz and Lumley [63]	1996	40	Right colectomy	180	130	28	20
		40	Anterior resection	240	150	38	20
Agachan et al. [64]	1997	175	Colon and rectal	201	141	30	70

[a]No homogeneous criteria applied.
[b]Average time in minutes.
[c]Derived from Fig. 15.1.
Adapted with permission from Stocchi and Nelson [59].

already fully trained in the traditional open technique. Conversely, it is expected that surgeons of the younger generation, being familiar with laparoscopy as part of their basic training, will learn more quickly and favor a more widespread application of LAC.

Conversion

The attitude toward conversion is also a key factor. If it seems evident that converting to open surgery results in a longer postoperative recovery and hospital stay when compared to a laparoscopically completed procedure, less obvious is the appropriate time when conversion should be considered. In addition, there is evidence from at least two studies that conversion can be associated with increased morbidity [24, 37]. Although a reduction in conversion rate has been considered a marker of increased experience, other issues should be taken into account to explain a crude conversion rate. It could be argued that surgeons accepting patients with a higher risk of requiring an open procedure and operating with a lower threshold for conversion will be more likely to increase not only their conversion rate but also the cost-effectiveness of laparoscopic surgery overall. In this regard, the value of early conversion is supported by Ramos and colleagues [38], who showed that converted procedures can be more expeditious than laparoscopic-completed counterparts. Therefore, it is probably safer for a surgeon to have a low threshold for conversion, since the timing of conversion is critical to reduce not only overall costs but also complications. There is increasing evidence of effective cost containment without any impairment in surgical outcomes when conversion is considered early during the procedure. It is apparent that each surgeon should develop the sensitivity to detect early in the procedure those conditions that would mandate conversion in any case and avoid any laparoscopic procedure completed at the expense of expeditiousness and straightforwardness.

Cancer Issues

Extent of Resection

Although follow-up is required to accurately examine cancer outcomes, there are a number of parameters that have been considered as indicative of an adequate cancer operation, including the length of the resected specimen, resection margins, and number of sampled lymph nodes. Initial trials revealed that LAC is comparable to OC when these comparative measurements

Table 14.2. Lymph node retrieval for open vs. laparoscopic colorectal surgery

Authors	Year	No. of patients (lap/open)	Type of operation	Laparoscopic (ranges, when reported)	Open
Hoffman et al. [6]	1994	32/31	Colon and rectal	8.0	6.1
Musser et al. [65]	1994	17/24	Colon and rectal	10.6	7.9
Van Ye et al. [43]	1994	14/20	Colon and rectal	10.5 (0–32)	7.6 (2–19)
Fine et al. [39]	1995	30/–	Colon and rectal	8.7–10[a]	10[a]
Tucker et al. [42]	1995	20/15[b]	Colon and rectal	8.7	6.4[b]
Saba et al. [15]	1995	20/25	Segmental colectomies	6 (0–21)	10 (2–27)
Franklin et al. [4]	1996	192/214	Colon and rectal	37	32
Gellman et al. [5]	1996	37/38	Colon and rectal	9.3	9.5
Lord et al. [11]	1996	13/19	Right colectomy	11.6	10.1
		19/30	Anterior resection	7.8	8.9
Moore et al. [40]	1996	30/34	Right colectomy	16.9 (4–56)	15.9 (4–30)
Stage et al. [41]	1997	15/14	Colon and rectal	7[c] (3–14)	8[c] (4–15)

[a]Three different surgeons are reported and compared to "average for similar cases."
[b]Comparison with patients converted to open procedures.
[c]Median.
Adapted with permission from Stocchi and Nelson [59].

are considered (Table 14.2) [4–6, 11, 13, 15, 39–43]. Most recent reviews and randomized clinical trials do not find any difference between the number of lymph nodes and length of specimen resection margins. One meta-analysis by Kuhry et al. [25] that reported on the long-term outcomes of laparoscopic surgery for colorectal cancer included six randomized controlled trials and found that in their review laparoscopic-assisted colectomy had a mean of one lymph node less than open colectomy ($p = 0.03$). This finding may have been influenced by the weighting of a relatively small randomized control trial with 30 patients and a significant difference in resected lymph nodes. Overall, the more recent large multicenter controlled trials all have revealed that there is no difference between the number of lymph nodes resected [21, 22, 44].

Tumor Staging

The magnified view offered by the laparoscope is an excellent method for intraperitoneal inspection. Findings at laparoscopy can be useful to plan the most appropriate management of the patient. In the case of detection of peritoneal carcinomatosis or non-resectable disease, a palliative procedure, being a resection or stoma creation, can follow. A bulky, locally advanced cancer or a perforating tumor can dictate conversion. In the case of apparently resectable disease, tumor staging is warranted. The traditional intraoperative tumor staging for open procedures includes inspection of the peritoneal cavity and palpation with particular emphasis on the liver, which is the most frequent location of distant metastases. This universally accepted approach can be complemented by preoperative computed tomography (CT), based on the preference of the surgeon. While inspection can be satisfactorily accomplished through the laparoscope, palpation is obviously not possible. The consequences of this new strategy are not known. Only prospective randomized trials will be able to establish whether preoperative CT staging of the liver alone results in a less accurate cancer staging and decreased survival. It is our impression that CT and ultrasound (US) imaging and laparoscopic viewing of the liver are complementary for intrahepatic and surface detection of metastases, respectively.

Alternative strategies to effectively examine the liver are being pursued. Laparoscopic ultrasonography (LUS) appears as a possible alternative for liver staging during laparoscopic surgery. Experimental [45] and initial clinical experiences have shown encouraging results. In a study of 60 patients randomized to either LAC or open colectomy, LUS was compared to CT scan and open intraoperative ultrasonography with bimanual palpation of the liver in a blinded fashion. After a median follow-up of 17 months, while staging modalities were comparably accurate in the detection of liver metastases, LUS was actually superior in the detection of benign hepatic lesions [46]. In another study of 76 consecutive patients undergoing LAC for cancer, LUS was less expensive and more sensitive than external ultrasonography and as sensitive as magnetic resonance imaging (MRI) [47]. Although these results would suggest a great potential for LUS, technical complexity still hampers a more widespread application of this novel modality, especially for surgeons who are not familiar with LAC.

Wound Recurrences

Alarming reports on tumor recurrences occurring at port sites have prompted concerns regarding the possibility that the use of pneumoperitoneum might be associated with a specific pattern of recurrence in addition to the traditional ones [48]. This is one of the factors that have prevented LAC initially from becoming a more popular procedure. However, when the incidence of port-site recurrence has been analyzed over longer time periods and on large numbers of patients, results have not been substantially dissimilar to the incidence of wound recurrence following open surgery (Table 14.3).

The pathogenesis of wound recurrences is still unclear. Although some experimental studies have suggested that cancer cells can be spread through the pneumoperitoneum, other reports have actually found that laparoscopy contributes to a slower tumor growth. Clinical studies have associated many of the wound recurrences to advanced tumor and a dismal prognosis. In contrast with that, a retrospective study conducted by the Clinical Outcomes of Surgical Therapy (COST) group has detected four cases of wound recurrence in 372 patients with adenocarcinoma of the colon and rectum treated by laparoscopic approach between 1991 and 1994 [49]. Only one of them resulted in a cancer-related death following a converted resection of a T4N1 colon cancer extended to the pancreas. In contrast, the other three port-site recurrences were successfully resected, with the patients having no evidence of disease at the time of the publication of the report. Although long-term follow-up was not available, this finding would suggest that wound recurrence does not necessarily portend a bad prognosis and might at least in some cases be less aggressive than what has been traditionally considered [49].

Table 14.3. Reported rates of wound tumor recurrences following laparoscopic colorectal surgery

Author	No. of wound recurrences/ No. of patients	Percent
Guillou et al. [66]	1/57	1.8
Berends et al. [48]	3/14	21
Drouard and Passone-Szerzyna [67]	12/507[a]	2.4
Boulez [18]	3/117	2.5
Fleshman et al. [49] (COST group)	4/372	1.1
Franklin et al. [4]	0/192	0
Gellman et al. [5]	1[b]/58	1.7
Hoffman et al. [68]	1/130	0.8
Kwok et al. [69]	1[b]/83	1.2
Lacy et al. [70]	0/106	0
Larach et al. [71]	0/108	0
Vukasin et al. [72]	5/451	1.1
Fielding et al. [73]	2[c]/149	1.3
Bouvet et al. [2]	0/91	0
Khalili et al. [7]	0/80	0
Milsom et al. [12]	0/55	0
Leung et al. [17]	1/179[a]	0.7

[a]Five cases of metastatic disease or carcinomatosis.
[b]After palliative procedure.
[c]After one palliative procedure.
Adapted with permission from Stocchi and Nelson [59].

Results of Randomized Trials and Meta-Analyses

A number of large multicenter trials have now been reported and are ongoing [44, 50–52]. In addition, meta-analysis and reviews of both the short-term and long-term outcomes of trials comparing laparoscopic vs. open approaches for the treatment of colon cancer have now been reported [21, 22, 25]. Comparing the two approaches, none of the studies reported a significantly shorter operating room time for the laparoscopic repair. The perioperative morbidity and mortality in the Barcelona, COST, CLASICC, and COLOR trials, however, are comparable. In addition, regarding the cancer recurrence, no difference has been found in survival between laparoscopic- and open colectomy-treated patients (Fig. 14.5). The rate and patterns of recurrence are comparable between the two approaches as well (Table 14.4). The short-term quality of life for a patient undergoing laparoscopic colectomy has been reported as improved compared to the laparoscopic group in the early assessment. However, 60 days after surgery in pooled data, there was no further advantage for the laparoscopic over the conventional technique. There appears to be no difference in survival either by cancer staged or by overall survival and for disease-free survival between the two approaches. The concern about the difference in trocar site recurrences and wound recurrences has meanwhile been reported to not be substantiated. In summary regarding the overall operative and cancer-specific outcomes, the overwhelming majority of the data revealed that LAC is a feasible and safe approach for the treatment of colon cancer.

Credentialing

A critical issue for the proper assessment of the effectiveness of laparoscopic technique in colon cancer is the quality control on the technical aspects of the procedure. In this view, surgeons are encouraged to participate in the trial, but are required to provide evidence of sufficient experience with submission of 20 documented LAC procedures. An appointed steering committee reviews videos of the procedure and accepts candidates as participating surgeons after ensuring that the basic oncologic principles that are routine parts of the open procedures are adhered to in the laparoscopic technique.

Table 14.4. COST Laparoscopic Trial – 5-year Cancer Outcomes

	Open $N = 428$ (%)	LAC $N = 435$ (%)	*p*-value
Overall survival	75	77	0.94
Disease-free survival	69	69	0.96
Local recurrence	2.6	2.3	0.79
Overall rates of recurrence	21.8	19.4	0.25

Outlook

Over the last several years, interest has been sparked in the use of natural orifices to enter the abdominal cavity or to retrieve specimen [53]. Most of those procedures are currently in investigational and experimental status; however, there has been a recent report of a transvaginal radical sigmoidectomy with the assistance of minilaparoscopic instrumentation from the Barcelona group [54].

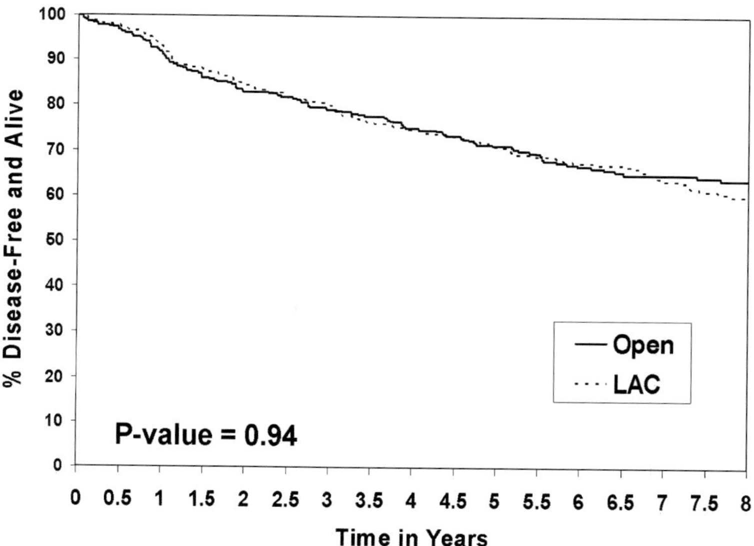

Figure 14.5

Five-year disease-free survival for patients with colon cancer (all stages) undergoing laparoscopic or open colectomy in the COST trial (Reprinted with permission from Fleshman et al. [74])

The theory behind using natural orifices is that the visceral innervation of the natural orifices allows for a more painless and less distressful access to the abdominal cavity. Currently, there is little data available comparing the natural orifice translumenal endoscopic surgical (NOTES) procedures with laparoscopic procedures. Anecdotal reports do suggest that less postoperative pain medication may be required in the patient undergoing NOTES [55]. The feasibility of experimental right hemicolectomy using NOTES has been demonstrated in a cadaveric model [56, 57]. While it is currently unclear whether the NOTES approach will truly revolutionize the minimally invasive surgical field and have significant impact on the treatment of colon cancer, the concept appears appealing and efforts should be made to investigate whether patient benefit is provided by the approach. In addition to the endoscopic translumenal procedures, endoluminal procedures are gaining more acceptance.

Conclusion

The initial skepticism for laparoscopic colectomy is gradually diminishing as patient-related benefits are being confirmed on an increasingly wide basis. Oncologic concerns regarding treatment of colorectal cancer with laparoscopic resection have now been investigated in prospective randomized trials. High-level evidence now supports the safety and feasibility of the laparoscopic approach for colon cancer.

References

1. Kemp J, Finlayson S (2008) Nationwide trends in laparoscopic colectomy from 2000 to 2004. Surg Endosc 22(5):1181–1187
2. Bouvet M et al (1998) Clinical, pathologic, and economic parameters of laparoscopic colon resection for cancer. Am J Surg 176(6):554–558
3. Falk PM et al (1993) Laparoscopic colectomy: a critical appraisal. Dis Colon Rectum 36(1):28–34
4. Franklin ME Jr. et al (1996) Prospective comparison of open vs. laparoscopic colon surgery for carcinoma. Five-year results. Dis Colon Rectum 39(10 Suppl):S35–S46
5. Gellman L, Salky B, Edye M (1996) Laparoscopic assisted colectomy. Surg Endosc 10(11):1041–1044
6. Hoffman GC, Baker JW, Fitchett CW, Vansant JH (1994) Laparoscopic-assisted colectomy. Initial experience. Ann Surg 219(6):732–740, discussion 740–3
7. Khalili TM et al (1998) Colorectal cancer: comparison of laparoscopic with open approaches. Dis Colon Rectum 41(7):832–838
8. Lacy AM et al (1995) Short-term outcome analysis of a randomized study comparing laparoscopic vs open colectomy for colon cancer. Surg Endoc 9(10):1101–1105
9. Leung KL et al (1997) Laparoscopic-assisted resection of rectosigmoid carcinoma. Immediate and medium-term results. Arch Surg 132(7):761–764, discussion 765
10. Liberman MA et al (1996) Laparoscopic colectomy vs traditional colectomy for diverticulitis. Outcome and costs [see comment]. Surg Endosc 10(1):15–18
11. Lord SA et al (1996) Laparoscopic resections for colorectal carcinoma. A three-year experience. Dis Colon Rectum 39(2):148–154
12. Milsom JW et al (1998) A prospective, randomized trial comparing laparoscopic versus conventional techniques in colorectal cancer surgery: a preliminary report [see comment]. J Am Coll Surg 187(1):46–54, discussion 54–5
13. Musser DJ et al (1994) Laparoscopic colectomy: at what cost? Surg Laparosc Endosc 4(1):1–5
14. Peters WR, Bartels TL (1993) Minimally invasive colectomy: are the potential benefits realized? Dis Colon Rectum 36(8):751–756
15. Saba AK et al (1995) Laparoscopic assisted colectomies versus open colectomy. J Laparoscop Surg 5(1):1–6
16. Senagore AJ et al (1993) Open colectomy versus laparoscopic colectomy: are there differences? Am Surg 59(8): 549–553, discussion 553–4
17. Leung KL et al (1999) Laparoscopic-assisted resection of colorectal carcinoma: five-year audit. Dis Colon Rectum 42(3):327–332, discussion 332–3
18. Boulez J (1996) Surgery of colorectal cancer by laparoscopic approach. Ann Chir 50(3):219–230
19. Schwandner O, Schiedeck TH, Bruch HP (1999) Advanced age–indication or contraindication for laparoscopic colorectal surgery? Dis Colon Rectum 42(3): 356–362
20. Stocchi L et al (2000) Safety and advantages of laparoscopic vs. open colectomy in the elderly: matched-control study. Dis Colon Rectum 43(3):326–332
21. Schwenk W et al (2005) Short term benefits for laparoscopic colorectal resection. Cochrane Database Syst Rev 20(3):CD003145
22. Lourenco T et al (2008) Laparoscopic surgery for colorectal cancer: safe and effective? – A systematic review. Surg Endosc 22(5):1146–1160
23. Schwenk W et al (1999) Pulmonary function following laparoscopic or conventional colorectal resection: a randomized controlled evaluation. Arch Surg 134(1):6–12, discussion 13
24. Stevenson AR et al (1998) Laparoscopically assisted anterior resection for diverticular disease: follow-up of 100 consecutive patients. Ann Surg 227(3):335–342
25. Kuhry E et al (2008) Long-term outcome of laparoscopic surgery for colorectal cancer: a cochrane systematic review of randomised controlled trials. Cancer Treat Rev 34(6):498–504
26. Levrant SG, Bieber EJ, Barnes RB (1997) Anterior abdominal wall adhesions after laparotomy or laparoscopy. J Am Assoc Gynecol Laparosc 4(3):353–356

27. Braga M et al (2005) Laparoscopic vs. open colectomy in cancer patients: long-term complications, quality of life, and survival. Dis Colon Rectum 48(12):2217–2223
28. Kloosterman T et al (1994) Unimpaired immune functions after laparoscopic cholecystectomy. Surgery 115(4): 424–428
29. Bessler M et al (1994) Is immune function better preserved after laparoscopic versus open colon resection? Surg Endosc 8(8):881–883
30. Harmon GD et al. (1994) Interleukin-6 response to laparoscopic and open colectomy. Dis Colon Rectum 37(8): 754–759
31. Delgado S et al (2001) Acute phase response in laparoscopic and open colectomy in colon cancer: randomized study. Dis Colon Rectum 44(5):638–646
32. Leung KL et al (2000) Systemic cytokine response after laparoscopic-assisted resection of rectosigmoid carcinoma: a prospective randomized trial. Ann Surg 231(4):506–511
33. Dean PA et al (1994) Laparoscopic-assisted segmental colectomy: early Mayo Clinic experience. Mayo Clin Proc 69(9):834–840
34. Radice E, Young-Fadok TM, Nelson H (1998) Benefits of laparoscopic stoma creation: a casematched series (Abstract # G0145). Gastroenterology 114(Suppl 1):A35
35. Kockerling F et al (1998) Prospective multicenter study of the quality of oncologic resections in patients undergoing laparoscopic colorectal surgery for cancer. The Laparoscopic Colorectal Surgery Study Group. Dis Colon Rectum 41(8):963–970
36. Rosser JC Jr., Rosser LE, Savalgi RS (1998) Objective evaluation of a laparoscopic surgical skill program for residents and senior surgeons [see comment]. Arch Surg 133(6): 657–661
37. Slim K et al (1995) High morbidity rate after converted laparoscopic colorectal surgery. Br J Surg 82(10): 1406–1408
38. Ramos JM et al (1995) Role of laparoscopy in colorectal surgery. A prospective evaluation of 200 cases.[see comment]. Dis Colon Rectum 38(5):494–501
39. Fine AP et al (1995) Laparoscopic colon surgery: report of a series. Am Surg 61(5):412–416
40. Moore JW et al (1996) Lymphovascular clearance in laparoscopically assisted right hemicolectomy is similar to open surgery. Aus NZ J Surg 66(9):605–607
41. Stage JG et al (1997) Prospective randomized study of laparoscopic versus open colonic resection for adenocarcinoma [see comment]. Br J Surg 84(3):391–396
42. Tucker JG et al (1995) Laparoscopically assisted bowel surgery. Analysis of 114 cases. Surg Endosc 9(3):297–300
43. Van Ye TM, Cattey RP, Henry LG (1994) Laparoscopically assisted colon resections compare favorably with open technique. Surg Laparosc Endosc 4(1):25–31
44. Clinical Outcomes of Surgical Therapy Study G (2004) A comparison of laparoscopically assisted and open colectomy for colon cancer [see comment]. N Engl J Med 350(20):2050–2059
45. Stocchi L et al (1999) Laparoscopic ultrasonography: a developmental model (Abstract). Dis Colon Rectum 42(4):A51
46. Milsom JW et al (2000) Prospective, blinded comparison of laparoscopic ultrasonography vs. contrast-enhanced computerized tomography for liver assessment in patients undergoing colorectal carcinoma surgery. Dis Colon Rectum 43(1):44–49
47. Hartley JE et al (2000) Laparoscopic ultrasound for the detection of hepatic metastases during laparoscopic colorectal cancer surgery. Dis Colon Rectum 43(3):320–324, discussion 324–5
48. Berends FJ et al (1994) Subcutaneous metastases after laparoscopic colectomy [see comment]. Lancet 344(8914):58
49. Fleshman JW et al (1996) Early results of laparoscopic surgery for colorectal cancer. Retrospective analysis of 372 patients treated by Clinical Outcomes of Surgical Therapy (COST) Study Group. Dis Colon Rectum 39 (10 Suppl):S53–S58
50. Guillou PJ et al (2005) Short-term endpoints of conventional versus laparoscopic-assisted surgery in patients with colorectal cancer (MRC CLASICC trial): multicentre, randomised controlled trial [see comment]. Lancet 365(9472):1718–1726
51. Lacy AM et al (2002) Laparoscopy-assisted colectomy versus open colectomy for treatment of non-metastatic colon cancer: a randomised trial [see comment]. Lancet 359(9325):2224–2229
52. Veldkamp R et al (2005) Laparoscopic surgery versus open surgery for colon cancer: short-term outcomes of a randomised trial. Lancet Oncol 6(7):477–484
53. Dozois E et al (2008) Transvaginal colonic extraction following combined hysterectomy and laparoscopic total colectomy: a natural orifice approach. Tech Coloproctol 12(3):251–254
54. Lacy AM et al (2008) MA-NOS radical sigmoidectomy: report of a transvaginal resection in the human. Surg Endosc 22(7):1717–1723
55. Zorron R. NOTES transvaginal cholecystectomy – comparative clinical study with Laparoscopy. Proceedings of the 3rd International Conference on NOTES, San Francisco, 2008.
56. Whiteford MH, Denk PM, Swanstrom LL (2007) Feasibility of radical sigmoid colectomy performed as natural orifice translumenal endoscopic surgery (NOTES) using transanal endoscopic microsurgery. Surg Endosc 21(10): 1870–1874
57. Young-Fadok TM et al (2007) NOTES right colectomy: a feasibility study (Abstract #790). Gastroenterology 132(4):A115
58. Young-Fadok TM, Nelson H (2000) Laparoscopic right colectomy: five-step procedure. Dis Colon Rectum 43(2):267–271
59. Stocchi L, Nelson H (1998) Laparoscopic colectomy for colon cancer: trial update. J Surg Oncol 68:255–267
60. Jansen A (1994) Laparoscopic-assisted colon resection. Evolution from an experimental technique to a standardized surgical procedure. Ann Chir Gynecol 83: 86–91
61. Simons AJ, Anthone GJ, Ortega AE et al (1995) Laparoscopic-assisted colectomy learning curve. Dis Colon Rectum 38:600–603
62. Wishner JD, Baker JW Jr, Hoffman GC et al (1995) Laparoscopic-assisted colectomy. The learning curve. Surg Endosc 9:1179–1183

63. Stitz RW, Lumley JW (1996) Laparoscopic colorectal surgery – new advances and techniques. Ann Acad Med Singapore 25:653–656
64. Agachan F, Joo JS, Sher M, Weiss EG, Nogueras JJ, Wexner SD (1997) Laparoscopic colorectal surgery. Do we get faster? Surg Endosc 11:331–335
65. Musser DJ, Boorse RC, Madera F, Reed JF 3rd. (1994) Laparoscopic colectomy: at what cost? Surg Laparosc Endosc 4:1–5
66. Guillou PJ, Darzi A, Monson JR (1993) Experience with laparoscopic colorectal surgery for malignant disease. Surg Oncol 2(Suppl 1):43–49
67. Drouard F, Passone-Szerzyna N. Les greffes neoplasiques parietales en chirurgie laparoscopique colo-rectale. Communication III Symposium SFCE, Bordeaux, 1995
68. Hoffman GC, Baker JW, DoxeyJ B, Hubbard GW, Ruffin WK, Wishner JA (1996) Minimally invasive surgery for colorectal cancer. Initial follow-up. Ann Surg 223:790–796
69. Kwok SP, Lau WY, Carey PD, Kelly SB, Leung KL, Li AK (1996) Prospective evaluation of laparoscopic-assisted large bowel excision for cancer. Ann Surg 223:170–176
70. Lacy AM, Garcia-Valdecasas JC, Delgado S et al (1997) Postoperative complications of laparoscopic-assisted colectomy. Surg Endosc 11:119–122
71. Larach SW, Patankar SK, Ferrara A, Williamson PR, Perozo SE, Lord AS (1997) Complications of laparoscopic colorectal surgery. Analysis and comparison of early vs. latter experience. Dis Colon Rectum 40:592–596
72. Vukasin P, Ortega AE, Greene FL et al (1996) Wound recurrence following laparoscopic colon cancer resection. Results of the American society of colon and rectal surgeons laparoscopic registry. Dis Colon Rectum 39: S20–S23
73. Fielding GA, Lumley J, Nathanson L, Hewitt P, Rhodes M, Stitz R (1997) Laparoscopic colectomy. Surg Endosc 11:745–749
74. Fleshman J, Sargent D, Green E et al (2007) Laparoscopic colectomy for cancer is not inferior to open surgery based on 5-year data from the cost study group trial. Ann Surg 246(4):655–664

Laparoscopic Resection of Rectal Cancer

Tonia M. Young-Fadok

Contents

The diagnosis, staging, and treatment of rectal cancer are well established and will be covered briefly. The main intent of this chapter is to describe laparoscopic techniques that adhere to oncologic requirements for the resection of rectal cancer. It is important to remember that the remainder of the complex treatment of rectal cancer should not be influenced by consideration of a laparoscopic approach.

Current Issues and Concerns

Resection of rectal cancer by open techniques is well standardized. Heald and others have demonstrated that complete excision of the lymphovascular mesorectal envelope associated with the rectum, in the procedure known as total mesorectal excision (TME), is associated with significantly reduced local recurrence rates [1, 2]. The technique has been accepted and adopted internationally. The issue is whether or not the stringent requirements of this approach can be achieved with laparoscopic instrumentation and techniques.

Randomized controlled trials [3–7] and a meta-analysis [8] have established that there are short-term benefits from laparoscopic resection of colon cancer when compared with open resection. In addition, despite early concerns regarding incisional tumor recurrences after a laparoscopic approach for colon cancer, the studies have demonstrated equivalent oncologic outcomes in terms of overall and disease-free survival. However, only one trial has included rectal cancer patients, the UK Medical Research Council Conventional vs. Laparoscopic-Assisted Surgery in Colorectal Cancer (UKMRC CLASICC) [6], and although 3 year oncologic outcomes were reported to be similar [9], there were concerns regarding high rates of circumferential positive margins, and high conversion rates, in addition to lack of standardization of the techniques and use of neoadjuvant therapy.

F.L. Greene, B.T. Heniford (eds.), *Minimally Invasive Cancer Management*,
DOI 10.1007/978-1-4419-1238-1_15,

Thus, although the oncologic adequacy of laparoscopic resection for colon cancer has been established, this has not been established for rectal cancer. Whether performed open or laparoscopically, TME is a more challenging procedure than colon resection, given the confines of the bony pelvis and the specific planes of dissection that must be followed.

A randomized controlled trial is underway comparing laparoscopic vs. open resection for rectal cancer, under the auspices of the American College of Surgeons Oncology Group (ACoSOG), trial Z6051 [10]. This chapter emphasizes some of the oncologic approaches approved for surgeon participation in this study. As always, resection of rectal cancer, whether laparoscopic or open, should only be performed by surgeons adequately trained in the relevant techniques.

Diagnosis and Staging

Initial diagnosis may be made on the basis of physical examination in the case of a distal rectal cancer or on endoscopic evaluation performed either for screening or for symptoms. Evaluation includes a complete history and physical examination; laboratory tests include a complete blood count, chemistries, liver function tests, and carcinoembryonic antigen (CEA) level; imaging includes chest radiograph (CXR), computed tomography (CT) scan of the abdomen and pelvis; and complete evaluation of the colon and rectum with colonoscopy and biopsies. The aim is to determine the characteristics of the primary tumor – size, distance from or involvement of the sphincter muscles, and mobility or fixation to circumferential structures (sacrum, coccyx, pelvic floor, vagina, prostate, or bladder). The CXR and CT help assess for distant metastases that may determine a curative vs. a palliative approach. Positron emission tomography may also be helpful in ruling out metastatic disease, but needs to be used selectively, as its use in Medicare patients may result in the patient being charged for the procedure.

Patients without evidence of systemic disease (stage IV) are further evaluated to determine the degree of penetration of the primary tumor through the rectal wall (T category) and absence or presence of involved lymph nodes. Endoscopic ultrasound (EUS) is most widely used for this in the United States; magnetic resonance imaging (MRI) is more widely used in Europe and is also used in the United States in cases of equivocal EUS findings, or in order to better delineate circumferential margins, particularly when involvement of the sacrum is suspected.

Full-thickness tumors (T3) and evidence of nodal involvement are generally treated with neoadjuvant chemoradiation, with a 6-week course of 5,040 Gy and a chemotherapy regimen that utilizes infusional 5-fluorouracil. Surgical intervention is then planned after a "cooling-off" period of approximately 6 weeks, allowing surrounding tissues to recover, and tumor response to chemoradiation to continue. T4 lesions that may require en-bloc resection of adjacent structures, if not down-sized by neoadjuvant therapy, are unlikely to be amenable to a laparoscopic approach and are not covered here. Likewise, the very few early lesions that are appropriate for local excision are not further covered.

Oncologic Principles and Operative Strategy

Laparoscopic resection of rectal cancer should adhere to the same oncologic principles that have been well established for open resection of rectal cancer [11]. The laparoscopic approach should not result in deviation from these principles, and inability to adhere to the standard operative approach is an indication for conversion to an open procedure.

A curative oncologic resection is widely considered to include the following technical and anatomic details:

- Rectal washout with tumoricidal solution.
- Preliminary examination of the liver and peritoneal surfaces to rule out metastatic disease.
- Minimal manipulation of the tumor.
- Proximal or high ligation of the inferior mesenteric artery (IMA). Some surgeons accept proximal ligation of the superior rectal artery.
- Total mesorectal excision for tumors of the mid and distal rectum and appropriate level of mesorectal excision for tumors of the proximal rectum.
- Clear circumferential margins.
- Adequate distal margin, 2 cm where possible, 1 cm for very distal lesions.
- Use of specimen extraction bag or wound protector during extraction of the specimen.

Only the last detail is specific to laparoscopic operations, the other details pertaining equally to laparoscopic and open procedures.

Indications and Contraindications

Careful patient selection is paramount in ensuring both patient safety and optimal oncologic outcomes. The first requirements are of the surgeon: he or she must be familiar with the demands of the TME approach and have the laparoscopic skills to be able to apply this technique without compromising the adequacy of the oncologic resection. Patient factors that contraindicate a laparoscopic approach are morbid obesity, known extensive adhesions, or bulky tumor filling the pelvis on CT scan. Coagulopathy and pregnancy are relative contraindications.

Preoperative Preparation

Preoperative preparation consists of several components: restaging the patient who has had neoadjuvant chemoradiation therapy, evaluation of the patient's medical fitness for a major abdominal operation, and planning for a potential stoma.

Restaging typically consists of physical examination (including a digital rectal examination to determine response of the tumor to chemoradiation), blood tests (complete blood count, electrolytes, renal and liver functions tests, and carcinoembryonic antigen), chest radiograph, and CT scan of the abdomen and pelvis. In selected patients, additional testing in the form of PET scan or MRI may be warranted, as indicated by concerns for metastatic disease or circumferential tumor margins, respectively.

All patients undergoing elective resection of rectal cancer in our institution have a full medical evaluation and examination. This ensures adequate cardiac and pulmonary reserves for these major resections. Comorbidities, such as diabetes, COPD, renal insufficiency, are elucidated and management is optimized. As resection is usually scheduled approximately 6 weeks after completion of chemoradiation, patients have usually recovered from any side effects, but if there are concerns regarding nutritional status, prealbumin levels are obtained.

Preoperative counseling includes a discussion of the operative risks, benefits, and alternatives. Typically the risks are those of bleeding, infection, anastomotic leak, ureteral injury, bladder and sexual dysfunction (especially urinary retention, impotence, and retrograde ejaculation in men), and standard perioperative risks of deep vein thrombosis (DVT), pulmonary embolus, stroke, and myocardial infarction. Counseling also includes consultation with an enterostomal therapist who initiates discussion about stoma care and marks the patient's abdomen for optimal stoma siting.

Perioperative Preparation

The patient is given a bowel preparation to be performed the day before operation. Options have become more limited since the withdrawal of phosphate-based laxatives. On the day before surgery, the patient consumes only clear liquids and in the afternoon takes a 2 l polyethylene glycol preparation, accompanied by two 10 mg bisacodyl tablets.

On the day of operation, DVT prophylaxis includes elastic stockings, sequential compression devices, and subcutaneous heparin. We follow the Surgical Infection Prevention (SIP) guidelines with administration of an appropriate antibiotic, within 60 min of the incision and discontinue prophylactic antibiotic coverage within 24 h of closure of the incision [12–15]. Adherence to SIP guidelines has been facilitated by moving the responsibility for preoperative antibiotic administration from the preoperative nursing staff to the anesthesia team and using Ertapenem 1 g iv, which affords 24 h coverage, and thus no postoperative antibiotic orders are required (unless the patient is allergic to penicillin in which case pre- and postoperative coverage is afforded by the approved combination of ciprofloxacin 500 mg iv and metronidazole 500 mg iv).

Some surgeons have a preference for epidural anesthesia. While it may reduce postoperative ileus, there is oftentimes hesitation in a busy operating room schedule to increase delay to incision time. There is also the disinclination to consider an epidural when there is the expectation from a laparoscopic case that the patient will have small incisions and less pain. This author does not have a strong preference for epidural anesthesia for laparoscopic cases.

Instruments

Table 15.1 lists our typical instruments for laparoscopic proctectomy. My preferred energy source for dissection is electrocautery scissors with a curved tip. These reproduce the use of cautery devices in the open

Table 15.1. Trocars and Instrumentation

Trocars
One 12 mm supraumbilical trocar for the laparoscope
One 12 mm right lower quadrant trocar for stapler
Two 5 mm trocars (suprapubic midline, left lower quadrant)
Instruments
30 degree 10 mm laparoscope
Two 5 mm atraumatic bowel graspers
Laparoscopic scissors with finger-operated cautery switch
Bowel sizers (used transanally to assist with retraction)
Vessel sealing energy device (surgeon preference)
Laparoscopic articulated linear stapler (30 and 45 mm cartridges)
Circular stapler
Suction irrigator
Smoke evacuator
Optional Additional Equipment
Additional 5 mm trocar if required to assist pelvic dissection

setting and the curved tip facilitates visualization. For tissue division I use a vessel sealing device, whereas others prefer the ultrasonic shears. I find the former faster than the ultrasonic shears and able to divide all the vessels encountered in the mesentery, including the IMA.

Positioning

Prior to induction of general endotracheal anesthesia, sequential compression devices are placed on the patient's lower extremities, over-graded compression stockings, and the device is started, prior to the vasodilatation that occurs with the onset of general anesthesia. After intubation, the patient is carefully positioned in the modified Lloyd-Davis position (referred to within Mayo Clinic as the combined synchronous position) (Fig. 15.1). The anus should be just beyond the end of the table to facilitate use of circular stapling instruments or potential need for hand sewn anastomosis. The legs are supported in padded mobile lithotomy stirrups, and the thighs *must* be within 5–10° of being level with the torso to prevent interference with the laparoscopic instruments deployed via the lower quadrant trocars during mobilization of the splenic flexure. We use pink foam padding, taped to the operating table, to prevent the patient slipping. After padding the hands with pink foam, a draw sheet placed under the patient is wrapped under and around the arms and then tucked under the torso to keep the arms closely aligned to the patient's body. Additional gel pads are placed under the elbows. It is important to tuck both arms, if possible, to facilitate operating in the pelvis. Some surgeons prefer the use of a moldable beanbag. We prefer not to use this: it takes longer to position the patient and injuries have been described with the beanbag. We have experienced no injuries associated with the above method of positioning. A catheter is placed within the bladder, and an orogastric tube is placed to decompress the stomach and is removed at the end of the case.

Rectal irrigation is performed with full-strength povidone–iodine solution which is left in place, theoretically to prevent tumor cell implantation in the anastomosis [16]. It is our preference to do this prior to commencement of the procedure rather than as the rectum is about to be transected, because adequacy of the bowel preparation can be confirmed and the solution remains in contact with the tumor for a greater period of time. Digital rectal exam confirms mobility of the tumor and its distance from the superior margin of the sphincter complex.

Port Placement

A supraumbilical cut down is employed in most patients to place the initial 12 mm blunt port and establish the pneumoperitoneum to 13 mmHg. In a teaching institution we believe the cut down technique is safer, and in the supraumbilical position the cut down is made easier by fusion of the anterior and posterior rectus fascia. If the patient has a prior midline incision, this technique can still be used, or an optical viewing port can be used beneath either costal margin. I never use a Veress needle.

Again to facilitate teaching, a standard pattern of port placement is used for all cases and adapted as indicated. A diamond-shaped pattern of ports is used: supraumbilical 12 mm port, two 5 mm ports in the left lower quadrant and the suprapubic midline, and a 10 mm port in the right lower quadrant. The lower quadrant ports can be placed within the rectus sheath, but the epigastric vessels must be visualized to

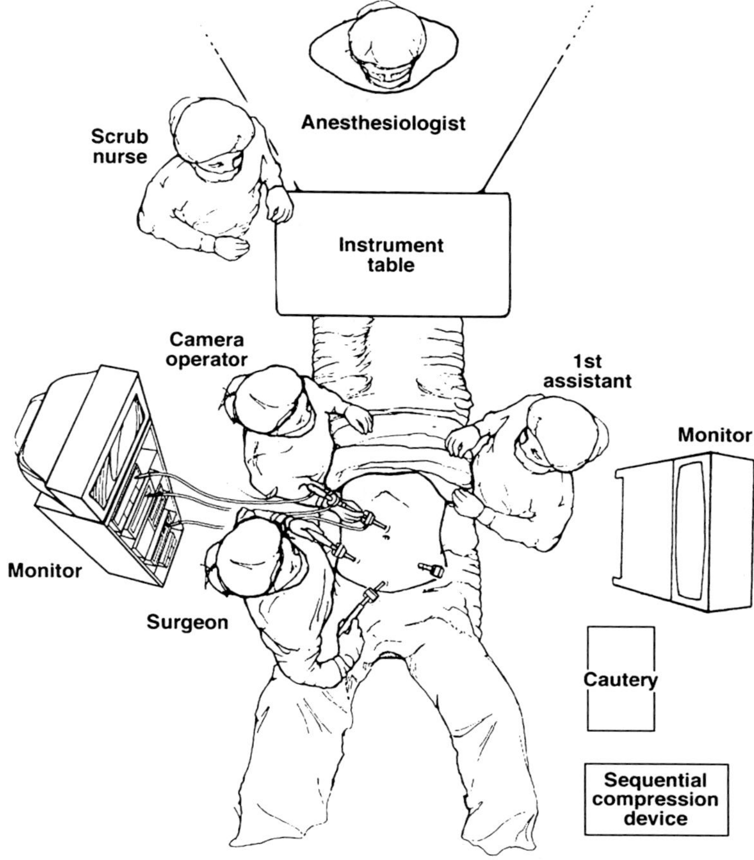

Figure 15.1

Typical operating room positioning and setup (Reprinted by permission of Mayo Foundation for Medical Education and Research. All rights reserved)

avoid injury. When it is definitely anticipated that an ileostomy will be created, the marked site is used for the right lower quadrant port, after excising a disc of skin and subcutaneous fat.

Procedure

Assessment and Tumor Localization

All four quadrants of the abdomen, and the pelvis, are viewed to exclude metastatic deposits and determine the feasibility of a laparoscopic approach. If the lesion in the rectum is above the reach of the examining finger, rigid, or flexible proctoscopy can be performed and the distal margin of the tumor marked if it is above the peritoneal reflection. If the tumor is below the peritoneal reflection this endoscopy may need to be repeated prior to transection of the rectum. The degree of insufflation required for this step is minimal as the lesion is in the rectum.

Liver Evaluation

Direct Inspection

As part of the initial evaluation of the peritoneal cavity the liver is inspected. For optimal views, the operating table should be in steep reverse Trendelenburg. Use of a 10 mm 30° scope allows the surfaces of the liver to be examined. We do not routinely perform liver ultrasonography. The COST randomized controlled trial of laparoscopic vs. open colectomy for colon cancer performed CT scans in all patients preoperatively and inspection of the liver intraoperatively [4]. There was no excess of liver metastasis in the laparoscopic arm, despite the inability to palpate the liver. Hence the assumption that CT scan of the liver plus inspection of the liver surface is equivalent to intraoperative palpation of the liver. In fact, laparoscopic visualization appears, if anything, to demonstrate small flat superficial lesions that are missed by CT scan. Whereas some surgeons perform routine intraoperative hepatic ultrasound, with our current CT scans affording resolution to 3 mm, it is doubtful that intraoperative ultrasound adds anything beyond expense to the procedure. In cases of indeterminate lesions within the liver, the case is scheduled concomitantly with one of our experienced ultrasonographers to perform intraoperative ultrasound of the liver. This is rare given the resolution of current CT scanners.

Overview of Laparoscopic Proctectomy

There are two main laparoscopic approaches: medial-to-lateral and lateral-to-medial. In the former, the base of the IMA is isolated and divided at the beginning of the procedure, and the dissection of the left colon off the retroperitoneum occurs in a medial-to-lateral fashion. Proponents note that this approach adheres to the Turnbull no-touch technique and that leaving division of the lateral attachments until the end of the mobilization helps to retract the colon out of the operative field.

The author is a proponent of the lateral-to-medial approach. With this technique, the starting point for the procedure is opening the lateral peritoneal attachments along the white line of Toldt alongside the sigmoid and descending colon and mobilizing the colon from the lateral aspect of the retroperitoneum. The IMA is divided toward the end of the procedure, after dissection and transection of the rectum. Such an approach has several advantages: the approach is similar to the open one, and thus the tissue planes are more readily recognized by trainees; the plane of dissection tends to be more bloodless, as the white line of Toldt is a natural embryological plane, almost like having a "dotted line"; there is no proven oncologic advantage to early division of the vessels; and there is no resultant section of ischemic colon sitting in the abdominal cavity while the rectal dissection is being performed.

Mobilization of the Left Colon and Splenic Flexure

The operating table is placed in Trendelenburg position with the left side inclined upward, using gravity to move loops of small bowel away from the operative field. The surgeon and camera assistant stand on the patient's left side facing a video monitor placed near the patient's left hip. The first assistant stands on the right using a monitor placed near the patient's right knee. The camera is used through the supraumbilical port. The surgeon uses a Babcock or other bowel grasper via the LLQ port and electrocautery scissors via the suprapubic port. The first assistant generally is not needed during this portion but may assist with retraction. Commencing at the left pelvic brim, the left lateral peritoneal reflection alongside the sigmoid colon is opened, staying *immediately* medial to the white line of Toldt, i.e., leaving the peritoneal reflection with the patient. By staying in this correct plane, the ureter is found at the base of the plane and can then be gently swept laterally (Fig. 15.2).

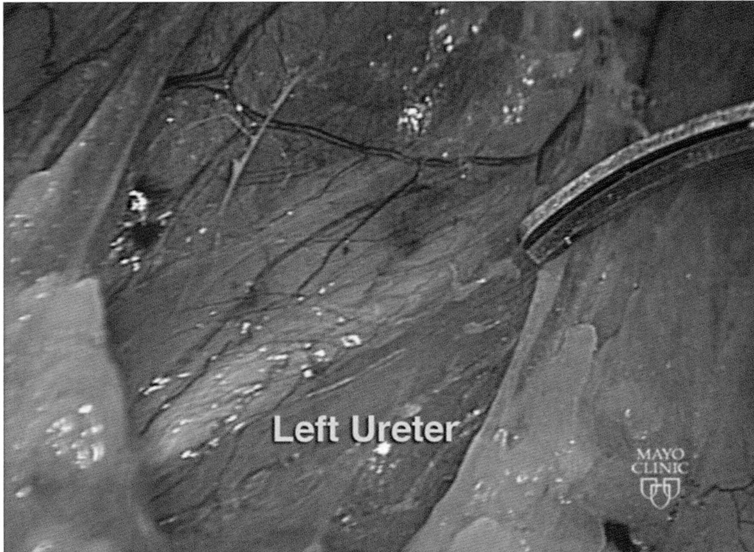

Figure 15.2

The left ureter is carefully identified and observed for movement to confirm its identity

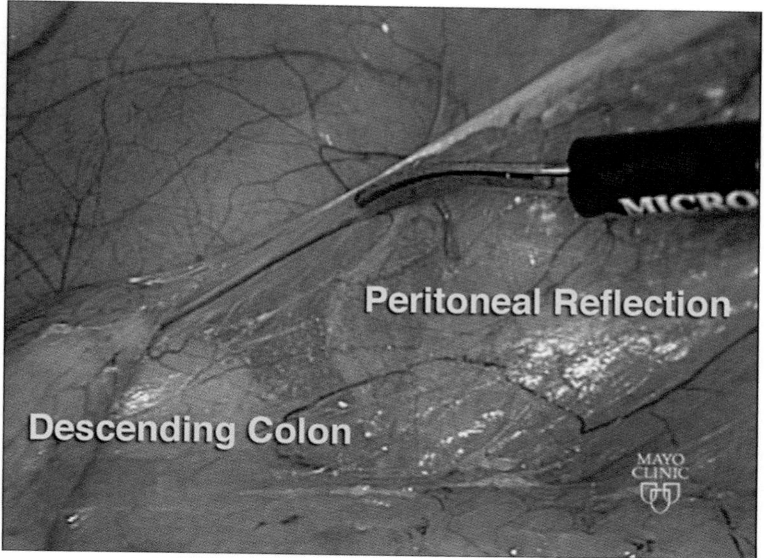

Figure 15.3

The left lateral peritoneal reflection alongside the descending colon is opened, immediately medial to the white line of Toldt

The left lateral peritoneal reflection alongside the descending colon is then opened and the descending colon mobilized medially to the full medial extent of the mesentery (Fig. 15.3). The plane typically becomes a little more fibrous or "sticky" as the dissection proceeds cephalad and medially over Gerota's fascia. Dissection proceeds as far toward the splenic flexure as this position allows.

We mobilize the splenic flexure on all cases of rectal resection. The table is then moved to reverse Trendelenburg, still with the left side inclined up. The surgeon stands between the legs using the RLQ and suprapubic ports. The first assistant stands on the left side, and all use the left-sided video monitor which is moved to the patient's left shoulder. It is often surprising how far the dissection has proceeded toward the splenic flexure. Laterally, dissection is performed behind the splenic flexure/proximal descending colon to lift it off the retroperitoneum and pancreas (Fig. 15.4). Dissection continues medially above the colon, entering the lateral aspect of the lesser sac to free the distal transverse colon (Fig. 15.5).

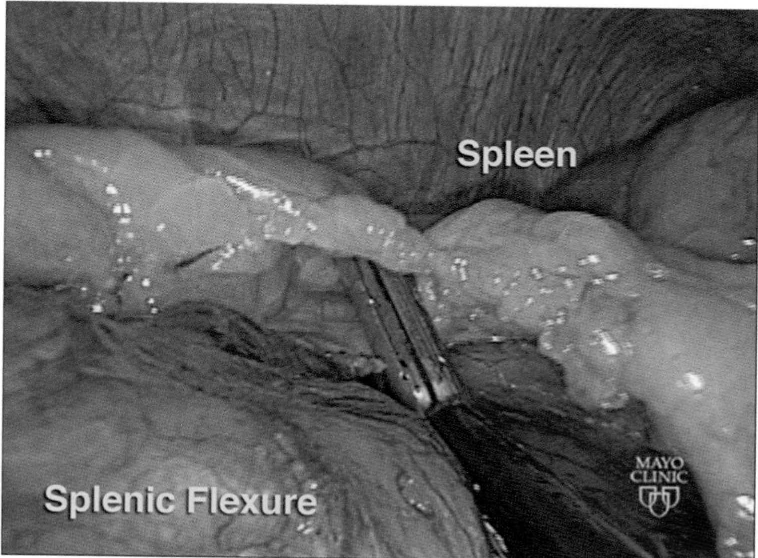

Figure 15.4

The lateral aspect of the splenic flexure is mobilized, dissecting the proximal descending colon off the retroperitoneum

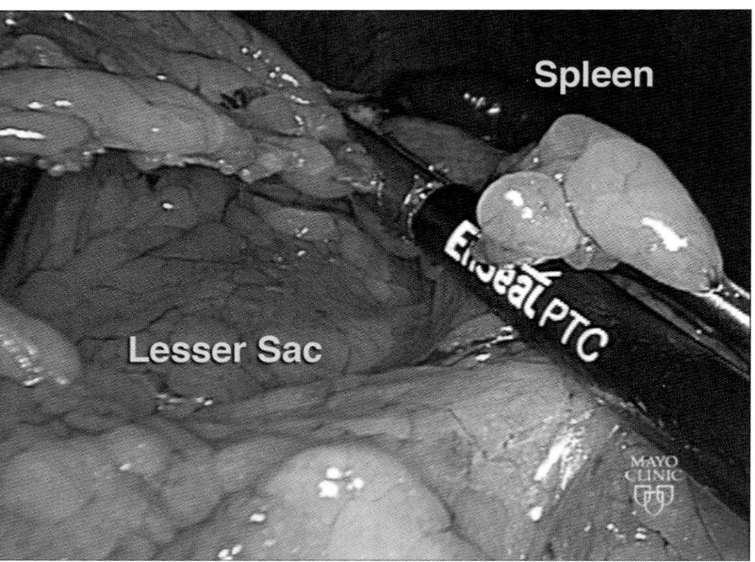

Figure 15.5

The medial aspect of the splenic flexure is mobilized, by entering the lesser sac

There are two methods of approaching the omentum. In a patient with normal body mass index (BMI), it is usually possible to elevate the omentum and dissect in the bloodless plane between the omentum and the superior border of the distal transverse colon in order to separate the omentum from the colon. In a heavier patient, this plane is often obscured, and it is easier to mobilize the distal transverse colon with the omentum still attached. This is achieved by reducing the degree of reverse Trendelenburg, moving the omentum inferiorly, and entering the lesser sac above the distal transverse colon (Fig. 15.5). The dissection is then continued laterally, dividing the splenocolic attachments until the splenic flexure is fully mobilized. Adequate mobilization is checked: if the splenic flexure can be moved down to a position below the umbilicus then the entire left colon can be exteriorized via a periumbilical incision.

Pelvic Dissection

Following full mobilization of the entire left colon to the midline, attention is then turned to the pelvis. The surgeon stands on the patient's left side, the first assistant on the right, and the two monitors at the patient's ankles. With the table in Trendelenburg and left side inclined up, the left ureter is identified prior to scoring the left pararectal peritoneum at approximately the level of the sacral promontory (Fig. 15.6). The presacral space is entered and is developed medially, laterally, and distally as far as visualization allows. The correct plane is a bloodless plane anterior to the hypogastric nerves, which are carefully identified and protected (Fig. 15.7). The magnification provided by the laparoscope aids in identification of the nerves.

After moving the table to slight right side up, and identifying the right ureter, the right pararectal peritoneum is scored (Fig. 15.8). The correct line of incision is often indicated by air in the tissues demarcating the plane already developed from the left side. The presacral space is entered and the dissection joined with that already performed from the left, again identifying and protecting the right hypogastric nerve. The plane is again developed medially, laterally, and distally.

By pulling the rectum out of the pelvis this now allows tension to be placed to expose the plane of dissection anteriorly. In female patients who have not had a hysterectomy the uterus may be elevated out of the pelvis by using a uterine manipulator, or more simply, by placing a transabdominal suture through the fundus of the uterus and tying the suture at skin level over a pledget. In all female patients, exposure of the rectovaginal septum can be enhanced by placing a sponge stick in the vagina and elevating the vagina anteriorly.

In this manner, complete circumferential dissection of the rectum can be performed in the correct TME plane (Fig. 15.9). For mid-rectal cancers, the distal margin should be evaluated with rigid or flexible endoscopy and a margin 2 cm distal to the tumor is the point where the mesorectum is divided. This is achieved in one of several ways such as using an energy

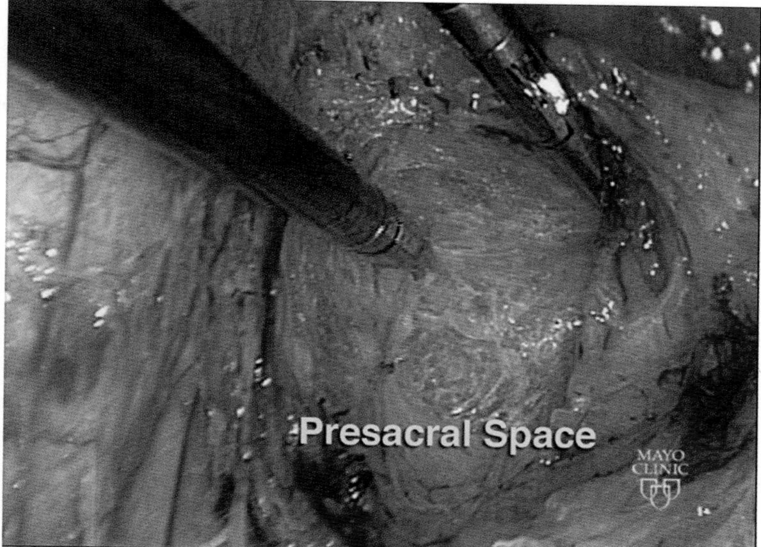

Figure 15.6

The left pararectal peritoneum is scored and the presacral space is entered

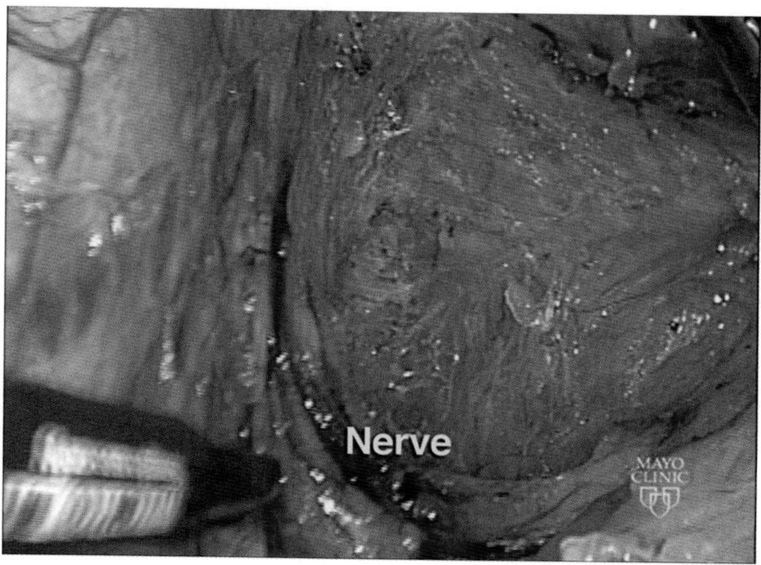

Figure 15.7

The left hypogastric nerve can clearly be seen with the magnification afforded by the laparoscope

source sufficient for dividing the superior rectal vessels; using cautery and then clips for the vessels; or separating the mesorectum by developing a plane between it and the posterior wall of the rectum, and then using the linear stapler to divide it. The rectum can then be divided with a laparoscopic articulated linear stapler. Another washout of the rectum is not necessary at this point as povidone–iodine was placed prior to the start of the procedure. The author finds it easier to deploy the stapler via the right lower quadrant port, pulling the rectum slightly toward the left of the pelvis to ensure a perpendicular transection line. Others prefer to place the 12 mm trocar in the suprapubic position and staple via this. I find that in very low tumors the correct placement of the stapler may be precluded by interference with the pubis. In a female patient it is often possible to use a 45 mm or sometimes even a 60 mm cartridge, so only one or two firings of the stapler are necessary. It is important to commence a subsequent firing of the stapler in the "vee" from the prior stapler application. In male patients, the narrower confines of the pelvis often mandate use of a 30 mm cartridge and multiple applications. Still other authors, especially those who use a hand-assist

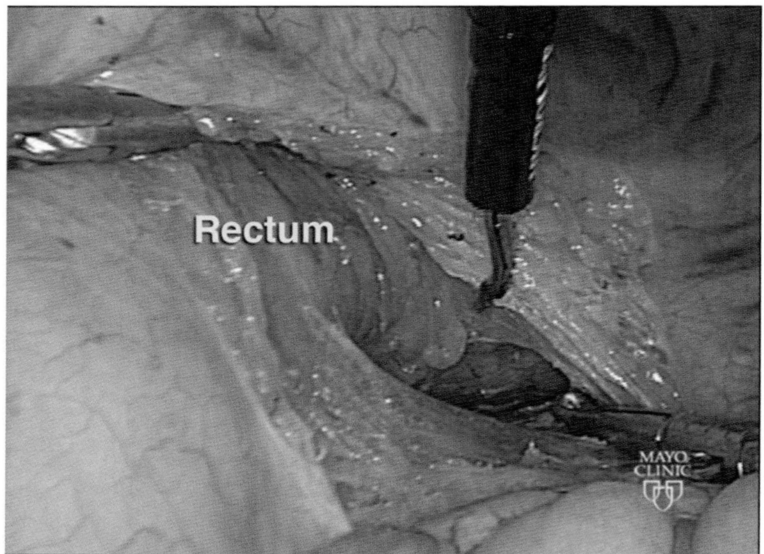

Figure 15.8

The right pararectal peritoneum is scored, and the dissection readily joined in the presacral space with the dissection already performed from the left

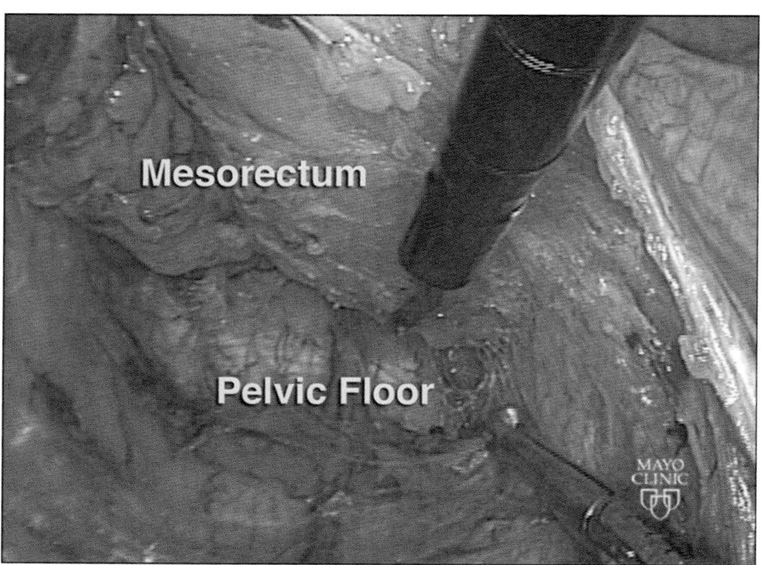

Figure 15.9

As the pelvic floor is reached, the "baby's bottom" appearance of the intact mesorectal specimen is noted

approach, will deploy a TA or transverse stapler via the incision used for the hand device. The author considers this "cheating"!

For distal rectal cancers, the dissection is carried to the pelvic floor and the distal margin is confirmed by digital examination (Fig. 15.10). At this point the mesorectum has tapered out and just the rectum is present. The stapler is deployed via the RLQ port. An assistant placing upward pressure on the perineum can be helpful in placing the stapler. If a 1 cm margin cannot be obtained in this fashion, then either mucosectomy or intersphincteric dissection can be performed from the perineum if a sphincter-preserving procedure is still considered oncologically appropriate.

Mesenteric Transection

Still in Trendelenburg and with the left side up, the distal sigmoid colon and rectum are elevated and fanned out to expose the base of the mesentery and the inferior mesenteric artery (IMA). The existing dissection in the presacral plane is carried through cephalad until

Figure 15.10

As the dissection nears completion the pelvic floor is clearly visible

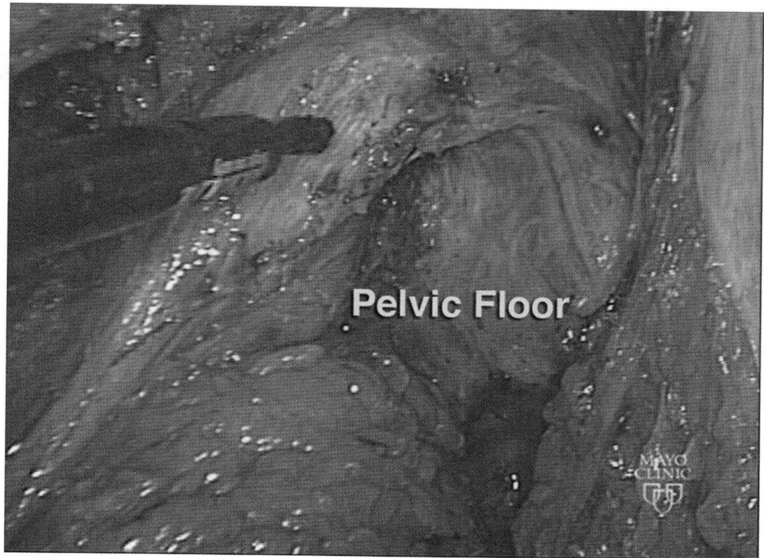

the base of the IMA is reached. The mesenteric window superior to this is opened and the vessel is isolated and then divided using the surgeon's method of choice (energy source that divides vessels up to 7 mm, clips, or vascular load in the linear stapler, Fig. 15.11). Division of the mesentery continues until there is sufficient length of the chosen resection margin to reach the chosen distal resection margin for the anastomosis. Division of the inferior mesenteric vein below the inferior border of the pancreas is sometimes necessary, but not in all cases, and is not routinely performed as it does not add to the oncologic appropriateness of the procedure.

Specimen Exteriorization

A Babcock clamp is placed on the transected edge of the rectum. The pneumoperitoneum is evacuated via the trocars to protect the incisions from the theoretical

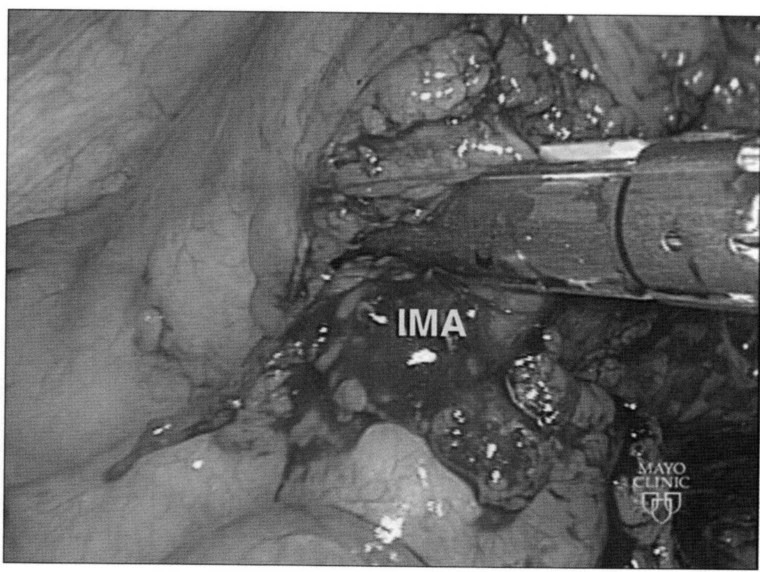

Figure 15.11

The inferior mesenteric artery is encircled at its base and divided with the laparoscopic linear stapler with a vascular cartridge

risk of implantation of tumor cells. A wound protector is placed (we have previously used a sterilized plastic bag, four cents per case, and currently use the sterile plastic sleeve that encloses the suction–irrigation device, for free!). The supraumbilical port is removed and the incision is enlarged around the umbilicus to 3–5 cm, veering around the left side of the umbilicus if a RLQ ileostomy is planned, so the incision does not interfere with placement of the back plate of the stoma device. The Babcock clamp passes the rectum up to the incision and the specimen is exteriorized from the transected end of the rectum to the descending colon.

A proximal resection margin is chosen, usually proximal- to mid-sigmoid, and the colon is transected, with a stapler if a J-pouch is to be created, or sharply with cautery for a straight anastomosis or coloplasty pouch. A colonic J-pouch or coloplasty pouch is constructed for a distal anastomosis. A purse string suture is placed in the cut edge of the colon/apex of the J-pouch and the head of a circular (EEA) stapler is inserted and secured with the suture.

Anastomosis

The abdominal cavity is irrigated and aspirated. The fascia of the periumbilical incision is closed with interrupted sutures, all of which are tied except the second and third most cephalad ones which are used to secure the blunt port back in the incision. The pneumoperitoneum is reestablished. The first assistant moves to the perineum. The anal sphincter is gently dilated with the sizers. The EEA stapler is inserted into the anus and carefully advanced to the transverse staple line in the rectum. The spike is brought out immediately adjacent to the staple line (Fig. 15.12). The head of the stapler is identified and the cut edge of the mesentery is carefully followed to ensure that the colon is not twisted (following the tenia is not as accurate as checking the cut edge of the mesentery). The head of the stapler is docked onto the handle, and the stapler is reapproximated, fired, and removed (Fig. 15.13). Both tissue donuts are inspected to ensure they are intact. Saline is irrigated into the pelvis, and with the lumen of colon above the anastomosis obliterated with a clamp, rigid proctoscopy with air insufflation is performed to rule out an air leak.

Creation of Ileostomy

The anterior fascia at the 12 mm trocar site/planned stoma site is incised in a cruciate fashion. The rectus muscle fibers are separated (and the inferior epigastric vessels divided only if traversing the site) and the posterior fascia is also incised in a cruciate manner. A loop of distal ileum, approximately 6–12 in. proximal to the ileocecal valve (depending on the patient's BMI), is brought up through this site under direct visualization with correct orientation and without tension. The

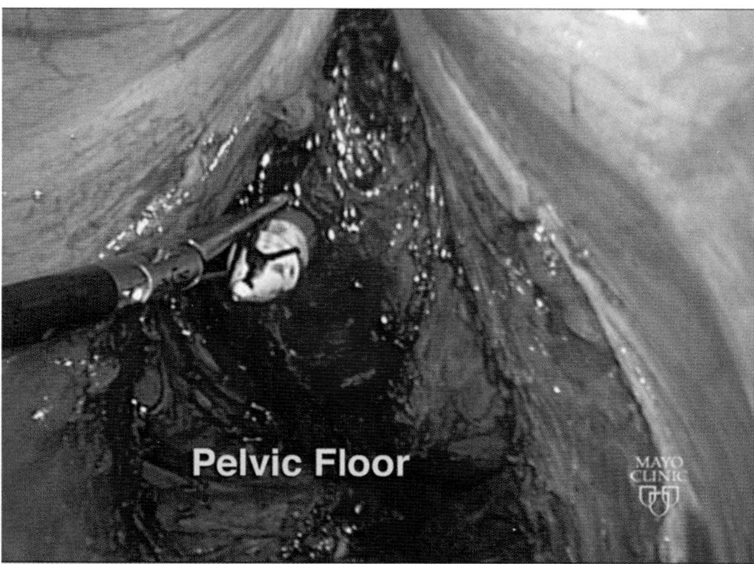

Figure 15.12
The EEA circular stapler is inserted and the spike brought out adjacent to the staple line, which is clearly seen at the level of the pelvic floor

Group (2007) Laparoscopically assisted vs. open colectomy for colon cancer: a meta-analysis. Arch Surg 142:298–303
9. Jayne DJ, Guillou PJ, Thorpe H et al (2007) Randomized trial of laparoscopic-assisted resection of colorectal carcinoma: 3-year results of the UK MRC Clasicc trial. J Clin Oncol 25:3061–3068
10. ACOSOG home page at http://www.acosog.org
11. Nelson H, Petrelli N, Carlin A, Couture J, Fleshman J, Guillem J, Meidema B, Ota D, Sargent D (2001) Guidelines 2000 for colon and rectal cancer surgery. J Natl C Inst 93(8):583–596
12. Bratzler DW, Hunt DR (2006) The surgical infection prevention and surgical care improvement projects: national initiatives to improve outcomes for patients having surgery. Clin Infect Dis 43:322–330
13. Bratzler DW, Houck PM, Surgical Infection Prevention Guidelines Writers Workgroup (2004) Antimicrobial prophylaxis for surgery: an advisory statement from the National Surgical Infection Prevention Project. Clin Infect Dis 38:1706–1715
14. Hospital Quality Alliance. Quality Measures. Accessed at http://www.hospitalqualityalliance.org/hospitalquality alliance/qualitymeasures/qualitymeasures.html
15. Centers for Medicare & Medicaid Services. Reporting hospital quality data for annual payment update fact sheet. Accessed at http://www.cms.hhs.gov/HospitalQualityInits/08_HospitalRHQDAPU.asp
16. Umpleby HC, Williamson RC (1984) The efficacy of agents employed to prevent anastomotic recurrence in colorectal carcinoma. Ann Surg Oncol 66:192–194
17. Porter GA, Soskolne CL, Yakimets WW, Newman SC (1998) Surgeon-related factors and outcome in rectal cancer. Ann Surg 227(2):157–167
18. Dorrance HR, Docherty GM, O'Dwyer PJ (2000) Effect of surgeon specialty interest on patient outcome after potentially curative colorectal cancer surgery. Dis Colon Rectum 43:492–498
19. Feliciotti F, Guerrieri M, Paganini AM, DeSanctis A et al (2003) Long term results of laparoscopic vs. open resections for rectal cancer for 124 unselected patients. Surg Endosc 17:1530–1535
20. Morino M, Parini U, Giraudo G et al (2003) Laparoscopic total mesorectal excision: a consecutive series of 100 patients. Ann of Surg 237:335–342
21. Leung KL, Kwok SPY, Lam SCW, Lee JFY, Yiu RTC, Ng SSM, Lai PBS, Lau WY (2004) Laparoscopic resection of rectosigmoid carcinoma: prospective randomized trial. Lancet 363:1187–1192
22. Fleshman JW, Wexner SD, Anvari M, LaTulippe J-F et al (1999) Laparoscopic vs. open abdominoperineal resection for cancer. Dis Colon Rectum 42:930–939
23. Kockerling F, Scheidbach H, Schneider C, Barlehner E, The Laparoscopic Colorectal Surgery Study Group et al (2000) Laparoscopic abdominoperineal resection: early postoperative results of a prospective study involving 116 patients. Dis Colon Rectum 43:1503–1511
24. Goh YC, Eu KW, Seow-Choen F (1997) Early postoperative results of a prospective series of laparoscopic vs. open anterior resections for rectosigmoid cancers. Dis Colon Rectum 40:776–780
25. Leroy J, Jamali F, Forbes L et al (2004) Laparoscopic total mesorectal excision (TME) for rectal cancer surgery. Surg Endosc 1:281–289
26. Leung KL, Kwok SPY, Lau WY et al (2000) Laparoscopic assisted abdominoperineal resection for low rectal adenocarcinoma. Surg Endosc 14:67–70
27. Breukink S, Pierie J, Wiggers T (2007) Laparoscopic versus open total mesorectal excision for rectal cancer (review). The Cochrane Collaboration IN: The Cochrane Library 2:1–40
28. Asbun HJ, Young-Fadok TM (eds) (2008) American college of surgeons multimedia atlas of surgery. Cine-Med, Inc, Woodbury, CT

Transanal Endoscopic Microsurgery (TEM)

John H. Marks

Contents

Introduction

The ultimate minimally invasive procedure for intra-abdominal neoplasia is one that avoids any abdominal incision. To this end, colonoscopy with polypectomy meets the criteria and stands as the first major step in minimally invasive therapy of colorectal neoplasia. NOTES (Natural Orifice Translumenal Endoscopic Surgery) holds open the promise for just such an approach. To date the only large experience in this type of natural orifice therapy is with transanal excision of rectal polyps and select rectal cancers. Unfortunately, limited reach transanally has significantly hampered this approach. TEM has addressed this problem. Nonetheless, limited experience of surgeons has impeded the widespread adoption of this approach. In addition, concerns about the adequacy of oncologic treatment of a rectal cancer with a full-thickness excision have properly minimized acceptance of this approach. High local recurrence rates using a transanal approach have been attributed to the inability to reach the cephalad aspect of the cancer's margin, working within the lumen potentially spreading viable cancer cells and the untreated lymphatic space.

In more advanced rectal cancers the use of radiation therapy has gained widespread acceptance to decrease local recurrence rates while improving survival and the ability to avoid the need for a permanent colostomy [1–3]. With higher doses of radiation therapy as well as the addition of chemotherapy a more pronounced response to radiotherapy has been noted. Complete pathologic response rates of 12% were found with radiotherapy alone, 16–18% with radiation therapy and a 5FU bolus, and 28–31% complete response rates with radiation and 5FU given as a continuous venous infusion [4–8]. These improved responses have led to an exploration of different surgical approaches. Gerald Marks in association with Mohammed Mohiuddin

F.L. Greene, B.T. Heniford (eds.), *Minimally Invasive Cancer Management*,
DOI 10.1007/978-1-4419-1238-1_16,

was the first to perform full-thickness local excision (FTLE) after high-dose radiation therapy at Thomas Jefferson University. Tumor downstaging after high doses of radiation allowed for local excision techniques in medically compromised patients [9]. This was later expanded to more aggressive radiation therapy followed by full-thickness local excision in an elective setting [10]. This approach has gained more acceptance as increased complete response rates and downstaging rates have been found with more aggressive chemoradiation therapy [11, 12]. However, with these new opportunities new challenges have evolved. Would the radiated bowel heal? Would there be adequate bowel function following this? Would one be able to gain access to everything but the most distal third of the rectum to apply this approach? The experience of Marks as well as Lezoche, Habr-Gama, and others has reinforced the ability of the area to heal after local excision chemotherapy [13, 14]. The application of TEM has markedly expanded the application of local excision to the middle and upper third of the rectum without the need for a transsphincteric or a transsacral approach. The equipment, technique, and application of this approach as well as some short- and long-term results will be presented in this chapter.

Development

TEM was first developed in Germany by Professor Gerhard Buess [15]. This operating system provides endoluminal insufflation with microscopic enhancement of the visual field increasing visibility with the ability to manipulate tissue, dissect, cauterize, and suture. Greater surgical access through the anus to the inside of the rectum up to 15–20 cm from the anal verge became possible.

Instrumentation

Operating proctoscope. The operating proctoscope comes in three variations, each of which is 40 mm in diameter and ranging from 12 to 20 cm in length. The longer shaft is utilized for the mid and upper rectum while the shorter shaft is utilized for the distal third of the rectum. The beveled end allows for mechanical as well as air distraction of the rectal wall. For lesions where the inferior margin comes down very close to the anus itself, a non-beveled 12 mm shaft is ideal for visualization without loss of the air seal (Fig. 16.1). The shafts themselves are attached and locked airtight to a handle, which serves as the footprint for the operating microscope to mount. The handle is then attached to the table itself via a Martin's arm which has one tightening handle that when turned allows for different angles to be maintained in three separate joints (Fig. 16.2). Initially the obturator is utilized to insert the instrument, similar to a large rigid sigmoidoscope. The open faceplate and attached light cord allow the surgeon to visualize the rectal lesion

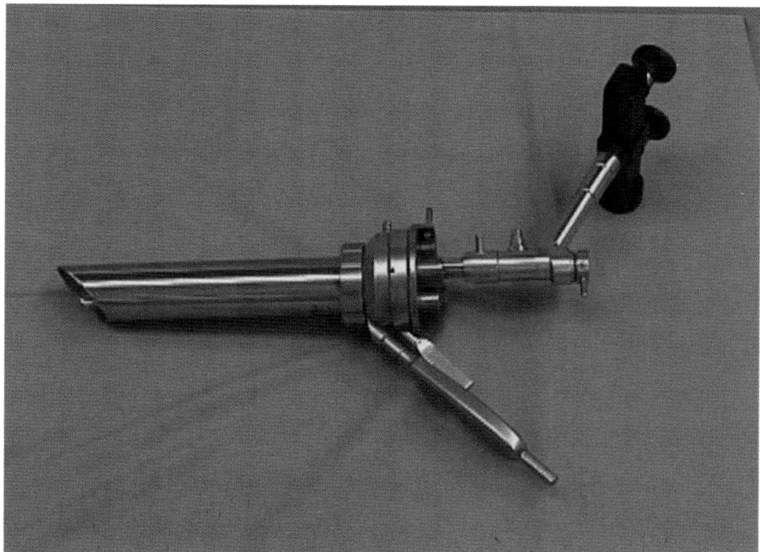

Figure 16.1

Twenty centimeters beveled proctoscope with attached working faceplate and stereoscope

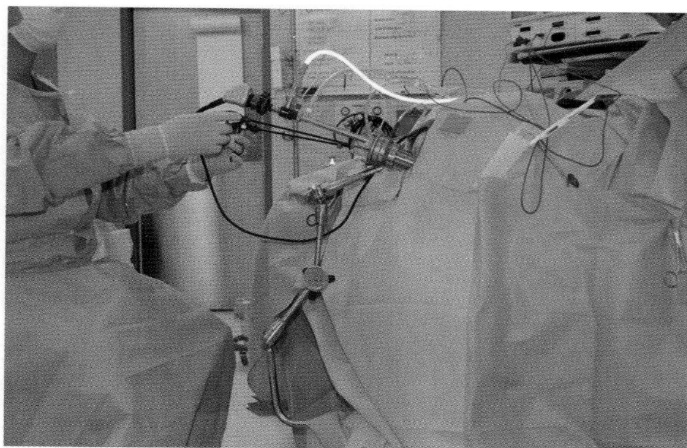

Figure 16.2
Proctoscope assembled with Martin's arm

and to assure that the lesion is positioned in the bottom 180° of the proctoscope (Fig. 16.3). The Martin's arm is attached and the second faceplate is attached. The second faceplate consists of an opening for the operating microscope and a bottom area with three openings, one for right-handed instruments, one for left-handed instruments, and a third one for suction (Fig. 16.4). In Europe the third opening is unnecessary as the ERBE unit has been developed with an instrument to both cauterize and suction. Unfortunately the company has not pursued making this device available to American patients and surgeons as they feel it is not cost-effective to pursue (Christian Erbe, 2002, personal communication). Hopefully this is something they will reassess as the technique becomes more popular in North America. The instruments are passed through two valves: first external stoppers with holes in them followed by an internal shutter valve mechanism which allows for the exchange of instrumentation with a minimal loss of intraluminal pressure. The air is insufflated through the operating microscope, which is attached along with a tube for irrigation and a tube to measure intraluminal pressure. There is an attached lens for a teaching scope that allows the assistant to see matters; however, the vision is different as the binocular vision provides roughly a 20% increase in visual field.

Surgical instruments. The instruments available are right- and left-handed graspers, which are angled so that they can lift the tissue through the long operating proctoscope. The instruments include (1) right- and left-handed graspers, angled and straight, (2) scissors, right and left handed, and (3) angled cautery knife utilized for dissection and electrocautery. Additionally there are clip appliers and straight and angled needle drivers as well (Fig. 16.5).

TEM insufflator. The insufflator is designed to deliver carbon dioxide at 8 l/min supplying constant steady flow to avoid over insufflation. There is also a built in suction mechanism that allows for the evacuation of smoke and blood. Water is automatically injected through a foot pedal in order to clean the lens. The suction pump is designed to evacuate air pressure beneath that of the inflow to avoid desufflating

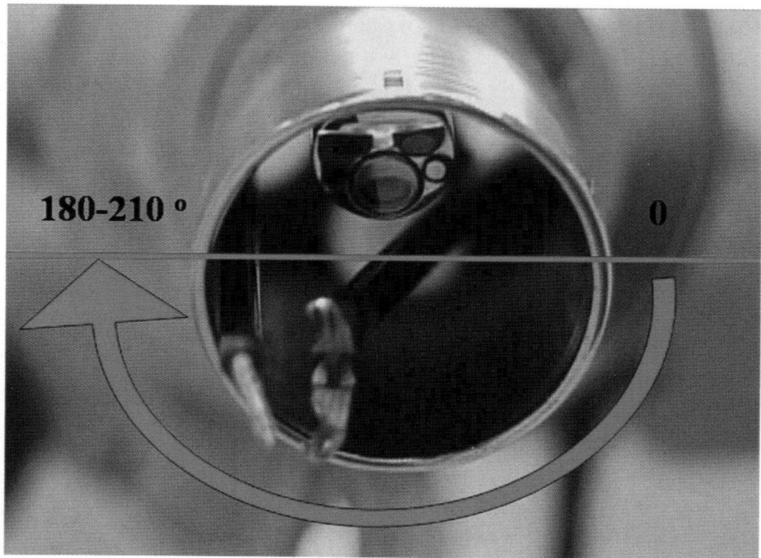

Figure 16.3
View of scope on end. *Arrow* demonstrating limited degree of motion

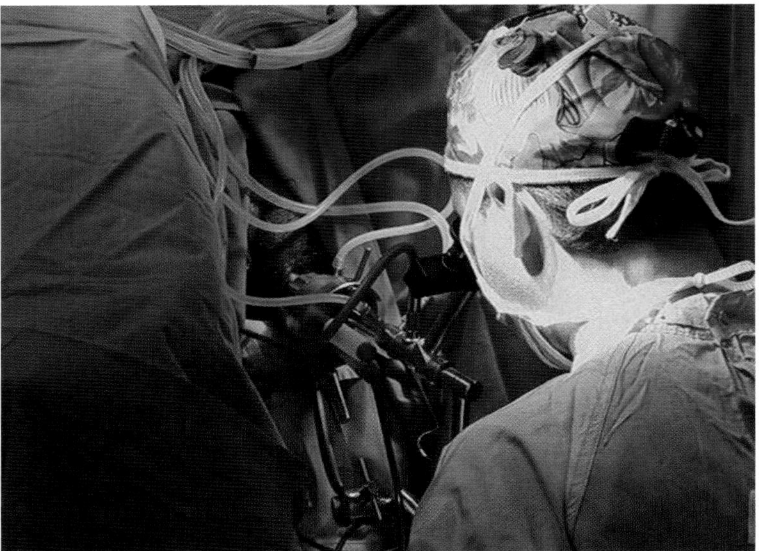

Figure 16.4

TEM operating system fully assembled in use

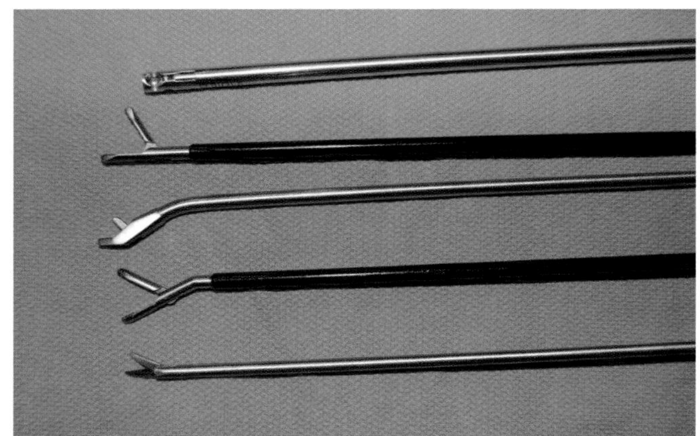

Figure 16.5

From *top* to *bottom*: angled grasping forceps, needle holder, straight scissors, and straight grasping forceps

completely the gas in the lumen of the rectum and creating a complete lack of exposure with collapse of the rectal wall (Fig. 16.6).

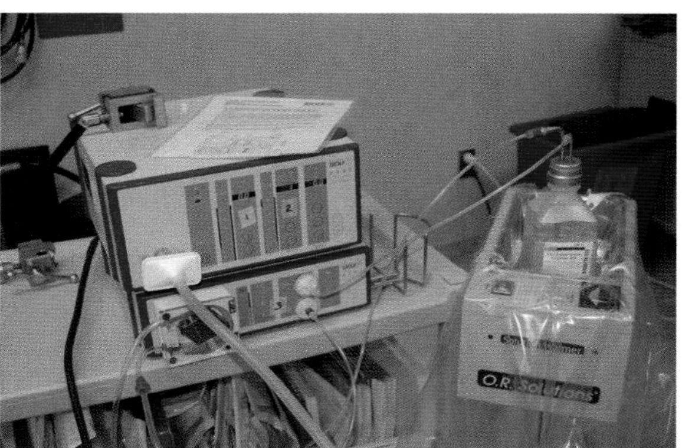

Figure 16.6

TEM combination system. CO_2 pneumoinsufflator and foot-controlled suction irrigation system

Evaluation and Patient Selection

While TEM is a tremendous tool in the treatment of sessile rectal polyps, the focus of this chapter remains the use of TEM in the treatment of cancer. To address this we will discuss the evaluation of a patient with a rectal mass.

Patients who present to the office with a rectal mass generally fit into three categories. First is an obvious rectal cancer, which is diagnosed or is clinically apparent. Second is a large lesion of which there is significant concern regarding an underlying cancer; however, this has not been demonstrated. Third is an obviously benign polyp, which can be removed straight away in a submucosal fashion using the TEM equipment.

On presentation, new patients are fully evaluated with a history and physical examination. In dealing with patients with rectal masses this includes a digital examination as well as flexible and rigid endoscopy in the office to determine for certain the characteristics of the mass and the quadrant in which the tumor is located. This becomes especially important when using TEM, as one is able only to operate on the bottom 180° of the lumen (as was shown in Fig. 16.3). Level of the lesion in the rectum relative to the anorectal ring is noted as this represents the anatomic distal margin of the rectum. Additionally, the size, shape, ulceration, fixity, clinical T category, and cephalad margin are also noted. The latter point is especially important when considering removal of the mass transanally. Unimportant in abdominal surgery, the cephalad margin is critical when considering transanal excision, as the inability to reach frequently results in positive margins and local recurrence. While digital examination is most useful if the lesion is palpable from below, flexible endoscopy adds a tremendous amount to the clinicians' understanding of the lesion regarding the morphology, size, and appearance. A rigid endoscopic exam is essential for lesions that are non-palpable to determine for certain the quadrant where the cancer resides.

Following this, additional staging is carried out with endorectal ultrasound and dedicated pelvic MRI. While arguments can be made for both modalities they both suffer from the difficulty of differentiating early T category lesions from each other as well as microscopic nodal involvement [16, 17]. Having said this, the opinion of an experienced clinician's examination in evaluating the cancer clinically is invaluable and plays as important a role as any of these more "objective methods." If, due to induration or appearance, the surgeon has a concern regarding an underlying cancer, the patient should be re-biopsied or taken to the operating room for examination under anesthesia. Biopsies should be taken from the indurated area of the mass with larger biopsy forceps. It is also essential for the surgeon to review with his or her pathologist the original readings of the biopsies to assure proper decisions are made.

Once this has been completed decisions need to be made as to how best to proceed. The general view in the literature regarding TEM is that cancers should be T1 lesions or selective T2 lesions less than 4 cm with no nodal involvement, well differentiated, and have no lymphovascular invasion. Furthermore, high anteriorly based lesions should be avoided, as this would allow entrance into the abdominal cavity.

Large polyps without evidence of cancer. Our approach is slightly different and is described as follows: These patients undergo resection of the polyp in a submucosal fashion. In elderly patients with severe comorbidities a full-thickness excision with repair is performed with the notion that in the event a small underlying invasive component is found, we might treat these patients with postoperative radiation.

Adenocarcinoma of the rectum. In known cancers, even T1 and T2 cancers must have chemoradiation therapy preoperatively if one is going to consider a local excision [3, 18, 19]. The data on these lesions is too unfavorable with local excision by itself. To this end, decisions regarding local excision are based on the cancer *after* completion of radiation therapy. The indications are for residual cancers less than 4 cm, T2 or less with no evidence of invasion of the lymph nodes. A preoperative PET scan is not routinely obtained; however, this is something that likely will play a larger role in this patient population as we move forward trying to differentiate small foci of disease extramurally. In describing the extent and size of the lesion, one must focus not only on the mucosal remnant after radiation therapy but also on the area of intramural induration around this area as all of this must be excised with a 1 cm margin. Following this, one must be able to technically close the defect in the rectal wall.

As a word of caution, complete responses following treatment can make it difficult to identify the original location of the lesion that needs to be excised. For this reason it is imperative that detailed description of the location is carried out on original presentation of the patient. Furthermore if concerns exist regarding the visibility of the cancer after radiotherapy, India ink should be injected around the area so that the position for excision can be determined. This is one of the primary reasons that we see the patients at 3-week intervals during treatment.

Patients are treated according to the algorithm shown in Fig. 16.7. In general at this time, patients with T3 lesions or node positivity, as well as those with cancers in the distal 6 cm of the rectum, are treated to 5,580 cGy radiation therapy with 5FU continuous venous infusion chemotherapy. The patient is examined at 3-week intervals during treatment, and surgery is performed between 8 and 12 weeks following completion of the radiation. All patients,

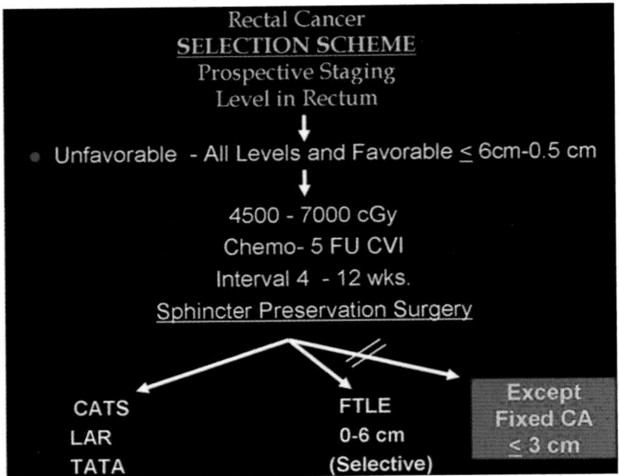

Figure 16.7

Rectal cancer management algorithm

except those with fixed cancer *after* radiation undergo sphincter preservation surgery. With this approach we have maintained an abdominoperineal resection (APR) rate of 7%. Operative approaches are either radical or local excisions, now with TEM. Local excision candidates fall into three groups: (1) the medically compromised patients unable to tolerate radical surgery; (2) the staged group where factors such as age, body habitus, medical status, or a compromised gastrointestinal tract make TEM a more attractive option after fully informed consent; (3) the elective group where, depending on tumor response and patient's intense desire to avoid an abdominal procedure, TEM is carried out after fully informed consent. In the staged and elective groups if pathology reveals a T3 or N+ cancer a radical resection is advised. Employing these guidelines we have elected to perform local excision in 18% of our overall rectal cancer patient group.

Procedure

Patients receive a full bowel prep and preoperative antibiotics. Again if any question exists regarding the position of the lesion, this must be determined before the patient is on the operating table, as it will determine patient positioning. This can be done by digital examination and/or rigid endoscopy. The patient will require a general endotracheal anesthetic. While theoretically the operation can be performed with generous local or regional block or a spinal anesthetic, the insufflation of the rectum and intestine leads to labored breathing and the need for intubation in over 60% of the cases in my experience, and therefore it is best to proceed with a general endotracheal approach from the start. Patients are positioned depending on the location of the cancer. Posterior cancers require the patient to be in lithotomy position, anterior cancers in the prone position, right-sided cancers with the patient in the right lateral decubitus position, and left-sided in the left lateral decubitus position (Fig. 16.8) Again, this is because the surgeon can only operate in the bottom 180° of the TEM lumen.

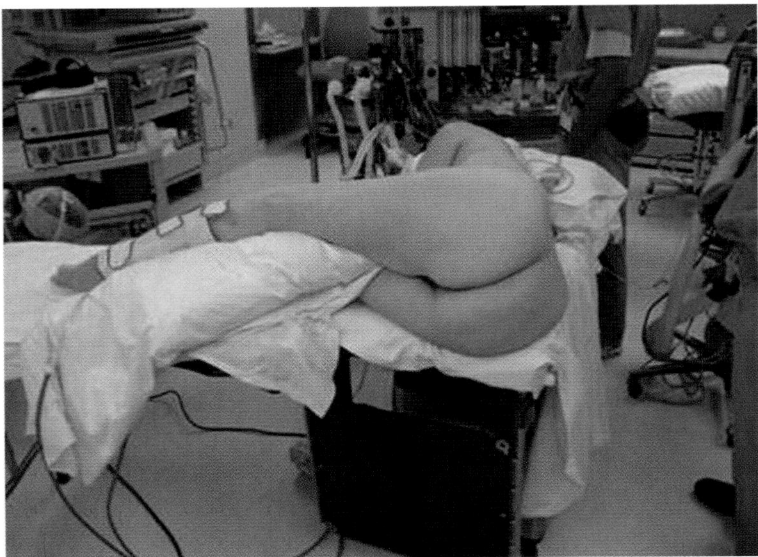

Figure 16.8

Patient positioned in right lateral decubitus position for right-sided lesion. Arm table extension supporting legs

When the patient is in the prone position it must be in a split leg arrangement so that the surgeon can get in between the patient's legs. When in lithotomy position, stirrups are appropriate. If the cancer is located on the right or the left side, the patient is placed in a L position lateral decubitus, with a hand table extension in order to support the weight of the legs.

Informed consent includes a discussion of the risk of entering the abdominal cavity and the need for laparotomy or laparoscopy with a temporary diverting stoma, a low anterior resection (LAR), or APR. Anterior perforation into the vagina and delayed rectovaginal or rectourethral fistula is also possible and should be mentioned. Additionally, injury to the sphincter muscle and the need for an anoplasty in someone with anal stenosis are also problems that must be discussed when obtaining informed consent for surgical technique.

The anal canal is gently dilated with one and two and then three fingers. This glove is lubricated with mineral oil. The obturator is placed through the anal canal. In 250 cases I have never had to do a formal anoplasty in order to allow introduction of the operating equipment. Sometimes in a tight anal canal the EEA sizers are used to gently dilate the anal canal and then this is progressed up to the TEM obturator and then the whole operating microscope is able to be placed.

The position of the lesion is ascertained by placing a faceplate on the operating proctoscope. Insufflating the rectum the surgeon examines the lumen and confirms the position of the lesion. The Martin's arm is attached to the table and to the operating proctoscope. The clear glass faceplate is then exchanged for the operating faceplate with the operating microscope in place. It should be noted there is also another device, which allows for a larger video portrayal of what is being seen with the teaching scope, but this sacrifices microscopic vision. While ergonomically superior for the surgeon, the video device results in a minor loss of visual field in order to utilize it. It is advantageous to use this approach when dealing with lesions that extend outside of just one quadrant.

Once the second faceplate of the operating microscope is in place, tubing is attached for insufflation, irrigation, pressure monitoring, and suction. The unit is turned on and fine adjustments regarding the positioning over the mass are performed. With these in place, one introduces three caps with small holes. The operating instruments are inserted through a flutter valve. These valves allow only a minimal drop in intraluminal pressure and loss of visualization. With the right- and left-handed grasper, the ability to reach around the lesion is determined. Electrocautery is then used to mark with a 1 cm margin circumferentially around the lesion to be excised (Fig. 16.9). After radiotherapy it is important to emphasize that the area to be resected is a 1 cm margin around the area of induration within the wall and not just the mucosal remnant, as the mucosal scar of this can be quite small.

The electrocautery is then used to incise in a full-thickness fashion through the mucosa and the muscularis down into the perirectal fat. The plan is for this to be definitive therapy, and thus a large volume of the underlying fat is taken with the specimen. The dissection is generally carried out circumferentially through the mucosa and muscularis propria in the perirectal fat circumferentially leaving the lesion itself freed as an island of tissue circumferentially. Special care must be taken when working anteriorly as extended use of

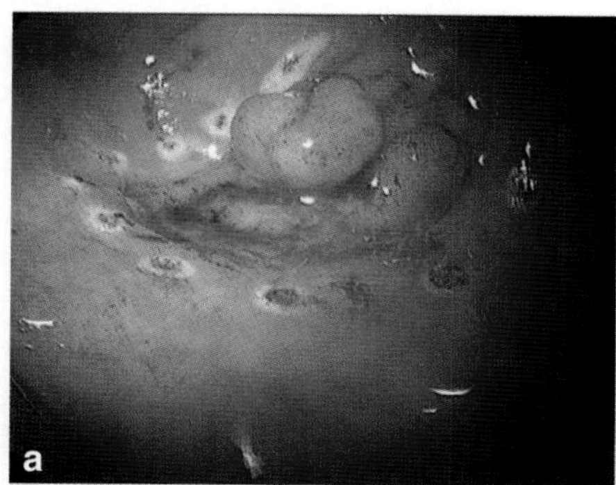

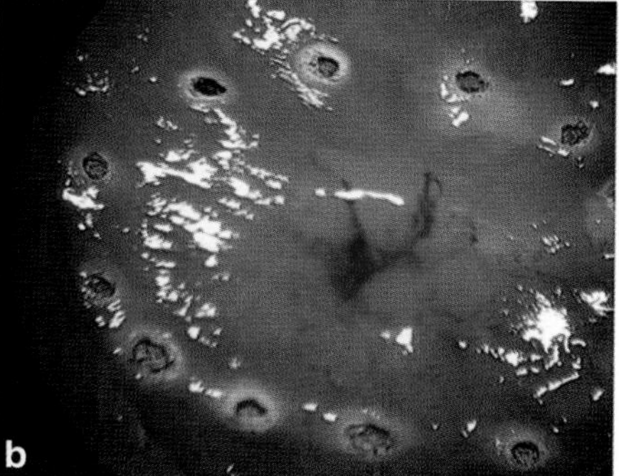

Figure 16.9

One centimeter resection margin marked with electrocautery prior to excision of lesion the cautery with electrocoagulation can lead to delayed thermal injury and development of a rectovaginal fistula. Bleeding points must be controlled immediately as they are encountered in order to maintain proper visualization in the operative field. Once this island is created, dissection is taken underneath this by going superiorly beneath the perirectal fat. A marking stitch is generally placed in the inferior border of the lesion to maintain orientation when the specimen is removed. As the resection is about to be completed, there is often a deep, penetrating vessel which is encountered. This large blood supply must be grasped and cauterized in order to avoid losing vascular control. If the peritoneal cavity is entered, depending on the size of the defect and the operator's comfort level, an appropriate strategy must be devised. A small defect can easily handle a 3-0 Vicryl stitch tied intraluminally. A larger defect might call in the question of the need for a temporary diverting stoma. This is a very rare occurrence and has been necessary only one time in over 250 cases.

Once the lesion is excised and removed from the operating scope it is pinned out separately on a corkboard. This is done to maintain orientation and to help the pathologists with their determination of margins. We hand this over to the pathologist with marking stitches in place pinned on the corkboard in order to minimize any possibilities for confusion (Fig. 16.10).

Once the excision is completed, all of the instruments are removed and washed in 50% dilute Betadine solution. The lumen itself is also irrigated with Betadine solution to minimize the possibility of any tumor implantation. Gloves are changed and closure of the defect is performed. This is carried out by first using a 4 cm 2-0 PDS stitch to divide the luminal defect in half. This stitch takes tension off of the wall and allows for an easier running suture to be carried out. One of the marked differences operating endoluminally, as opposed to laparoscopically, is that there is only an in and out motion. There is very little lateral and diagonal movement of the instrumentation. To avoid having to tie intraluminally, malleable silver clips are applied to the ends of the suture and tightened in order to maintain the closure (Fig. 16.11). The defect is closed starting on the right side and then going to the left. Generally a 10 cm stitch of 2-0 PDS is what is used to start. If the suture is too long, it is very difficult to manipulate. If it is too short, multiple sutures are necessary in order to complete the closure. A running full-thickness stitch is carried out starting inferiorly on the right-hand side and going from right to left. Depending on the size of the lesion itself, it may take two or three sutures in order to fully close the defect. Once the closure is completed, by pulling up on the suture the closure can be tightened and an additional clip applied if needed. This is necessary as the surgeon is unable to have an assistant following the closure as would normally be the case to maintain proper tautness in a running closure. Once this is done, the area is inspected assuring no defects are present. If a defect is noted, additional sutures may be applied.

It should be noted there is a school of surgeons who advocate leaving the wound entirely open and

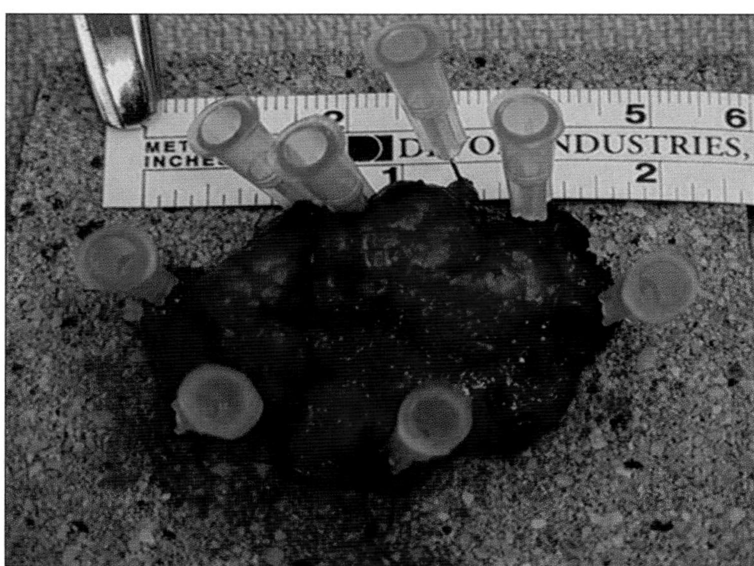

Figure 16.10
Specimen pinned on cork board with marking stitch and properly oriented prior to pathological assessment

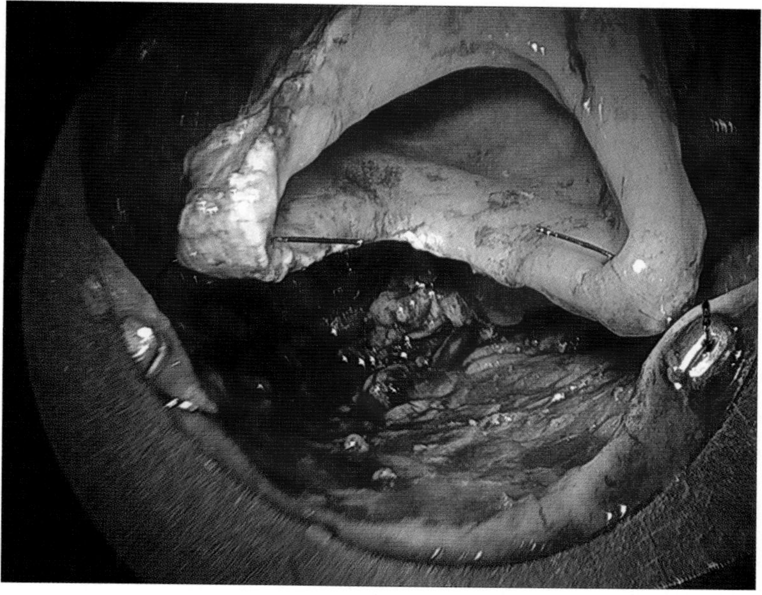

Figure 16.11

Anchoring stitches with silver suture clips facilitating closure of rectal wall defect

granulating in [20]. Concerns exist regarding bleeding, development of abscesses, and position of a large defect. In the radiated field there is no experience at all in doing this and I think it would be ill advised to leave these wounds open because of the difficulty of healing in radiated tissue.

Postoperative Care

In all cancer cases a Foley catheter is placed and is left in place overnight. Patients are generally started on liquids either later that day or the next morning. Following radiation therapy, antibiotics (doxycycline) are used long term. Diet is slowly advanced as patients tolerate. Activity is only limited to avoid Valsalva or bending as this puts pressure on the anastomosis. Milk of Magnesia is used in a one ounce dose, which is increased or decreased in order to maintain a loose, but not explosive, bowel movement. This is generally continued for approximately 1 week. Diet is advanced as the patient is capable and generally patients are discharged home 1 or 2 days following surgery. Most commonly patients are completely asymptomatic following surgery. The development of increased drainage and/or pain 1–3 weeks after surgery is indicative of a wound disruption. While it has been my experience this occurs 21% of the time, the vast majority of the time this is treatable with long-standing oral antibiotics, which is generally doxycycline and when severe, narcotics for pain [10]. On a rare occasion, when patients are incapacitated by the pain or threaten to become septic, a diverting stoma is necessary.

A small amount of blood seen is not uncommon and not something that needs to be of concern. If it were to increase in volume one would consider reevaluating this in the operating room, but this has occurred in less than 1% of our patients. Delayed problems include development of stenosis and incontinence. The issue of stenosis is protected against by the large operating lumen of the operating TEM microscope. Regarding incontinence, we have had no long-standing problems of incontinence. We have had four patients who have had temporary control issues that have improved over time likely from stretch of the sphincter mechanism. This is similar to that described using other methods. Studies showed no significant manometric problems following TEM surgery [21].

Results

Local therapy in the form of full-thickness local excision has been performed for the small select rectal cancer since the early 1900s. However, a closer look at the data raises serious questions in that regard. Theoretically the failure of local excision can stem from either the incomplete excision of the luminal component of the cancer or failure to address cancer in the lymph nodes. From a technical standpoint the challenge of operating transanally has to do with the cephalad reach from below and difficulty with obtaining a clear view. This results in the frequent performance of a piecemeal excision with inferior results [21, 22]. The TEM approach addresses this and this too explains the superior local recurrence rates reported with TEM [23, 24]. In the most favorable lesions, T1 cancers, the University of Minnesota reported failure rates of 21% and the Cleveland Clinic found local recurrence rates of 29% [3, 18]. This calls into question not only the possibility of an incomplete excision but also the idea of implantation of viable cancer cells in the closure at the time of surgery. Winde's group treated 50 patients with pT1 carcinomas with either TEM ($n = 24$) or anterior resection ($n = 26$) and found no difference in 5 year survival or local recurrence. Survival was 96% in both groups and there was only a 4.6% local recurrence rate in patients treated with TEM [25]. The stark difference in results argues for the improved outcomes in patients treated with TEM, as one would hypothesize because of the superior optics and reach.

The second issue confounding the greater use of local excision for rectal cancer is the lack of treatment of the lymph nodes. The high incidence of local failure is understandable with the information that 12% of T1 and 22% of T2 cancers are associated with lymph node involvement in the Memorial study of 1992 [26]. These nodes are entirely untreated in a local excision approach. Local recurrence in this situation is really a local persistence of untreated rectal cancer. Furthermore, the possibility of tumor cell implantation may occur during surgical excision when perirectal tissues are exposed to viable shed cancer cells.

The initial data of our prospective program of FTLE following high-dose preoperative radiation alone gave us reason to believe that radiation, by its downstaging of the rectal cancer and the sterilization of the perirectal microlymphatics, avoids the aforementioned causes of local recurrence with FTLE. Viable tumor cells within the lumen are nonexistent. The local recurrence rate in the first 44 FTLE patients of 14% and then in a subsequent group of 10% with an 83.5% overall 5 year actuarial survival attested to the benefit of preoperative radiation [27, 28]. Upon refinement of the selection scheme employing chemoradiation exclusively and utilizing TEM, the first 43 patients in that group had an impressive local recurrence rate of 4.7% and a 5 year actuarial survival of 93% [29]. The total number of rectal cancer patients treated by FTLE which includes conventional surgery and radiation alone ($n = 58$) and TEM patients with chemoradiation is approaching 200 patients. There has not been a mortality. In the group of TEM patients, the rate of wound separation is 21% and only 9% of patients required a temporary stoma [29]. Lezoche expanded on this work performing a prospective randomized study comparing TEM to radical surgery for T2 cancers. Their work showed a 5.7% local recurrence in the TEM group and no difference in recurrence, metastases, or survival in the two groups [8].

An increasing number of cancers are noted to undergo complete disappearance in what is labeled a "complete response." Our rate of complete responders is 28% which is consistent with many other reports. Professor Angelita Habr-Gama of Sao Paulo, Brazil, reports that with the use of extended chemotherapy, the total response rate is greater than 50% (Dr. Angelita Habr-Gama, 2008, personal communication). With a complete or nearly complete response there is an added challenge regarding the precise site of the original tumor. Because of the need to know the exact site, we insist upon examining patients at no greater than 3-week intervals while under therapy. This enables us to follow the regression of the tumor and accurately note its position in the event of total disappearance. We have employed the use of India ink tattooing as an aid in localization but have found this to be less than a totally reliable means of identifying the tumor site where there has been a complete response.

References

1. Swedish Rectal Cancer Trial (1997) Improved survival with preoperative radiotherapy in respectable rectal cancer. N Engl J Med 336(14):980–987
2. Mohiuddin M et al (1990) High-dose preoperative irradiation for cancer of the rectum. Int J Radiat Oncol Biol Phys 20:37–43
3. Madbouly KM et al (2005) Recurrence after transanal excision of T1 rectal cancer: should we be concerned? Dis Colon Rectum 48(4):711–719, discussion 719–21
4. Marks G et al (1991) High-dose preoperative radiation and radical sphincter-preserving surgery for rectal cancer. Arch Surg 126:1534–1540
5. Cambray I, Amenós M et al (2007) Preoperative radiochemotherapy (RT-CT) in rectal cancer. Prospective study with postoperative RT-CT control group. Clin Transl Oncol 9(3):183–191
6. Chao M et al (2005) Preoperative chemotherapy and radiotherapy for locally advanced rectal cancer. ANZ J Surg 75:286–291

7. Habr-Gama A et al (2005) Long-term results of preoperative chemoradiation for distal rectal cancer correlation between final stage and survival. J Gastrointest Surg 9(1):90–101
8. Lezoche E et al (2008) A prospective randomized study with a 5 year minimum follow-up of TEM vs. laparoscopic total mesorectal excision in T2 N0 low rectal cancer after neoadjuvant therapy. Surg Endosc 22(2):352–358
9. Marks G et al (1990) High-dose preoperative radiation and full- thickness local excision: a new option for patients with select cancers of the rectum. Dis Colon Rectum 33: 735–739
10. Marks J et al (2003) Transanal endoscopic microsurgery in the treatment of select rectal cancers or tumors suspicious for cancer. Surg Endosc 17(7):1114–1117
11. Lezoche E et al (1998) Transanal endoscopic microsurgical excision of irradiated and nonirradiated rectal cancer. A 5-year experience. Surg Laparosc Endosc 8(4):249–256
12. Habr-Gama A et al (1998) Low rectal cancer: impact of radiation and chemotherapy on surgical treatment. Dis Colon Rectum 41(9):1087–1096
13. Habr-Gama A et al (2006) Assessment and management of the complete clinical response of rectal cancer to chemoradiotherapy. Colorectal Dis 8(Supp 3):21–24
14. Lezoche E et al (2005) Long-term results in patients with T2-3 N0 distal rectal cancer undergoing radiotherapy before transanal endoscopic microsurgery. Br J Surg 92:1546–1552
15. Buess G et al (1988) Technique of transanal endoscopic microsurgery. Surg Endosc 2(2):71–75
16. Schaffzin DM, Wong WD (2004) Endorectal ultrasound in the preoperative evaluation of rectal cancer. Clin Colorectal Cancer 4(2):124–132
17. Brown G et al (2004) High-resolution MRI of the anatomy important in total mesorectal excision of the rectum. Am J Roentgen 182(2):431–439
18. Mellgren A et al (2000) Is local excision adequate therapy for early rectal cancer? Dis Colon Rectum 43(8):1064–1071, discussion 1071–4
19. Killingback M (1992) Local Excision of Carcinoma of the Rectum: Indications. World J Surg 16:437–446
20. Maslekar S et al (2007) Transanal endoscopic microsurgery for carcinoma of the rectum. Surg Endosc 21(1):97–102
21. Cataldo PA et al (2005) Transanal endoscopic microsurgery: a prospective evaluation of functional results. Dis Colon Rectum 48(7):1366–1371
22. Moore JS et al (2008) Transanal endoscopic microsurgery is more effective than traditional transanal excision for resection of rectal masses. Dis Colon Rectum 51(7):1026–1030
23. Saclarides TJ (1998) Transanal endoscopic microsurgery: a single surgeon's experience. Arch Surg 133:595–599
24. Buess G et al (2001) Transanal endoscopic microsurgery. Surg Onc Clin North Am 10(3):709–731, xi
25. Winde G et al (1996) Surgical cure for early rectal carcinomas (T1). Transanal endoscopic microsurgery vs. anterior resection. Dis Colon Rectum 39(9):969–976
26. Brodsky JT et al (1992) Variables correlated with the risk of lymph node metastasis in early rectal cancer. Cancer 69(2):322–326
27. Bannon JP et al (1995) Radical and local excisional methods of sphincter-sparing surgery after high-dose radiation for cancer of the distal 3 cm of the rectum. Ann Surg Oncol 2(3):221–227
28. Mohiuddin M et al (1994) High-dose preoperative radiation and full thickness local excision: a new option for selected T3 distal rectal cancers. Int J Radiat Oncol Biol Phys 30(4):845–849
29. Valsdottir EB et al. Transanal endoscopic microsurgery (T.E.M.) treatment of rectal cancer: a comparison of outcomes with and without neoadjuvant radiation therapy. SAGES, 2008, Abstract.

Laparoscopic Ablation of Liver Tumors

David A. Iannitti, David Sindram

Contents

Introduction

Ablation, or destruction, of tumors is a broadly accepted therapy in the treatment of a variety of soft tissue tumors, including tumors in the lungs, liver, kidney, and other organs. Significant improvements in ablative strategies, both operative and non-operative, have resulted in a growing body of literature demonstrating significant improvement in patient survivals in various tumor processes.

Ablation has become an important strategy in the treatment of hepatocellular carcinoma and is increasingly applied to liver metastases from colorectal carcinoma, as well as tumors from other origins. Initial experience was obtained with ethanol ablation [1]. However, thermoablative strategies have currently largely replaced ethanol injections. As experience using these modalities has grown, the thermocoagulative strategies, such as radiofrequency and microwave ablation, have proven to be superior to ethanol injections in the treatment of hepatocellular carcinoma. Although niche applications for cryoablation, freezing of tumors, may still exist, initial enthusiasm has waned in the past several years, particularly in liver cancer, due to a comparatively higher complication rate [2].

This field is in constant flux, and several ablative modalities are currently in development and remain to be clinically proven. Examples of such techniques are cellular reprogramming with irreversible electroporation [3], high-frequency focused ultrasound ablation [4], laser ablation [5], and radiation ablation with external beam stereotactic surgery or internal radiation with yttrium microsphere infusions. This chapter primarily focuses on the minimally invasive approach for thermal coagulation with radiofrequency and microwave technologies.

F.L. Greene, B.T. Heniford (eds.), *Minimally Invasive Cancer Management*,
DOI 10.1007/978-1-4419-1238-1_17,

Spectrum of Disease

Tumor ablation can be used to treat a variety of hepatic malignancies. The majority of patients presently undergoing ablation therapy have liver metastases from colorectal carcinoma or primary hepatocellular carcinoma. However, thermal ablation could also be used to treat a variety of pathologies including intrahepatic cholangiocarcinoma, hepatic adenoma, and metastatic renal cell, breast, and neuroendocrine tumors. Outcomes for local therapy for these diseases have been not as well studied; however, ablation therapy for liver-only disease may have a survival and symptomatic benefit. Pathologies including metastatic sarcoma, gastric, pancreas, esophageal, and lung cancers have not traditionally demonstrated improvement in long-term survival with liver-directed therapy and should only be considered for ablative therapy in highly selected cases. The prevalence, natural history, and outcomes of non-ablative therapies for metastatic colorectal carcinoma and hepatocellular carcinoma are reviewed.

Liver Metastases from Colorectal Cancer

The liver is a common site for metastatic cancer. The liver is the second-most common site, after the regional lymph nodes, of metastasis from organs drained by the portal venous system. The United States reports approximately 150,000 new cases of colorectal cancer per year. Up to 25% of the cases have liver metastases at the time of presentation and 50% develop liver metastases within 5 years. Therefore, 75,000 patients per year are at risk of developing liver metastases from colorectal cancer. Twenty percent of patients with liver metastases (15,000 cases/year) have disease limited to this organ. This is the group of patients that interventional therapies may potentially cure or provide improved survival.

The natural history of colorectal metastases to the liver has been well described. If untreated, patient survival averages 6–21 months. The extent of metastatic disease is the single most important factor for survival. Patients with a solitary metastasis to the liver have a median survival of 21 months. Twenty percent of these patients are alive at 3 years; however, there are few, if any, 5-year or long-term survivors. Patients with multifocal unilobar and bilobar disease have median survivals of 15 and 5 months, respectively. Patients with primary malignancies of the pancreas or stomach with metastatic disease to the liver have a dismal mean survival of only 2–3 months.

Systemic chemotherapy has seen significant improvement in recent years [6]. Traditional first-line chemotherapy with 5-fluorouracil (5-FU) alone or in combination with leucovorin for the treatment of metastatic colorectal cancer had a response rate of less than 30%. Current chemotherapy regimens for metastatic colorectal carcinoma include oxaliplatin, 5-FU, and leucovorin (FOLFOX) with bevacizumab which has demonstrated significant improvement in tumor response and disease-free and long-term survival [7]. Second-line regimens include irinotecan, cetuximab, and capecitabine. Regional therapy with hepatic artery infusion (HAI) with 5-fluoro-2′-deoxyuridine (FUDR) has resulted in some improvement in tumor control as well as disease-free survival when used in the adjuvant setting [8]. A variety of other chemotherapeutic agents have been studied for transarterial therapy with mixed response rates. The most significant improvement in hepatic arterial infusional therapy is the use of yttrium microsphere therapy. These 25–35 μm-sized radioactive particles are selectively taken up by hepatic tumors to deliver intratumoral radiation. Dramatic tumor responses have been documented; however, number of administrations and long-term response rates have yet to be determined.

Hepatic resection for metastatic colorectal cancer to the liver offers the best opportunity for long-term survival. Of the 15,000 cases in the United States per year with liver-only colorectal metastases, 3,750 cases are candidates for surgical resection. Long-term survival at 3, 5, and 10 years following hepatic resection is estimated to be 40, 30, and 20%, respectively. Patients with fewer than four metastatic lesions, greater than 1 cm surgical margins, and no extrahepatic disease have 5-year survival rates up to 40% [9]. Clearly, medically fit patients with liver-only disease and surgically attainable 1 cm margins should undergo hepatic resection for the treatment of metastatic colorectal [10].

Recurrence of metastatic disease is seen in 38% of patients following hepatic resection. The liver is involved in 45–75% of these cases. Recurrent metastatic disease involves the liver only in 40% of cases. Only one-third of these patients are candidates for a second hepatic resection [11]. Although the overall number of reported patients undergoing repeat hepatic resection for recurrent liver-only disease is small, acceptable outcomes have been reported. Operative mortality and postoperative morbidity are 5 and 15–40%, respectively. Median survival can be greater than 30 months and 5-year survival is 16–32%. It can be concluded that patients with recurrent hepatic metastases are still candidates for a local therapy and can have acceptable long-term results.

Although outcomes for patients undergoing surgical treatment for metastatic and recurrent metastatic colorectal cancer to the liver are favorable surgical resection can be offered to only a small percentage of patients with metastatic disease. Seventy-five percent of patients with liver-only metastases, accounting for 11,250 cases per year, are not candidates for hepatic resection. There are a number of factors that would preclude patients from undergoing hepatic resection: multifocal unilobar lesions, bilobar disease, invasion, or juxtaposition to various anatomic structures not allowing 1 cm surgical margins, cirrhosis, and comorbid medical conditions. It is this group of patients with potentially "curative" disease that is the focus of interstitial therapies such as radiofrequency ablation or microwave ablation. Similarly, patients with recurrent liver-only metastatic colorectal cancer may be considered for an ablative approach.

Hepatocellular Carcinoma

Hepatocellular carcinoma (HCC) is a prevalent problem on a worldwide basis, particularly in Asia and South Africa. An estimated 1,000,000 cases of HCC develop yearly in the world. The incidence of HCC in the United States is much less than in endemic areas, at 1.8 per 100,000 people; however, this incidence is rapidly rising. The development of HCC is linked to alcoholic cirrhosis, hepatitis C virus (HCV) infection, hepatitis B virus (HBV) infection, and other etiologies for chronic hepatitis and cirrhosis.

Patients with HCC generally have poor outcomes. Untreated patients with small (less than 3 cm) lesions are expected to have a median survival of 2 years. These tumors exhibit a widely variable growth rate, having a mean doubling time of 4 months. Patients with more advanced stage of disease have median survivals of only 6–9 months. Alcoholic cirrhosis and impaired liver function have an adverse effect of patient survival with HCC. More than half of patients with HCC in North America have alcoholic cirrhosis associated with it. Median survival in this group of patients is 9 months, regardless of the stage of disease [12].

Systemic chemotherapy for hepatocellular carcinoma traditionally has yielded minimal benefits. The standard agent for decades has been doxorubicin, a highly toxic chemotherapeutic agent. More recent agents have included liposomal doxorubicin, thalidomide, octreotide, and many others again with mixed results. The first systemic agent to show a modest 2–3 months survival improvement is sorafenib, a multi-target tyrosine kinase inhibitor [13]. Currently, multiple clinical trials using sorafenib are ongoing.

Surgical resection had traditionally been the treatment of choice for patients with HCC, particularly for small (<4 cm), single lesions. Conversely, diffuse metastatic disease is beyond surgical cure and should be triaged toward the best medical therapy, e.g., sorafenib treatment. For tumor burden between these parameters, strategies are less defined. Recurrence or progression of disease remains an issue in patients treated surgically for HCC. Within 5 years, 80% of patients will develop recurrence. Approximately two-thirds of patients will have a recurrence in the liver only; however, only 10% are candidates for further surgical treatment. With their landmark paper in 1996, Mazzaferro et al. arbitrarily chose a set of criteria in HCC at which point an important survival benefit in transplanted patients was demonstrated over resected liver lesions [14]. These criteria were coined the "Milan criteria," and suggest triage to transplantation, if the patient is a transplant candidate, with up to 3 HCC lesions that are less than 5 cm in diameter. Subsequent studies in the following years have demonstrated the validity of this strategy, also by intention to treat analysis. However, local issues such as organ availability may alter the favorable outcome due to interval tumor progression. Hence, strategies to bridge patients to transplant have become acceptable. Either by means of chemo/radio embolization, and/or thermoablation, patients are treated while waiting for transplantation [15].

If a patient is not a transplantation candidate, several strategies are currently being investigated. Single lesions <4 cm should be resected, although non-inferiority has been suggested in initial trials comparing resection to thermocoagulative treatment. The ablative strategy is currently being validated in various clinical trials, and we believe may be the treatment of choice for this disease process. Lesions >4 cm appear to benefit from chemoembolization, prior to resection, ablation, or transplantation. Controversy exists in this area and results from various clinical trials are eagerly anticipated.

Physics of Thermal Ablation

Normally perfused tissues can tolerate temperatures up to 45°C. Heating tissue at 50–55°C for 4–6 min produces irreversible cellular damage. At temperatures between 60°C and 100°C, almost immediate coagulation of tissue is induced, with irreversible damage to mitochondrial and cytosolic proteins of the cells. Above this temperature, tissue vaporizes and carbonizes. An important factor that affects the success of thermal ablation of tumors is the ability to ablate all viable tumor tissue and an adequate tumor-free margin. The ideal diameter of an ablation is 2 cm larger than the diameter of the tumor. This ensures that all microscopic invasions around the tumor have been destroyed. Therefore a 5 cm ablation zone is needed to treat a 3 cm diameter tumor. Otherwise, multiple overlapping ablations must be performed.

Radiofrequency ablation (RFA) is based on the interaction of an alternating electric current with living tissue. At a high-frequency setting (460–480 kHz), the current causes agitation of ions in the adjacent tissue. This generates frictional heat that extends into the tissue by conduction. RFA is the most widely used thermal ablation technology worldwide for the treatment of liver cancer. The AngioDynamics® (Queensbury, NY) system (formerly RITA Medical generator) was the first commercially available RFA system for liver utilized a 50 W generator. The current system is a 250 W RF generator. The Boston Scientific (Natick, MA) system (formerly RadioTherapeutics generator) was used in most reported RFA studies, with a 200 W output generator, and is also impedance based. The Valleylab (Boulder, CO) system (formerly Radionics generator) uses actively cooled tip electrodes and is output based with a 200 W generator. Actively cooling the electrodes keeps the local tissue temperature and impendence lower, thus allowing for more energy delivery into the tumor. The above systems are designed to create ablation diameters up to 4–5 cm with a single or multiple electrodes, although local factors including "heat sink" effect may limit the actual size. Using a switching controller attached to the output generator along with up to three separate shaft-cooled electrodes permits larger sized ablations without the need for sequential overlapping ablations and decreases the risk of undertreating tumors. Newer developments in RFA technology include saline perfusion RF electrodes and bipolar RF electrode configurations which do not need grounding pads.

Microwave ablation (MWA) relies on high-frequency electromagnetic radiation that is generated to heat the intracellular water molecules of the surrounding tissue and involves the use of devices with a frequency of 900 MHz to 10 GHz. The passage of microwaves "broadcasted" into tissue causes rapid rotation of water molecules. The water molecule itself is polarized as is the electromagnetic wave; when the wave hits the water molecule, the molecule oscillates, thereby creating movement resulting in heat. It is this heat that causes coagulative necrosis and ultimately tumor ablation. This generated heat is uniformly, instantaneously, and continuously distributed until the radiation from the microwave field is stopped.

Microwave technology has several (theoretical) advantages over RFA, such as absence of electrical current through the patient, negating the need for a grounding pad, faster ablation times, and the option to use multiple probes simultaneously. Depending on the energy (wattage) and frequency of the transmitted signal into the tumor higher intratumor temperatures can be achieved compared to RFA. Also, the broadcasted microwave field is not significantly interfered by blood flow through vessels during the application of the signal. This is an important difference between MWA and RFA, as RFA is entirely dependent on heat originating from the tip of the probe and high-frequency currents and, as such, much more susceptible to a heat sink effect of blood flow and charring of the tissues immediately surrounding the tip of the probe. Charring impedes subsequent alternating current through the patient and results in reduced ablation areas. Additionally, as a result of the higher temperatures, and reduced heat sink effect with MWA, the subsequent conduction of the heat into the surrounding tissues at the end of the application allows for much larger and more homogeneous ablation zones, even surrounding larger blood vessels. This technology has been used in open surgical, laparoscopic, and percutaneous therapeutic approaches for tumors of the liver.

Microtaze (Heiwa Electronics Industry, Inc., Tokyo, Japan) developed the first MWA needle antenna, capable of producing 1.5 cm size ablation; this was found in early studies not to be clinically useful, due to the small size [16]. The ValleyLab (Boulder, CO) VivaWave™ system (formerly Vivant generator) generates up to 45 W per antenna at 915 MHz; 13-gauge needle-type multiple antennae are used to synergistically create a 5 cm zone of thermocoagulation. Clustering the small diameter antennae promotes a synergistic amplification of the fields and larger ablation volumes. The cooled shaft version is designed for percutaneous and laparoscopic approaches to liver tumors. The Acculis V MTA^{TM} microwave system (Microsulis Medical Ltd, Hampshire, UK) operates at 2.45 GHz frequency with single 5 mm applicator which can create 5 cm size ablation in 4 min and 7–8 cm ablation in 8 min in a single application. The 30 cm length antenna is particularly useful for laparoscopic ablations. Both systems have been launched commercially in 2008 in the United States. MicroTherm X-100 (MTX-100) system developed by the BSD Medical Corp (Salt Lake City, UT) is unique in that it allows synchronized energy output from multi-antennae configurations. This 915 MHz generator was FDA approved in 2008. In principle, synchronizing the microwave waveform output through multiple antennae may reduce the wattage to achieve similar-sized ablations in target tissues, potentially decreasing the unwanted side effects of over-heating of antennae associated with high-wattage output models. 9.2 GHz generators are currently being developed for treatment of small ($\leq$1 cm) tumors.

Surgical Technique for Laparoscopic Ablation

Equipment needed to perform laparoscopic thermoablation of liver tumors varies only slightly per chosen energy modality. The general setup remains the same, regardless of the energy source. Standard laparoscopic equipment, a laparoscopic ultrasound probe, and the probes and energy source of the chosen system are required. It is preferable to have two video towers with the added capability to show the ultrasound images as a picture-in-picture, using a video image splitter. This allows for simultaneous viewing of the ultrasound and the probe placement in real time, enhancing the precision of the procedure. Probes for laparoscopic thermoablation are available in various lengths and sizes, largely depending on the type of energy source and their manufacturer. Most systems have specific smaller diameter probes, suited for laparoscopic application. The 5 mm MTA antenna fits down a standard 5 mm trocar.

Laparoscopic ultrasound has been demonstrated to be useful for a variety of purposes in laparoscopic surgery. This is particularly true during the performance of any thermoablative procedure. Ultrasound guidance is essential to identify and localize the target lesions; to assess the relationship to surrounding tissue, ducts, and vessels; and to monitor the progression of the thermoablative effect during the application of the energy. Developments in laparoscopic ultrasound probes have produced flexible, more maneuverable probes with a number of features. Various modes, including B-mode, M-mode, spectral Doppler, and color-flow monitoring, provide useful information used to distinguish various structures, such as biliary structures from blood vessels. Dexterity with laparoscopic ultrasound and understanding of ultrasonographic anatomy of the liver, particularly when viewing from varying angles and positions, are essential when performing laparoscopic ablative procedures.

Patient positioning is dependent on the location of the hepatic tumors to be treated. The supine position is most often adequate. Patients with lesions in the posterior sector of the right lobe of the liver (segments VI and VII) can be placed in an oblique position with the right side elevated up to 45° and the right arm elevated and across the chest. This position provides added exposure to the flank and facilitates placement of probes posteriorly (Fig. 17.1).

Most patients undergoing laparoscopic thermoablation of hepatic tumors will have had previous abdominal surgery. Since adherence of abdominal viscera to the anterior abdominal wall is a concern, the initial port is placed in an area distant from previous incisions and dissections. The open method of initial port placement using a blunt-tipped trocar is preferred.

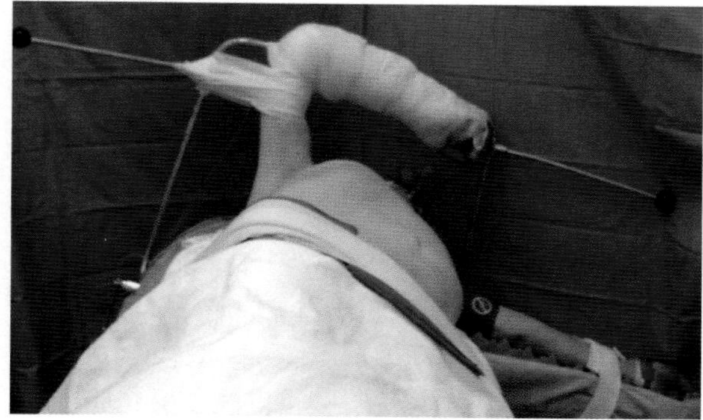

Figure 17.1

Patient positioning for ablation of a right posterior sector lesion. The patient is placed supine at a 45° angle with the right side up. The right arm is supported across the chest as shown. This allows the patient position to range from 0°–90° with bed rotation

A minimum of two ports is needed. However, several additional ports may be used to perform an adequate lysis of adhesions. The liver should be freed from adherent structures to its anterior surface, as well as adhesions to the diaphragm. The falciform and round ligaments may or may not need to be divided, depending on the exposure required.

After the adhesiolysis, the entire abdominal cavity is carefully explored for the presence of extrahepatic recurrence of metastatic disease not identified by preoperative radiographic studies. Suspicious tissue should be biopsied and submitted to pathology for immediate diagnosis. Extrahepatic disease would potentially preclude local treatment for the hepatic lesions. Next, the liver is evaluated in a complete and systematic fashion by ultrasound. All liver segments, portal tracts, hepatic veins, and inferior vena cava are carefully evaluated. All hepatic lesions are noted, particularly with reference to size, shape, and location relative to hepatic and vascular structures.

The lesion to be treated is approached in the following way: The location of the lesion is confirmed with ultrasound from multiple angles. The therapy probe is inserted through the capsule under ultrasound guidance, with the ultrasound and energy probes parallel (Fig. 17.2). This will provide a longitudinal image of the probe by ultrasound as it courses through the tissue. If the ultrasound and energy probes are oblique or perpendicular to each other, then a cross-sectional view of the probe, only a dot on the screen, will be seen. This may lead to inaccurate probe positioning or inadvertent puncture of adjacent structures. When proper placement of the probe is confirmed, the energy can be applied. Depending on the device, the energy delivery process is constantly monitored to ensure appropriate delivery, as per the devices' parameters. Progressive development of the ablation zone is monitored by ultrasound. Depending on the energy used, a typical ultrasound image is recorded. Once the energy delivery parameters are reached, the probe is carefully removed. The exit site of the probe should be inspected for bleeding and bile leakage. Hemostatic agents, electrocautery, or suturing of the hepatic capsule may be required. Larger tumors may require multiple passes or simultaneous application of probes in different positions to completely ablate the lesion with appropriate margins. A general strategy for larger tumors is to place the first puncture to the deep-medial margin of the tumor. As the ablation is carried out, microbubble formation will obscure the deeper aspects of the ablation (Fig. 17.3). Subsequent punctures are directed more superficially and laterally.

Follow-up consists of serial evaluations of tumor markers and abdominal computed tomography (CT) or magnetic resonance imaging (MRI) scans within 1 month of the ablation, then every 3–6 months thereafter (Fig. 17.4).

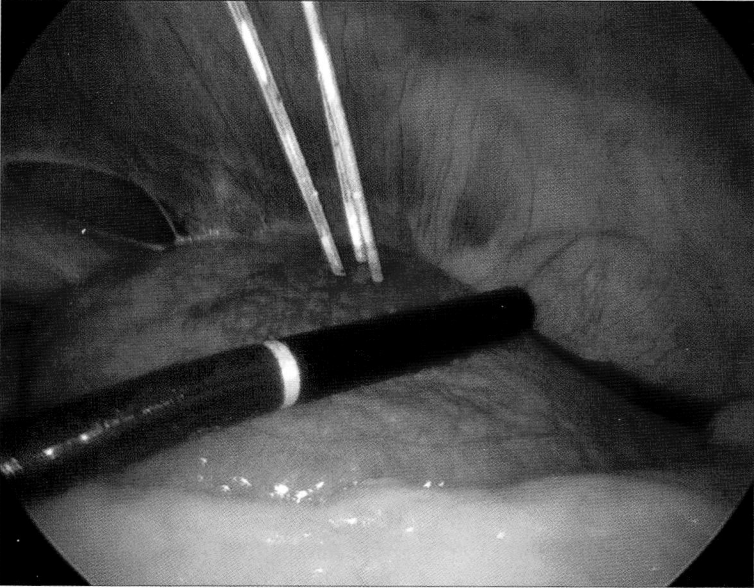

Figure 17.2

Laparoscopic view of a microwave ablation of a segment II liver tumor using three 915 MHz cooled shaft transcutaneous antennae

Part IV

Laparoscopic Management of Other Solid Organs

Laparoscopic Splenectomy for Malignant Diseases

R. Matthew Walsh, B. Todd Heniford

Contents

Since Delaitre and Maignien [1] reported the first laparoscopic splenectomy in 1991, the utility of laparoscopic splenectomy in the treatment of hematologic diseases such as hereditary spherocytosis, immune thrombocytopenic purpura, and autoimmune hemolytic anemia has been well established. Thousands of cases in the surgical literature have documented laparoscopic splenectomy as safe and effective in the management of these benign hematologic disorders. As with other minimally invasive surgical techniques, when compared to conservative or open surgery, patients appear to benefit from rapid advancement of diet, reduced postoperative pain and analgesic requirements, a shorter postoperative hospital stay, and an improved cosmetic result. Additionally, the period of convalescence is brief with an early return to work and normal activities. Although no prospective, randomized, controlled trials comparing open splenectomy with laparoscopic splenectomy have been completed, or are ever likely to be done, retrospective case–control series in both children and adults consistently favor the laparoscopic approach [2–9]. Although the minimally invasive method for splenic resection is now considered the "gold standard" for the treatment of benign hematologic diseases, a long-term evaluation of its hematologic benefits needs to be completed [10] and is ongoing in ours and several other centers.

A variety of malignant diseases involving the spleen, both primary and metastatic, may require splenectomy for either diagnostic or therapeutic reasons. The role of minimally invasive surgery in the management of malignant diseases involving the spleen is better defined with increased experience with laparoscopic splenectomy. The frequency of laparoscopic splenectomy for malignancy remains small compared to benign disease indications at most centers. In a large collective review of 946 patients by Gigot et al. [10] in which indications for laparoscopic splenectomy were clearly defined, malignancies involving the spleen

F.L. Greene, B.T. Heniford (eds.), *Minimally Invasive Cancer Management*,
DOI 10.1007/978-1-4419-1238-1_18,

represented only 11% of the cases. This may reflect a relatively small incidence of malignant splenic disease, or a reluctance to perform laparoscopic splenectomy due to technical and oncologic challenges that often accompany malignant splenic diseases. Splenomegaly, peri-splenitis, hilar lymphadenopathy, and the surgeon's concern for splenic disruption and tumor spillage may contribute to a hesitancy to perform laparoscopic splenectomy. These conditions are typically not present in benign hematologic disorders and add to the difficulty and potential complications of a minimally invasive approach. These patients may also have associated cytopenias and generalized debilitation that can result in an operative mortality historically as high as 23% in the open splenectomy era [11]. This chapter reviews the indications, selection criteria, and perioperative management for laparoscopic splenectomy for malignant diseases and the technique of laparoscopic splenectomy with contributory technical factors for splenomegaly and summarizes the experience with laparoscopic splenectomy with an assessment of its applicability and safety.

Indications

Malignancies involving the spleen can be grouped into lymphoproliferative diseases, myeloproliferative diseases, metastatic diseases, and primary (nonlymphoma) malignancies. Lymphoproliferative diseases include known or suspected diagnosis of Hodgkin's/non-Hodgkin's lymphoma, chronic B-cell lymphocytic leukemia, and hairy cell leukemia. Myeloproliferative disorders originate as a bone marrow problem and include myelofibrosis, chronic or acute myelogenous leukemia, and essential thrombocytosis [12]. Depending on the nature of the malignant disease, laparoscopic splenectomy may be performed for diagnosis, staging, or therapy. Primary cancers that metastasize to the spleen include colonic, gastric, ovarian, endometrial, lung, breast, prostatic, skin (melanoma), and esophageal [13, 14]. Splenic metastases are uncommon and usually occur in the setting of widespread visceral metastases. Patients with an isolated metastasis should be considered for laparoscopic splenectomy for palliation or in conjunction with additional adjuvant therapy. Splenectomy is also the treatment for patients with primary (nonlymphoma) malignancies of the spleen such as angiosarcomas, plasmacytomas, and malignant fibrous histiocytomas [15, 16]. These tumors are extremely uncommon, but these patients should be considered candidates for laparoscopic splenectomy if the lesion remains confined to the spleen. The more common reasons for splenectomy in malignancy are described below.

Lymphoproliferative Disease

Hodgkin's Disease

In 1832, Thomas Hodgkin first described the clinical and postmortem features of the disease that would bear his name, Hodgkin's lymphoma. The approach to the treatment of patients with Hodgkin's disease has changed markedly and continues to evolve. Initially, all treatments were considered palliative, including the first treatments with radiation therapy. Encouraging preliminary results of radiation therapy led to progressively higher and curative doses of radiation [17]. The addition of chemotherapeutic agents has resulted in curative therapy for the majority of patients. The achievements made in treatment have not been devoid of significant, late post-treatment complications, which include infection, pulmonary fibrosis, cardiac failure, and, most importantly, secondary malignancy. Secondary malignancies are a leading cause of morbidity and death among long-term survivors of Hodgkin's [18]. Most of these cancers are solid tumors and typically occur after a minimal latency of 5–10 years, with breast and lung cancers accounting for the largest absolute risk. The current emphasis on treating Hodgkin's disease is to maintain a high degree of freedom from relapse and to reduce the late sequelae [19]. A more tailored approach to treatment with less risk of complications from chemotherapy and/or radiation therapy is being considered for early-stage Hodgkin's disease in patients with favorable prognostic indicators [20].

Critical in the treatment decisions is an accurate staging of the disease. The Ann Arbor staging system has been a popular and useful method of categorizing patients for more than 25 years. Cotswold's modifications also have proven useful in incorporating the bulk of disease [21]. The stage of disease has a strong prognostic value. Ann Arbor stages I, II, and IIIA are in prognostically favorable groups, whereas stages IIIB and IV are unfavorable. Additional independent prognostic factors include age, gender, erythrocyte sedimentation rate, blood lymphocyte counts, and the presence of systemic symptoms. Female patients, those less than 70 years of age, the lack of constitutional ("B") symptoms, an erythrocyte sedimentation rate of less then 30, and lymphocyte count greater than 1,000 all show some advantage to the patient [22]. Prognostic value of histologic subtype is of little current value, although lymphocyte-predominant, nodular patients have a greater risk for disease recurrence.

Fundamental in an effective strategy toward a tailored, less aggressive treatment protocol is an accurate determination of the disease stage. Noninvasive procedures predominate in the workup, but are variably applied. Investigational studies include computed tomography (CT) of the chest and abdomen, magnetic resonance imaging (MRI) of the spleen and bone marrow, gallium scanning, technetium bone scanning, immunoscintigraphy, and positron emission tomography (PET) with fluorodeoxyglucose. The current state of the art of treating Hodgkin's is the use of PET scanning for staging and prognosis. Assessment of treatment response by PET in early restaging, or even mid-treatment, has resulted in tailoring of therapy. It is becoming clear that PET has strong potential to improve clinical outcomes by sparing good-risk patients from overly aggressive treatments and by more accurately identifying poor-risk patients to guide changes in management [23, 24].

Combining prognostic variables can be useful in predicting patients with the lowest risk for occult abdominal involvement. This is commonly done in Europe to determine treatment groups [25, 26]. Patients should be considered for staging laparotomy and splenectomy only if the outcome of the procedure influences treatment. This approach is based on the philosophy that in some patients extensive staging reduces both the initial treatment needed and the subsequent treatment-related complications, both in the short and in the long term. The historical morbidity and mortality of a laparotomy in these patients, 32 and 6.8%, respectively [27], had to be subtracted from the benefits of improved staging. Laparoscopic staging with splenectomy can reduce the morbidity of surgical staging through the utilization of minimally invasive techniques while ensuring comparable operative staging.

Surgical staging for Hodgkin's disease should include splenectomy, a wedge and three core biopsies of the liver, and lymph node samples from the left and right paraaortic, iliac, celiac, porta hepatis, and mesenteric regions. Staging laparotomy or laparoscopy is not justified unless care is taken to ensure that patients are staged completely. The most significant finding gained from abdominal staging is the presence or absence of splenic involvement. Further, in patients with clinical stages I and II disease who are found to have positive nodes at operation, the nodes are typically located in the paraaortic region. Only 4% will have occult disease in the porta hepatis lymph nodes. The complications of staging laparotomy are not innocuous and are an important factor in considering its role in the evaluation of patients. Staging laparoscopy may positively impact on the rate of postoperative complications in these patients. To date, no major change in the management of Hodgkin's disease in the hematology community has occurred and staging laparoscopy with laparoscopic splenectomy is rarely utilized.

Non-Hodgkin's Lymphoma (NHL)

The spleen is involved in 30–40% of patients with NHL; usually it is a consequence of advanced disease [28]. Manifested by splenomegaly, this may be a direct result of tumor (lymphomatous) invasion or parenchymal expansion due to an increased sequestration of cellular blood components (Fig. 18.1). Treatment is directed at local symptoms attributed to splenomegaly or the hematologic consequences of sequestration. Although many patients with splenomegaly are asymptomatic, those who become symptomatic complain of abdominal fullness and pain, early satiety, pleuritic chest pain (Kehr's sign), weakness, malaise, or easy bruisability. Local symptoms are typically related to splenic enlargement, but splenic infarctions can occur. Hematologic manifestations include thrombocytopenia, neutropenia, and anemia that are difficult to treat medically and may prevent the administration of adequate chemotherapy [29]. Splenectomy can reliably alleviate local symptoms of splenomegaly and reverse cytopenias, which may predict improved survival. These benefits can be achieved via laparotomy with a mortality and morbidity of less than 5 and 30%, respectively, even with advanced disease [29, 30]. Infections are the most commonly reported complications of splenectomy, including sepsis, wound infection, and subphrenic abscess. The use of preoperative pneumococcal, hemophilus, and meningococcal vaccines and prophylactic antibiotics, meticulous surgical technique, and avoidance of intraabdominal drains can decrease infectious complications [31].

Primary splenic lymphoma refers to lymphoma confined to the spleen, with or without hilar

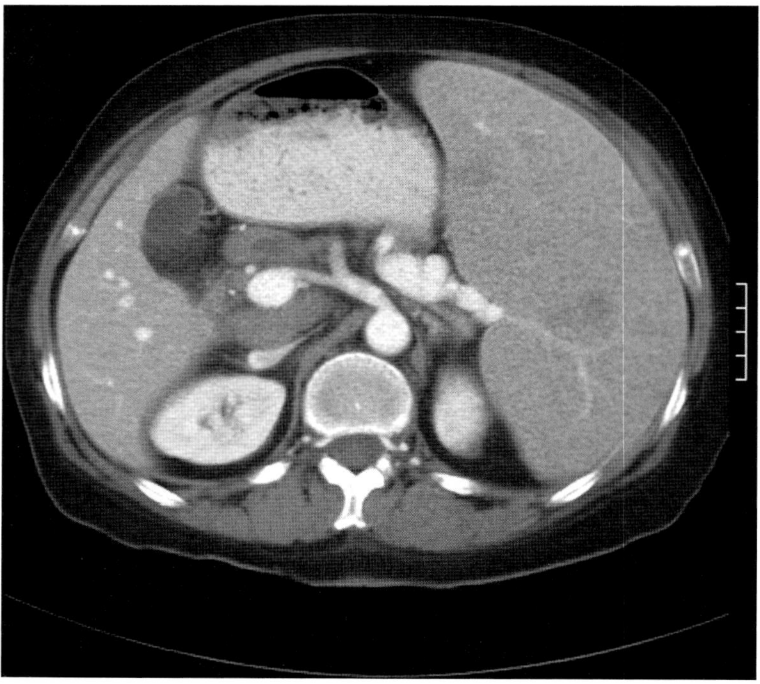

Figure 18.1

Massive splenectomy on a preoperative computed tomography (CT) image of a patient with primary splenic lymphoma

lymphadenopathy. When strictly defined, this is an uncommon manifestation of NHL, representing 1% of all patients with malignant lymphoma [32]. The presentation of primary splenic lymphoma commonly includes left upper quadrant abdominal pain, weight loss, fatigue, anorexia, fever, and night sweats. Although splenomegaly is discernible on physical exam, asymptomatic splenomegaly is not typical of the disease.

Noninvasive radiologic investigations such as liver–spleen and gallium scanning and ultrasound are useful in documenting splenomegaly, but they are not accurate in diagnosing lymphomatous splenic involvement. Lymphomatous nodules of less than 1 cm can be visualized with current CT imaging. The differential diagnosis of large solitary or multiple splenic masses with low-attenuation foci includes abscesses, hematomas, cysts, Hodgkin's disease, angiosarcoma, and metastatic carcinoma.

Splenectomy is indicated for suspected isolated splenic lymphoma to alleviate the symptoms, confirm the diagnosis, and treat the disease [33]. Splenectomy alone for primary splenic lymphoma is associated with improved survival as compared to patients with diffuse NHL and splenomegaly [32]. The mean weight of spleens primarily involved with lymphoma is over 1 kg, which does not necessarily preclude consideration of laparoscopic splenectomy. We have successfully performed laparoscopic splenectomy for spleens weighing greater than 4.5 kg. We have found preoperative measurement of craniocaudal splenic length to be useful in predicting the feasibility of laparoscopic splenectomy [34].

Hairy Cell Leukemia

Hairy cell leukemia is an uncommon B-cell lymphoproliferative disorder characterized by severe splenomegaly and circulating and bone marrow lymphocytes displaying prominent cytoplasmic projections ("hairy cells"). The disease is chronic and progressive, but patients generally require no specific therapy until they develop neutropenia, thrombocytopenia, anemia, or recurrent infections. Most patients will eventually require some form of treatment. Until the introduction of interferon-2, splenectomy was the treatment of choice for hairy cell leukemia. Although this technique did not cause disease remission, 40–75% of patients had an improvement or normalization of peripheral blood cells, with a median response duration of 5–20 months, and 60–70% survived 5 years [35]. In a large retrospective analysis, patients undergoing splenectomy lived longer than patients without surgery [36].

The clinical benefit of splenectomy is clear, but the impact on survival remains uncertain. With the purine analogues cladribine and pentostatin, response rates are even better than with interferon-2 and long-lasting remissions can be achieved in most patients. Splenectomy should be considered for the rare patient who is refractory to medical treatment and have splenomegaly that is symptomatic or results in severe cytopenia [37].

Myeloproliferative Disease

Chronic myelogenous leukemia represents up to 30% of all adult leukemias and presents usually in the fifth and sixth decades of life. The Philadelphia translocation between chromosomes 9 and 22 is pathognomonic for the disease. Approximately 50–75% of patients will present with splenomegaly. A peripheral blood smear will show leukocytosis with a wide spectrum of myelogenous differentiation and basophilia. The degree of splenomegaly correlates with the total body granulocyte mass and blood granulocyte count [38]. Although there is some correlation between the size of the spleen and the time to blast crisis, splenectomy has not been shown to improve or delay the onset of blast transformation [39]. However, splenectomy during the blast or accelerated phase can lead to improved quality of life by decreasing transfusion requirements.

Myelofibrosis is fortunately a rare disorder that occurs predominantly in males, usually after the seventh decade. Universally fatal, the mean survival is 5 years. Splenectomy may be considered with caution for palliation aimed at decreasing transfusion requirements and symptoms of splenomegaly. The severity of complications during or following laparoscopic splenectomy due to bleeding can be higher when operating for myelofibrosis [40]. It appears that survival following splenectomy for myeloproliferative diseases is worse than for lymphoproliferative diseases [41].

Selection Criteria

The choice of operative approach for patients with malignant splenic disease is particularly important as it typically involves patients with a varying degree of splenomegaly. The potential operative approaches should include open laparotomy, standard laparoscopic splenectomy, and hand-assisted laparoscopic splenectomy (HALS) [38, 42]. No randomized data exists to provide definitive conclusions, but hopefully patients can be offered expertise in all of these options so the most appropriate procedure selected based on reasonable surgical judgment. Provided adequate surgical experience is available, very few patients require open laparotomy. Nonrandomized comparative trials of open vs. laparoscopic splenectomy in splenomegaly show that while laparoscopic splenectomy is associated with longer operative times, it also results in lower mortality and morbidity rates, earlier return to normal activity, less narcotic use, and shorter hospital stay [40, 43]. Excluding other disease and patient factors, splenomegaly should not be considered a contraindication for a laparoscopic technique.

Having selected a laparoscopic approach in the setting of splenectomy does require a high level of proficiency in advanced laparoscopic skills. Fortunately skill acquisition for laparoscopic splenectomy for splenomegaly is rapid when the surgeon has advanced laparoscopic skills and familiarity with normal-sized spleens [44]. Other than splenomegaly there are additional patient factors that may alter your surgical approach. Body habitus can be a subtle factor that influences the experienced surgeon. Splenic size alone is not the sole predictor of successful laparoscopic outcome since the size and configuration of the abdominal cavity, laxity of the abdominal wall, and response to muscle relaxation are important, yet difficult to predict prior to operation. Obesity is not a specific contraindication to laparoscopic splenectomy, and obese patients are expected to reap the benefits of a laparoscopic procedure compared to conventional surgery [45]. Somewhat surprisingly the underlying hematologic disease has little documented effect on the operative approach. It is intuitive that preoperative platelet count significantly impacts amount of operative blood loss [46], and close interaction with a hematologist is fruitful in reducing the severity of cytopenias preceding operation. Patients with myelofibrosis may be also prone to intraoperative bleeding risk [40]. Multiple adhesions located in the epigastrum and left upper quadrant from prior abdominal surgery may also impact a laparoscopic approach. Portal hypertension is now a relative contraindication provided you have sufficient expertise and are well prepared for the challenge [47, 48].

Having opted for a laparoscopic approach a decision needs to be made whether a standard laparoscopy or HALS procedure is most appropriate. Factors which may impact this decision and operative time include bagging time, operative blood loss, conversion to open, and perioperative morbidity. Ideally the need to utilize HALS would be made at the outset of operation to minimize the length of unproductive operative time. The principle criteria which impact the operative outcomes relate to the size and configuration of the spleen. Unfortunately, preoperative data are often lacking with retrospective series determining outcomes based on post-operative morcellated weights. While it is possible to estimate preoperative splenic weights [49], the most valuable reproducible variables are splenic width, length, depth, and volume which are known from a preoperative CT scan. Craniocaudal length is the easiest to measure, and we have defined splenomegaly as >11 cm, massive splenomegaly as >17 cm, and super massive splenomegaly >22 cm [34]. Splenic size and conversion has been shown in a small number of patients to relate with operative outcomes [46]. Patients who underwent laparoscopic splenectomy for massive splenectomy were significantly more likely to be converted to open based on mediolateral length, increased intraoperative bleeding due to high body mass index, and splenic volume. Significant predictive factors for bleeding during HALS included high splenic volume and anteroposterior splenic length and significant increase in postoperative morbidity due to craniocaudal length. It has been our practice to initiate the operation with a hand-assisted device for supermassive splenomegaly and to use standard laparoscopy for smaller spleens with conversion to hand-assisted as necessary.

Relative contraindications for laparoscopic splenectomy include lymphadenopathy at the splenic hilum and inflammation effecting the spleen and surrounding tissues. In Hodgkin's and non-Hodgkin's lymphoma, large lymph nodes may be present at the splenic hilum, which can increase the difficulty of the dissection and thus the risk of vascular or pancreatic injury [50]. Perisplenic inflammation secondary to malignant disease or splenic infarction will increase the risk for capsular tear when mobilizing the spleen.

Preoperative Preparation

All patients undergoing elective splenectomy should receive vaccinations for the encapsulated bacteria 2 weeks prior to surgery. The current pneumococcal vaccine, which is composed of 23 capsular types of pneumococcus, the second generation of the *Haemophilus influenza* type b (Hib) vaccine, and the meningococcal vaccine should be administered. Because they cannot produce adequate antibody levels in response to it, children under 2 years of age should not receive the vaccines. Instead such children should receive prophylactic penicillin until the age of 2, at which time they may be administered the vaccine (Table 18.1). Some physicians advocate penicillin prophylaxis in children until the age of 18 years or for life [51].

All patients should be typed and cross-matched for blood, and those with thrombocytopenia should also have platelets available. Sufficient time should be allotted during the preoperative period to acquire the blood products because typing and crossing may be difficult. Preoperative platelet administration is not performed due to rapid platelet destruction within the spleen. In patients with lymphoma or leukemia, preparation is made to have a blood warmer in the operating room; it is used with all transfusions to reduce the incidence of cryoglobulinemia. Preoperative embolization of the splenic artery has been proposed for patients with splenomegaly to reduce operative blood loss and decrease the size of the spleen. We have not used this option due to the post-procedural pain, cost, embolization-related complications, and our ongoing success without it.

As for every operation, preoperative discussions with the patient and family include possible risks and complications. This discussion should include the incidence of postsplenectomy sepsis (PSS). Unfortunately, the majority of data predate the widespread use of the polyvalent pneumococcal vaccine. Over the last

Table 18.1. Current recommendations for penicillin prophylaxis and pneumococcal vaccination in children[a]

Age (years)	Daily antibiotic	Pneumococcal vaccination
0–2	Yes	No
2–5	Yes	Yes
5–18	Optional	Every 6 years
>18	No	Every 6–10 years

[a]The initial vaccine should be administered at 2 years of age, but not before. Revaccination should begin at the age of 5 years

15–20 years, there have been few isolated case reports of patients who, after having received the pneumococcal vaccine, went on to develop PSS. Konradsen reported that no patient who underwent splenectomy between 1979 and 1987 in Demark, and received the pneumococcal vaccine, developed PSS [52]. Similarly, there have been a paucity of cases described in patients who were prescribed daily penicillin prophylaxis.

Operative Technique

Lateral positioning for laparoscopic splenectomy is our preferred approach and is particularly well suited for patients with modest splenomegaly [42, 53, 54]. Enlargement of the spleen can result in unusual and abnormal configurations that, along with the increased size, makes the spleen difficult to maneuver [55]. Perisplenitis, adhesion, or enlarged lymph nodes may also limit exposure. After the patient is placed in a lateral position, gravity helps to expose the retroperitoneal and perihilar attachments. Less direct manipulation and retraction allows for a safer dissection with a reduced risk of capsular injury even in the presence of dense adhesions.

Prophylactic antibiotics, usually a first-generation cephalosporin, are given perioperatively. General endotracheal anesthesia is administered and while the patient is in the supine position, a Foley catheter, orogastric tube, and any additional monitoring devices are placed. The patient is rolled into a right lateral decubitus position with the arms extended and secured to an arm board. Protective rolls are placed between the legs, under the right axilla, and beneath the flank at the level of the umbilicus. Patients are positioned so that their umbilicus lies over the break in the table. After proper positioning, the table is flexed, lengthening the distance between the iliac crest and the costal margin. The surgeon and assistant position themselves on the right side of the table facing the patient's abdomen (Fig. 18.2). The video monitor is viewed over the patient's left shoulder. The patient is placed in reverse Trendelenburg's position to allow for caudal displacement of small bowel, colon, and omentum and to promote the collection of blood and irrigation fluid in the pelvis away from the operative field.

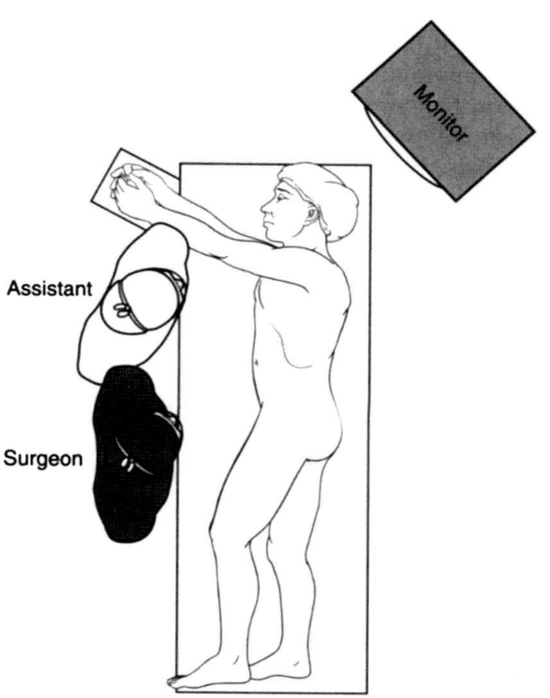

Figure 18.2

Organization of the operating room for laparoscopic splenectomy. The surgeons stand facing the abdomen with a video monitor directly across from them. The scrub nurse stands across the table toward the patient's foot

Three left subcostal ports are typically used, but occasionally a fourth trocar is required for larger spleens (Fig. 18.3). A lateral trocar (5 or 10 mm) is placed below the level of the 11th rib, a medial trocar (5 or 10 mm) is placed below the level of the 11th rib, a medial trocar (5 or 10 mm) is placed close to the midline, and a middle trocar (10 or 5/12 mm) is placed an equal distance between the medial and the lateral trocars. Optimal positioning of the ports would be 4 cm below the inferior tip of the spleen parallel to the left costal margin, but within reach of the diaphragm. If the spleen is extremely large, the trocars may have to be placed substantially more inferior than normal, creating the need to place one additional port posteriorly to facilitate access to the diaphragm. The middle trocar is placed first, utilizing an open technique. All additional ports are placed under direct laparoscopic guidance. It is necessary to

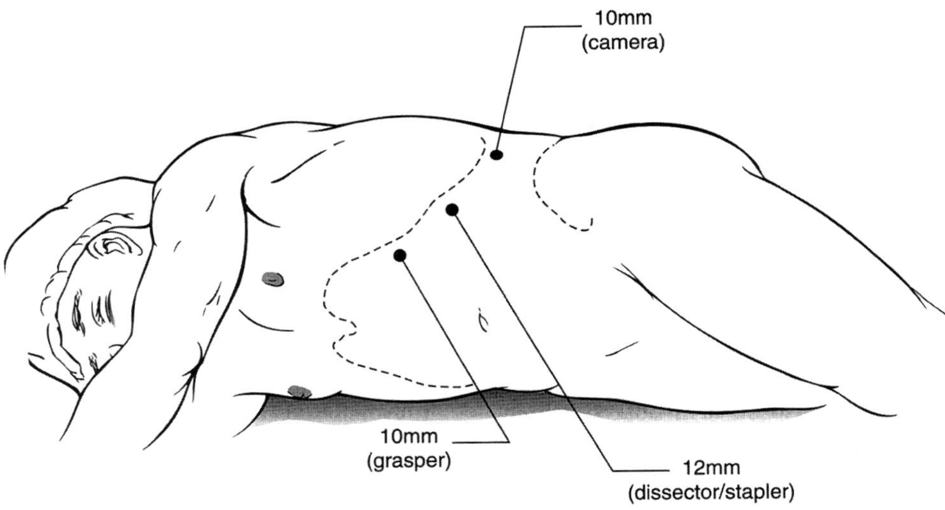

Figure 18.3

Trocar placements for the laparoscopic splenectomy. Three subcostal trocars are typically required; a fourth port may be placed further laterally if needed

use a 5 or 10 mm, 30° and/or 45° laparoscope to ensure adequate visualization. The operation proceeds best when the camera is exchanged between the medial and the lateral ports and the surgeon operates with both hands.

The splenic flexure of the colon is mobilized when exposure of the inferior pole of the spleen is obscured. Proceeding in an inferior to superior direction, the posterior peritoneal attachments are incised approximately 1 cm away from the spleen. The dissection continues lateral to medial until the tail of the pancreas and splenic hilar vessels are visualized. Medial retraction and rotation of the spleen is facilitated by grasping the 1-cm leaf of peritoneum still attached to the spleen with a blunt grasper. If a hand-assisted device is used, it is placed in the position of the medial port through a vertical paramedian incision. The hand will provide medial retraction and rotation of the spleen instead of a blunt grasper (Fig. 18.4). The gastroepiploic branches along the inferior pole of the spleen are divided between clips or with the harmonic scalpel (Ethicon Endo-Surgery, Cincinnati, Ohio). Care is taken when mobilizing the superior pole of the spleen to identify the short gastric vessels and the greater curvature of the stomach. Once all of the attachments have been removed, the hilar pedicle is divided with a gastrointestinal anastomosis stapler with a vascular cartridge (Fig. 18.5). Several firings of the stapler are usually required to transect the splenic hilum. The stapler can also be used to divide the short gastric vessels. If the spleen is exceptionally large, the superior attachments to the diaphragm are left intact to assist in placing the spleen into a retrieval bag. After the hilar vessels and short gastric vessels have been transected, the spleen is placed into an appropriately sized impermeable retrieval bag. This bag must be strong and flexible so that it will not rupture during extraction.

Placing the spleen into the retrieval bag can be one of the most time-consuming and challenging aspects of the operation. The closed end of the retrieval bag should be placed at the diaphragm, with the bag opened widely facing the lateral trocar (Fig. 18.6). The posterior lip of the bag should be grasped with a left-handed instrument while grasping the stapled edge of the splenic hilum with a right-handed instrument. The patient is placed into Trendelenburg position and the spleen is gradually directed into the bag. If a hand-assist is required, it is usually done at the time of extraction of a massive spleen to assist in bagging and splenic morcellation. The apparatus is placed in an enlarged trocar site for use of the nondominant hand. After the spleen is within the retrieval bag, the opening of the bag is delivered through the largest port site and

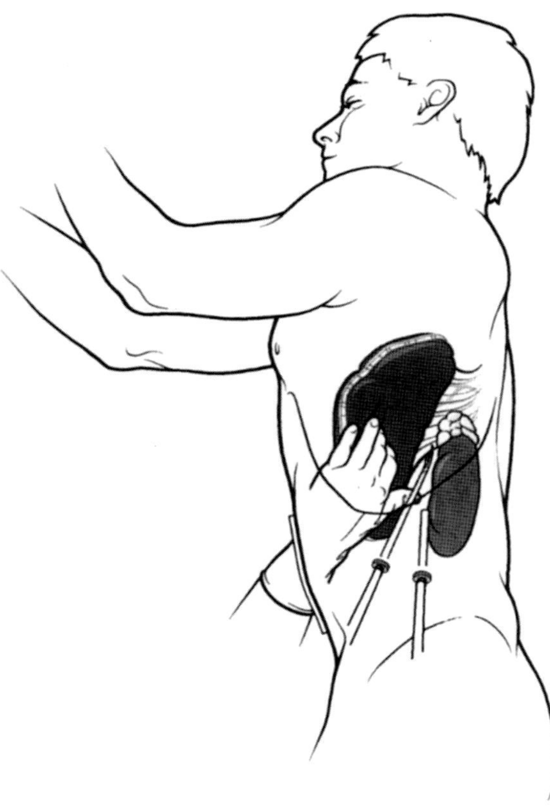

Figure 18.4
Hand-assisted laparoscopic splenectomy. The hand port replaces the medial port and provides the reaction to expose the tail of the pancreas and splenic hilum

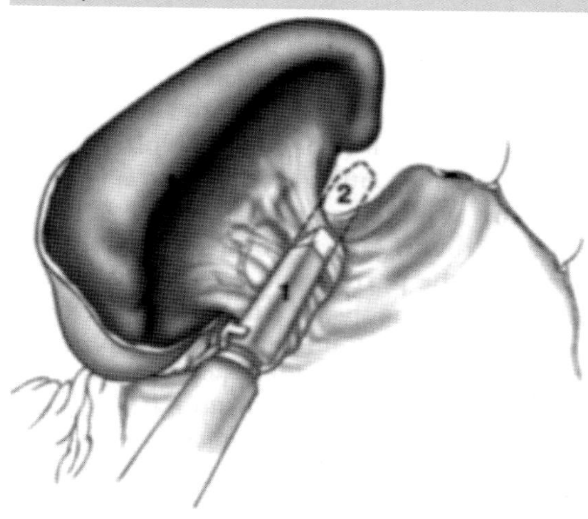

Figure 18.5
Applying a laparoscopic stapler to the hilum of the spleen. Typically two to four stapler loads will be required to completely transect the splenic vasculature

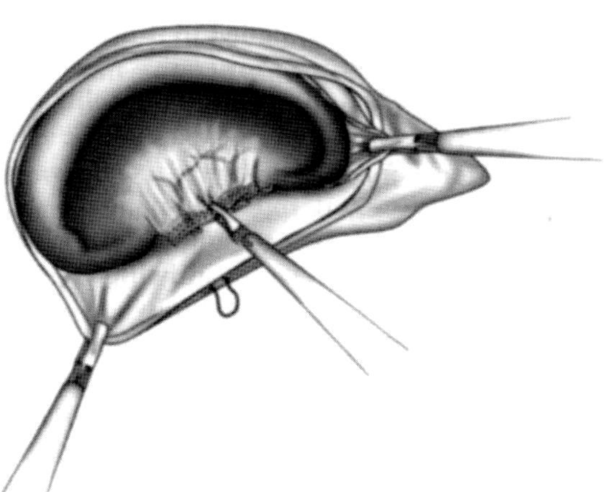

Figure 18.6
Placing the spleen into an impermeable bag inside the abdomen

the spleen is morcellated with ringed forceps. A spleen of suitable size can be placed in a 15 mm Endo-catch bag (Ethicon Endo-Surgery), but extra care must be taken to not disrupt this thinner bag at manual morcellation extraction. The abdomen is then reinsufflated, the operative site is irrigated, and meticulous hemostasis obtained. A drain is placed if a pancreatic injury is suspected.

The patient's orogastric tube and Foley catheter are removed in the operating room. A clear liquid diet is initiated the evening of surgery and advanced to a regular diet on the first postoperative day. Patients are encouraged to ambulate beginning the day of surgery. Laboratory tests are obtained only as needed or indicated by the preoperative malignant hematologic disease.

Outcomes

The historical data of splenectomy for malignancy showed a high operative mortality ranging from 18 to 23% [11, 56]. Recent mortality rates following open splenectomy for hematologic malignancy have improved to 8–9%, this despite high morbidity rates of 41–52% [41, 57]. These series also demonstrated that splenic size is an independent risk factor for postoperative complications and that pulmonary complications predominate following open splenic resection. Laparoscopic splenectomy for malignancy compared favorably to open splenectomy and is the current standard providing adequate expertise exists. Multiple series have shown mortality rates between 0 and 2% and morbidity rates of 6–22% [34, 57, 58]. Compared to other indications for laparoscopic splenectomy, patients operated for hematologic malignancy have the highest perioperative mortality of 1.5% and highest long-term mortality of 22% [59].

The ability to achieve satisfactory outcomes in patients operated laparoscopically for malignancy likely relates to the technical conduct of the operation. A safe completion of the laparoscopic operation is the factor which confers low morbidity and shortened hospitalization without major blood loss or injury to organs in proximity such as the pancreas [60]. Achieving safe patient outcomes may require conversion to HALS or open splenectomy for bleeding of limited exposure. Conversion rates of 41% have been reported in cases of splenomegaly [61]. A high conversion rate has been shown to decrease from 33 to 0% with increased experience [44], and most large series demonstrate a conversion rate of 12–23% for standard laparoscopic splenectomy for splenomegaly [46]. The use of HALS has been shown to decrease the rate of conversion to laparotomy when used to salvage a laparoscopic procedure or as the initial operative approach. A HALS approach should be utilized judiciously based on surgeon experience and comfort. Direct comparative data are hard to find since the HALS technique is often applied selectively to the largest spleens [62]. When HALS has been employed it has been shown to have similar morbidity rates compared to standard laparoscopic splenectomy [62, 63]. Recent data have also shown a decrease in length of operation, operative blood loss, and rate of conversion [58, 63]. Table 18.2 summarizes the largest and most recent studies comparing standard laparoscopy and HALS. The length of stay following a HALS ranges from 5 to 7 days. These data suggest that HALS should be used in patients with massive splenomegaly particularly from the outset when the spleen is > 22 cm in craniocaudal length or long mediolateral splenic length [34, 46].

The outcomes of laparoscopic splenectomy for hematologic malignancy can also be viewed in comparison to patients operated for benign disease, typically ITP. These data are summarized in Table 18.3 and generally convey that patients operated for malignancy are significantly older and require a long operative time with higher blood loss. The operative mortality, morbidity, and length of stay are both similar and excellent.

The recognized benefits of laparoscopic splenectomy appear to be attainable for patients operated for malignancy. Excellent outcomes can be achieved in patients operated for lymphoproliferative myeloproliferative disease, as well as metastatic or primary splenic neoplasms. A careful approach to laparoscopic splenectomy including proper positioning, vascular control, and appropriate mobilization of the spleen

Table 18.2. Laparoscopic vs. hand-assisted laparoscopic splenectomy

	Rosen et al. [62]		Targarona et al. [65]		Wang et al. [63]	
	LAP	HALS	LAP	HALS	LAP	HALS
Number	31	14	40	37	16	20
Spleen wt (g)	1,031	1,516[a]	1,576	1,785	1,185	1,346
Operative time	186	177	165	141[a]	195	141[a]
Conversion (%)	23	7	18	8	25	0
Mortality (%)	0	0	0	1	0	0
Morbidity (%)	16	35	38	20	13	0
Length of stay (days)	4.2	5.4	6	6	5.3	7.4[a]

[a] Statistical significance, $p < 0.05$

Table 18.3. Laparoscopic splenectomy for benign and malignant disease

	Targarona et al. [66]		Torelli et al. [67]		Walsh et al. [12]	
	Benign	Malignant	Benign	Malignant	Benign	Malignant
Number	100	37	23	15	86	73
Age (years)	37	60[a]	42	57	46	61
Operative time (min)	138	161	122	128	126	148
Spleen wt (g)	279	1,210[a]	300	1,270[a]	162	680[a]
Conversion (%)	5	14	0	0	1	12
Mortality (%)	0	0	0	1	0	0.6
Morbidity (%)	13	22	4	3	8	8
Length of stay (days)	3.7	5[a]	4.8	6.8	2	3[a]

[a] Statistical significance, $p<0.05$

including use of a hand-assist allows a minimally invasive approach to be successful [64, 65].

Conclusion

Laparoscopic splenectomy has emerged as the standard treatment in patients requiring splenectomy for benign hematologic diseases. Experience with laparoscopic splenectomy for malignant disease is limited, and the role of minimally invasive surgery in the management of these patients is still evolving. Our experience, as well as that of others, has demonstrated its feasibility and safety despite the fact that malignant hematologic diseases are frequently associated with splenomegaly. Hand-assisted laparoscopy is an alternative approach to overcome the technical challenges of splenomegaly. This device should be considered by those with little experience with laparoscopic splenectomy for malignant diseases and when abdominal CT scanning demonstrates a spleen that is greater than 19 cm in width and greater than 23 cm in craniocaudal length. Although laparoscopic splenectomy for malignant diseases is feasible, the role of minimally invasive surgery in the staging of Hodgkin's lymphoma is still experimental. During the next decade, surgeons will gain more experience with laparoscopic splenectomy and as they expand its indications to malignant diseases of the spleen, laparoscopic splenectomy's role in malignant hematologic disease will more clearly be defined.

References

1. Delaitre B, Maignien B (1991) Splenectomy by the laparoscopic approach. Report of a case. Presse Med 20:2263
2. Huber MR, Kumar S, Tefferi A (2003) Treatment advances in adult immune thrombocytopenic purpura. Ann Hematol 82:723–737
3. Rescorla FJ (2002) Laparoscopic splenectomy. Semin Pediatr Surg 11:226–232
4. Park A, Targarona EM, Trias M (2001) Laparoscopic surgery of the spleen: state of the art. Langenbecks Arch Surg 386:230–239
5. Brunt LM, Langer JC, Quasebarth MA et al (1996) Comparative analysis of laparoscopic vs. open splenectomy. Am J Surg 173:596–601
6. Smith CD, Meyer TA, Goretsky MJ et al (1996) Laparoscopic splenectomy by the lateral approach: a safe and effective alternative to open splenectomy for hematologic diseases. Surgery 120:789–794
7. Walsh RM, Heniford BT, Brody F, Ponsky J (2001) The ascendance of laparoscopic splenectomy. Am Surg 67:48–53
8. Janu PG, Rogers DA, Lobe TE (1996) A comparison of laparoscopic and traditional open splenectomy in childhood. J Pediatr Surg 31:109–114
9. Friedman RL, Fallas MJ, Carroll BJ et al (1996) Laparoscopic splenectomy for ITP: the gold standard. Surg Endosc 10:991–995
10. Gigot JF, Lengele B, Gianello P et al (1998) Present status of laparoscopic splenectomy for hematologic diseases: certitudes and unresolved issues. Semin Laparosc Surg 5: 147–167
11. Mittelman A, Stutzman L, Grace JT (1968) Splenectomy in malignant lymphoma and leukemia. Geriatrics 23:142–149
12. Walsh RM, Brody F, Brown N (2004) Laparoscopic splenectomy for lymphoproliferative disease. Surg Endosc 18: 272–275

13. Giulliani A, Caporale A, DiBari M et al (1999) Isolated splenic metastasis from endometrial carcinoma. J Exp Clin Cancer Res 18:93–99
14. Kyzer S, Koren R, Klein B et al (1998) Giant splenomegaly caused by splenic metastases of melanoma. Eur J Surg 24:336–337
15. Colovic MD, Jankovic GM, Golovic RB et al (1998) Non-secretory solitary plasmacytoma of the spleen. Med Oncol 15:286–288
16. Mallipudi BV, Chawdhery MZ, Jeffery PJ (1998) Primary malignant fibrous histiocytoma of spleen. Eur J Surg Oncol 24:448–449
17. Tubiana M (1991) Hodgkin's disease: historical perspective and clinical presentation. In: Bailliere's clinical hematology, vol 9. Balliere Tindall, Philadelphia, pp 503–530
18. Hodgson DC (2008) Hodgkin lymphoma: the follow-up of long-term survivors. Hematol Oncol Clin North Am 22(2):233–244
19. Mauch PM (1996) Management of early stage Hodgkin's disease. In: Bailliere's clinical hematology, vol 9. Balliere Tindall, Philadelphia, 531–541
20. Klimm B, Engert A, Diehl V (2005) First-line treatment of Hodgkin's lymphoma. Curr Hematol Rep 4:15–22
21. Lister TA, Crowther D, Sutcliffe SB et al (1989) Report of a committee convened to discuss the evaluation and staging of patients with Hodgkin's disease. J Clin Oncol 7:1630–1636
22. Sprecht L, Lauritzen AF, Nordentoft AM et al (1990) Tumor cell concentration and tumor cell burden in relation to histopathologic subtype and other prognostic factors in early stage Hodgkin's disease. The Danish National Hodgkin's Study Group. Cancer 65:2594–2601
23. Kasamon YL, Wahl RL (2008) FDG PET and risk-adapted therapy in Hodgkin's and non-Hodgkin's lymphoma. Curr Opin Oncol 20:206–219
24. Bartlett NL (2008) Modern treatment of Hodgkin lymphoma. Curr Opin Hematol 14:408–414
25. Leibenhaut M (1989) Prognostic indicators of laparotomy findings in clinical stage I-II supradiaphragmatic Hodgkin's disease. J Clin Oncol 7:81–91
26. Mauch P, Larson D, Osteen R et al (1990) Prognostic factors for positive staging in patients with Hodkin's disease. J Clin Oncol 8:257–265
27. Jockovick M, Mendenhall NP, Sombeck MD et al (1994) Long-term complications of laparotomy in Hodgkin's disease. Ann Surg 219:615–624
28. Lehne G, Hannisdal E, Langholm R, Nome OA (1994) 10-year experience with splenectomy in patients with malignant non-Hodgkin's lymphoma. Cancer 74:933–939
29. Delpero JR (1990) Splenectomy for hypersplenism in chronic lymphocytic leukemia and malignant non-Hodgkin's lymphoma. Br J Surg 77:443–449
30. Brodsky J, Abcar A, Styler M (1996) Splenectomy for non-Hodgkin's lymphoma. Am J Clin Oncol 19:558–561
31. Konradsen HB (1996) Humoral immune response to pneumococcal vaccination: prevention of infections with Streptococcus pneumonia by immunization. APMIS 60: 1–28
32. Brox A, Bishinski JI, Berry G (1991) Primary non-Hodgkin's lymphoma of the spleen. Am J Hematol 38: 95–100
33. Xiros N, Economopoulos T, Christodoulidis C et al (2000) Splenectomy in patients with malignant non-Hodgin's lymphoma. Eur J Haematol 64:145–150
34. Kercher KW, Matthews BD, Walsh RM et al (2002) Laparoscopic splenectomy for massive splenomegaly. Am J Surg 183:192–196
35. Saven A, Piro LD (1992) Treatment of hairy cell leukemia. Blood 79:111–1120
36. Jansen J, Hermans J (1981) Splenectomy in hairy cell leukemia: a retrospective multice analysis. Cancer 47: 2066–2076
37. Ulrich M, Strehl J, Gorschluter M et al (2003) Advances in the treatment of hairy-cell leukemia. Lancet Oncol 4: 86–94
38. Burch M, Misra M, Phillips EH (2005) Splenic malignancy: a minimally invasive approach. Cancer J 11:36–42
39. Baccarani M (1984) Results of a prospective randomized trial of early splenectomy in chronic myeloid leukemia. The Italian Coopertive Study Group on chronic myeloid leukemia. Cancer 54:333–338
40. Feldman LS, Demyttenaere SV, Polyhronopoulos GN et al (2008) Refining the selection criteria for laparoscopic \ open splenectomy for splenomegaly. J Laparoendosc Adv Surg Tech A 1:13–19
41. Nelson E, Mone M (1999) Splenectomy in high risk patients with splenomegaly. Am J Surg 178:581–586
42. Heniford BT, Park A, Walsh RM et al (2001) Laparoscopic splenectomy in patients with normal-sized spleens versus splenomegaly: does size matter? Am Surg 67:865–867, discussion 857–858
43. Owera A, Hamade Am, Ol B, Ammori BJ (2006) Laparoscopic versus open splenectomy for massive splenomegaly: a comparative study. J Laparoendosc Adv Surg Tech A 16:241–246
44. Grahn SW, Alvarez J, Kirkwood K (2006) Trends in laparoscopic splenecomy for massive splenomegaly. Arch Surg 141:755–762
45. Dominguez EP, Choi EP, Scott YU et al (2007) Impact of morbid obesity on outcome of laparoscopic splenectomy. Surg Endosc 21:422–426
46. Berindoague R, Targarona EM, Balague C et al (2007) Can we predict immediate outcome after laparoscopic splenectomy for splenomegaly? Multivariate analysis of clinical, anatomic, and pathologic features after 3D reconstruction of the spleen. Surg Innov 14:243–251
47. Cobb WS, Heniford BT, Burns JM et al (2005) Cirrhosis is not a contraindication to laparoscopic surgery. Surg Endosc 19:418–423
48. Kercher KW, Carbonell AM, Heniford BT et al (2004) Laparoscopic splenectomy reverses thrombocyto[penia] in patients with hepatitis C cirrhosis and portal hypertension. J Gast Surg 8:120–126
49. Walsh RM, Chand B, Brodsky J, Heniford BT (2003) Determination of intact splenic weight based on morcellated weight. Surg Endosc 17:1266–1268
50. Nicholson IA, Falk GI, Muligan SC (1998) Laparoscopically assisted massive splenectomy: a preliminary report of the technique of early hilar devascularization. Surg Endosc 12:73–75
51. Price VE, Dutta S, Blanchette VS et al (2006) The prevention and treatment of bacterial infections in children with

asplenia or hyposplenia: practice considerations at the hospital for sick children, Toronto. Pediatr Blood Cancer 46: 597–603
52. Winther TN, Kristensen TD, Kaltoft MS, Konradsen HB, Knudsen JD, Hogh B (2009) Invasive pneumococcal disease in Danish children, 1996-2007, prior to the introduction of heptavalent pneumococcal conjugate vaccine. Acta Paediatr 98:328–331
53. Poulin EC, Thibault C (1993) The anatomical basis for laparoscopic splenectomy. Can J Surg 36:484–488
54. Park A, Gagner M, Pomp A (1997) The lateral approach to laparoscopic splenectomy. Am J Surg 173:126–130
55. Dawson AA, Jones PF, King DJ (1987) Splenectomy in the management of hematological disease. Br J Surg 74: 353–357
56. Horowitz J, Smith JL, Weber TK et al (1996) Post-operative complications after splenectomy for hematologic malignancies. Ann Surg 223:290–296
57. Friedman RL, Hiatt JR, Korman JL et al (1997) Laparoscopic or open splenectomy for hematologic disease: which approach is superior? J Am Coll Surg 185:49–54
58. Rosen M, Brody F, Walsh RM et al (2002) Outcome of laparoscopic splenectomy based on hematologic indication. Surg Endosc 16:272–279
59. Balague C, Targarona EM, Cerdan G et al (2004) Long-term outcome after laparoscopic splenectomy related to hematologic diagnosis. Surg Endosc 18:1283–1287
60. Chand B, Walsh RM, Ponsky J, Brody F (2001) Pancreatic complications following laparoscopic splenectomy. Surg Endosc 15:1273–1276
61. Berman RS, Yahanda AM, Mansfield PF et al (1999) Laparoscopic splenectomy in patients with hematologic malignancies. Am J Surg 178:530–536
62. Rosen M, Brody F, Walsh RM, Ponsky J (2002) Hand-assisted laparoscopic splenectomy vs. conventional laparoscopic splenectomy in cases of splenomegaly. Arch Surg 137:1348–1352
63. Wang K, Hu S, Zhang G et al (2007) Hand-assisted laparoscopic splenectomy for splenomegaly: a comparative study with conventional laparoscopic splenectomy. Chin Med J 120:41–45
64. Walsh RM, Heniford BT (1999) Role of laparoscopy for Hodgkin's and non-Hodgkin's lymphoma. Semin Surg Oncol 16:284–292
65. Targarona EM, Balague C, Trias M (2007) Is the laparoscopic approach reasonable in cases of splenomegaly? Sem Laparosc Surg 11:185–190
66. Park A, Targarona EM, Trias M (2001) Laparoscopic surgery of the spleen: state of the art. Langenbecks Arch Surg 386:230–239
67. Torelli P, Cavaliere D, Casaccia M, Panaro F, Grondona P, Rossi E, Santini G, Truini M, Gobbi M, Bacigalupo A, Valente U (2002) Laparoscopic splenectomy for hematological diseases. Surg Endosc 16:965–971

Table 19.1. Instrumentation for hand-assisted laparoscopic radical nephrectomy

Position	Operative side up	Beanbag
Supplies	Pillows × 5	Axillary roll
	Video monitor at head of bed	3″ cloth tape
	Green sheet under beanbag	Blankets and towels
	Ioban™ #6640	Marking pen
	Scope warmer	Hand control Bovie
	Foley kit with urometer	Harmonic scalpel LCS 5 mm
	Skin stapler	4 × 8 sponges
	Suction tubing (for beanbag)	Hand-assisted device
	12-mm trocar × 2	5-mm trocar × 1 (right nephrectomy)
Instruments	10-mm Endo Clip applier	
	Endo-GIA (vascular 2.0-mm staples – 30 and 45 mm length)	
	Endo-GIA reloads (reticulating – 30 and 45 mm)	
	10-mm 30° scope	10-mm 45° scope (available)
	Harmonic scalpel	Light cord
	5-mm laparoscopy set	
Suture	0 Vicryl × 2 (cut needle off; use with Storz suture passer to close ports)	
	#1 PDS CT X 2	
	4-0 Monocryl PS-2 × 2	
Drugs	0.25% Marcaine, plain	
	Surgicel	
	Mannitol (25 g) – anesthesia	

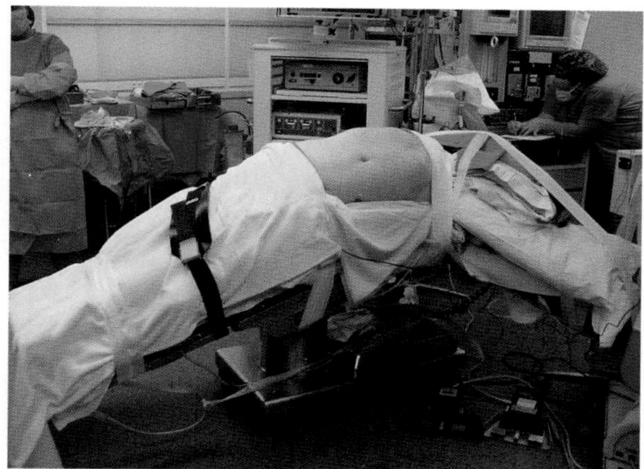

Figure 19.1

Lateral patient positioning for laparoscopic right radical nephrectomy. Note that the operating table is flexed and the patient is well-secured to the table

(instrument) port is placed approximately four fingerbreadths medial and inferior to the left iliac crest along the lateral border of the rectus muscle (Figs. 19.4 and 19.5). The wrist and forearm of the surgeon's intra-abdominal hand is wrapped with an Ioban™ drape to facilitate passage of the hand through the hand-assisted device (Fig. 19.6).

Hand-Assisted Laparoscopic Left Radical Nephrectomy

When pneumoperitoneum has been established, the peritoneal cavity is surveyed for the presence of adhesions and evidence of altered anatomy or metastatic disease. The splenic flexure of the colon is initially mobilized away from the kidney along the avascular plane between the colon mesentery and the Gerota's fascia. The left colon is mobilized from lateral to medial along the white line of Toldt. This same plane of dissection is carried cephalad, allowing for medial visceral rotation of the colon, spleen, and the tail of

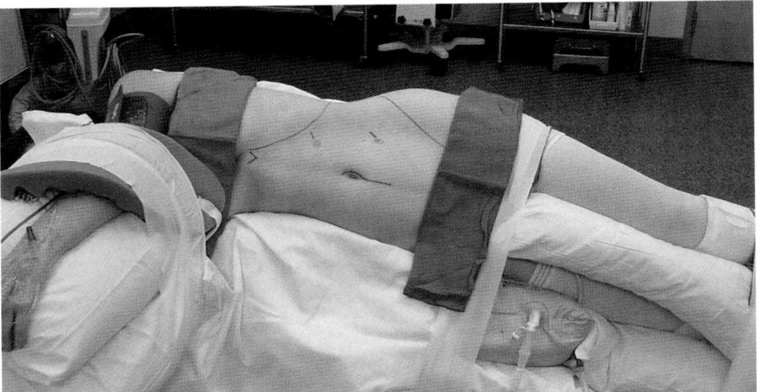

Figure 19.2

Patient position for laparoscopic left nephrectomy. All extremities are secured and padded

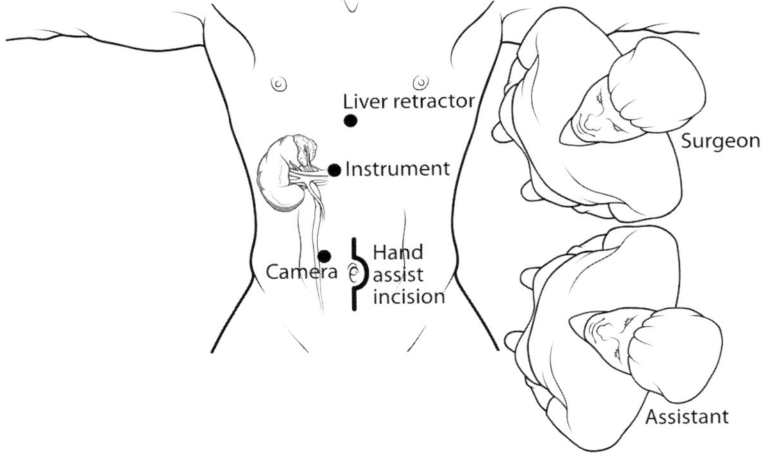

Figure 19.3

Port placement and surgeon/ assistant position for hand-assisted laparoscopic right nephrectomy (printed with permission of Carolinas HealthCare System)

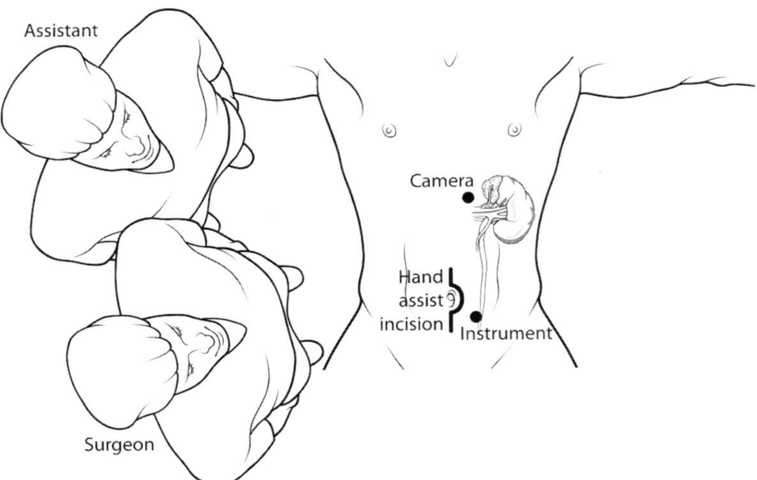

Figure 19.4

Port placement and surgeon/ assistant position for hand-assisted laparoscopic left radical nephrectomy (printed with permission of Carolinas HealthCare System)

the pancreas up to the level of the diaphragm. During this portion of the dissection, care must be taken to avoid injury to the gastric fundus as the stomach lies very close to the superior pole of the spleen. Similarly, the splenic vessels course along the lateral aspect of the pancreas; caution should be exercised during mobilization of the pancreatic tail to avoid hemorrhage from the splenic vessels. With complete division of

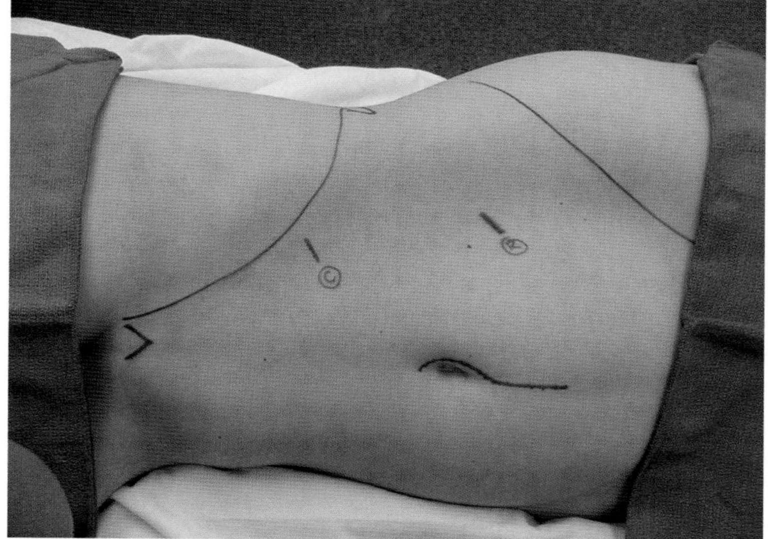

Figure 19.5

Port strategy for HAL left nephrectomy. The surgeon's left hand is inserted through a 7-cm periumbilical hand-assisted incision. The camera (C) and right-hand working port (R) are located lateral to the rectus muscle

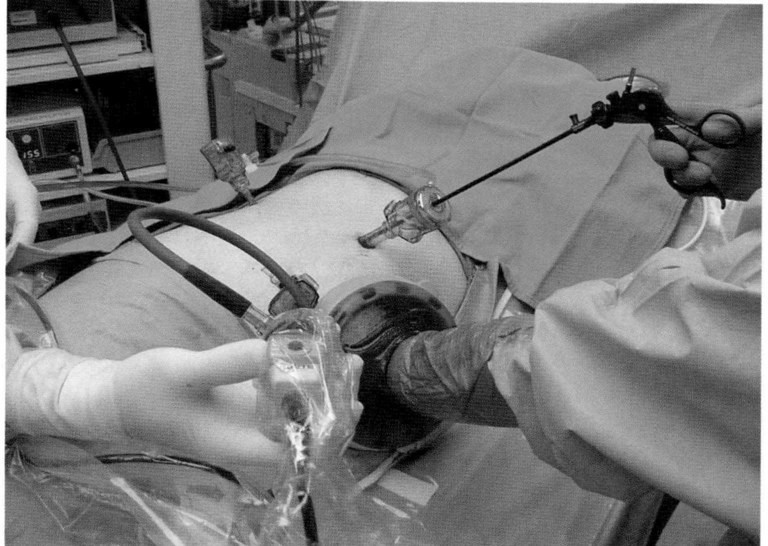

Figure 19.6

The surgeon's wrist is wrapped with an Ioban drape to facilitate passage of the nondominant hand through the hand-assisted device

the splenorenal attachments, gravity facilitates medial rotation of the adjacent viscera. No additional retraction of these structures is required.

Using hook electrocautery, Gerota's fascia is opened approximately 4–5 cm caudal to the lower pole of the kidney. Initially, this is done by opening Gerota's in a longitudinal fashion along the lateral border of the aorta (which is palpable using the intraperitoneal hand) and just medial and inferior to the gonadal vein. The gonadal vein and ureter are then identified and elevated up away from the psoas muscle along the avascular plane located superficial to the psoas fascia. The gonadal vein and ureter can be divided at this point using a 45-mm endovascular GIA stapler (2.0-mm vascular load). Division of these two structures facilitates subsequent medial rotation of the kidney and exposure of the renal hilum.

Starting at the lower pole, the posterior (retroperitoneal) renal attachments are divided with electrocautery or harmonic scalpel. Dissection is carried up to the diaphragm, allowing for complete lateral to medial mobilization of the upper pole of the kidney, including the upper pole fat and left adrenal gland. All perinephric fat is left on the kidney, allowing for resection of the tumor, the kidney, and the associated adipose tissue as a single en bloc specimen. With the kidney rotated medially, the lumbar vein(s) and the renal artery can be identified. If early division of the renal artery can be achieved safely, it is divided at this point with an endo-GIA vascular stapler.

Attention is turned to the medial aspect of the left kidney. The kidney is rotated laterally, allowing for Gerota's fascia to be opened along the medial, inferior edge of the gonadal vein. The gonadal vein can then be followed cephalad along its course into the left renal vein. The renal vein and adrenal vein are identified. The adrenal vein is dissected circumferentially, controlled proximally and distally with clips, and divided. By providing for additional renal vein mobility and length, we believe that division of the adrenal vein greatly facilitates subsequent division of the renal vein (regardless of whether or not adrenalectomy is planned).

Due to the theoretical risk of arterial–venous fistula, an attempt is made to separate the renal artery and vein to allow for stapling of the vessels with separate staple loads. If isolation of the vessels cannot be achieved easily and safely, then the hilum can be divided en masse with a single firing of the stapler. Ideally, this stapler application is done in such a manner that the vessels are divided "serially" (one followed by the other) as the vascular staple line is formed. In theory, we believe that this may minimize the potential for fistula formation. In most cases, the artery originates from the aorta cephalad to the renal vein and the two can be divided serially with one firing of the GIA 45-mm stapler. This maneuver is facilitated by elevation of the kidney using the intra-abdominal hand. The stapler is brought in through the left lower quadrant port and the hilar pedicle divided just lateral to the aorta.

For adrenal-sparing nephrectomy, a plane of dissection is developed between the medial aspect of the adrenal gland and the upper pole of the kidney. Attachments between the two organs are divided with the harmonic scalpel. If the adrenal is to be taken along with the kidney, the renal vessels are first divided using an endovascular GIA stapler. The plane between the aorta and the adrenal gland is then dissected and divided with a combination of clips and harmonic scalpel. Occasionally, a vascular stapler is used to divide the medial attachments between the adrenal gland and the retroperitoneum, as multiple small arteries often supply the adrenal gland and originate directly from the aorta. Once the remaining attachments to the diaphragm are divided, the kidney is extracted through the hand-assisted device. The hand-assisted incision is closed with slowly absorbable suture, and the port sites are closed with a suture passer.

Hand-Assisted Laparoscopic Right Radical Nephrectomy

For HAL right radical nephrectomy, the dissection begins with mobilization of the hepatic flexure and right colon away from the lower pole of the kidney. The duodenum can then be mobilized medially to allow for clear visualization of the vena cava and right renal vein. Starting 3–4 cm caudad to the lower pole of the right kidney, Gerota's fascia is opened in a longitudinal fashion just lateral to the IVC. This maneuver allows for identification of the right gonadal vein and ureter. Both structures are elevated up away from the psoas muscle and divided with a vascular stapler. The posterior renal attachments are then divided as described on the left.

With the kidney elevated and retracted laterally, Gerota's fascia is opened medially along the lateral border of the IVC. Care is taken to identify and protect the right renal vein. This plane of dissection is carried cephalad in a longitudinal fashion adjacent to the lateral aspect of the liver, up to the interface of the liver with the right hemi-diaphragm. After Gerota's fascia is opened, the right lobe of the liver can be retracted medially without difficulty. With the kidney elevated by the surgeon's left hand, the renal hilum can be dissected and the vessels divided, either individually or en masse. For right nephrectomy, the division of the short right renal vein and artery occasionally requires that the utilization of the camera/instrument ports be reversed during transection of the renal hilum. For this portion of the procedure, the camera is brought in through the superior port and the articulating linear vascular stapler (2.0 mm/gray load endo-GIA) is brought in through the inferior port, allowing for improved trajectory of the stapler (in parallel with the vena cava) during division of the renal vessels. The right adrenal gland is generally spared, except in cases of large (T2) tumors, upper pole lesions immediately adjacent to the adrenal gland, or in patients with preoperative adrenal abnormalities on CT scan. Removal of the right adrenal gland can be challenging, as dissection and division of the short right adrenal vein is potentially hazardous. Right adrenalectomy requires complete mobilization of the right lobe of the liver and definitive delineation of the vena cava. Great care must be taken during right adrenalectomy to avoid injury to the vena cava or avulsion of the right adrenal

overlying adipose tissue. Hook electrocautery is then used to circumscribe the tumor along the intended line of resection by scoring the renal capsule circumferentially with a 5-mm margin around the tumor. If needed, intraoperative ultrasound can be used to evaluate the depth of penetration of endophytic tumors [41]. We use a laparoscopic vascular bulldog clamp (Aesculap, Inc., Tuttlingen, Germany) to occlude the renal artery prior to tumor resection. Prior to clamp application, mannitol and sodium bicarbonate are administered intravenously to increase urine output and to limit ischemic damage to renal tubules [42]. Sharp tumor resection (without cautery) is performed using laparoscopic scissors, to allow for clear visualization of normal parenchyma during excision and to avoid cautery artifact at the resection margin.

Following resection, the specimen is extracted through the hand-assisted incision and immediately evaluated by an in-room pathologist for gross assessment of margins. If the margin is positive grossly, a deeper margin is excised prior to repair of the renal defect. Hemostasis is achieved with a combination of suture ligation, cautery, and application of topical hemostatic agents. For lesions that appear to penetrate the collecting system on CT scan, a ureteral catheter is placed preoperatively. Prior to tumor resection, methylene blue is injected into the catheter. Obvious defects in the collecting system are closed with absorbable 3-0 Vicryl suture. The renal defect is then closed over Surgicel bolsters (Ethicon, Inc, Somerville, NJ) and a flowable gelatin mixed with thrombin, using absorbable 2-0 Vicryl sutures placed through the adjacent renal capsule. A fibrin sealant is applied to the repair prior to removal of the vascular clamp.

Outcomes for Hand-assisted Partial Nephrectomy

Our group has analyzed its experience using the above technique and compared the results with a contemporary group of patients undergoing open partial nephrectomy. The data for our first 70 HALPNs (versus 40 open partial nephrectomies) are described. For each group, mean tumor size was equivalent at 2.6 cm (range 1–4 cm), while HALPN was associated with shorter operative times, blood loss, and warm ischemia times compared with open partial nephrectomy (OPN) (Table 19.3).

Table 19.3. Intraoperative data

Variable	HALPN ($n = 70$)	OPN ($n = 40$)	p value
Mean operative time (min)	161	191	0.027
Mean warm ischemia time (min)	27.0	33.1	0.035
Mean blood loss (ml)	120	353	0.0003

HALPN: hand-assisted laparoscopic partial nephrectomy, OPN = open partial nephrectomy.

In four HALPN cases (5.7%), an intraoperative positive margin determination was made on gross inspection by the in-room pathologist, and a deeper re-excision into the renal tumor bed was made. As a result, the final positive margin rate for the HALPN series was 0% compared with 5% for OPN. An essential aspect of our HALPN methodology is the presence of a pathologist in the operating room at the time of tumor excision. The in-room pathologist, not the surgeon, assesses the gross tumor margins immediately after renal tumor excision, which minimizes warm ischemia time as the pathologist examines the tumor immediately, rather than waiting for a frozen section. This compares favorably with other HALPN series which report 0–1% final positive margins [35] and pure laparoscopic partial nephrectomy studies with slightly higher rates of 2–3% [43].

Using the technique described, major complications have been rare (Table 19.4). We experienced one acute postoperative bleed (into the collection system/ureter) in the HALPN cohort and one delayed bleed in the OPN group. Both were managed conservatively without transfusion or reoperation. Urine leaks occurred in four patients managed by HALPN (5.7%) and two by OPN (5%). In two cases, we converted from planned partial nephrectomy to hand-assisted laparoscopic radical nephrectomy due to alterations in anatomy in one patient with a prior gunshot wound to the kidney and in one case of hilar vascular encasement by tumor. No conversions from HALPN to an open technique have been required. Patients undergoing HALPN have had an average length of stay of 4.9 days compared with 6.9 days for those undergoing OPN ($p = 0.007$).

Table 19.4. Perioperative outcomes

Variable	HALPN ($n = 70$)	OPN ($n = 40$)	p value
Major complications (%)	7.1	7.5	0.1
Postoperative bleed	1 (1.4%)	1 (2.5%)	
Urine leak	4 (5.7%)	2 (5.0%)	
Conversions (n)			
To HAL radical nephrectomy	2	n/a	
To open	0	n/a	
Length of hospital stay (days)	4.9	6.9	0.007
Tumor recurrence (n)	1	1	

We have experienced one renal tumor recurrence in each group. Both occurred in patients with T3 lesions at the time of initial resection. One was subsequently treated with percutaneous cryoablation in a patient with known metastatic disease. The second was treated with hand-assisted laparoscopic radical nephrectomy. The HALPN tumor recurrence was recognized 2 years postoperatively, and the patient is alive without evidence of disease following radical nephrectomy. The OPN recurrence was identified 2.5 years postoperatively; the patient died from cardiac disease with nonprogressive metastatic renal cell carcinoma 3 years post open partial nephrectomy.

Conclusion

Laparoscopic radical nephrectomy provides the distinct perioperative advantages of minimally invasive surgery when compared with the traditional open approach. More importantly, intermediate and long-term data confirm that the technique offers equivalent oncologic outcomes for renal cell carcinoma. Early data regarding the applicability of the laparoscopic approach to locally advanced disease as well as cytoreductive nephrectomy for metastatic patients is encouraging, but long-term outcomes will need to be evaluated. For favorably located lesions measuring <4 cm, laparoscopic partial nephrectomy is safe and effective, though technically challenging. While varying laparoscopic operative approaches have been advocated, all are effective and all maintain the benefits of minimally invasive surgery while providing long-term outcomes which are comparable to the traditional open approach. Ultimately, the individual surgeon should use the approach with which he/she has the most comfort and experience.

Acknowledgments The authors offer special thanks to Mrs. Cissy Swartz for her editorial assistance with this chapter.

References

1. Greene FL, Kercher KW, Nelson H, Teigland CM, Boller AM (2007) Minimal access cancer management. CA Cancer J Clin 57:130–146
2. Dunn MD, Portis AJ, Shalhav AL et al (2000) Laparoscopic versus open radical nephrectomy: a 9-year experience. J Urol 164:1153–1159
3. Flowers JL, Jacobs S, Cho E et al (1997) Comparison of open and laparoscopic live donor nephrectomy. Ann Surg 226:483–489, discussion 489–490
4. Jacobs JK, Goldstein RE, Geer RJ (1997) Laparoscopic adrenalectomy. A new standard of care. Ann Surg 225: 495–501, discussion 501–502
5. Park A, Marcaccio M, Sternbach M, Witzke D, Fitzgerald P (1999) Laparoscopic vs. open splenectomy. Arch Surg 134:1263–1269
6. Cadeddu JA, Ono Y, Clayman RV et al (1998) Laparoscopic nephrectomy for renal cell cancer: evaluation of efficacy and safety: a multicenter experience. Urology 52:773–777
7. Kercher KW, Heniford BT, Matthews BD et al (2003) Laparoscopic versus open nephrectomy in 210 consecutive patients: outcomes, cost, and changes in practice patterns. Surg Endosc 17:1889–1895
8. Robson CJ, Churchill BM, Anderson W (1969) The results of radical nephrectomy for renal cell carcinoma. J Urol 101:297–301
9. Colombo JR Jr, Haber GP, Jelovsek JE, Lane B, Novick AC, Gill IS (2008) Seven years after laparoscopic radical nephrectomy: oncologic and renal functional outcomes. Urology 71:1149–1154
10. Bandi G, Christian MW, Hedican SP, Moon TD, Nakada SY (2008) Oncological outcomes of hand-assisted laparoscopic radical nephrectomy for clinically localized renal cell carcinoma: a single-institution study with >or=3 years of follow-up. BJU Int 101:459–462
11. Henderson A, Murphy D, Jaganathan K, Roberts WW, Wolf JS Jr, Rane A (2008) Hand-assisted laparoscopic nephrectomy for renal cell cancer with renal vein tumor thrombus. Urology 72:268–272
12. Catalano C, Fraioli F, Laghi A et al (2003) High-resolution multidetector CT in the preoperative evaluation of patients with renal cell carcinoma. AJR Am J Roentgenol 180: 1271–1277
13. Sadler GJ, Anderson MR, Moss MS, Wilson PG (2007) Metastases from renal cell carcinoma presenting as gastrointestinal bleeding: two case reports and a review of the literature. BMC Gastroenterol 7:4
14. Toprak U, Erdogan A, Gulbay M, Karademir MA, Pasaoglu E, Akar OE (2005) Preoperative evaluation of renal anatomy

and renal masses with helical CT, 3D-CT and 3D-CT angiography. Diagn Interv Radiol 11:35–40
15. Spahn M, Portillo FJ, Michel MS et al (2001) Color Duplex sonography vs. computed tomography: accuracy in the preoperative evaluation of renal cell carcinoma. Eur Urol 40:337–342
16. Choyke PL, Walther MM, Wagner JR, Rayford W, Lyne JC, Linehan WM (1997) Renal cancer: preoperative evaluation with dual-phase three-dimensional MR angiography. Radiology 205:767–771
17. Beer AJ, Dobritz M, Zantl N, Weirich G, Stollfuss J, Rummeny EJ (2006) Comparison of 16-MDCT and MRI for characterization of kidney lesions. AJR Am J Roentgenol 186:1639–1650
18. Heary RF, Bono CM (2001) Metastatic spinal tumors. Neurosurg Focus 11:e1
19. Nelson CP, Wolf JS Jr (2002) Comparison of hand assisted versus standard laparoscopic radical nephrectomy for suspected renal cell carcinoma. J Urol 167:1989–1994
20. Gill IS, Schweizer D, Hobart MG, Sung GT, Klein EA, Novick AC (2000) Retroperitoneal laparoscopic radical nephrectomy: the Cleveland clinic experience. J Urol 163:1665–1670
21. Ono Y, Kinukawa T, Hattori R et al (1999) Laparoscopic radical nephrectomy for renal cell carcinoma: a five-year experience. Urology 53:280–286
22. Permpongkosol S, Chan DY, Link RE et al (2005) Long-term survival analysis after laparoscopic radical nephrectomy. J Urol 174:1222–1225
23. Rassweiler J, Tsivian A, Kumar AV et al (2003) Oncological safety of laparoscopic surgery for urological malignancy: experience with more than 1,000 operations. J Urol 169:2072–2075
24. Tanaka K, Hara I, Takenaka A, Kawabata G, Fujisawa M (2008) Incidence of local and port site recurrence of urologic cancer after laparoscopic surgery. Urology 71:728–734
25. Glazer AA, Novick AC (1996) Long-term followup after surgical treatment for renal cell carcinoma extending into the right atrium. J Urol 155:448–450
26. Desai MM, Gill IS, Ramani AP, Matin SF, Kaouk JH, Campero JM (2003) Laparoscopic radical nephrectomy for cancer with level I renal vein involvement. J Urol 169: 487–491
27. Walther MM, Lyne JC, Libutti SK, Linehan WM (1999) Laparoscopic cytoreductive nephrectomy as preparation for administration of systemic interleukin-2 in the treatment of metastatic renal cell carcinoma: a pilot study. Urology 53:496–501
28. Jordan GH, Winslow BH (1993) Laparoendoscopic upper pole partial nephrectomy with ureterectomy. J Urol 150:940–943
29. Permpongkosol S, Bagga HS, Romero FR, Sroka M, Jarrett TW, Kavoussi LR (2006) Laparoscopic versus open partial nephrectomy for the treatment of pathological T1N0M0 renal cell carcinoma: a 5-year survival rate. J Urol 176: 1984–1988, discussion 1988–1989
30. Porpiglia F, Volpe A, Billia M, Scarpa RM (2008) Laparoscopic versus open partial nephrectomy: analysis of the current literature. Eur Urol 53:732–742, discussion 742–743
31. Bhayani SB (2008) Laparoscopic partial nephrectomy: fifty cases. J Endourol 22:313–316
32. Allaf ME, Bhayani SB, Rogers C et al (2004) Laparoscopic partial nephrectomy: evaluation of long-term oncological outcome. J Urol 172:871–873
33. Wolf JS Jr, Seifman BD, Montie JE (2000) Nephron sparing surgery for suspected malignancy: open surgery compared to laparoscopy with selective use of hand assistance. J Urol 163:1659–1664
34. Stifelman MD, Sosa RE, Nakada SY, Shichman SJ (2001) Hand-assisted laparoscopic partial nephrectomy. J Endourol 15:161–164
35. Strup S, Garrett J, Gomella L, Rowland R (2005) Laparoscopic partial nephrectomy: hand-assisted technique. J Endourol 19:456–459, discussion 459–460
36. McClean JM, Kercher KW, Mah NA et al (2008) Strategies in the management of renal tumors amenable to partial nephrectomy. Surg Endosc 23(9):2161–2166, Epub ahead of print
37. van Ophoven A, Tsui KH, Shvarts O, Laifer-Narin S, Belldegrun AS (1999) Current status of partial nephrectomy in the management of kidney cancer. Cancer Control 6:560–570
38. Patard JJ, Shvarts O, Lam JS et al (2004) Safety and efficacy of partial nephrectomy for all T1 tumors based on an international multicenter experience. J Urol 171: 2181–2185
39. Hafez KS, Fergany AF, Novick AC (1999) Nephron sparing surgery for localized renal cell carcinoma: impact of tumor size on patient survival, tumor recurrence and TNM staging. J Urol 162:1930–1933
40. Uzzo RG, Novick AC (2001) Nephron sparing surgery for renal tumors: indications, techniques and outcomes. J Urol 166:6–18
41. Fazio LM, Downey D, Nguan CY et al (2006) Intraoperative laparoscopic renal ultrasonography: use in advanced laparoscopic renal surgery. Urology 68: 723–727
42. Merten GJ, Burgess WP, Rittase RA, Kennedy TP (2004) Prevention of contrast-induced nephropathy with sodium bicarbonate: an evidence-based protocol. Crit Pathw Cardiol 3:138–143
43. Breda A, Stepanian SV, Liao J et al (2007) Positive margins in laparoscopic partial nephrectomy in 855 cases: a multi-institutional survey from the United States and Europe. J Urol 178:47–50

Laparoscopic Adrenalectomy for Metastatic Cancer

Kent W. Kercher

Contents

Introduction

During the past decade, laparoscopic adrenalectomy has become the standard surgical approach for most adrenal tumors. When compared with the traditional open approach, laparoscopic solid organ surgery has been associated with substantial reductions in perioperative morbidity, length of stay, and convalescence [1–4]. As experience with minimally invasive surgical techniques has evolved, more aggressive approaches have lead to laparoscopic resection of larger tumors, bilateral pathology, and metastatic disease. Functional adrenal lesions including pheochromocytoma, laparoscopic adrenalectomy have been shown to be safe and effective, with significant advantages over the traditional open approach. However, laparoscopic management of malignant adrenal tumors remains somewhat controversial. This chapter reviews the current status of laparoscopic adrenalectomy for metastatic disease and focuses on the technical aspect of the operation.

Adrenalectomy for Metastatic Disease: Literature Review and Oncologic Outcomes

Although the adrenal glands represent relatively common sites of metastatic disease for a number of primary cancers, isolated (and potentially curable) metastasis to the adrenal is rare. In most cases, the finding of an adrenal metastasis is a manifestation of a more systemic process and does not lend itself to surgical resection for cure or even long-term disease control. Yet, there is growing evidence that resection of isolated (adrenal only) spread of melanoma, lung, kidney, colon, and breast cancer may improve survival in select patients. In series of open adrenalectomy for metastatic lesions, median survival rates of up to 30 months have been reported, compared with

F.L. Greene, B.T. Heniford (eds.), *Minimally Invasive Cancer Management*,
DOI 10.1007/978-1-4419-1238-1_20,

historical survival ranges of 6–8 months without resection [5]. The Memorial Sloan–Kettering experience supports adrenalectomy for metastases in patients with isolated disease in which complete resection is feasible, particularly in patients with disease-free intervals of greater than 6 months [6].

Metastases of renal cell carcinoma (RCC) to the ipsilateral adrenal gland accounts for 10–15% of metastatic disease in RCC [7]. Metastasis to the contralateral adrenal gland is a relatively uncommon phenomenon, representing only a small fraction of RCC metastases. Yet, adrenalectomy for metastases from RCC has been associated with some of the most favorable results [8]. In an early review of the literature by Heniford, 35 patients with contralateral adrenal metastasis underwent curative resection. Over an average follow-up period of 26 months, 62% of patients had no evidence of residual or recurrent RCC [9].

More recent literature has similarly suggested that, with aggressive surgical management of contralateral adrenal metastasis, patients may enjoy a survival benefit. Ito et al. reviewed 256 patients with RCC who had undergone radical nephrectomy with ipsilateral adrenalectomy and evaluated these patients for ipsilateral and contralateral adrenal metastases [10]. Of these, 4.5 % had ipsilateral adrenal metastases from RCC and 1.5 % had contralateral adrenal metastases. Lau et al. retrospectively reviewed 11 patients who had surgery for metastatic RCC to the contralateral adrenal gland treated with adrenalectomy (two with synchronous and nine with metachronous metastases) [11]. Seven patients died from RCC at a mean of 3.9 years after adrenalectomy; one died from other causes at 3.4 years, one from an unknown cause at 1.7 years, and two were still alive at the last follow-up. This short case series describing synchronous metastases suggests that resection of RCC adrenal metastases may prolong survival.

Our group has had a similarly favorable experience with the management of renal cell metastases to the adrenal [12]. Over the past 8 years, we have performed 300 laparoscopic radical nephrectomies for RCC. Nine percent presented with metastatic disease, either to the lungs, bone, or adrenal gland(s). Of these patients, six patients were diagnosed with isolated (solitary) contralateral adrenal metastases: four synchronous and two metachronous (ranging from 30 months to 26 years postradical nephrectomy). Mean adrenal tumor size was 10.4 cm (range 4–19 cm). Five have undergone contralateral adrenalectomy (one purely laparoscopic, two hand-assisted laparoscopic, two open). There were no major perioperative complications. One patient was deemed radiographically unresectable and succumbed to his disease within 3 months. Of patients undergoing adrenalectomy, four are disease free at an average of 3 years (range 18 months to 5 years) postadrenalectomy. One patient who developed boney and pulmonary metastases has experienced stabilization of metastatic disease with interleukin-2 therapy and is alive 3 years after laparoscopic contralateral adrenalectomy for an 11 cm locally expansive adrenal implant. Based on this limited experience, our belief is that although adrenal metastasis from RCC often portends a poor prognosis, aggressive surgical management may yield a significant survival benefit in select patients. Our experience would also suggest that laparoscopic resection can be performed with relatively low rates of morbidity.

Long-term disease-free survival after resection of isolated adrenal metastases from non-small cell lung cancer has also been reported. In Luketich's retrospective series of 14 patients, chemotherapy followed by surgical resection was superior to chemotherapy alone in select patients [13]. All patients subject to medical management alone were dead by 21 months. In the surgically resected group, the 3-year actuarial survival was 38%. Other authors have reported similarly favorable outcomes, with 5-year survival rates of 25–40% in selected patients undergoing adrenal metastasectomy for lung cancer. Disease-free survival rates have ranged from 42 to 91% over a mean follow-up interval of 8–26 months [14–16]. Regardless of tumor pathology or origin, all authors point to careful patient selection for successful outcomes. These include complete control of the primary tumor, a metastatic survey which confirms isolated adrenal disease, and complete surgical resection of the involved adrenal.

Several factors support the minimally invasive resection of adrenal metastases. One is the dramatic increase in surgeon experience with advanced laparoscopic techniques over the past decade. With the growth of laparoscopic solid organ surgery, surgeon comfort levels with organ dissection, atraumatic retraction, vascular control, and specimen retrieval in the treatment of both benign and malignant lesions of the kidney, adrenal, spleen, and pancreas have become standard practice. Minimally invasive techniques offer excellent visualization, early vascular control, and the ability to effectively evaluate for peritoneal spread of disease that might preclude resection. These features, along with the general consensus that laparoscopy can be safely applied to cancer, have made the transition from open to laparoscopic adrenal metastasectomy a natural progression.

One feature that provides substantial support for the laparoscopic approach is the recognition that most malignancies metastasize to the medullary portion (center) of the gland rather than to the adrenal cortex. Adrenal metastases rarely penetrate through the capsule of the gland, making laparoscopic surgical resection much less likely to result in tumor fracture, which could potentially predispose to increased rates of local recurrence or intraperitoneal dissemination [14]. To date, the use of laparoscopic adrenalectomy for metastasis has been associated with only three reports of port-site recurrence following resection of isolated disease [17–19]. These included two lung cancers and one case of metastatic melanoma.

Gill and Moinzedah described 31 patients who underwent laparoscopic adrenalectomy for malignancy: 26 with isolated adrenal metastasis, 6 with primary (incidentally discovered) adrenal cortical carcinoma (ACC), and 1 with malignant pheochromocytoma [15]. In this series, the overall local recurrence rate was 23%, including 5 of 26 (19%) patients with adrenal metastases and 2 of 6 (33%) with ACC. There were no port-site recurrences in any patient and there were no positive margins in patients with adrenal metastasis. One patient with metastatic RCC developed carcinomatosis. The remainder of patients with local recurrence also recurred at other (systemic) sites. Notably, patients with local recurrence had a shorter 3-year survival than those without local recurrence (17% vs. 66%, $p = 0.016$). Overall 5-year actuarial survival was 40% at a median follow-up of 26 months. These data compare favorably with a similar series of 37 patients who underwent open resection of adrenal metastases with a 5-year actuarial survival of 24% and a median survival of 21 months [6]. Other authors have published similar results in small series of patients, with no differences in the incidence of positive resection margins or survival compared with similar groups undergoing open resection of adrenal metastases and no reports of port-site recurrences [16, 20].

Preoperative Evaluation

While incidental adrenal lesions (nonfunctional adrenal adenomas) are quite common (occurring in 5–7% of the adult population), any patient presenting with a newly diagnosed adrenal nodule should undergo a biochemical evaluation to rule out a functional adrenal lesion. This evaluation consists of serum and urine studies to rule out hyperaldosteronism, Cushing's syndrome, and pheochromocytoma. Biochemical evaluation includes serum electrolytes, aldosterone, renin, cortisol, and metanephrines. Twenty-four-hour urine levels for cortisol and metanephrines are also obtained in the majority of cases. Planned removal of functional lesions requires preoperative medical preparation, which may include alpha/beta-blockade and consultation with an endocrinologist, particularly in patients with Cushing's syndrome.

In patients with suspected metastasis to the adrenal gland(s), functional studies can be expected to be normal, although our routine is to obtain a baseline biochemical evaluation as describe above. Radiographic imaging studies provide the most valuable information in these patients. Direct assessment of the adrenal glands and adjacent organs is most effectively obtained through a dedicated intravenous contrast CT scan through the adrenal glands. In addition to assessing the size and extent of adrenal disease, a complete metastatic survey is critical to rule out spread of disease to other organs. Depending on the nature of the primary tumor, PET/CT of the chest, abdomen, and pelvis is generally the most comprehensive method of assessing for other distant spread of disease and may be combined with bone scan. Brain CT or MRI is also recommended. For indeterminate lesions either in the adrenal or in other locations, percutaneous biopsy may be helpful in establishing the diagnosis, particularly if this information would change the management plan.

Given the potential for rapid interval development of additional sites of metastatic spread in some patients, it is most advantageous to update the metastatic survey in close proximity to planned adrenal metastasectomy. The finding of other lesions outside of the adrenal gland would preclude curative resection of an adrenal metastasis. Of course, any decision to proceed with surgery should be coordinated with the patient's medical oncologist and a strategy for postoperative monitoring and/or adjuvant therapy devised. Patients should be strongly cautioned that adrenalectomy for metastatic disease may not be curative and that careful monitoring for the metachronous development of additional disease will be required.

Operative Technique

Laparoscopic Trans-abdominal Left Adrenalectomy

Patient Position, Port Strategy, and Establishment of Pneumoperitoneum

Following the induction of general endotracheal anesthesia, a Foley catheter and orogastric tube are placed. Sequential compression devices are placed on both lower extremities. A single preoperative intravenous dose of a first-generation cephalosporin is given. The patient is placed in the lateral decubitus position on a bean bag, with the left side up. The umbilicus is positioned just below the break in the table. An axillary roll is inserted. Prior to applying suction to the bean bag, the table is flexed. This maneuver increases the distance between the costal margin and the iliac crest, providing adequate working space for the laparoscopic ports (Fig. 20.1). All extremities are secured and padded with multiple pillows and ulnar pads, and a warming blanket is positioned over the upper body. The abdomen and left flank are prepped and draped widely to include the left chest and the midline from the xiphoid to the pubis anteriorly and to the vertebral column posteriorly.

The port strategy for left adrenalectomy is illustrated in Figs. 20.2 and 20.3. A minimum of three subcostal ports (two 12-mm and one 5-mm) are required. The center port (12-mm) is used for the laparoscope (camera), with a 5-mm working port for the left hand and a 12-mm port for the surgeon's right hand. Ports are centered on the costal margin and spaced 5–6 cm apart. The camera port is placed first at the mid-point between the xiphoid process and the tip of the 11th rib. A fourth (5-mm) port can be added in the flank (just medial to the tip of the 11th rib) for retraction of larger tumors. A 10-mm 30° laparoscope is used for all cases. A 10-mm clip applier and/or endo-vascular GIA stapler can be inserted through the right-hand (12-mm) working port for control and division of the left adrenal vein.

Access to the abdomen for establishment of pneumoperitoneum is most efficiently and safely carried out with either an open "cutdown" approach or through the use of an optical port following pre-insufflation with a Veress needle. For the open approach, a muscle-splitting technique is used and each layer of fascia and the peritoneum are opened under direct vision. A blunt 5-mm port is inserted, pneumoperitoneum established, and then exchanged for a 12-mm port. Accessory ports are placed under direct laparoscopic vision. In patients without prior left upper quadrant surgery, the Veress needle can be used selectively for initial insufflation of the abdomen. An optical trocar is then inserted (with the aid of a 10-mm 0-degree laparoscope), allowing for visualization of the layers of the abdominal wall as the port enters the peritoneal cavity.

Operative Steps

Survey of the abdominal cavity is performed to assess for adhesions, alterations in anatomy, or evidence of peritoneal spread of disease. The left adrenal lies along the superior medial aspect of the left kidney, within the confines of Gerota's fascia. The left adrenal gland is

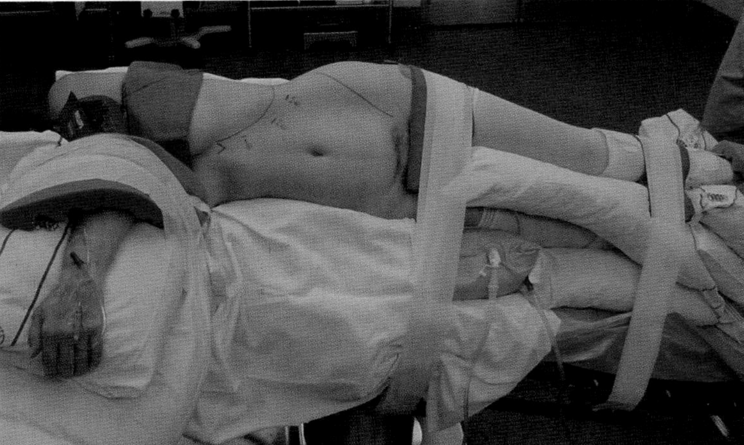

Figure 20.1

Lateral patient positioning for laparoscopic left adrenalectomy. Table is flexed and all extremities are padded and secured

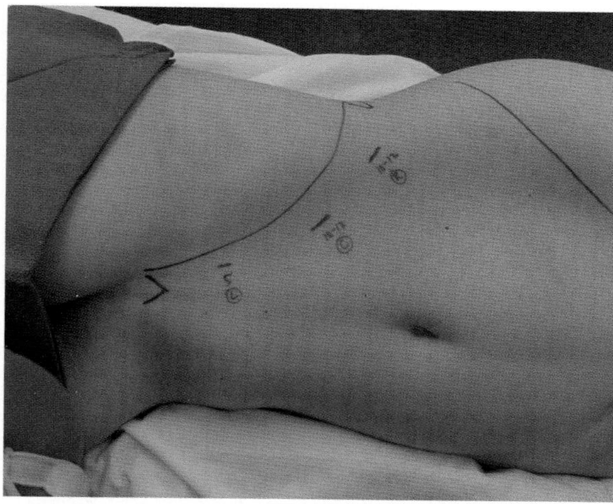

Figure 20.2

Port locations for laparoscopic left adrenalectomy. Left (L)-hand working port (5-mm), camera (C) 12-mm port, and right (R)-hand working port (12-mm) are inserted along the costal margin

situated deep in the retroperitoneum, posterior to the splenic flexure of the colon, and lateral to the tail of the pancreas and the spleen (Fig. 20.4). Mobilization of adjacent structures is therefore required to access the adrenal gland. The splenic flexure of the colon and the spleen is mobilized first. Once the native attachments between the flexure and the anterior abdominal wall are taken down, a plane of dissection is developed between the colonic mesentery and Gerota's fascia. Identification of this relatively avascular plane allows for medial visceral rotation of the colon, the spleen, and the tail of the pancreas. This plane is followed cephalad to the level of the diaphragm, allowing for the spleen and tail of the pancreas to be rotated medially away from the left kidney and left adrenal gland. While mobilizing the spleen, care must be taken to recognize that the greater curvature of the stomach, the tail of the pancreas, and the splenic vessels lie in very close proximity to the plane of dissection. Care must be taken to avoid injury to these structures. Following complete division of the splenorenal attachments, gravity facilitates medial rotation of the adjacent viscera. No additional retraction of the adjacent organs should be required.

In thin patients, the adrenal gland, kidney, and associated venous anatomy can be seen relatively well prior to opening Gerota's fascia. Frequently, the renal vein and adrenal vein can be visualized as well. In heavier patients who have large amounts of perinephric adipose tissue, identification of the adrenal gland and the adjacent vascular structures can be more difficult and may be facilitated by the use of laparoscopic ultrasound. However, in these cases, we have generally found it more helpful to open Gerota's fascia to identify the left renal vein, which is usually quite large and prominent. The left adrenal vein confluence with the renal vein can then be found along the superior border of the renal vein, and the adrenal vein is traced cephalad to the gland. Access to the adrenal gland is initially obtained by opening Gerota's fascia along the inferomedial aspect of the gland, between the renal vein and the adrenal gland. The adrenal vein runs in a caudal to cranial direction, perpendicular to the renal vein. In order to perform the operation safely, a clear understanding of the venous anatomy of the adrenal gland is critical. In almost all cases, the left adrenal gland is drained by a single vein that joins with the inferior phrenic vein prior to draining into

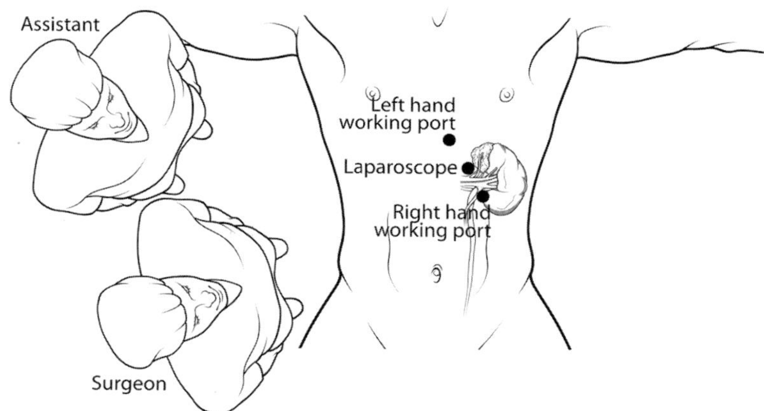

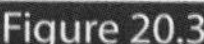
Figure 20.3

Port strategy and surgeon/assistant positions for laparoscopic left adrenalectomy (printed with permission of Carolinas HealthCare System)

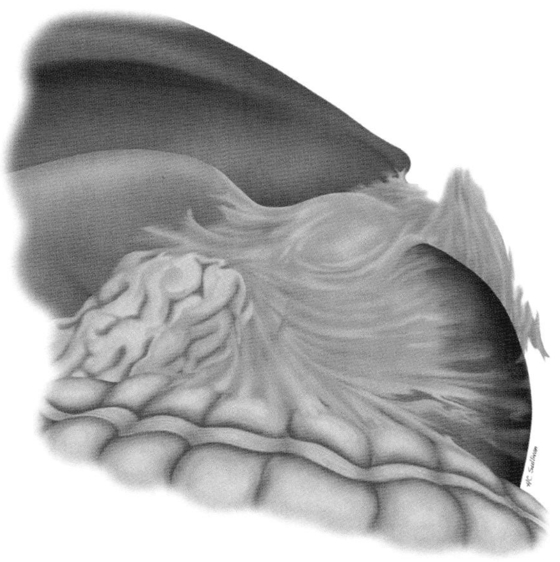

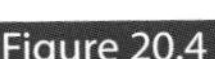

Figure 20.4

Left retroperitoneal anatomy prior to mobilization of the splenic flexure and division of splenorenal attachments (printed with permission of Carolinas HealthCare System)

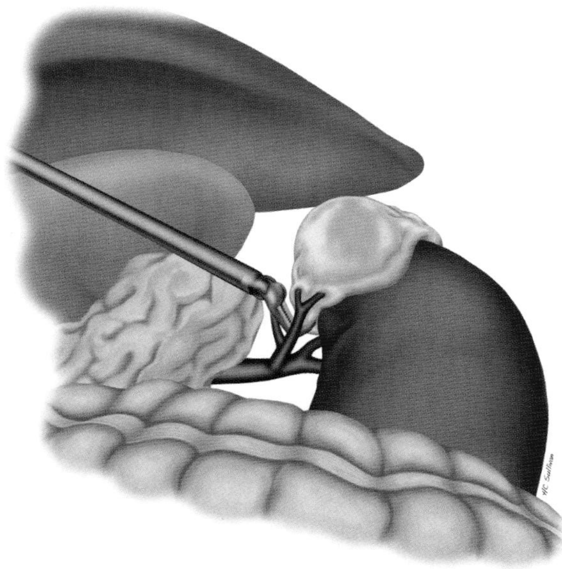

Figure 20.5

Venous anatomy of the left adrenal gland. The confluence of the left adrenal vein and inferior phrenic vein is seen entering the left renal vein. Right angle dissector isolates the left adrenal vein (printed with permission of Carolinas HealthCare System)

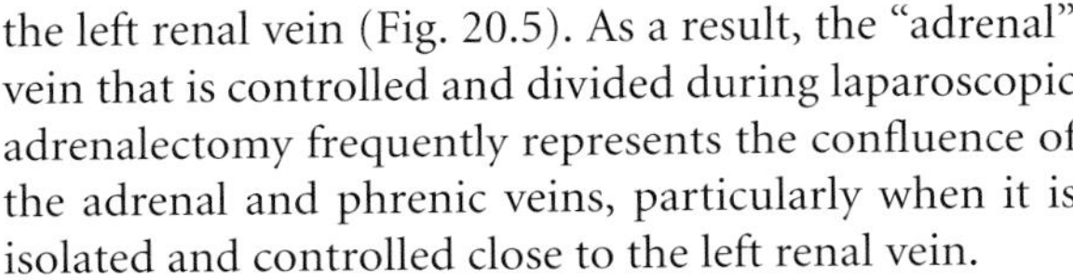

the left renal vein (Fig. 20.5). As a result, the "adrenal" vein that is controlled and divided during laparoscopic adrenalectomy frequently represents the confluence of the adrenal and phrenic veins, particularly when it is isolated and controlled close to the left renal vein.

Once the adrenal vein is identified, early control can be achieved with clips. Ideally, the vein should be traced to the adrenal gland (cephalad) and to the renal vein (caudad). The phrenic vein usually continues on in a cephalad direction to the diaphragm along the medial aspect of the adrenal gland. For division of the adrenal vein, three clips are placed on the patient (renal vein) side and two clips on the specimen side. The vessel is then divided with laparoscopic scissors. For adrenal veins too large to be controlled with clips, an endo-GIA stapler with a vascular (2.0-mm) cartridge can be used. In these instances, care must be taken to ensure that the venous anatomy is clearly delineated and that the vein being divided is truly the adrenal vein rather than a branch of the renal vein. If the structure believed to be the adrenal vein does not run perpendicular to the renal vein, then one must rule out the possibility that the vessel either represents an accessory adrenal vein or that it actually drains the upper pole of the kidney.

Following division of the adrenal vein, the attachments between the medial aspect of the adrenal gland and the upper pole of the kidney are divided. Using hook electrocautery, Gerota's fascia is first opened along the plane between the two organs. The harmonic scalpel is used to divide the deeper attachments, as this plane of dissection is often associated with oozing from multiple small vessels that enter the lateral edge of the gland. In most patients, division of this plane also requires transection of the adipose tissue that overlies the superior pole of the kidney. As long as the lateral edge of the adrenal gland/tumor is visualized, the superior pole fat can be divided safely with the harmonic scalpel. Care should be taken to stay lateral enough (along the superior pole of the kidney) to avoid injury to the gland or rupture of the tumor. However, extreme caution must be taken to recognize that the renal artery and vein lie immediately adjacent to the lateral aspect of the adrenal gland. Superior pole branches of the renal artery and vein are at risk for injury if the proximity of these structures is not recognized. Particularly with larger adrenal tumors, the normal anatomy can be altered, and the tumor will often encroach upon the renal vessels. Careful review of the patient's imaging studies prior to and during surgery can be helpful in delineating the pertinent vascular anatomy. A CT scan with intravenous contrast is usually the most helpful in this regard, with coronal reconstructions being particularly valuable in most cases.

The arterial anatomy of the adrenal gland is more variable than the venous anatomy. On the left, the gland is supplied by multiple small arterial branches arising from the renal artery (inferior suprarenal arteries), the aorta (left middle suprarenal arteries), and the inferior phrenic (left superior suprarenal arteries). In most cases, these vessels can be controlled effectively with the harmonic scalpel or electrocautery. Larger vessels (particularly those arising from the aorta) are controlled with clips.

Following dissection of the plane between the adrenal gland and the upper pole of the left kidney, attention is turned to the inferior, medial edge of the adrenal gland. The gland must be retracted up away from the renal hilum and retroperitoneal attachments to allow for safe dissection. During elevation of the gland, it is important to use Gerota's fascia or peri-adrenal fat as a "handle," rather than grasping the gland itself. Even minor trauma to the gland by laparoscopic instruments can cause obscurative venous bleeding that makes subsequent dissection and visualization difficult and frustrating. Minor oozing can be controlled by gentle pressure along with the assistance of topical hemostatic agents or laparoscopic sponges. Elevation of the inferior pole of the adrenal gland will allow for access to the plane between the adrenal gland and the retroperitoneum. The aorta lies along the medial aspect of this plane, while the gland lies on the psoas muscle and diaphragm posteriorly. Branches of the left middle suprarenal arteries supply the medial aspect of the adrenal gland and arise directly from the aorta. These vessels can be reliably controlled with clips on the aortic side followed by division with the harmonic scalpel on the specimen side. The plane between the gland and the psoas is relatively avascular and can be divided using an energy source with or without clips. As dissection proceeds along the superior, medial edge of the gland, the continuation of the left inferior phrenic vein should be identified and controlled with clips prior to dividing the final attachments between the diaphragm and the gland. Once all attachments are divided, the gland is placed in an impervious extraction bag and removed through one of the 12-mm port sites. The operative field is inspected for hemostasis. Port sites are closed with absorbable suture using a laparoscopic suture passer.

Laparoscopic Trans-abdominal Right Adrenalectomy

Patient Position and Port Strategy

For laparoscopic right adrenalectomy, the patient is positioned in the lateral decubitus position with the right side up. Otherwise, patient positioning and establishment of pneumoperitoneum are identical to that described previously. The port strategy for right adrenalectomy is illustrated in Figs. 20.6 and 20.7. On

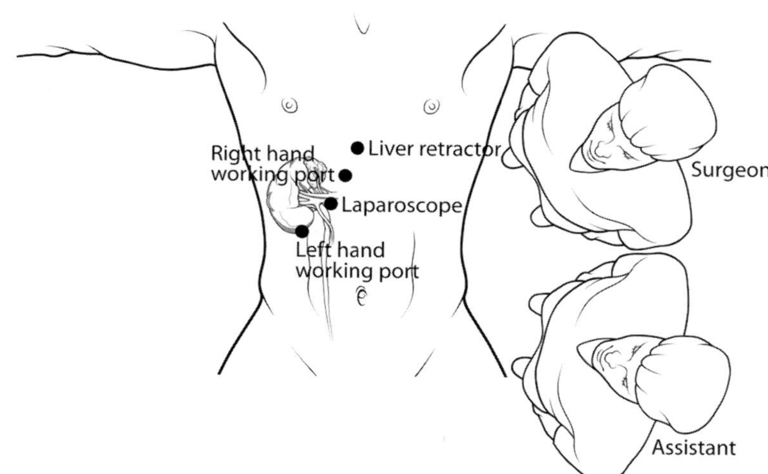

Figure 20.6

Port strategy and surgeon/assistant positions for laparoscopic right adrenalectomy (printed with permission of Carolinas HealthCare System)

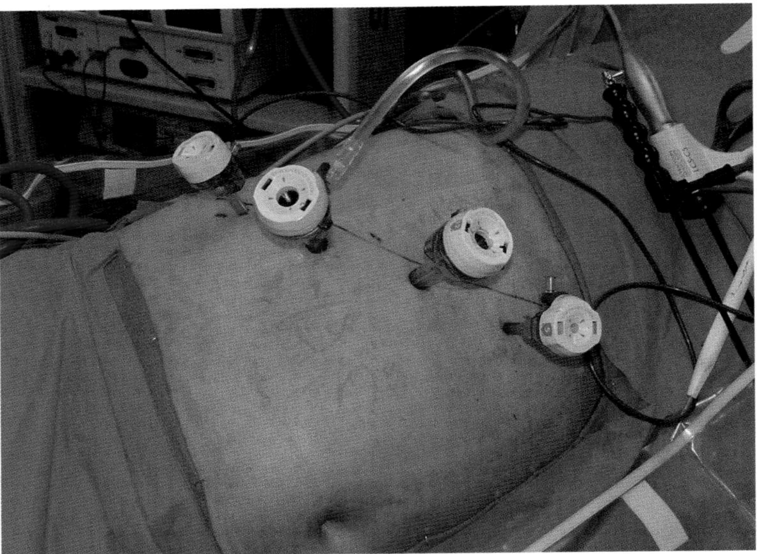

Figure 20.7

Four subcostal ports are required for laparoscopic left adrenalectomy: two 12-mm and two 5-mm ports are shown

the right, four subcostal ports are required (two 12-mm and two 5-mm). Ports are centered on the costal margin and spaced 5–6 cm apart. The 12-mm ports are used for the laparoscope and the right-hand working instrument, with a 5-mm working port for the left hand. A 10-mm clip applier and/or endo-vascular GIA stapler can be inserted through the right-hand working port for control and division of the right adrenal vein. A 5-mm port placed in the epigastrium just lateral to the falciform ligament is used for retraction of the right lobe of the liver.

Operative Steps

The right adrenal gland lies superior to the upper pole of the right kidney, deep to Gerota's fascia, and lateral to the right lobe of the liver and vena cava (Fig. 20.8). The right lobe of the liver is elevated and retracted medially, and the triangular ligament of the liver is divided with electrocautery. Attachments between the liver and the diaphragm are taken down to allow for complete medial retraction of the right lobe. Care should be taken to identify and avoid injury to the inferior phrenic vein during this dissection. Intermittent cessation of positive pressure ventilation will prevent excursion of the diaphragm during this portion of the procedure and will minimize the risk of injury to the diaphragm itself. This dissection is critical for safe right adrenalectomy, as it allows for complete exposure of the retrohepatic vena cava, right adrenal vein, and the medial edge of the adrenal gland. In most patients

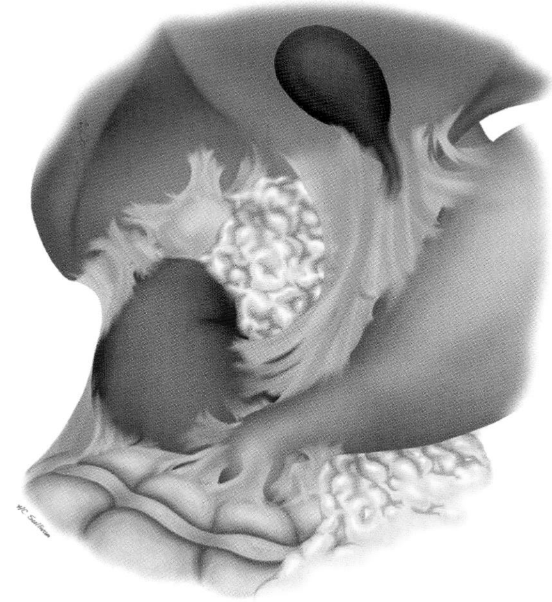

Figure 20.8

Right retroperitoneal anatomy prior to division of the right triangular ligament and prior to opening of Gerota's fascia (printed with permission of Carolinas HealthCare System)

(even those who are obese), the vena cava can be visualized just lateral to the inferior edge of the right lobe of the liver, at the interface between the liver and Gerota's

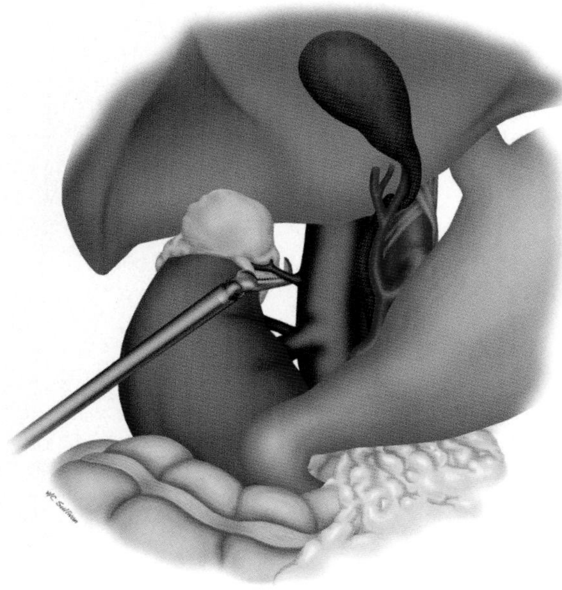

Figure 20.9

Anatomy of the right retroperitoneum demonstrating the relationship between the right adrenal gland, upper pole of the kidney, and the vena cava. Right angle dissector isolates the right adrenal vein (printed with permission of Carolinas HealthCare System)

fascia. The second portion of the duodenum is also visible slightly more inferiorly, but does not generally require mobilization for access to the vena cava or adrenal gland (Fig. 20.9). Retroperitoneal dissection is initiated at the lateral margin of the vena cava, just cephalad to the right renal vein. Gerota's fascia is opened with hook electrocautery, providing access to the retroperitoneal space. This plane of dissection is carried cephalad to the level of the diaphragm, opening Gerota's fascia in a longitudinal fashion approximately 1 cm lateral to the interface of the right lobe of the liver with the retroperitoneum. The liver can then be more effectively retracted and the retrohepatic vena cava exposed along its lateral edge. In larger tumors, and especially those that are highly vascular, care must be taken to elevate Gerota's fascia up away from the tumor as it is divided. Failure to do so can result in injury to the underlying tumor or to the vessels that run along its surface. Injury of the gland or tumor is often associated with persistent oozing that can make subsequent dissection difficult and potentially dangerous.

Once the liver is mobilized, a plane of dissection is established between the lateral margin of the vena cava and the medial edge of the adrenal gland, beginning at the lower pole of the gland and working cephalad. The gland/tumor is gently retracted laterally with the left-hand working instrument, while the attachments between the gland and the cava are dissected, then divided with hook cautery (Fig. 20.10). Care must be taken to avoid injury to the lateral wall of the vena cava while carefully approaching the right adrenal vein from inferiorly. The vein is typically quite short (1–2 cm), relatively wide (8–10 mm), and runs in a perpendicular direction from the gland directly into the lateral aspect of the vena cava. One should be careful to avoid mistaking one of the multiple small accessory veins or arteries for the adrenal vein. To confirm that the vein is indeed the right adrenal vein, control should require the use of a full 10-mm clip (Fig. 20.11).

Prior to circumferential dissection of the adrenal vein, we have found that mobilization of the adrenal gland cephalad to the adrenal vein can be helpful in obtaining mobility of the gland/tumor as well as length on the adrenal vein. When the attachments between the liver and the diaphragm have been completely divided, the liver can be retracted medially to a sufficient extent to allow for access to the medial aspect of the superior pole of the adrenal gland. Small arteries entering the gland from the aorta (medially) can be divided with electrocautery or harmonic scalpel. Dissection is carried from cranial to caudal along the medial aspect of the gland down to the level of the previously identified right adrenal vein.

With the medial attachments of the gland divided cranial and caudal to the vein, circumferential dissection of the adrenal vein is achieved with a right-angle dissector. This is perhaps the most critical aspect of the operation as injury to the right adrenal vein can result in massive hemorrhage, which can be very difficult to control laparoscopically. If the vein can be well visualized, then a single clip is placed on the patient side (immediately adjacent to the vena cava) to control the caval side of the vein prior to any further dissection. Additional dissection of the vein can then be undertaken to allow for complete control with proximal and distal clips. Our practice is to leave 2–3 clips on the patient (vena cava) side and one or two clips on the specimen side, prior to dividing the vein. Occasionally the vein is too large to be controlled with clips. In these cases, an endo-GIA stapler with a vascular load (2.0 mm/gray cartridge) is used to divide the vein.

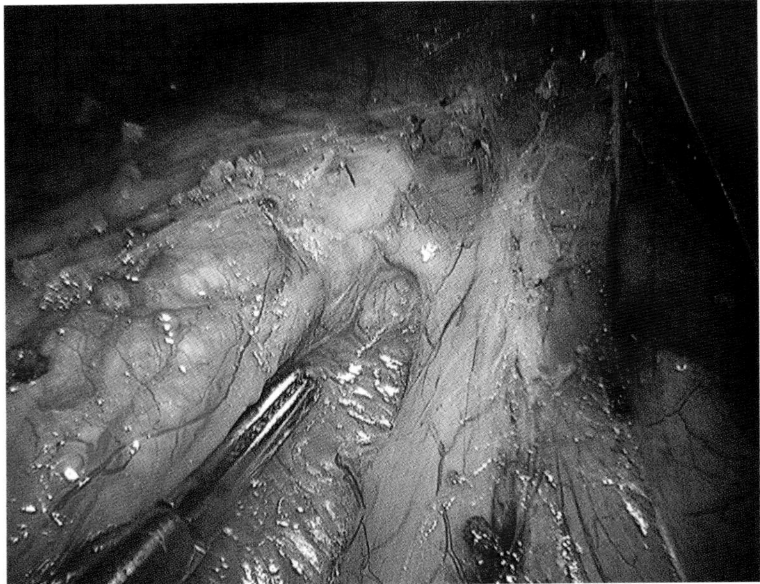

Figure 20.10

A plane of dissection is developed between the adrenal gland and the vena cava. The right adrenal vein can be seen entering the lateral wall of the vena cava

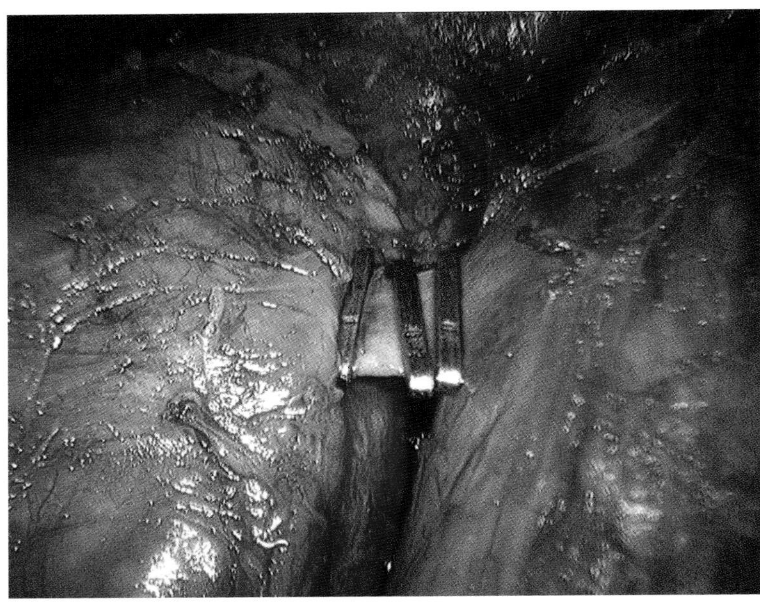

Figure 20.11

The right adrenal vein is controlled with multiple clips

Following division of the adrenal vein, the inferior pole of the gland is elevated, and the attachments between the gland and the upper pole of the kidney are divided. Typically, multiple small arteries and small veins enter the lower pole of the gland. This is usually the area most at risk for troublesome oozing. These vessels usually respond poorly to electrocautery and are more effectively controlled with harmonic scalpel and/or clips. In most patients, there is a layer of adipose tissue (upper pole renal fat) between the inferior-lateral aspect of the adrenal gland and the upper pole of the kidney. In patients with large right adrenal tumors, the surgeon must be aware that the lower pole of the gland may encroach upon the right renal vessels. Elevation of the adrenal gland is usually effective in avoiding injury to the renal vessels and the upper pole of the kidney during this portion of the dissection. Retroperitoneal attachments between the gland, the psoas muscle, and the diaphragm are divided with an energy source. When the gland is free, it is placed in an impervious extraction bag and extracted through one of the 12-mm port sites. The port site may need to be enlarged slightly for the removal of larger tumors. Otherwise, morcellation of the specimen within the extraction bag can facilitate removal.

Hand-Assisted Laparoscopic Adrenalectomy

In some cases, purely laparoscopic adrenalectomy can be challenging or even contraindicated due to large tumor size, adherence to adjacent structures, or concerns that a potentially malignant tumor may be prone to rupture. Metastatic lesions are frequently more vascular and more adherent to adjacent structures, making minimally invasive surgery potentially quite challenging when compared with adrenalectomy for benign disease. Depending on the surgeon's level of experience and laparoscopic skills, an open approach may be more appropriate in these cases. Hand-assisted laparoscopy (HAL) is another potential option, which restores the tactile feedback of open surgery while maintaining many of the benefits of minimally invasive surgery. In difficult cases, hand-assisted laparoscopy can be used either at the outset of the case or as an alternative to open conversion.

The trocar strategy for HAL right adrenalectomy is illustrated in Fig. 20.12. Port placement for the left side is a mirror image of that shown for the right. Patient positioning is identical to that described for purely laparoscopic adrenalectomy. The hand-assist device is inserted through a 7-cm peri-umbilical midline incision. The surgeon's left hand is place intraperitoneal. Two 12-mm ports (one for the right-hand laparoscopic instrument and one for the laparoscope) are required. For right adrenalectomy, a 5-mm epigastric port is used for liver retraction.

While HAL adrenalectomy is used relatively infrequently, this technique can allow for successful removal of larger lesions, which may not be amenable to a purely laparoscopic approach. Of our group's most recent 159 laparoscopic adrenalectomies, eight (5%) were performed using a hand-assisted approach. A concomitant radical nephrectomy was performed in two cases; one for an unrelated RCC tumor and the other for an adrenal lesion that invaded or encroached upon the renal hilum. The remainder required the use of a HAL approach due to large tumor size (mean 8.8 cm, range 6–13 cm) with inability to safely mobilize the tumor away from adjacent structures without the use of tactile feedback and blunt retraction provided by the intraperitoneal hand. When compared with a purely laparoscopic approach, HAL adrenalectomy was associated with longer operative times (190 min vs. 165 min), more blood loss (188 ml vs. 70 ml), and increased length of stay (10.8 days vs. 4 days). Clinical information on patients managed with a hand-assisted laparoscopic approach are detailed in Table 20.1.

If the entire adrenal gland along with its adjacent adipose tissue cannot be safely resected without compromising tumor margins or avoiding penetration of the adrenal capsule, then conversion to either a hand-assisted approach or open approach is indicated. In these cases, resection of adjacent organs may be required to obtain negative surgical margins. To this

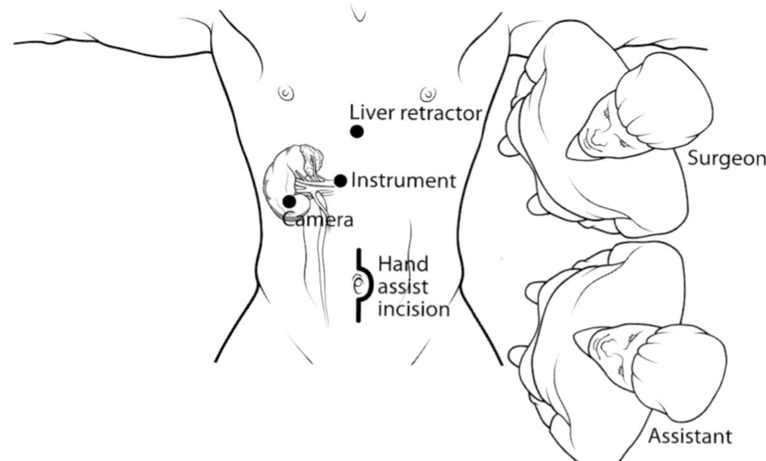

Figure 20.12

Port strategy for hand-assisted laparoscopic right adrenalectomy (printed with permission of Carolinas HealthCare System)

Table 20.1. Hand-assisted laparoscopic adrenalectomy ($n = 8$) vs. purely laparoscopic adrenalectomy ($n = 151$)

Clinical diagnosis	Pathology	Side	Tumor size (cm)	EBL (ml)	OR time (min)	LOS (days)
Metastasis	RCC	R	11	350	295	5
Metastasis	Lung	R	7	600	245	43
Pheo	Pheo	R	6	100	230	5
Pheo	Pheo	L	13	200	259	6
Metastasis	RCC	L	9.5	75	196	4
Adrenal mass	Myelolipoma	L	8	25	85	9
Metastasis	ACC	R	7.5	50	120	5
Pheo	Pheo	R	8.5	100	149	9
HAL (mean)	–	–	8.8	188	190	10.8
Purely laparoscopic (mean)	–	–	3.8	70	165	4.0

EBL, estimated blood loss; OR, operating room; LOS, length of stay; RCC, renal cell carcinoma; Pheo, pheochromocytoma; ACC, adrenal cortical carcinoma; HAL, hand-assisted laparoscopic

end, hand-assisted laparoscopy can aid in tactile assessment of tumor extent and/or adherence to adjacent organs and may facilitate en bloc resection of adjacent structures, including the spleen, kidney, and tail of pancreas. On a number of occasions, we have used the hand-assisted technique to successfully resect the kidney and adrenal gland en bloc, when encroachment upon the renal vessels has prevented adrenalectomy alone and would have compromised renal blood supply and/or oncologic margins.

Conclusions

Laparoscopic adrenalectomy for metastatic disease is technically feasible and offers potential advantages over the traditional open approach. In selected patients, an aggressive approach to adrenal resection can be associated with long-term disease-free survival and prolonged overall survival. Yet, solitary metastases are rare. Careful preoperative evaluation is required to rule out more widespread metastatic disease to other sites prior to embarking upon adrenalectomy. For patients who are deemed to be appropriate candidates for laparoscopic adrenalectomy, each surgeon must assess his or her technical skills in approaching malignant adrenal tumors. Malignant adrenal lesions are frequently associated with larger size, peri-adrenal desmoplastic response, and increased vascularity. Each of these factors makes the resection of malignant tumors technically more difficult than that required for benign disease. Inadvertent disruption of malignant lesions has the potential to result in local or port recurrence and may adversely impact oncologic outcomes. If the tumor cannot be safely dissected and resected without compromising tumor margins or avoiding tumor spillage, then conversion to either a hand-assisted or open approach is warranted.

Despite arguments in favor of applying minimally invasive approaches to the majority of adrenal lesions, the laparoscopic resection of metastatic and primary adrenal malignancies remains controversial. Long-term disease-free survival after adrenal metastasectomy for isolated metastases from renal, colorectal, lung, and melanoma primaries shows promise in select patients. By reducing the trauma of surgical access, minimally invasive adrenalectomy has clear advantages over an open approach. Yet, improvements in patient satisfaction and early postoperative outcomes should not overshadow the primary goals of patient safety and the performance of an accepted and established oncologic resection. While existing data are encouraging, only through careful staging and appropriate patient selection can the long-term efficacy of the laparoscopic approach be assessed in these patients.

Acknowledgments Special thanks to Cissy Moore-Swartz for her editorial assistance with this chapter.

References

1. Dunn MD, Portis AJ, Shalhav AL et al (2000) Laparoscopic versus open radical nephrectomy: a 9-year experience. J Urol 164:1153–1159
2. Flowers JL, Jacobs S, Cho E et al (1997) Comparison of open and laparoscopic live donor nephrectomy. Ann Surg 226:483–489, discussion 489–490
3. Jacobs JK, Goldstein RE, Geer RJ (1997) Laparoscopic adrenalectomy. A new standard of care. Ann Surg 225: 495–501, discussion 501–502
4. Park A, Marcaccio M, Sternbach M, Witzke D, Fitzgerald P (1999) Laparoscopic vs. open splenectomy. Arch Surg 134:1263–1269
5. Higashiyama M, Doi O, Kodama K, Yokouchi H, Imaoka S, Koyama H (1994) Surgical treatment of adrenal metastasis following pulmonary resection for lung cancer: comparison of adrenalectomy with palliative therapy. Int Surg 79: 124–129
6. Kim SH, Brennan MF, Russo P, Burt ME, Coit DG (1998) The role of surgery in the treatment of clinically isolated adrenal metastasis. Cancer 82:389–394
7. Sagalowsky AI, Molberg K (1999) Solitary metastasis of renal cell carcinoma to the contralateral adrenal gland 22 years after nephrectomy. Urology 54:162
8. Lo CY, van Heerden JA, Soreide JA et al (1996) Adrenalectomy for metastatic disease to the adrenal glands. Br J Surg 83:528–531
9. Heniford BT, Pratt B (2001) Laparosopic adrenalectomy for metastatic cancer. In: Greene FL, Heniford BT (eds) Minimally invasive cancer management. Springer, New York, NY, pp 319–332
10. Ito A, Satoh M, Ohyama C et al (2002) Adrenal metastasis from renal cell carcinoma: significance of adrenalectomy. Int J Urol 9:125–128
11. Lau WK, Zincke H, Lohse CM, Cheville JC, Weaver AL, Blute ML (2003) Contralateral adrenal metastasis of renal cell carcinoma: treatment, outcome and a review. BJU Int 91:775–779
12. Greene FL, Kercher KW, Nelson H, Teigland CM, Boller AM (2007) Minimal access cancer management. CA Cancer J Clin 57:130–146
13. Luketich JD, Burt ME (1996) Does resection of adrenal metastases from non-small cell lung cancer improve survival? Ann Thorac Surg 62:1614–1616
14. Ayabe H, Tsuji H, Hara S, Tagawa Y, Kawahara K, Tomita M (1995) Surgical management of adrenal metastasis from bronchogenic carcinoma. J Surg Oncol 58: 149–154
15. Moinzadeh A, Gill IS (2005) Laparoscopic radical adrenalectomy for malignancy in 31 patients. J Urol 173:519–525
16. Sarela AI, Murphy I, Coit DG, Conlon KC (2003) Metastasis to the adrenal gland: the emerging role of laparoscopic surgery. Ann Surg Oncol 10:1191–1196
17. Weyhe D, Belyaev O, Skawran S, Muller C, Bauer KH (2007) A case of port-site recurrence after laparoscopic adrenalectomy for solitary adrenal metastasis. Surg Laparosc Endosc Percutan Tech 17:218–220
18. Saraiva P, Rodrigues H, Rodrigues P (2003) Port site recurrence after laparoscopic adrenalectomy for metastatic melanoma. Int Braz J Urol 29:520–521
19. Rassweiler J, Tsivian A, Kumar AV et al (2003) Oncological safety of laparoscopic surgery for urological malignancy: experience with more than 1,000 operations. J Urol 169:2072–2075
20. Valeri A, Borrelli A, Presenti L et al (2001) Adrenal masses in neoplastic patients: the role of laparoscopic procedure. Surg Endosc 15:90–93

Minimally Invasive Approaches to Lung Cancer

David P. Mason, Sudish C. Murthy, Jang Wen Su, Thomas W. Rice

Contents

Background

Minimally invasive thoracic surgical techniques appear to reduce important morbidity and facilitate return to normal activity when compared with standard open approaches [1–3]. Mechanisms for this benefit likely include reduction in pain, earlier ambulation, and decreased inflammatory response to injury [3–6]. Before such techniques are routinely adopted, however, it is incumbent upon thoracic surgeons to demonstrate that therapeutic benefit of the procedure is not compromised. For resection of lung cancer, this means there must be comparable completeness of resection with appropriate lymph node sampling or lymphadenectomy [2, 7–9].

Video-assisted thoracic surgery (VATS) has proven to be a safe and effective minimally invasive technique in the management of numerous thoracic disease conditions. Little debate exists among surgeons regarding the appropriateness of VATS for pleural biopsies, bullectomy, pleurodesis, and lung biopsy [10, 11]. However, VATS lobectomy for lung cancer remains a controversial procedure and has met resistance [7, 12–15]. This is in part attributable to technical challenges of the procedure and what appears to be a steep learning curve [16–19]. In addition, until recently, there has not been a uniform definition of what actually constitutes a VATS lobectomy [15]. Finally, and perhaps most importantly, because VATS lobectomy for lung cancer is a relatively new technique, data remain sparse regarding important oncologic outcomes, such as cancer-free survival and risk of recurrence [20, 21]. For this reason, the majority of lobectomies in the United States are still performed by thoracotomy. However, data showing that VATS lobectomy is the procedure of choice for stage IA lung cancer [1, 2, 20, 22–24] are emerging, and it is routinely performed in this setting at Cleveland Clinic. In this chapter, we describe the diagnostic and therapeutic

F.L. Greene, B.T. Heniford (eds.), *Minimally Invasive Cancer Management*,
DOI 10.1007/978-1-4419-1238-1_21,

VATS procedures available for diagnosing and managing lung cancer and emphasize our own techniques for VATS lobectomy.

Diagnosis and Staging

Diagnosis

VATS surgical diagnostic techniques are important and necessary tools in the thoracic surgeon's armamentarium. A principal role is diagnosis of the solitary pulmonary nodule. A benefit of a VATS diagnostic approach compared with percutaneous or bronchoscopic sampling is that an excisional biopsy is obtained and thus false-positive and false-negative examinations are virtually eliminated. A diagnosis thus obtained is accurate with excellent positive and negative predictive value. A major concern has been localization of the nodule and successful excision biopsy.

Unlike bimanual palpation afforded by thoracotomy, palpation at VATS diagnostic procedures is limited to instrument "palpation" or single-digit palpation via an enlarged thoracoport. It has been estimated that if a nodule is more than 5 mm from the pleural surface and 10 mm or less in diameter, there is 63% failure in localization by palpation [25]. To overcome the problem of localization by palpation, multiple techniques have been suggested. Gonfiotti and colleagues explored different localization techniques in patients with pulmonary nodules less than 2 cm in diameter and 1.5–3 cm from the pleural surface [26]. In 25 patients, CT-guided hook-wire insertion successfully localized nodules in 21 (84%), while finger localization identified nodules in only 7 (28%). Dislodging of the needle was reported in 6 (16%) patients, and pneumothorax complicated 6 (16%) hook-wire localizations. In 25 patients, CT needle identification and injection of a radionucleotide tracer successfully localized nodules in 24 (96%), whereas finger palpation was successful in 6 (24%). Contamination of the pleural space with the tracer caused localization failure in one patient and one pneumothorax was reported. Sortini and colleagues compared different means of localization in a patient population with a mean nodule size of 1.26±0.22 cm and mean distance from the pleura of 2.6±0.5 cm [27]. Intraoperative ultrasound localization (96% successful) and radionucleotide localization (80% successful) were no different from finger localization (76 and 80% successful).

Subcentimeter pulmonary nodules are increasingly common with widespread use of modern CT equipment and represent the maximum challenge of localization. There are no reports of populations composed solely of subcentimeter pulmonary nodules; however, there are reports in which mean/median size of nodules is subcentimeter. Burdine and colleagues used radionucleotide and methylene blue techniques in 17 patients with newly diagnosed or previously treated malignancy to successfully locate and resect all nodules (mean nodule size 9.2±3.6 mm, mean depth 9.4±5.2 mm) using VATS techniques [28]. Stiles and colleagues used radionucleotide techniques to successfully localize and excise by VATS techniques 44 of 46 nodules (mean size 9 mm, range 3–22 mm; median depth 5 mm, range 0–50 mm) [29].

Ground glass opacities (GGO) are potentially more difficult to localize than solid nodules. However, in practice, current preoperative localization techniques have proven highly effective. Forty-five of 174 nodules successfully localized by CT-guided lipiodol marking and fluoroscopy-assisted VATS excision were GGO [30]. GGO was not a determinant of localization using a hook-wire technique in 150 patients with 168 nodules [31].

Staging

VATS staging is complementary to conventional and evolving staging techniques. VATS excision of pulmonary nodules in lobes other than the lobe in which the primary cancer is situated is necessary to confirm M1 classification. VATS sampling of lymph nodes that are not accessible to mediastinoscopy mediastinotomy, and endobronchial ultrasound, typically R8, L8, R9, and L9 stations, is indicated when confirmation of N2/N3 classification of these stations will influence therapy. The unparalleled access to the pleural space offered by VATS is invaluable in staging patients with suspected malignant pleural effusions (T4/M1) and pleural involvement associated with primary lung cancers (T4). It has a limited role in staging T3 lung cancers with direct invasion of the chest wall, mediastinal, or diaphragm.

Pulmonary Resection

Sublobar Resection

For patients with T1N0M0 lung cancer who are able to tolerate lobectomy, survival is improved and local recurrence reduced compared with patients receiving sublobar resection [32–34]. Inaccuracies of clinical staging caused high failure (45%) of attempted thoracoscopic wedge resection of clinical T1 (20% failure to perform VATS wedge) and T2 (50% failure to perform VATS wedge) lung cancers [35]. However, for cancers of 2 cm or less in diameter, segmentectomy and possibly wedge resection may be indicated and performed with outcome similar to lobectomy [36].

Theoretically, sublobar resections may not provide adequate resection of the primary cancer and regional lymph nodes. However, local recurrence has been reported to decrease by half (15–7.5%) if resection margins more than 1 cm from the primary cancer are obtained in patients undergoing sublobar resections for stage I lung cancer [37]. The addition of brachytherapy to sublobar resection has been associated with few local recurrences [38]. Segmentectomy may better encompass and contain lung cancers 2 cm or less and regional lymph nodes than wedge resection [39, 40]. Of 91 clinical stage I lung cancer patients undergoing sublobar resection, 11 (12%) had regional lymph node metastases; 10 of these had intersegmental metastases (five confined to the segment resected) [41]. Of the 10 patients with intersegmental lymph node metastases, 7 had metastases in both hilar/lobar and mediastinal lymph nodes. If sublobar resections are to be considered for lung cancers 2 cm or less, adequate resection margins and appropriate regional lymph node sampling/resection are necessary.

The combination of severe pulmonary impairment and presence of a lung cancer 2 cm or less has been used as an indication for VATS sublobar resection. This is not yet a proven use for VATS sublobar resection. It must be remembered that comorbidities may dominate survival in these patients, and outcome may not be predictably influenced by pulmonary function [42]. In matched "high-risk" patient groups receiving either sublobar resection or three-dimensional conformal radiation therapy for stage I lung cancers, overall and disease-free survivals were not statistically different [43]. Advanced radiosurgery techniques are available and being investigated in this group of patients. Currently, VATS sublobar resection of lung cancers 2 cm or less in "high-risk" patients is a therapeutic alternative, but it has not been demonstrated to be superior to other forms of therapy.

Lobectomy

Indications for VATS lobectomy are identical to lobectomy via thoracotomy: localized lung cancer with pulmonary function adequate to tolerate resection and absence of prohibitive medical comorbidities. While VATS lobectomy has been reported in patients with advanced local stage disease [44], our practice is to perform VATS lobectomy in patients who demonstrate clinical and surgical staging suggestive of stage I lung cancer. Finally, we prefer that the cancer or nodule be relatively peripheral and less than or equal to 3 cm in diameter. Relative contraindications to VATS lobectomy include prior ipsilateral chest surgery or pleurodesis, previous lobectomy, inability to tolerate single-lung ventilation, obesity that prevents adequate manipulation of VATS instruments, mediastinal radiation, and coexisting granulomatous disease of the mediastinum.

Definition of VATS Lobectomy

Until recently, there has not been a standardized definition of VATS lobectomy. However, a true VATS lobectomy is an anatomic pulmonary resection that is performed with individual identification, isolation, and transaction of pulmonary artery, vein, and bronchus with accompanying hilar and mediastinal lymph node sampling or dissection [15, 20]. This must be performed without rib spreading and typically utilizes two to three 1-cm thoracoports and a 3- to 8-cm access (utility) incision.

Preoperative Evaluation

CT scan, positron emission tomography (PET) scan, and brain magnetic resonance imaging (MRI) are routinely performed in all patients with suspected lung cancer [45–48]. Patient fitness for surgery is determined by history, physical exam, and spirometry. In general, patients with good performance status and pulmonary function studies, including DLCO, who demonstrate a predicted post-resection FEV_1 >40% are candidates for lobectomy [49–52]. Cardiopulmonary exercise testing and quantitative ventilation–perfusion scans should be ordered when adequacy of pulmonary reserve is in question [53]. Cardiac stress testing and echocardiography should be utilized to rule out unexpected but likely concomitant cardiac disease or to quantify known cardiac comorbidity. It is our experience that older patients and those with marginal pulmonary function and fitness are the best candidates for

VATS lobectomy because of decreased postoperative pain and reduced surgical trauma [22, 54–56].

Techniques

Surgical Procedure. Because even small, peripheral lesions hold risk for mediastinal lymph node metastases, we recommend and routinely perform cervical mediastinoscopy at the same setting as VATS lobectomy [57]. This adds little time to the operation and prevents futile resection. We recommend initial bronchoscopy be performed through a single lumen tube to evaluate airway anatomy, rule out endobronchial cancer that precludes use of VATS, and clear airway secretions. When mediastinoscopy and frozen-section lymph node assessment rule out N2 or N3 cancer, the patient is reintubated with a double-lumen endotracheal tube and positioned into lateral decubitus position with careful positioning and extremity padding to avoid peroneal nerve and brachial plexus injury. The chest is widely prepped for full thoracotomy should this be necessary. The operating table is slightly flexed at the patient's waist level to increase the range of maneuverability of instruments and thoracoscope.

Instruments. No specialized instrumentation is necessary for VATS lobectomy, although a small assortment of minimally invasive surgical instruments can be useful. Standard sponge-stick holders are used to retract the lung and standard angled clamps to isolate vessels. We have found that coaxial forceps and scissors facilitate working between the narrow intercostal spaces. Thoracoscopic Kittner dissectors facilitate blunt dissection. Otherwise, instrumentation is no different from that of open lobectomy. All vessels are divided with an endoscopic linear cutting stapler with a vascular cartridge (2.5-mm staple height, hereinafter called endoscopic vascular stapler), and if their caliber is small, they are either clipped or ligated. The bronchus is transected with an endoscopic linear cutting stapler with a tissue cartridge (3.5- or 4.8-mm staple height, depending on tissue thickness, hereinafter called endoscopic stapler). A large, sturdy, endoscopic retrieval bag must be used to remove the lobe from the chest cavity to prevent seeding of the incision.

Thoracoport Placement. The importance of careful port placement cannot be overemphasized. Well-positioned thoracoports allow a controlled and safe VATS lobectomy, while poorly placed thoracoports lead to technical difficulties and surgeon frustration. As a general rule, ports should be widely spaced to prevent instruments from interfering with each other or "chop-sticking." A 1-cm camera thoracoport is placed in the eighth interspace, midaxillary line. Typically two additional thoracoports are placed in the sixth interspace anterior axillary line and posteriorly 3 cm below the tip of the scapula (Fig. 21.1). Additionally, a 3-cm midaxillary line access incision is created, which can be widened as necessary. The intercostal muscles in the access incision are undercut several centimeters anteriorly and posteriorly to allow specimen removal. No rib spreading is performed. A soft-tissue protector is used in the access incision

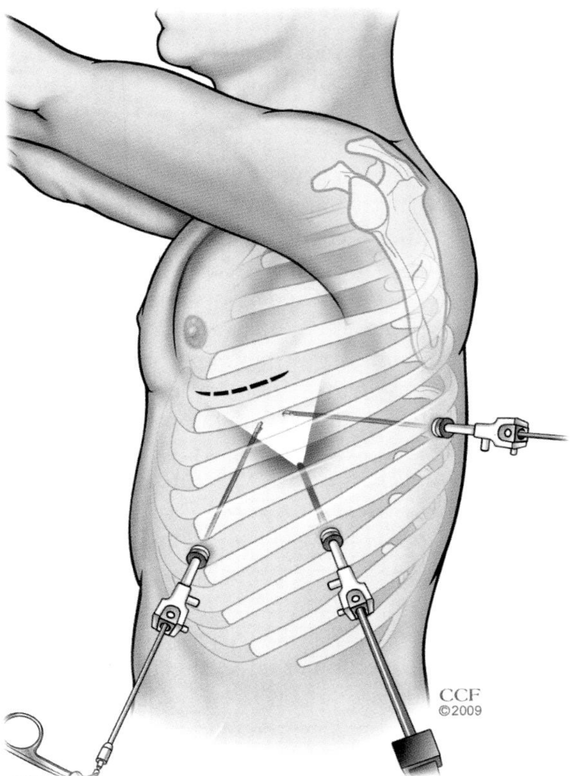

Figure 21.1

Typical thoracoport and access incision placements for left VATS lobectomy. Triangulation of the thoracoports permits convergence (working distance) of the camera and instruments at the pulmonary hilum (underlying the access incision) without interference between the camera and instruments (reprinted with the permission of The Cleveland Clinic Center for Medical Art & Photography © 2009. All Rights Reserved)

to minimize tissue injury. Differences in body habitus and the lobe being resected necessitate slight variations in port position. We prefer that the access incision be placed directly over the superior pulmonary vein for upper lobectomy and inferior pulmonary vein for lower lobectomy.

Mobilization of the Lung. Before making the access incision, CO_2 insufflation speeds atelectasis and commencement of dissection. Incomplete atelectasis may create unsafe working conditions and increases the likelihood of retraction-induced pulmonary injury and subsequent air leak. The lobe containing the cancer is carefully identified. Preferably, the cancer is palpated to confirm its location. All lobes are palpated as best possible through the thoracoports or access incision to rule out previously undetected metastases or synchronous primary lung cancer. Any uncertainty of cancer location or surgical anatomy mandates thoracotomy. Incomplete fissures do not preclude VATS lobectomy.

Unlike in open lobectomy, repositioning the lobe for optimal exposure during VATS lobectomy can be time consuming, and maximal dissection should be carried out during each exposure. Vascular and bronchial anatomy must be carefully identified. VATS dissection for lobectomy commences with sharp, circumferential division of the mediastinal pleura and mobilization of the inferior pulmonary ligament. The inferior pulmonary ligament is exposed through upward traction on the lower lobe through the posterior port. Next, the anterior hilum is exposed with posterior traction through the posterior port. The posterior hilum is exposed with anterior traction through the anterior port and access incision.

Management of the Hilar Vessels. After full division of the mediastinal pleura, methodical hilar dissection is carried out with careful identification of the pulmonary artery and superior and inferior pulmonary veins. The venous drainage of each lobe must be confirmed and anatomic anomalies identified before any structures are divided. Particular attention should be paid to the right middle lobe vein, which can become compromised during right upper lobectomy. Technical errors due to inadequate identification of the anatomy must be avoided. At open lobectomy, order of dissection is typically pulmonary vein, then pulmonary artery, then fissures, and finally the bronchus, significant variability exists for VATS lobectomy. Most dissection in a VATS lobectomy is from the anterior port and access incision. For upper lobectomy, frequently it is helpful to divide the pulmonary vein first (Fig. 21.2) to facilitate exposure of the pulmonary artery (Fig. 21.3).

Mobilization of the pulmonary artery starts with sharp dissection. A beginner's error is to attempt blunt dissection of the pulmonary artery without first dividing the peri-adventitial tissue and cutting down sharply to the "egg-shell white" adventitia (Fig. 21.4). If dissected in the wrong plane, the artery becomes difficult to encircle, rendering the operation hazardous. Adequate lengths of vessels must be mobilized in this dissection plane to prevent injury during ligation and division. If dissection of the pulmonary artery is particularly difficult because of inflammation, VATS should be abandoned and the pulmonary artery controlled proximally by encircling the main pulmonary artery and placing vessel loops around it. The pulmonary veins can tolerate vigorous dissection during isolation. It is imperative that the endoscopic vascular stapler be placed at an appropriate angle to prevent

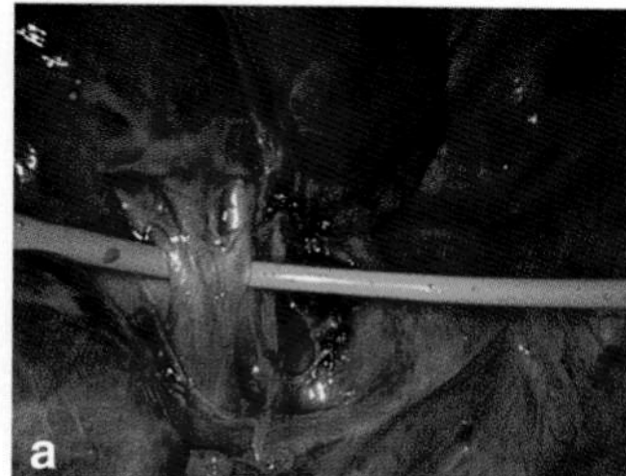

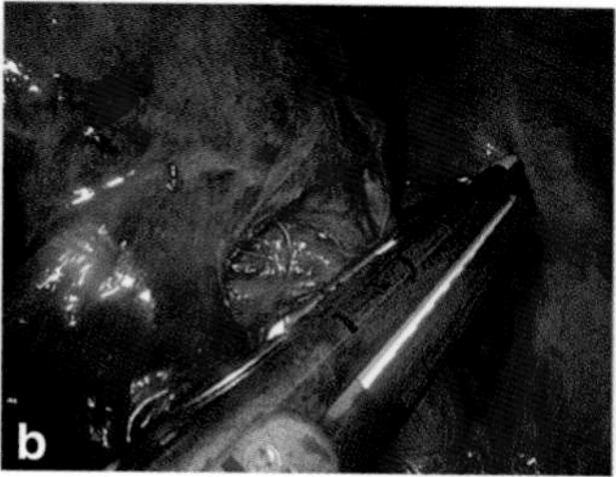

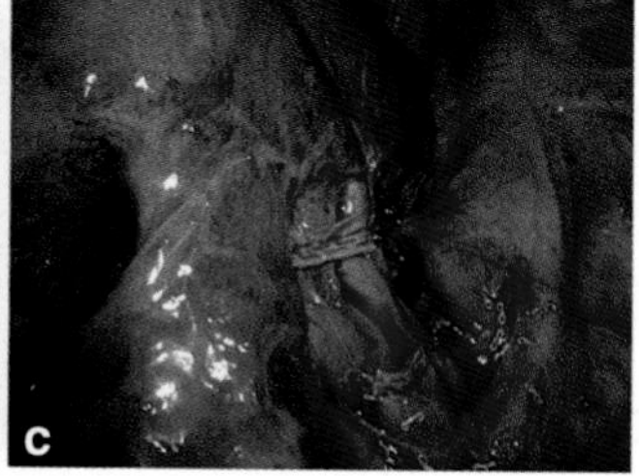

Figure 21.2

(**a**) The upper lobe branches of the right superior pulmonary vein have been dissected and circumferentially mobilized. A red rubber catheter ("endo-leader") has been passed behind the vein and will be used to guide the endoscopic vascular stapler into place. (**b**) The endoscopic vascular stapler both staples and divides the right upper lobe vein. (**c**) Division of the right upper lobe vein exposes the underlying pulmonary artery and its branches to the right upper lobe

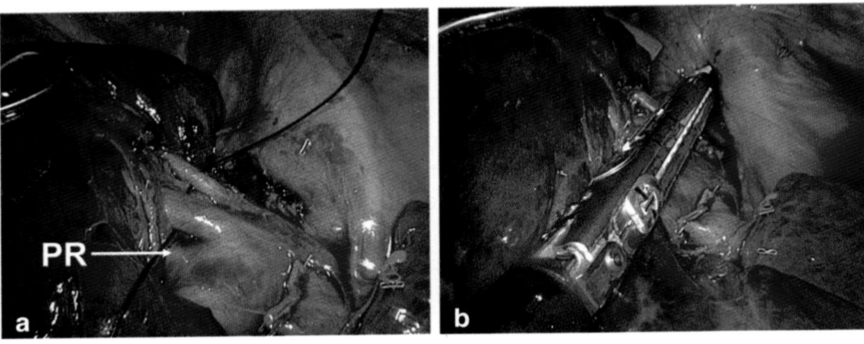

Figure 21.3

(**a**) The truncus arteriosus branches of the pulmonary artery are dissected and circumferentially mobilized. A silk suture is passed behind the artery to guide the "endo-leader" and then the endoscopic vascular stapler into place. The posterior recurrent branch of the pulmonary artery (PR) that supplies the posterior segment of the right upper lobe can be seen. After division of the truncus arteriosus, it will be the next artery to be divided. (**b**) The endoscopic vascular stapler both staples and divides the truncus arteriosus branches of the right upper lobe pulmonary artery

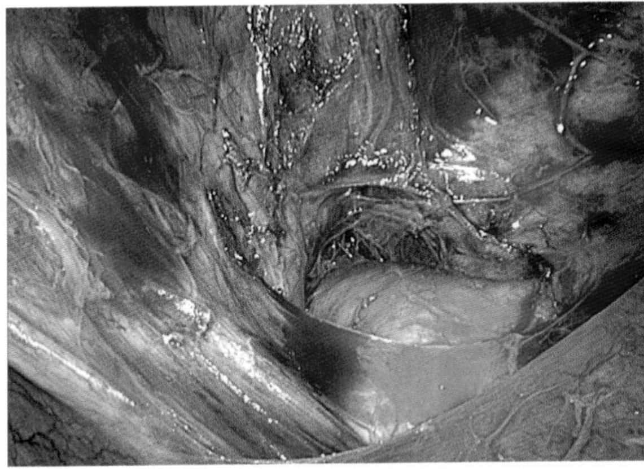

Figure 21.4

Exposure of the interlobar portion of the left pulmonary artery. Careful sharp dissection has been carried down to the adventitia of the artery. Further dissection in this plane permits safe mobilization of pulmonary arterial branches

undue torque and injury to the vessels. Passage of the stapler behind the dissected vessel is facilitated by using an "endo-leader" fashioned from a red rubber catheter and placed over the anvil of the stapler (Fig. 21.2a). Positioning of the endovascular stapler is also improved by using a reticulating-type model and choosing the thoracoport that affords the best stapler approach.

Management of the Bronchus. The bronchus must be divided with endoscopic linear cutting staplers in VATS lobectomy (Fig. 21.5), as opposed to right-angle staplers typically used during thoracotomy. This is generally performed from an anterior approach, even in right upper lobectomy, where traditionally, the airway is dissected and encircled from behind. After dissection of the bronchus, all peribronchial lymph nodes are swept toward the specimen to avoid incorporating lymph nodes in the bronchial margin. The endoscopic stapler is closed over the bronchus. Gentle, hand bagging (inflation) of the lung is then performed by the anesthesiologist to confirm that the remaining lobes expand before the airway is divided. Bronchoscopy should be performed to confirm anatomy if lung expansion is not adequate. We recommend routine frozen-section evaluation of the bronchial margin and any parenchymal margin close to the cancer. The stump is tested by inflation to 30 cm of water pressure.

Management of the Fissure. Although a more complete fissure certainly facilitates lobectomy, VATS lobectomy can be carried out with incomplete or absent fissures. Fissures can be divided either early or late during VATS lobectomy, whatever facilitates exposure, dissection, and manipulation of the lobe. For a completely fused fissure, we typically divide all hilar structures and then create a long continuous multiple stapled parenchymal closure along a tangent that approximates the location of the fissure (Fig. 21.6).

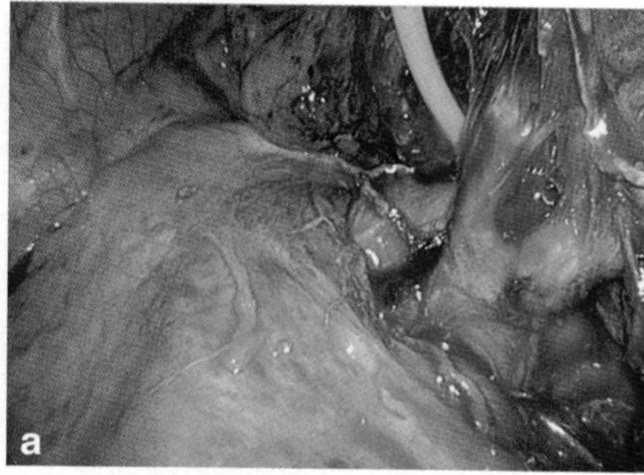

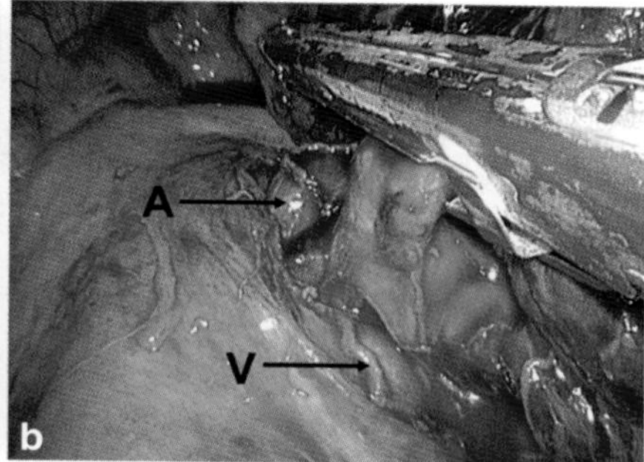

Figure 21.5

(a) The left upper lobe bronchus has been circumferentially mobilized and an "endo-leader" has been passed behind it after division of the upper lobe vein (V) and truncus arteriosus branch of the pulmonary artery (A). (b) The left upper lobe bronchus is stapled and divided with an endoscopic stapler (thick tissue cartridge, 4.8-mm staple height)

Figure 21.6

The inferior portion of the right major fissure is taken in a step-wise fashion with serial fires of an endoscopic stapler (tissue cartridge, 4.8-mm staple height)

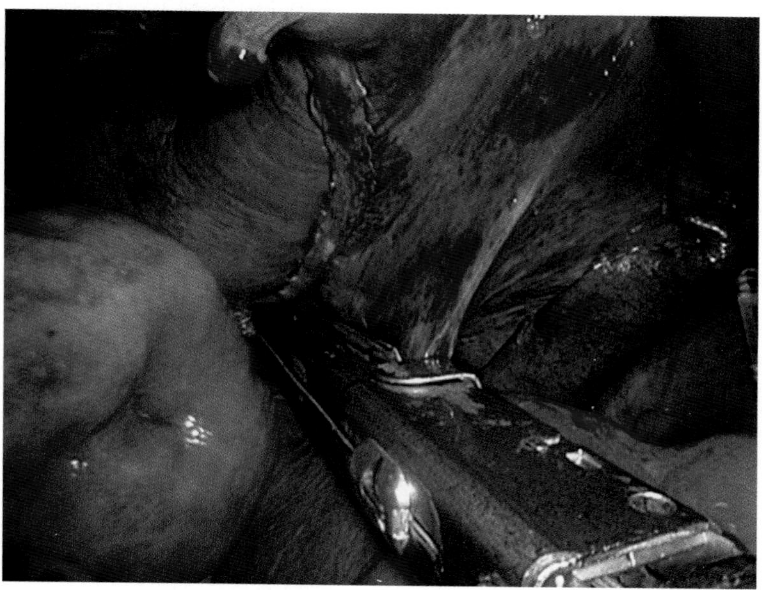

Emphysematous lung should be divided with an endoscopic stapler buttressed with pericardial or polytetrafluoroethylene strips.

Lymphadenectomy. Lymph node sampling or lymphadenectomy should not be compromised by VATS. Identical techniques are used, although more patience is generally required for thorough lymphadenectomy. We are able to perform ipsilateral lymphadenectomy with careful removal of all lobar, hilar, and mediastinal lymph node stations, including levels 2R, 4R, 3, 7, 8R, 9R, 10R, 11R, and 12R in the right chest and levels 5, 6, 7, 8L, 9L, 10L, 11L, and 12L in the left.

Completion of the Operation. The lobe is placed into an endoscopic retrieval bag and removed through the access incision (Fig. 21.7). The staple lines are inspected and tested for both hemostasis and pneumostasis (Fig. 21.8). A soft drain is placed through a separate small incision or one of the thoracoports (Fig. 21.9). The incisions are closed (Fig. 21.10).

Right Upper Lobectomy

The right upper lobe is retracted posteriorly using a sponge-stick holder passed through the most posterior thoracoport. Hilar dissection is begun with identification and dissection of the upper lobe branch

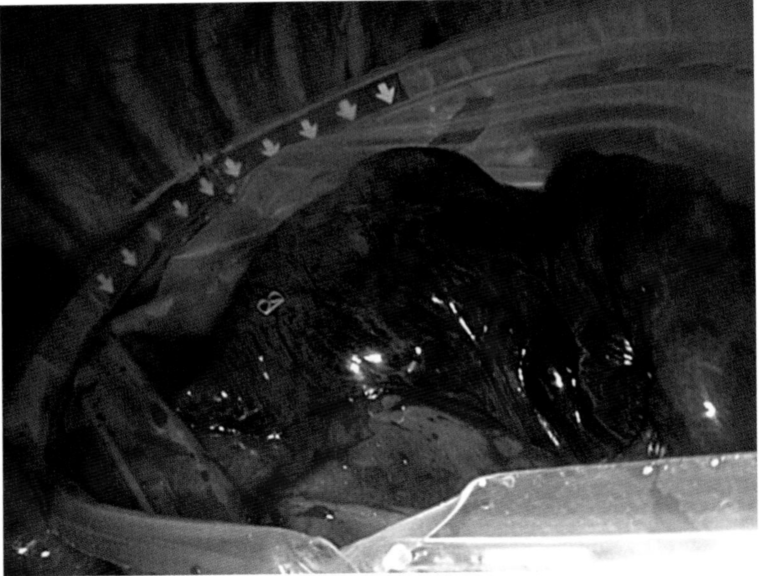

Figure 21.7

The right upper lobe is placed into a sturdy endoscopic retrieval bag for removal through the access incision

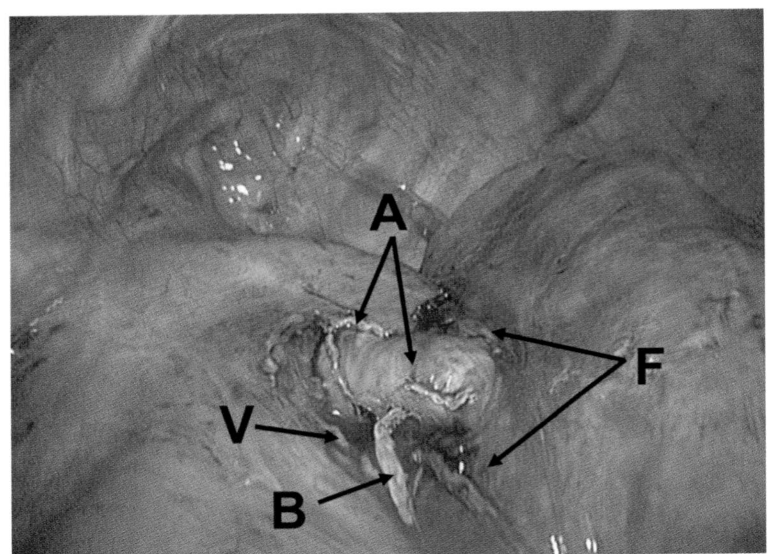

Figure 21.8

After removal of the left upper lobe, the pulmonary artery (A) and vein (V) closures are inspected and hemostasis ensured. Closures of the bronchus (B) and fissure (F) are also inspected and tested

of the superior pulmonary vein and right main pulmonary artery. Forceps passed through the access incision lift the perivascular tissue that is divided by scissors brought through the anterior thoracoport. The superior pulmonary vein is dissected from surrounding tissue using a combination of sharp and blunt dissection. The venous drainage of the middle lobe vein must be carefully identified and preserved. A right-angled clamp is then brought through the access port and passed behind the upper lobe portion of the superior pulmonary vein. Next, an endoscopic vascular stapler is passed through the anterior port and used to divide the vein.

Once the superior pulmonary vein is transected, the pulmonary artery and its branches are better visualized. The truncus arteriosus is encircled through the access incision and transected with an endoscopic vascular stapler brought through the anterior thoracoport. The ongoing pulmonary artery (pars interlobaris) is dissected sharply and the recurrent branch to the posterior segment identified. This arterial branch is best divided from an anterior approach, again bringing

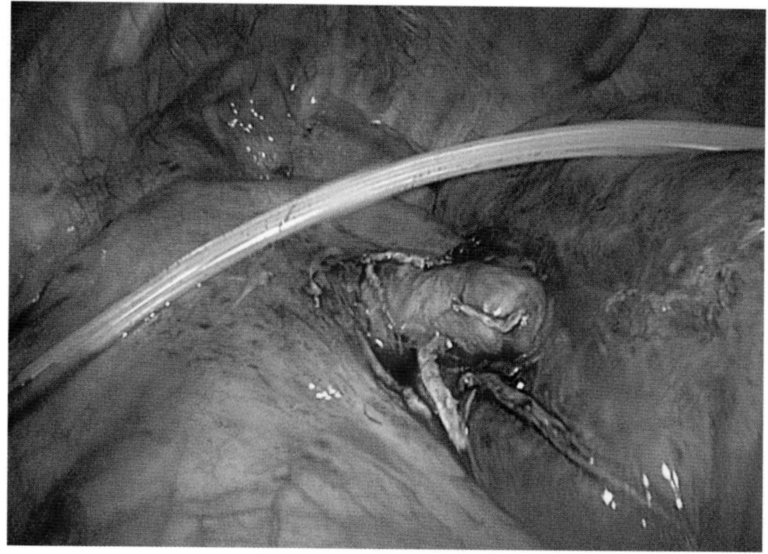

Figure 21.9

A soft drain is inserted through the posterior thoracoport and looped over the lower lobe to drain the space previously occupied by the left upper lobe

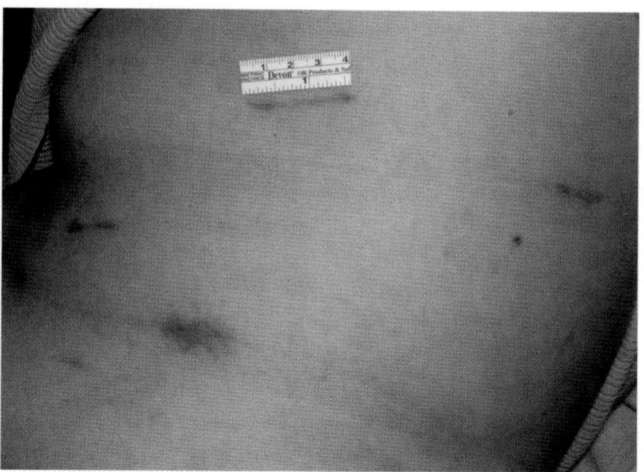

Figure 21.10

The incisions used for left VATS lobectomy. A ruler is placed above the 4-cm access incision

the endoscopic vascular stapler through the anterior thoracoport. Depending on anatomy, this can be done before or after dividing the right upper lobe bronchus. Unlike right upper lobectomy via posterolateral thoracotomy, we find that the bronchus is best approached anteriorly. It is dissected sharply through the access incision and divided with an endoscopic stapler through the anterior thoracoport. After bronchial division, the lobe remains attached only by the fissure, which can then be divided using serial application of an endoscopic stapler passed through the anterior thoracoport. Alternatively, the bronchus can be circumferentially dissected and used as a landmark for completion of the fissure and divided last. The resected lobe is placed into a large endoscopic bag and removed through the access incision. The bronchial stump and parenchymal staple lines are then pressurized and tested for air leak by immersing them in saline, which is instilled through the access incision.

Right Middle Lobectomy

Right middle lobectomy can be done by an approach through the fissure or an anterior approach. A fissure approach commences with dissection at the confluence of the minor (horizontal) and major fissures. This exposes the interlobar portion of the pulmonary artery. The middle lobe is retracted anteriorly through the anterior thoracoport and arterial dissection carried out through the access incision. The middle lobe artery, which may have one or two branches, is encircled and transected with an endoscopic vascular stapler. The bronchus is then exposed, dissected, and transected through the posterior port. Next, the lobe is reflected posteriorly and the middle lobe vein transected through the anterior port. Care must be taken when separating it from the upper lobe vein. Finally, the fissure is completed and the lobe placed in an endoscopic retrieval bag and removed through the access incision.

When an anterior approach is chosen, the sequence of exposure and division is reversed, with division first of the middle lobe vein followed by airway, bronchus, and fissure.

Right Lower Lobectomy

The lower lobe is retracted superiorly through the access incision, facilitating division of inferior pulmonary ligament and mediastinal pleura. The inferior pulmonary vein can then be easily dissected through the anterior thoracoport. After confirming the presence of a superior pulmonary vein, the inferior vein is encircled and transected using an endoscopic vascular stapler through the anterior thoracoport.

Blunt dissection at the confluence of the major and minor fissures is followed by sharp scissor dissection that identifies the plane over the basilar trunks of the pulmonary artery. Next, the superior segmental artery is identified, sharply dissected, and encircled. The middle lobe artery is identified and spared. The basilar and superior segmental branches are then individually transected with serial fires of an endoscopic vascular stapler passed through the anterior thoracoport. The fissure is completed with an endoscopic stapler placed through the anterior thoracoport. Finally, the superior segmental and basal segmental bronchi are individually transected to avoid impingement on the middle lobe bronchus. The specimen is placed in an endoscopic retrieval bag and removed.

Left Upper Lobectomy

The left upper lobe tends to have the most variable arterial blood supply, so vascular dissection should be carried out with attention to anatomic irregularities. After sharp division of the mediastinal pleura, dissection of the superior pulmonary vein and pulmonary artery is carried out through the access incision while retracting the lung posteriorly through the posterior access port. Through the access incision, the pulmonary vein is encircled with a right-angled clamp and then divided with an endoscopic vascular stapler passed through the anterior thoracoport. Division of the superior pulmonary vein exposes the first, short, anterior branch of the pulmonary artery and the more distal apicoposterior trunk. These are encircled and divided sequentially with the endovascular stapler placed through the anterior port. The distal ongoing pulmonary artery, as well as the upper lobe bronchus, becomes increasingly exposed with division of successive arterial branches. At this point, the anterior portion of the fissure can be divided using serial applications of an endoscopic stapler. The lingular branches of the pulmonary artery are now identified and divided. Alternatively, while reflecting the lobe posteriorly and depending upon the angle, the upper lobe bronchus may be divided first through the anterior access incision or thoracoport. Finally, the posterior aspect of the fissure is completed and the specimen removed.

Left Lower Lobectomy

The lung is mobilized and the inferior pulmonary ligament transected. The inferior pulmonary vein is dissected and transected with an endoscopic vascular stapler passed through the anterior thoracoport. The pulmonary artery is then exposed in the fissure using a combination of blunt and sharp dissection while the lower lobe is retracted inferiorly through the posterior thoracoport. Once the basilar trunk and the superior segmental branches of the pulmonary artery are identified, they are serially encircled and transected using an endoscopic vascular stapler passed through the anterior thoracoport. Division of the posterior aspect of the fissure through the anterior thoracoport facilitates arterial exposure. The anterior aspect of the fissure is then divided with an endoscopic stapler passed through the anterior thoracoport. Next, the lower lobe bronchus is dissected and transected using an endoscopic stapler. The specimen is placed in an endoscopic retrieval bag and extracted through the access incision.

Indications for Open Conversion

VATS lobectomy must sometimes be converted to open thoracotomy. As surgeon experience and comfort with VATS techniques increase, this should become an infrequent event [15–18]. We believe that there are several indications for conversion to thoracotomy, including major hemorrhage, uncertainty in identifying the location of a lesion, unclear surgical anatomy, and positive surgical margin. Major hemorrhage is clearly the most feared complication by surgeons. However, rapid placement of a sponge-stick through the access incision successfully tamponades most bleeding and allows controlled thoracotomy and repair. The location and nature of vascular injury dictate the choice of thoracotomy. We recommend posterolateral thoracotomy in the event of a proximal pulmonary artery injury. Otherwise, bleeding can typically be controlled via extension of the access incision and limited anterolateral thoracotomy.

Other problems requiring conversion to thoracotomy are less frequent. If the lobe in which the cancer is located is not identified with certainty on preoperative imaging and cannot be identified at VATS, a thoracotomy is necessary and clearly mandated. Similarly, if vascular or bronchial anatomy is not clearly identifiable, conversion to thoracotomy must be performed. Positive bronchial or parenchymal staple-line margins should be explored by thoracotomy and re-resection carried out to obtain a negative margin.

Palliation

Malignant pleural effusion complicating lung cancer is a terminal finding, with median survival in the range of 2–6 months [58, 59]. Effective palliation is paramount, and repeated thoracentesis has fortunately given way to more definitive management strategies. In fit patients in whom the lung is not entrapped, VATS drainage and talc pleurodesis can effectively palliate malignant pleural effusion. However, VATS talc pleurodesis was found to be no more effective in palliation of malignant pleural effusions than bedside talc instillation via a chest tube [60]. Pleural symphysis requires lung expansion. When the lung is entrapped or where general anesthesia and VATS are not indicated, percutaneous placement of an indwelling pleural catheter (PleurX®, Denver Biomedical, Golden, CO) is highly effective in managing malignant pleural effusions [61]. Outpatient management of malignant pleural effusions with chronic indwelling catheters reduces treatment costs [62]. Removal of pleural catheters is possible, but is highly unlikely in lung cancer patients [63]. Many physicians now use permanent indwelling pleural catheters as the treatment of choice regardless of patient status or expected median survival. However, in patients with lung cancer and malignant pleural effusions, there are many management options, and treatment personalization is necessary.

Conclusions

Minimally invasive approaches to lung cancer are available for diagnosis, staging, definitive treatment, and palliation. Application of VATS techniques requires training, dedication to their use, and thoughtful application to ensure equivalent or superior outcome to open surgery. We have chosen to focus this chapter on VATS lobectomy because it is a significant technological advance in the treatment of lung cancer that has taken almost 20 years to gain acceptance [64, 65]. It represents what can be accomplished with thoughtful application of new technology, patience, and persistence [20, 66].

Acknowledgments Supported by the Daniel and Karen Lee Endowed Chair in Thoracic Surgery, Cleveland Clinic, Cleveland, OH.

References

1. Whitson BA, Andrade RS, Boettcher A et al (2007) Video-assisted thoracoscopic surgery is more favorable than thoracotomy for resection of clinical stage I non-small cell lung cancer. Ann Thorac Surg 83(6):1965–1970
2. Whitson BA, Groth SS, Duval SJ, Swanson SJ, Maddaus MA (2008) Surgery for early-stage non-small cell lung cancer: a systematic review of the video-assisted thoracoscopic surgery versus thoracotomy approaches to lobectomy. Ann Thorac Surg 86(6):2008–2016, discussion 16–18
3. Grogan EL, Jones DR (2008) VATS lobectomy is better than open thoracotomy: what is the evidence for short-term outcomes? Thorac Surg Clin 18(3):249–258
4. Yim AP, Wan S, Lee TW, Arifi AA (2000) VATS lobectomy reduces cytokine responses compared with conventional surgery. Ann Thorac Surg 70(1):243–247
5. Ng CS, Wan S, Hui CW et al (2007) Video-assisted thoracic surgery lobectomy for lung cancer is associated with less immunochemokine disturbances than thoracotomy. Eur J Cardiothorac Surg 31(1):83–87
6. Ng CS, Lee TW, Wan S et al (2005) Thoracotomy is associated with significantly more profound suppression in lymphocytes and natural killer cells than video-assisted thoracic surgery following major lung resections for cancer. J Invest Surg 18(2):81–88
7. Sagawa M, Sato M, Sakurada A et al (2002) A prospective trial of systematic nodal dissection for lung cancer by video-assisted thoracic surgery: can it be perfect? Ann Thorac Surg 73(3):900–904
8. Kaseda S, Hangai N, Yamamoto S, Kitano M (1997) Lobectomy with extended lymph node dissection by video-assisted thoracic surgery for lung cancer. Surg Endosc 11(7):703–706

9. Watanabe A, Koyanagi T, Ohsawa H et al (2005) Systematic node dissection by VATS is not inferior to that through an open thoracotomy: a comparative clinicopathologic retrospective study. Surgery 138(3):510–517
10. Kaiser D, Ennker IC, Hartz C (1993) Video-assisted thoracoscopic surgery–indications, results, complications, and contraindications. Thorac Cardiovasc Surg 41(6): 330–334
11. Sedrakyan A, van der Meulen J, Lewsey J, Treasure T (2004) Video assisted thoracic surgery for treatment of pneumothorax and lung resections: systematic review of randomised clinical trials. BMJ 329(7473):1008
12. Nakamura H (2007) Controversies in thoracoscopic lobectomy for lung cancer. Ann Thorac Cardiovasc Surg 13(4):225–227
13. Nicastri DG, Wisnivesky JP, Litle VR et al (2008) Thoracoscopic lobectomy: report on safety, discharge independence, pain, and chemotherapy tolerance. J Thorac Cardiovasc Surg 135(3):642–647
14. Kirby TJ, Mack MJ, Landreneau RJ, Rice TW (1995) Lobectomy–video-assisted thoracic surgery versus muscle-sparing thoracotomy. A randomized trial. J Thorac Cardiovasc Surg 109(5):997–1001, discussion 2
15. Swanson SJ, Herndon JE 2nd, D'Amico TA et al (2007) Video-assisted thoracic surgery lobectomy: report of CALGB 39802 – a prospective, multi-institution feasibility study. J Clin Oncol 25(31):4993–4997
16. McKenna RJ Jr (2008) Complications and learning curves for video-assisted thoracic surgery lobectomy. Thorac Surg Clin 18(3):275–280
17. Reed MF, Lucia MW, Starnes SL, Merrill WH, Howington JA (2008) Thoracoscopic lobectomy: introduction of a new technique into a thoracic surgery training program. J Thorac Cardiovasc Surg 136(2):376–381
18. Wan IY, Thung KH, Hsin MK, Underwood MJ, Yim AP (2008) Video-assisted thoracic surgery major lung resection can be safely taught to trainees. Ann Thorac Surg 85(2):416–419
19. Ng T, Ryder BA (2006) Evolution to video-assisted thoracic surgery lobectomy after training: initial results of the first 30 patients. J Am Coll Surg 203(4):551–557
20. McKenna RJ Jr, Houck W, Fuller CB (2006) Video-assisted thoracic surgery lobectomy: experience with 1,100 cases. Ann Thorac Surg 81(2):421–425, discussion 5–6
21. Flores RM, Alam N (2008) Video-assisted thoracic surgery lobectomy (VATS), open thoracotomy, and the robot for lung cancer. Ann Thorac Surg 85(2):S710–S715
22. Shaw JP, Dembitzer FR, Wisnivesky JP et al (2008) Video-assisted thoracoscopic lobectomy: state of the art and future directions. Ann Thorac Surg 85(2):S705–S709
23. Shigemura N, Akashi A, Funaki S et al (2006) Long-term outcomes after a variety of video-assisted thoracoscopic lobectomy approaches for clinical stage IA lung cancer: a multi-institutional study. J Thorac Cardiovasc Surg 132(3):507–512
24. Alam N, Flores RM (2007) Video-assisted thoracic surgery (VATS) lobectomy: the evidence base. JSLS 11(3):368–374
25. Suzuki K, Nagai K, Yoshida J et al (1999) Video-assisted thoracoscopic surgery for small indeterminate pulmonary nodules: indications for preoperative marking. Chest 115(2):563–568
26. Gonfiotti A, Davini F, Vaggelli L et al (2007) Thoracoscopic localization techniques for patients with solitary pulmonary nodule: hookwire versus radio-guided surgery. Eur J Cardiothorac Surg 32(6):843–847
27. Sortini D, Feo CV, Carcoforo P et al (2005) Thoracoscopic localization techniques for patients with solitary pulmonary nodule and history of malignancy. Ann Thorac Surg 79(1):258–262, discussion 62
28. Burdine J, Joyce LD, Plunkett MB, Inampudi S, Kaye MG, Dunn DH (2002) Feasibility and value of video-assisted thoracoscopic surgery wedge excision of small pulmonary nodules in patients with malignancy. Chest 122(4): 1467–1470
29. Stiles BM, Altes TA, Jones DR et al (2006) Clinical experience with radiotracer-guided thoracoscopic biopsy of small, indeterminate lung nodules. Ann Thorac Surg 82(4): 1191–1196, discussion 6–7
30. Watanabe K, Nomori H, Ohtsuka T, Kaji M, Naruke T, Suemasu K (2006) Usefulness and complications of computed tomography-guided lipiodol marking for fluoroscopy-assisted thoracoscopic resection of small pulmonary nodules: experience with 174 nodules. J Thorac Cardiovasc Surg 132(2):320–324
31. Dendo S, Kanazawa S, Ando A et al (2002) Preoperative localization of small pulmonary lesions with a short hook wire and suture system: experience with 168 procedures. Radiology 225(2):511–518
32. Warren WH, Faber LP (1994) Segmentectomy versus lobectomy in patients with stage I pulmonary carcinoma. Five-year survival and patterns of intrathoracic recurrence. J Thorac Cardiovasc Surg 107(4):1087–1093, discussion 93–94
33. Ginsberg RJ, Rubinstein LV (1995) Randomized trial of lobectomy versus limited resection for T1 N0 non-small cell lung cancer. Lung Cancer Study Group. Ann Thorac Surg 60(3):615–622, discussion 22–23
34. Kodama K, Doi O, Higashiyama M, Yokouchi H (1997) Intentional limited resection for selected patients with T1 N0 M0 non-small-cell lung cancer: a single-institution study. J Thorac Cardiovasc Surg 114(3):347–353
35. Shennib H, Bogart J, Herndon JE et al (2005) Video-assisted wedge resection and local radiotherapy for peripheral lung cancer in high-risk patients: the Cancer and Leukemia Group B (CALGB) 9335, a phase II, multi-institutional cooperative group study. J Thorac Cardiovasc Surg 129(4):813–818
36. Okada M, Koike T, Higashiyama M, Yamato Y, Kodama K, Tsubota N (2006) Radical sublobar resection for small-sized non-small cell lung cancer: a multicenter study. J Thorac Cardiovasc Surg 132(4):769–775
37. El-Sherif A, Fernando HC, Santos R et al (2007) Margin and local recurrence after sublobar resection of non-small cell lung cancer. Ann Surg Oncol 14(8):2400–2405
38. McKenna RJ Jr, Mahtabifard A, Yap J et al (2008) Wedge resection and brachytherapy for lung cancer in patients with poor pulmonary function. Ann Thorac Surg 85(2): S733–S736
39. Yoshikawa K, Tsubota N, Kodama K, Ayabe H, Taki T, Mori T (2002) Prospective study of extended segmentectomy for small lung tumors: the final report. Ann Thorac Surg 73(4):1055–1058, discussion 8–9

40. Okada M, Yoshikawa K, Hatta T, Tsubota N (2001) Is segmentectomy with lymph node assessment an alternative to lobectomy for non-small cell lung cancer of 2 cm or smaller? Ann Thorac Surg 71(3):956–960, discussion 61
41. Yamanaka A, Hirai T, Fujimoto T, Ohtake Y, Konishi F (2000) Analyses of segmental lymph node metastases and intrapulmonary metastases of small lung cancer. Ann Thorac Surg 70(5):1624–1628
42. Bernard A, Brondel L, Arnal E, Favre JP (2006) Evaluation of respiratory muscle strength by randomized controlled trial comparing thoracoscopy, transaxillary thoracotomy, and posterolateral thoracotomy for lung biopsy. Eur J Cardiothorac Surg 29(4):596–600
43. Yendamuri S, Komaki RR, Correa AM et al (2007) Comparison of limited surgery and three-dimensional conformal radiation in high-risk patients with stage I non-small cell lung cancer. J Thorac Oncol 2(11):1022–1028
44. Iwasaki A, Shirakusa T, Shiraishi T, Yamamoto S (2004) Results of video-assisted thoracic surgery for stage I/II non-small cell lung cancer. Eur J Cardiothorac Surg 26(1): 158–164
45. Rankin S (2008) PET/CT for staging and monitoring non small cell lung cancer. Cancer Imaging 8(Suppl A):S27–S31
46. Kernstine KH, Stanford W, Mullan BF et al (1999) PET, CT, and MRI with Combidex for mediastinal staging in non-small cell lung carcinoma. Ann Thorac Surg 68(3): 1022–1028
47. Lardinois D, Weder W, Hany TF et al (2003) Staging of non-small-cell lung cancer with integrated positron-emission tomography and computed tomography. N Engl J Med 348(25):2500–2507
48. Shim SS, Lee KS, Kim BT et al (2005) Non-small cell lung cancer: prospective comparison of integrated FDG PET/CT and CT alone for preoperative staging. Radiology 236(3):1011–1019
49. Ferguson MK, Little L, Rizzo L et al (1988) Diffusing capacity predicts morbidity and mortality after pulmonary resection. J Thorac Cardiovasc Surg 96(6):894–900
50. Ferguson MK, Reeder LB, Mick R (1995) Optimizing selection of patients for major lung resection. J Thorac Cardiovasc Surg 109(2):275–281, discussion 81–83
51. Filaire M, Bedu M, Naamee A et al (1999) Prediction of hypoxemia and mechanical ventilation after lung resection for cancer. Ann Thorac Surg 67(5): 1460–1465
52. Kocabas A, Kara K, Ozgur G, Sonmez H, Burgut R (1996) Value of preoperative spirometry to predict post-operative pulmonary complications. Respir Med 90(1): 25–33
53. Mazzone PJ, Arroliga AC (2005) Lung cancer: preoperative pulmonary evaluation of the lung resection candidate. Am J Med 118(6):578–583
54. Garzon JC, Ng CS, Sihoe AD et al (2006) Video-assisted thoracic surgery pulmonary resection for lung cancer in patients with poor lung function. Ann Thorac Surg 81(6):1996–2003
55. Cattaneo SM, Park BJ, Wilton AS et al (2008) Use of video-assisted thoracic surgery for lobectomy in the elderly results in fewer complications. Ann Thorac Surg 85(1):231–235, discussion 5–6
56. Jaklitsch MT, DeCamp MM Jr, Liptay MJ et al (1996) Video-assisted thoracic surgery in the elderly. A review of 307 cases. Chest 110(3):751–758
57. Kim K, Rice TW, Murthy SC et al (2004) Combined bronchoscopy, mediastinoscopy, and thoracotomy for lung cancer: who benefits? J Thorac Cardiovasc Surg 127(3): 850–856
58. Sugiura S, Ando Y, Minami H, Ando M, Sakai S, Shimokata K (1997) Prognostic value of pleural effusion in patients with non-small cell lung cancer. Clin Cancer Res 3(1): 47–50
59. Mott FE, Sharma N, Ashley P (2001) Malignant pleural effusion in non-small cell lung cancer–time for a stage revision? Chest 119(1):317–318
60. Dresler CM, Olak J, Herndon JE 2nd et al (2005) Phase III intergroup study of talc poudrage vs. talc slurry sclerosis for malignant pleural effusion. Chest 127(3):909–915
61. Murthy SC, Okereke I, Mason DP, Rice TW (2006) A simple solution for complicated pleural effusions. J Thorac Oncol 1(7):697–700
62. Putnam JB Jr, Walsh GL, Swisher SG et al (2000) Outpatient management of malignant pleural effusion by a chronic indwelling pleural catheter. Ann Thorac Surg 69(2): 369–375
63. Warren WH, Kim AW, Liptay MJ (2008) Identification of clinical factors predicting Pleurx catheter removal in patients treated for malignant pleural effusion. Eur J Cardiothorac Surg 33(1):89–94
64. Kirby TJ, Rice TW (1993) Thoracoscopic lobectomy. Ann Thorac Surg 56(3):784–786
65. Kirby TJ, Mack MJ, Landreneau RJ, Rice TW (1993) Initial experience with video-assisted thoracoscopic lobectomy. Ann Thorac Surg 56(6):1248–1252, discussion 52–53
66. Onaitis MW, Petersen RP, Balderson SS et al (2006) Thoracoscopic lobectomy is a safe and versatile procedure: experience with 500 consecutive patients. Ann Surg 244(3):420–425

of a uterine manipulator during the procedure. In a retrospective review of cases at Memorial Sloan Kettering it was noted that women who had minimally invasive surgery including a LAVH for endometrial cancer were more than three times more likely to have positive peritoneal cytology than those having abdominal surgery [31]. However, the significance of this finding is unknown. Also, other studies have examined this issue and not reported an increase in positive peritoneal cytology [32]. A single prospective study did not demonstrate any difference in positive cytology rates [33]. Because intraabdominal recurrence is rare for endometrial adenocarcinomas it is doubtful that tanstubal spread poses a significant risk.

Despite the fact that laparoscopy offers shorter recovery times, less wound morbidity, and better quality of life, acceptance of minimally invasive surgery into the practice of gynecologic oncology has been slow. A survey of the members of the Society of Gynecologic Oncologists suggested that only 45% of full members utilize this technique at all and only 6% state that they offer laparoscopic staging to more than 50% of their patients with endometrial cancer [17]. Although these numbers are low, this does represent a significant increase over the past 5 years [12]. Some of the resistance to adopting a minimally invasive approach to endometrial cancer surgery has been the need for retraining and increased operative times. The average increase in operative time is about 40 min, but there is a learning curve with a significant decrease in operative time, and an increase in the number of lymph nodes obtained during surgery after the first 25 cases [22]. As training and experience in these techniques increase it is likely that interest in minimally invasive surgery in endometrial cancer will increase. There is also interest in the use of robot-assisted surgery in endometrial cancer. While there is no proven patient benefit to the use of robotically assisted techniques, this may allow some surgeons to feel more comfortable performing minimally invasive surgery.

Ovarian Tumors

Benign Masses

The diagnosis of a pelvic mass is a common indication for surgery in gynecology. While the majority of these masses are benign, it is difficult to completely exclude malignancy prior to surgery. Removal of a pelvic mass is indicated in a premenopausal woman if the mass is greater than 10 cm in size or there is abdominal pain suggestive of ovarian torsion. For masses less than 10 cm, a functional cyst must be excluded prior to surgery. To exclude a functional cyst or hemorrhagic corpus luteum as the cause of the mass delay of 6 weeks with a repeat ultrasound is indicate [34]. For postmenopausal women, all masses should be removed unless the mass is less than 5 cm, completely simple, has no septations, and the Ca-125 is in the normal range [35, 36]. For masses that meet all these criteria, reassessment in 3 months is sufficient to ensure that the mass is not enlarging with routine examinations every 6–12 months afterward.

The traditional approach to a pelvic mass has been through a midline laparotomy. However, with sufficient laparoscopic expertise many masses can be safely approached with a minimally invasive approach. A Cochrane review has evaluated the utility of a laparoscopic approach to benign ovarian masses [37]. In this review it was noted that the surgical time for laparoscopy was longer. However, the increase in the laparoscopy group was only 11 min. Not surprisingly, the febrile morbidity (OR 0.34; 95% CI 0.13–0.88) and postoperative discomfort were significantly less in the laparoscopy group. The overall complication rate (OR 0.26; 95% CI 0.12–0.55) was also less. The length of hospital stay was reduced by an average of 2.8 days with an overall cost reduction of $1,045.00 per case. However, the authors caution that there was a limited sample size on which to draw these conclusions.

The American College of Obstetrics and Gynecology and the Society of Gynecologic Oncologists have published guidelines for referral of masses to a gynecologic oncologist. These include premenopausal women with a pelvic mass who have evidence of metastatic ovarian cancer, ascites, a Ca-125 over 200, or a strong family history. For postmenopausal women, referral should be made for similar indications but with any elevation of the Ca-125 level [38]. These guidelines have been reviewed in a multiinstitutional study and were shown to have a sensitivity of 70% in premenopausal women and 94% in postmenopausal women with a negative predictive value of over 90% in both groups [39].

The ACOG and SGO referral guidelines perform well except in premenopausal women with early ovarian cancer. While the sensitivity of these guideline for early ovarian cancer in postmenopausal women is 80%, the sensitivity in premenopausal women is only 56% [40]. It has been noted that the incidence of ovarian cancer in the population rises sharply at age 40. Therefore when evaluating an ovarian mass, it is prudent to have a high suspicion in the perimenopausal age group between age 40 and 50, even in the presence of a normal Ca-125 level. In this group ultrasound evaluation can be used as another screening tool. A number of ultrasound criteria have been proposed based on the size of the mass, the presence of mural nodules, and presence and characteristics of the internal septae. It was noted that one such ultrasound screening system was 89% sensitive with a negative predictive value of 96% [41].

If a malignant ovarian mass is encountered at the time of laparoscopy, careful documentation of findings in the upper abdomen including the omentum, diaphragm, peritoneal surfaces, and lymph nodes should be made. Saline can be used to obtain pelvic washings. If the mass has been removed at laparoscopy and gynecologic oncology consultation is not available, there is no need for an immediate laparotomy. The patient is best served by completing the intended laparoscopic operation with expedient referral to an expert in gynecologic oncology.

Risk of Rupture

Ideally, abdominal masses should be removed from the abdominal cavity without rupture or spillage in case of malignancy. One of the major concerns over laparoscopic removal of ovarian masses is the possibility that rupture of a mass might result in seeding of the abdominal cavity. The risk of rupture can be reduced if masses are placed in a protective bag and brought out through the umbilical incision or alternatively through the vagina at the time of a hysterectomy. Bags manufactured for use in spleenectomy that are made of nylon and coated with polyurethane are ideal for this purpose and come in sizes up to 8″ × 10″ which is large enough to remove a 10–12 cm mass [42].

One of the concerns about the use of laparoscopy for the removal of pelvic masses has been the risk of rupture. With the exclusion of endometriomas, it is not entirely clear that the risk of rupture is higher with laparoscopy. Randomized trials have demonstrated rupture rates of between 25 and 30% for both laparotomy and laparoscopy [43, 44]. In a study that excluded endometriomas, the risk of rupture with laparoscopy was 6% compared to 2% with endometriomas [45] (see Table 22.2).

When laparoscopic spillage does occur in cases of a malignant mass, it is not clear that the long-term prognosis is worse. With a malignant mass, rupture can change the stage. If the mass is unruptured and there is no extra-ovarian spread the FIGO and TNM stage is IA. However, a ruptured mass is to be classified as a FIGO and TNM stage IC with a note that the rupture is iatrogenic [46]. Women with stage IA grades 1 and 2 tumors normally do not need adjuvant chemotherapy. However, the standard of care is to give at least three cycles of chemotherapy to women with iatrogenic stage IC ovarian cancers. However, after postoperative chemotherapy there is no convincing evidence that the risk of recurrence is any different than if the tumor had not ruptured. In the largest retrospective series that attempted to examine this issue it was noted that the risk of recurrence was higher in women with ruptured masses in low-grade tumors with rupture (9% vs. 6%) and in high-grade tumors (28% vs. 31%) [47]. However, dense adhesions between the tumor and other pelvic structures have also been noted to be a risk factor for recurrence and may be the cause for tumor rupture at the time of surgery. In their series, the risk of recurrence was higher in low-grade tumor with adhesions (6% vs. 31%) and in high-grade tumors with adhesions (26% vs. 42%). It was theorized that women

Table 22.2. Randomized trials of laparoscopy vs. open surgery for the removal of pelvic masses

Author	Year	*n*	OR time (min)		Rupture	
			Open	Laparoscopy	Open	Laparoscopy
Fanfani et al. [45]	2004	100	87	72	2%[a]	6%[a]
Yuen et al. [91]	1995	102	52	59	30%	27%
Deckardt et al. [110]	1994	192	116	97	Not reported	

[a] Excluded endometriomas

with dense adhesions were at higher risk of rupture and the adhesions were actually a surrogate for more aggressive or higher stage tumors. When women with dense adhesions were excluded from the analysis, the risk of recurrence with rupture of the tumor was identical to that in unruptured tumors. It should be noted that most of the women in this study did not undergo a systematic staging procedure. Therefore, it is unclear how applicable these data are to women who have had a complete staging procedure. Other retrospective series have found that recurrence does not increase recurrence or that the prognostic significance is lost when a multivariate analysis is performed [48, 49].

Low Malignant Potential (Atypically Proliferating) Tumors of the Ovary

Tumors that display atypical architectural features that do not meet the criteria for invasive malignancy are referred to as tumors of low malignant potential. These tumors are often confined to one ovary, but advanced disease is occasionally present. Overall, the prognosis is excellent for these tumors. In a series of 146 stage I low malignant potential tumors followed by the GOG for a median of 42 months, there were no recurrences [50]. Even when disease is present outside the ovary the prognosis is excellent with a 95% 5-year survival with noninvasive implants and a 66% 5-year survival in the presence of invasive implants [51]. Optimal therapy is complete resection of all visible disease.

During open cases, a staging procedure is often performed in women with low malignant potential tumors. Staging can detect invasive implants in these women and might indicate a group that would benefit from adjuvant chemotherapy. However, the risk of invasive implants is small. More often this procedure is done because some of these women will be determined to have an overtly malignant ovarian tumor on the final pathology report. Thus, a staging procedure can potentially prevent the need for chemotherapy or a second staging operation in women who turn out to have an early ovarian carcinoma. It is more difficult to justify the staging of all women with low malignant potential tumors when the surgery is being performed laparoscopically due to length of the procedure and the technical difficulty of staging. If the patient is having an open procedure, there is a chance that a second laparotomy will be needed, which is not the case if the initial surgery is being performed laparoscopically.

In a review of the use of laparoscopy in women with low malignant potential tumors, it was noted the risk of rupture and recurrence was higher with laparoscopic surgery (see Fig. 22.1) [52]. However, most of these tumors recurred as low malignant potential tumors and the overall mortality was not different. Conservative therapy can also be contemplated in these women with a unilateral oophorectomy or

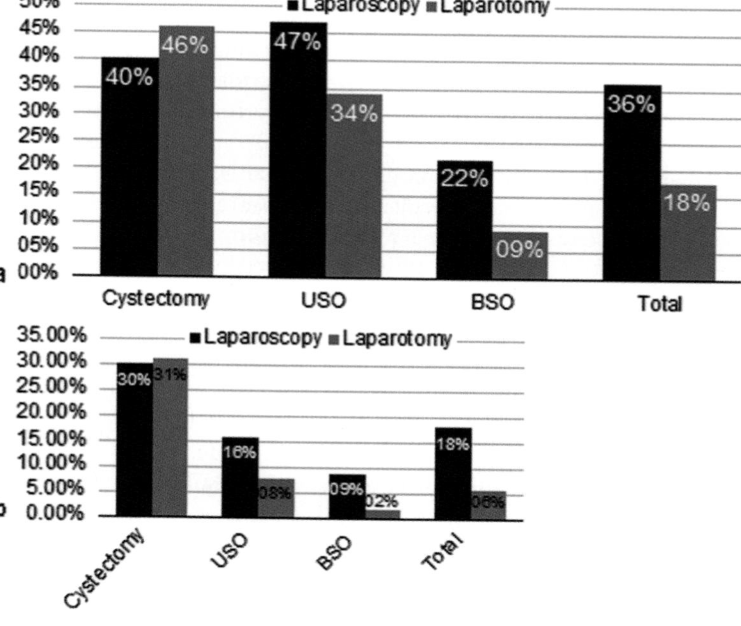

Figure 22.1

(**a**) Risk of rupture by type of surgery in atypically proliferating tumors of the ovary. From Poncelet et al. [52] (**b**) Risk of recurrence by type of surgery in atypically proliferating tumors of the ovary (reprinted with permission from Poncelet et al. [52]). USO = Unilateral Salpingo-oophorectomy, BSO = [Bilateral salpingo-oophorectomy

even a cystectomy. While the cure rate is higher with oophorectomy, a cystectomy can be performed without compromising overall survival if only one ovary is present or the tumor is small. In a large series of women with low malignant potential tumors the risk of recurrence was about 6% and the mortality was 0.2% after conservative therapy [53]. Overall, the fertility in this group was 60% after surgery.

Staging in Early Ovarian Cancer

For early ovarian cancer, adjuvant therapy may not be necessary in grade 1 or grade 2 tumors if the tumor is limited to the ovary. However, staging information in this situation is critical, as it has been demonstrated that treatment decisions in absence of staging information negatively impacts survival [11]. It has been shown that when ovarian cancer is apparently confined to one ovary there is extraovarian disease in over one third of patients [54]. Of the women with presumed stage I ovarian cancer, 13% were demonstrated to have aortic lymph node metastases, 8% pelvic lymph node metastases, and 33% malignant peritoneal washings. Serous tumors have been noted to have a very high incidence of para-aortic nodal metastasis with rates of isolated spread to this nodal group in over 20% of cases [55].

The first case report of laparoscopic staging of early ovarian cancer was by Riech in 1990 [56]. He performed a vaginal hysterectomy and removed an early ovarian cancer intact. He then used the laparoscope to complete the staging with an omentectomy and lymphadenectomy. While laparoscopic staging has now gained acceptance, it should only be performed by surgeons skilled in laparoscopic retroperitoneal dissection.

There has been concern about using laparoscopy to stage ovarian cancer. Difficulty with exposure can make a complete para-aortic lymphadenectomy difficult with a transperitoneal approach, especially on the left side. Anatomically, the lymphatic drainage follows the ovarian vessels, and lymphatic dissection should include tissue to the level of these vessels, and preferably to just below the renal vessels. It has been noted that 75% of positive para-aortic nodes are above the level of the inferior mesenteric vessels [55]. Several authors have reported results both laparoscopic transperitoneal and laparoscopic retroperitoneal lymphadenectomy in testicular cancer with results that are comparable to open procedures [57–59]. Retroperitoneal exposure is maximized with mobilization of the colon, but may require repositioning the patients after hysterectomy and bilateral oophorectomy. Visualization with a retroperitoneal approach can be excellent. However, it also requires special positioning and ideally needs to be done prior to any intraperitoneal laparoscopic procedure. In patients with early ovarian cancer, the diagnosis is often not known until after the ovary is removed. However, for restaging of patients who had an incidental cancer noted at a previous hysterectomy, the retroperitoneal approach is attractive.

As many as 10–15% of women with ovarian cancer are younger than 40 years old [60]. Conservative therapy for women who wish to maintain fertility can be contemplated if the tumor is apparently limited to one ovary. In this case, a unilateral oophorectomy, contralateral ovarian biopsy and complete surgical staging including omentectomy, unilateral pelvic and para-aortic lymphadentectomy, and careful inspection of all peritoneal surfaces. There is some controversy over whether or not a normal appearing contralateral ovary should be biopsied. Originally it was felt the incidence of bilaterality was high enough to justify this procedure. However, this can adversely effect fertility. Pathologic examination of biopsies from contralateral ovaries in completely staged women with tumors limited to the ovary documented disease in only 2% of cases and the risk of recurrence in the contralateral ovary is reported to be between 4 and 7% [61, 62]. Outcomes after conservative surgery have been good. A summary of all of the European trials with conservative surgery suggest that the cancer-related mortality is under 6% after conservative therapy of early ovarian cancer [61]. In a summary of the pregnancy outcomes it was noted that 53 of the 152 (35%) women conceived, resulting in 38 full-term pregnancies. No larger series have compared the effectiveness of laparoscopic conservative therapy to laparotomy. However, if retention of fertility is an option, fecundity may be better after laparoscopic surgery as compared to open surgery as the possibility of severe pelvic adhesions is lessened with a minimally invasive approach.

Advanced Ovarian Cancer

Survival in advanced ovarian cancer depends on the concept of maximal surgical effort. Although advanced ovarian cancer can rarely be completely resected at the time of surgery, there is significant survival benefit if the majority of disease can be removed. Ideally, all visible disease should be resected but there is still significant survival benefit if the largest residual focus of disease is less than 1 cm. Advanced ovarian cancer is challenging to manage through the laparoscope and is often not amenable to a minimally invasive approach. Significant s and bulky disease cannot be easily manipulated with small laparoscopic instruments and radical procedures for ovarian cancer delbulking are often required. However, laparoscopy can be used for diagnostic purposes, to gauge if patients are candidates for optimal cytoreduction, and can be used to remove upper abdominal disease in some cases [63, 64]. Laparoscopy has also been used to restage patients with ovarian cancer after neoadjuvant chemotherapy [65]. In cases with good therapeutic response to neoadjuvant therapy, the surgery can be completed without a laparotomy.

Second Look Surgery in Ovarian Cancer

Second look surgery in ovarian cancer was a concept originally introduced in colon cancer by Wangensteen for revaluation of patients [66]. In ovarian cancer this operation was performed to determine if patients who had a complete clinical response to chemotherapy could discontinue treatment since the chemotherapy was leukogenic and typically recommended for up to a year after the original surgery. Later, second look surgery was used to evaluate response in clinical trials as the surgical complete response rate to chemotherapy was an excellent surrogate for survival when comparing chemotherapy regimens. However, because of the significant morbidity of this surgery and a lack of data that would suggest that this surgery provides a survival advantage, this procedure is no longer routinely performed [67]. However, there are situations where surgical evaluation after primary therapy is still appropriate such as for the women who has completed therapy and has a normal CT scan but has persistently elevated tumor markers.

Minimally invasive techniques were applied to second look surgery in an attempt to lessen the morbidity and recovery from this procedure. Unfortunately, the morbidity of laparoscopy in women who have had previous radical surgery is significant. In a large series it was noted that the bowel injury rate exceeded 10% [68]. In addition to relatively high complication rates there are other challenges with laparoscopic surgery for second look assessment including the inability to palpate intraabdominal organs and visualize all of the peritoneal surfaces including the bowel mesentary and peritoneal gutters. Overall the false-positive rate of second look laparoscopy has been reported to be as high as 55% [69]. However, in patients having a second look procedure it has been noted that laparoscopy is positive 40–50% of the time and could allow the omission of a laparotomy for diagnosis of recurrent disease [69, 70]. Increasing experience with advanced laparoscopic techniques as well as better equipment have overcome some of these challenges but true second look surgeries are rarely performed today. However, in more recent series it has been shown that laparoscopy for second look surgery was associated with fewer complication, less blood loss, reduced hospital stay, and cost as compared to laparotomy [71].

Secondary Resection of Ovarian Cancer

With advances in laparoscopic surgical techniques, more advanced surgery has been performed. Occasionally women with ovarian cancer will have a limited recurrence that can be resected laparoscopically. If this cannot be removed with conventional laparoscopy, a hand-assisted port can be placed to facilitate resection. In a small series, it was noted in women with persistent or recurrent ovarian cancer in the spleen, the disease could be removed using conventional or a hand-assisted laparoscopic technique [72, 73]. In all cases this was accomplished in a reasonable amount of time with no significant complications. The only conversion in this series was for advanced carcinomatosis.

Cervical Cancer

The modern abdominal radical hysterectomy for cervical cancer was first described by Clarke in 1895 [74]. As a resident at Johns Hopkins he devised the operation that involved removal of the uterus, cervix, and parametrial tissues after extensive anatomic study. Later, a radical vaginal hysterectomy was described by Pavlic and was popularized by Shauta as they demonstrated that the vaginal approach had a lower mortality that the radical abdominal operation [75]. However, the vaginal approach was technically difficult and never achieved widespread popularity. As the concept of lymphadenectomy was incorporated into the treatment of cervical cancer there was little advantage to a radical vaginal hysterectomy since the lymphadenectomy would still require one or more abdominal incisions.

One of the earliest uses of laparoscopy in gynecologic oncology was for lymphatic assessment in women with cervical cancer at the time of radical hysterectomy [4]. While this initial attempt only retrieved an average of eight pelvic nodes, it did show that this procedure was technically feasible with minimal postoperative morbidity. Subsequently it was demonstrated that a laparoscopic lymphadenectomy could remove approximately 75% of the lymph nodes harvested at laparotomy and that nodal counts improved significantly after the first six cases [76]. As surgeons have become more comfortable with laparoscopy, there has been an increase in lymph node counts and many studies now demonstrate superior lymph node counts at the time of laparoscopic surgery [77–80].

Although exact numbers are not available, the majority of radical hysterectomies in the Untied States are still performed through an abdominal incision, although minimally invasive procedures are becoming more common with several large series have been reported (Table 22.3). Currently, the three approaches to minimally invasive hysterectomy have included vaginal radical hysterectomy, laparoscopic-assisted radical vaginal hysterectomy (LARVH), and total laparoscopic radical hysterectomy (TLRH). Currently, most surgeons prefer at least a partial laparoscopic approach to radical hysterectomy as laparoscopy is required in almost all cases to perform the lymphadenectomy. As expected, TLRH and LAVRH are associated with lower blood loss and shorter hospital stays (see Table 22.4). However, the operative times for minimally invasive surgery are generally longer than for abdominal hysterectomy. Currently, no randomized trial comparing these modalities has been conducted.

Many surgeons have adopted robotic assistance for the radical hysterectomy as dissection of the ureter during this procedure can be challenging. Proponents claim that robotic assisted technology will facilitate the use of minimally invasive technology for the treatment of cervical cancer. However, it is unclear if the cost of this technology is justified. Although there is no proven patient benefit to robotic assistance, many surgeons claim that robotic assisted surgery is faster. However, in the limited published intrainstitutional series an advantage of about 45 min was noted. A disadvantage over traditional laparoscopy is the larger incisions for the robot arms and an increased turnover time for the robotic equipment. In addition, the large ports are traditionally placed outside of the umbilicus leading to a less desirable cosmetic appearance.

Laparoscopic Sentinel Nodes

Dargent first reported his experience with laparoscopic sentinel lymphadenectomy in cervical cancer [81]. Using dye alone he was able to identify a sentinel node in 90% of patients and correctly identified all 11 women with positive lymph nodes. Subsequent studies utilizing a combination of dye and lymphoscintigraphy. The radioactive colloid is usually injected first and the blue dye is injected right before the incision as it will be cleared from the sentinel node in about 30 min [82]. Using this technique a sentinel node can be identified in about 85% of patients with operable cervical cancer. Most studies show that a sentinel node is more likely to be identified in smaller tumors

Table 22.3. Large published reports of laparoscopic radical hysterectomy

Author	Year	*n*	EBL (ml)	Node count	OR time	Convert rate (%)	Fistula rate (%)	LOS (days)
Spirtos et al. [111]	2002	78	225	34	205	6.4	1.3	
Pomel et al. [112]	2003	50	200	13	258	0	0	7.5
Gil-Moreno et al. [30]	2005	12	445	19	271	0	0	5.3
Rameriz et al. [113]	2006	20	200	13	332	0	0	1
Xu et al. [114]	2007	317				1.2	2.8	12
Malzoni et al. [115]	2007	65	55	31	196			
Weighted mean		542	162	26	229	1.9	2.1	

Table 22.4. Series of abdominal (A) radical abdominal hysterectomies compared to laparoscopic (L) and robotic assisted (R) radical hysterectomies

Author	Year	*N*			EBL			OR time			Nodes		
		A	L	R	A	L	R	A	L	R	A	L	R
Vidal et al. [116]	1996	47	15		600	250		180	270		25	25	
Abu-Rustum et al. [117]	2003	195	19		693	301		295	371		30	25	
Zakashansky et al. [118]	2007	30	30		520	200		318	424		21	31	
Shafer et al. [119]	2007	48		31	562		119	251		240	22		38
Li et al. [120]	2007	90	35		250	370		217	262		19	21	
Kim and Moon [121]	2007			10			355			231			27
Magrina et al. [122]	2008	35	31	27	444	208	133	167	220	190	28	26	26
Fanning et al. [123]	2008			20			300			390			18
Totals		445	130	20	548	268	191	254	306	257	26	26	29

with rates of up to 90% [82–84]. Some small studies have reported very low false-negative rates, but it is likely that the true false-negative rate for this procedure is 10–20% with higher false-negative rates in larger tumors [83, 84]. It is possible that sentinel lymphangiography could potentially identify unusual patterns of lymphatic drainage.

The routes of lymphatic drainage have been described from the cervix and have been reviewed by Dargent [81]. The main route follows the uterine artery to an external pelvic node which lies between the external iliac artery and vein. Two collateral routes have also been described. One follows the ureter and ends in a node along the internal iliac system adjacent to one of the branches of this vessel including the obturator or superior gluteal artery. The second collateral lymphatic system follows the superior hypogastric nerve plexus and terminates in a common iliac node that lies along the common iliac vein at the level of the sacral-iliac joint. Alternative lymphatic drainage has been reported to occur up to 20% of the time [82].

Radical Trachelectomy

The incidence of cervical cancer has declined due to effective screening for this disease. Although screening for cervical cancer has drastically decreased the incidence of this disease, women at childbearing age can develop this cancer due to lack of screening or screening failures. The traditional surgical treatment of women with stage I cervical cancer is a radical hysterectomy and often fertility is an issue for these women. In an effort to preserve fertility in young women, Dargent developed the radical trachelectomy as an alternative to radical hysterectomy and reported his findings in 1986. A radical trachelectomy removed the cervix and surrounding parametrium in a manor similar to a radical hysterectomy. The uterus is then re-anastomosed to the vaginal cuff and a permanent cerclage is placed. Successful pregnancies have been reported after this procedure. Because of the nature of the surgery, this operation is generally limited to women with tumors $\leq$2 cm and negative lymph nodes.

Although recent reports have described a laparoscopic approach to trachelectomy, the operation was first performed vaginally in conjunction with a laparoscopic pelvic node dissection [85]. In one of the largest series looking at the safety of this operation 118 patients who had a radical vaginal trachelectomy were compared to 139 who had a laparoscopic radical hysterectomy. There was no significant difference between the two populations in terms of complication rates and recurrence rates suggesting that this is a reasonable option for women with small cervical cancers who whish to retain their fertility.

Laparoscopic Radical Parametrectomy

Occasionally cervical cancer can develop after a supracervical hysterectomy or cervical cancer is discovered in the final pathology report after a simple hysterectomy.

In this situation one can still deliver curative radiation. However, the complication rates of radiation increase after hysterectomy as the presence of the uterus serves to keep the bowel away from the intracavitary implant that is a necessary component of treatment. A surgical option in these patients is radical trachelectomy with a parametrectomy with a pelvic lymphadenectomy. In this situation is rare and the largest series that has attempted this procedure laparoscopically included only six patients [86]. The authors reported the feasibility of this procedure with an operative time of 180 min and an average blood loss of 220 ml. In this small series no major complications were reported.

Pelvic Exenteration

Laparoscopic surgery has advanced to the point where a laparoscopic pelvic exenteration is now possible. A series of 16 patients undergoing laparoscopic anterior exenteration has been reported with a mean operative time of 240 min, estimated blood loss of 200 ml, and a postoperative stay of only 3.5 days [87]. There were no conversions to open surgery and the surgical margins were negative in all cases. Complications included an internal iliac artery injury that was managed laparoscopically and two patients with delayed return of bowel function.

Fistula Management

Hand-assisted laparoscopic development of a continent urinary diversion has been reported in association with an exenteration for recurrent cervical cancer with a vesico-vaginal fistula [88]. The surgery lasted for 6 h but with a perioperative blood loss of only 200 ml. Postoperatively the patient had return of normal bowel function by day three and recovered without major complications. This case demonstrates the rapid recovery from such extensive surgery when performed laparoscopically. However, due to the complexity of this type of surgery and the expertise required this type of operation is only done at a few centers that specialize in very advanced laparoscopic procedures.

Rectovaginal fistulas most often occur in women treated with radiation or who have recurrent cervical cancer. The rectovaginal fistula rate is reported to be 2–3% after full pelvic radiation and intracavitary implants [89, 90]. These patients are often managed with an end colostomy which can often be performed laparoscopically.

References

1. Kilgore LC, Partridge EE, Alvarez RD et al (1995) Adenocarcinoma of the endometrium: survival comparisons of patients with and without pelvic node sampling. Gynecol Oncol 56:29–33
2. Merrill RM (2008) Hysterectomy surveillance in the United States, 1997 through 2005. Med Sci Monit 14:CR24–CR31
3. Keshavarz H, Hillis SD, Kieke BA, Marchbanks PA (2002) Hysterectomy surveillance – Untied States, 1994–1999. MMWR 51:1
4. Querleu D, Leblanc E, Castelain B (1991) Laparoscopic pelvic lymphadenectomy in the staging of early carcinoma of the cervix. Am J Obstet Gynecol 164:579–581
5. Childers JM, Brzechffa PR, Hatch KD, Surwit EA (1993) Laparoscopically assisted surgical staging (LASS) of endometrial cancer. Gynecol Oncol 51:33–38
6. Makinen J, Johansson J, Tomas C et al (2001) Morbidity of 10 110 hysterectomies by type of approach. Hum Reprod 16:1473–1478
7. O'Hanlan KA, Lopez L, Dibble SL et al (2003) Total laparoscopic hysterectomy: body mass index and outcomes. Obstet Gynecol 102:1384–1392
8. Wang PH, Lee WL, Yuan CC et al (2001) Major complications of operative and diagnostic laparoscopy for gynecologic disease [see comment]. J Am Assoc Gynecol Laparosc 8:68–73
9. Johnson N, Barlow D, Lethaby A et al (2005) Methods of hysterectomy: systematic review and meta-analysis of randomised controlled trials. BMJ 330:1478
10. Koh CH (1998) A new technique and system for simplifying total laparoscopic hysterectomy. J Am Assoc Gynecol Laparosc 5:187–192
11. Le T, Adolph A, Krepart GV et al (2002) The benefits of comprehensive surgical staging in the management of early-stage epithelial ovarian carcinoma. Gynecol Oncol 85:351–355
12. Naumann RW, Higgins RV, Hall JB (1999) The use of adjuvant radiation therapy by members of the Society of Gynecologic Oncologists. Gynecol Oncol 75:4–9
13. Roland PY, Kelly FJ, Kulwicki CY et al (2004) The benefits of a gynecologic oncologist: a pattern of care study for endometrial cancer treatment. Gynecol Oncol 93:125–130
14. Spirtos NM, Eisekop SM, Boike G et al (2005) Laparoscopic staging in patients with incompletely staged cancers of the uterus, ovary, fallopian tube, and primary peritoneum: a Gynecologic Oncology Group (GOG) study. Am J Obstet Gynecol 193:1645–1649
15. Jemal A, Siegel R, Ward E et al (2008) Cancer statistics, 2008. CA Cancer J Clin 58:71–96
16. FIGO (1989) Annual report on the results of treatment in gynecologic cancer. Int J Gynecol Obstet 28:189–193
17. Naumann RW, Coleman RL (2007) The use of adjuvant radiation therapy in early endometrial cancer by members of the Society of Gynecologic Oncologists in 2005. Gynecol Oncol 105:7–12
18. Chan JK, Wu H, Cheung MK et al (2007) The outcomes of 27,063 women with unstaged endometrioid uterine cancer. Gynecol Oncol 106:282–288

19. American College of Obstetricians and Gynecologists (2005) ACOG practice bulletin, clinical management guidelines for obstetrician-gynecologists, number 65, August 2005: management of endometrial cancer. Obstet Gynecol 106:413–425
20. Childers JM, Surwit EA (1992) Combined laparoscopic and vaginal surgery for the management of two cases of stage I endometrial cancer. Gynecol Oncol 45:46–51
21. Melendez TD, Childers JM, Nour M et al (1997) Laparoscopic staging of endometrial cancer: the learning experience. JSLS 1:45–49
22. Eltabbakh GH (2000) Effect of surgeon's experience on the surgical outcome of laparoscopic surgery for women with endometrial cancer. Gynecol Oncol 78:58–61
23. Abu-Rustum NR, Alektiar K, Iasonos A et al (2006) The incidence of symptomatic lower-extremity lymphedema following treatment of uterine corpus malignancies: a 12-year experience at Memorial Sloan-Kettering Cancer Center. Gynecol Oncol 103:714–718
24. Spirtos NM, Schlaerth JB, Gross GM et al (1996) Cost and quality-of-life analyses of surgery for early endometrial cancer: laparotomy versus laparoscopy. Am J Obstet Gynecol 174:1795–1799, discussion 1799–800
25. Walker J, Mannel R, Piedmonte M et al (2006) Phase III trial of laparoscopy versus laparotomy for surgicalresection and comprehensive surgical staging of uterine cancer: A Gynecologic Oncology Group study funded by the National Cancer Institute. Gynecol Oncol 101:S
26. Kornblith A, Walker J, Huang H, Cella D (2006) Quality of life of patients in a randomized clincal trial of laparoscopy versus open laparotomy for the surgical resection and stagin of uterine cancer: a Gynecologic Oncology Group study. Gynecol Oncol 101:S22
27. Eltabbakh GH (2002) Analysis of survival after laparoscopy in women with endometrial carcinoma. Cancer 95:1894–1901
28. Malur S, Possover M, Michels W, Schneider A (2001) Laparoscopic-assisted vaginal versus abdominal surgery in patients with endometrial cancer – a prospective randomized trial. Gynecol Oncol 80:239–244
29. Leiserowitz G, Xing G, Parihk-Patel A et al (2007) Survival of endometrial cancer patients after laparoscopically assisted vaginal hysterectomy or total abdominal hysterectomy: Analysis of risk factors. Gynecol Oncol 104:S
30. Gil-Moreno A, Diaz-Feijoo B, Morchon S, Xercavins J (2006) Analysis of survival after laparoscopic-assisted vaginal hysterectomy compared with the conventional abdominal approach for early-stage endometrial carcinoma: a review of the literature. J Minim Invasive Gynecol 13:26–35
31. Sonoda Y, Zerbe M, Smith A et al (2001) High incidence of positive peritoneal cytology in low-risk endometrial cancer treated by laparoscopically assisted vaginal hysterectomy [see comment]. Gynecol Oncol 80:378–382
32. Kalogiannidis I, Lambrechts S, Amant F et al (2007) Laparoscopy-assisted vaginal hysterectomy compared with abdominal hysterectomy in clinical stage I endometrial cancer: safety, recurrence, and long-term outcome. Am J Obstet Gynecol 196(248):e1–e8
33. Eltabbakh GH, Mount SL (2006) Laparoscopic surgery does not increase the positive peritoneal cytology among women with endometrial carcinoma. Gynecol Oncol 100:361–364
34. Spanos WJ (1973) Preoperative hormonal therapy of cystic adnexal masses. Am J Obstet Gynecol 116:551–556
35. ACOG Practice Bulletin (2007) Management of adnexal masses. Obstet Gynecol 110:201–214
36. Rulin MC, Preston AL (1987) Adnexal masses in postmenopausal women. Obstet Gynecol 70:578–581
37. Medeiros LR, Fachel JMG, Garry R et al (2005) Laparoscopy versus laparotomy for benign ovarian tumours. Cochrane Database of Syst Rev 3:CD004751
38. (2000) Guidelines for referral to a gynecologic oncologist: rationale and benefits. The Society of Gynecologic Oncologists. Gynecol Oncol 78:S1–S13
39. Im SS, Gordon AN, Buttin BM et al (2005) Validation of referral guidelines for women with pelvic masses. Obstet Gynecol 105:35–41
40. Dearking AC, Aletti GD, McGree ME et al (2007) How relevant are ACOG and SGO guidelines for referral of adnexal mass? Obstet Gynecol 110:841–848
41. DePriest PD, Varner E, Powell J et al (1994) The efficacy of a sonographic morphology index in identifying ovarian cancer: a multi-institutional investigation. Gynecol Oncol 55:174–178
42. Eichel L, Abdelshehid C, Lee DI et al (2004) In vitro comparison of burst tension and puncture pressure in commonly used organ retrieval bags. J Am Coll Surg 199:166–169
43. Havrilesky LJ, Peterson BL, Dryden DK et al (2003) Predictors of clinical outcomes in the laparoscopic management of adnexal masses. Obstet Gynecol 102:243–251
44. Yuen PM, Yu KM, Yip SK et al (1997) A randomized prospective study of laparoscopy and laparotomy in the management of benign ovarian masses. Am J Obstet Gynecol 177:109–114
45. Fanfani F, Fagotti A, Ercoli A et al (2004) A prospective randomized study of laparoscopy and minilaparotomy in the management of benign adnexal masses. Hum Reprod 19:2367–2371
46. Staging Announcement (1986) FIGO cancer committee. Gynecol Oncol 25:383–385
47. Dembo AJ, Davy M, Stenwig AE et al (1990) Prognostic factors in patients with stage I epithelial ovarian cancer. Obstet Gynecol 75:263–273
48. Kodama S, Tanaka K, Tokunaga A et al (1997) Multivariate analysis of prognostic factors in patients with ovarian cancer stage I and II. Int J Gynaecol Obstet 56:147–153
49. Sevelda P, Dittrich C, Salzer H (1989) Prognostic value of the rupture of the capsule in stage I epithelial ovarian carcinoma. Gynecol Oncol 35:321–2
50. Barnhill DR, Kurman RJ, Brady MF et al (1995) Preliminary analysis of the behavior of stage I ovarian serous tumors of low malignant potential: a Gynecologic Oncology Group study. J Clin Oncol 13:2752–2756
51. Seidman JD, Kurman RJ (2000) Ovarian serous borderline tumors: a critical review of the literature with emphasis on prognostic indicators. Hum Pathol 31:539–557
52. Poncelet C, Fauvet R, Boccara J, Darai E (2006) Recurrence after cystectomy for borderline ovarian tumors: results

of a French multicenter study. Ann Surg Oncol 13: 565–571
53. Swanton A, Bankhead CR, Kehoe S (2007) Pregnancy rates after conservative treatment for borderline ovarian tumours: a systematic review. Eur J Obstet Gynecol Reprod Biol 135:3–7
54. Piver MS, Barlow JJ, Lele SB (1978) Incidence of subclinical metastasis in stage I and II ovarian carcinoma. Obstet Gynecol 52:100–104
55. Takeshima N, Hirai Y, Umayahara K et al (2005) Lymph node metastasis in ovarian cancer: difference between serous and non-serous primary tumors. Gynecol Oncol 99:427–431
56. Reich H, McGlynn F, Wilkie W (1990) Laparoscopic management of stage I ovarian cancer. A case report. J Reprod Med 35:601–604, discussion 604–5
57. Correa JJ, Politis C, Rodriguez AR, Pow-Sang JM (2007) Laparoscopic retroperitoneal lymph node dissection in the management of testis cancer. Cancer Control 14: 258–264
58. Janetschek G, Hobisch A, Holtl L, Bartsch G (1996) Retroperitoneal lymphadenectomy for clinical stage I nonseminomatous testicular tumor: laparoscopy versus open surgery and impact of learning curve. J Urol 156:89–93, discussion 94
59. Steiner H, Peschel R, Janetschek G et al (2004) Long-term results of laparoscopic retroperitoneal lymph node dissection: a single-center 10-year experience. Urology 63:550–555
60. Plante M (2000) Fertility preservation in the management of gynecologic cancers. Curr Opin Oncol 12:497–507
61. Colombo N, Parma G, Lapresa MT et al (2005) Role of conservative surgery in ovarian cancer: the European experience. Int J Gynecol Cancer 15(Suppl 3): 206–211
62. Zanetta G, Chiari S, Rota S et al (1997) Conservative surgery for stage I ovarian carcinoma in women of childbearing age. Br J Obstet Gynaecol 104:1030–1035
63. Deffieux X, Castaigne D, Pomel C (2006) Role of laparoscopy to evaluate candidates for complete cytoreduction in advanced stages of epithelial ovarian cancer. Int J Gynecol Cancer 16(Suppl 1):35–40
64. Fagotti A, Ferrandina G, Fanfani F et al (2006) A laparoscopy-based score to predict surgical outcome in patients with advanced ovarian carcinoma: a pilot study. Ann Surg Oncol 13:1156–1161
65. Ansquer Y, Leblanc E, Clough K et al (2001) Neoadjuvant chemotherapy for unresectable ovarian carcinoma: a French multicenter study. Cancer 91:2329–2334
66. Wangensteen OH, Lewis FJ, Tongen LA (1951) The "second-look" in cancer surgery; a patient with colic cancer and involved lymph nodes negative on the "sixth-look". J Lancet 71:303–307
67. Ozols RF, Bundy BN, Greer BE et al (2003) Phase III trial of carboplatin and paclitaxel compared with cisplatin and paclitaxel in patients with optimally resected stage III ovarian cancer: a Gynecologic Oncology Group study. J Clin Oncol 21:3194–3200
68. Berek JS, Griffiths CT, Leventhal JM (1981) Laparoscopy for second-look evaluation in ovarian cancer. Obstet Gynecol 58:192–198
69. Ozols RF, Fisher RI, Anderson T et al (1981) Peritoneoscopy in the management of ovarian cancer. Am J Obstet Gynecol 140:611–619
70. Piver MS, Lele SB, Barlow JJ, Gamarra M (1980) Second-look laparoscopy prior to proposed second-look laparotomy. Obstet Gynecol 55:571–573
71. Abu-Rustum NR, Barakat RR, Siegel PL et al (1996) Second-look operation for epithelial ovarian cancer: laparoscopy or laparotomy? Obstet Gynecol 88: 549–553
72. Chi DS, Abu-Rustum NR, Sonoda Y et al (2006) Laparoscopic and hand-assisted laparoscopic splenectomy for recurrent and persistent ovarian cancer. Gynecol Oncol 101:224–227
73. Krivak TC, Elkas JC, Rose GS et al (2005) The utility of hand-assisted laparoscopy in ovarian cancer. Gynecol Oncol 96:72–76
74. Clarke JG (1895) A more radical method for performing hysterectomy for cancer of the uterus. Bull Johns Hopkins Hosp 6:120
75. Sonoda Y, Abu-Rustum NR (2007) Schauta radical vaginal hysterectomy. Gynecol Oncol 104:20–24
76. Fowler JM, Carter JR, Carlson JW et al (1993) Lymph node yield from laparoscopic lymphadenectomy in cervical cancer: a comparative study. Gynecol Oncol 51:187–192
77. Johnson N (1994) Laparoscopic versus conventional pelvic lymphadenectomy for gynaecological malignancy in humans. Br J Obstet Gynaecol 101:902–904
78. Lanvin D, Elhage A, Henry B et al (1997) Accuracy and safety of laparoscopic lymphadenectomy: an experimental prospective randomized study. Gynecol Oncol 67: 83–87
79. Possover M, Krause N, Plaul K et al (1998) Laparoscopic para-aortic and pelvic lymphadenectomy: experience with 150 patients and review of the literature. Gynecol Oncol 71:19–28
80. Roy M, Plante M, Renaud MC, Tetu B (1996) Vaginal radical hysterectomy versus abdominal radical hysterectomy in the treatment of early-stage cervical cancer [see comment]. Gynecol Oncol 62:336–339
81. Dargent D, Martin X, Mathevet P (2000) Laparoscopic assessment of the sentinel lymph node in early stage cervical cancer. Gynecol Oncol 79:411–415
82. Kushner DM, Connor JP, Wilson MA et al (2007) Laparoscopic sentinel lymph node mapping for cervix cancer–a detailed evaluation and time analysis. Gynecol Oncol 106:507–512
83. Barranger E, Coutant C, Cortez A et al (2005) Sentinel node biopsy is reliable in early-stage cervical cancer but not in locally advanced disease. Ann Oncol 16:1237–1242
84. Coutant C, Morel O, Delpech Y et al (2007) Laparoscopic sentinel node biopsy in cervical cancer using a combined detection: 5-years experience. Ann Surg Oncol 14: 2392–2399
85. Marchiole P, Benchaib M, Buenerd A et al (2007) Oncological safety of laparoscopic-assisted vaginal radical trachelectomy (LARVT or Dargent's operation): a comparative study with laparoscopic-assisted vaginal radical hysterectomy (LARVH). Gynecol Oncol 106:132–141
86. Liang Z, Xu H, Chen Y et al (2006) Laparoscopic radical trachelectomy or parametrectomy and pelvic and

para-aortic lymphadenectomy for cervical or vaginal stump carcinoma: report of six cases. Int J Gynecol Cancer 16:1713–1716
87. Puntambekar S, Kudchadkar RJ, Gurjar AM et al (2006) Laparoscopic pelvic exenteration for advanced pelvic cancers: a review of 16 cases. Gynecol Oncol 102:513–516
88. Pomel C, Castaigne D (2004) Laparoscopic hand-assisted Miami Pouch following laparoscopic anterior pelvic exenteration. Gynecol Oncol 93:543–545
89. Lanciano RM, Martz K, Montana GS, Hanks GE (1992) Influence of age, prior abdominal surgery, fraction size, and dose on complications after radiation therapy for squamous cell cancer of the uterine cervix. A patterns of care study. Cancer 69:2124–2130
90. Matsuura Y, Kawagoe T, Toki N et al (2006) Long-standing complications after treatment for cancer of the uterine cervix–clinical significance of medical examination at 5 years after treatment. Int J Gynecol Cancer 16:294–297
92. Hidlebaugh DA, Orr RK (1997) Staging endometrioid adenocarcinoma. Clinical and financial comparison of laparoscopic and traditional approaches. J Reprod Med 42:482–488
93. Bajaj PK, Barnes MN, Robertson MW et al (1999) Surgical management of endometrial adenocarcinoma using laparoscopically assisted staging and treatment. South Med J 92:1174–1177
94. Gemignani ML, Curtin JP, Zelmanovich J et al (1999) Laparoscopic-assisted vaginal hysterectomy for endometrial cancer: clinical outcomes and hospital charges [see comment]. Gynecol Oncol 73:5–11
95. Eltabbakh GH, Shamonki MI, Moody JM, Garafano LL (2001) Laparoscopy as the primary modality for the treatment of women with endometrial carcinoma. Cancer 91:378–387
96. Scribner DR Jr, Walker JL, Johnson GA et al (2001) Laparoscopic pelvic and paraaortic lymph node dissection: analysis of the first 100 cases. Gynecol Oncol 82:498–503
97. Holub Z, Jabor A, Bartos P et al (2002) Laparoscopic pelvic lymphadenectomy in the surgical treatment of endometrial cancer: results of a multicenter study. J Soc Laparoendosc Surg 6:125–131
98. Langebrekke A, Istre O, Hallqvist AC et al (2002) Comparison of laparoscopy and laparotomy in patients with endometrial cancer. J Am Assoc Gynecol Laparosc 9:152–157
99. Manolitsas TP, Fowler JM (2001) Role of laparoscopy in the management of the adnexal mass and staging of gynecologic cancers. Clin Obstet Gynecol 44: 495–521
100. Kuoppala T, Tomas E, Heinonen PK (2004) Clinical outcome and complications of laparoscopic surgery compared with traditional surgery in women with endometrial cancer. Arch Gynecol Obstet 270:25–30
101. Obermair A, Manolitsas TP, Leung Y et al (2004) Total laparoscopic hysterectomy for endometrial cancer: patterns of recurrence and survival. Gynecol Oncol 92: 789–793
102. Barwijuk A, Jankowska S (2005) Is laparoscopic or abdominal hysterectomy with bilateral salpingo-oophorectomy more efficient in operative treatment of endometrial cancer? J Obstet Gynaecol 25:703–705
103. Kim R, Rose PG (2005) Surgical staging of gynecologic malignancies: the role of laparoscopy and sentinel node technology. Surg Oncol Clin North Am 14: 267–288
104. Tozzi R, Malur S, Koehler C, Schneider A (2005) Analysis of morbidity in patients with endometrial cancer: is there a commitment to offer laparoscopy? [see comment]. Gynecol Oncol 97:4–9
105. Wong CK, Wong YH, Lo LSF et al (2005) Laparoscopy compared with laparotomy for the surgical staging of endometrial carcinoma. J Obstet Gynaecol Res 31: 286–290
106. Zorlu CG, Simsek T, Ari ES (2005) Laparoscopy or laparotomy for the management of endometrial cancer. J Soc Laparoendosc Surg 9:442–446
107. Frigerio L, Gallo A, Ghezzi F et al (2006) Laparoscopic-assisted vaginal hysterectomy versus abdominal hysterectomy in endometrial cancer. Int J Gynaecol Obstet 93: 209–213
108. Cho Y-H, Kim D-Y, Kim J-H et al (2007) Laparoscopic management of early uterine cancer: 10-year experience in Asan Medical Center. Gynecol Oncol 106: 585–590
109. Eisenhauer EL, Wypych KA, Mehrara BJ et al (2007) Comparing surgical outcomes in obese women undergoing laparotomy, laparoscopy, or laparotomy with panniculectomy for the staging of uterine malignancy. Ann Surg Oncol 14:2384–2391
91. Yuen PM, Lo KW, Rogers MS (1995) A comparison of laparotomy and laparoscopy in the management of ovarian masses. J Gynecol Surg 11:19–25
110. Deckardt R, Saks M, Graeff H (1994) Comparison of minimally invasive surgery and laparotomy in the treatment of adnexal masses. J Am Assoc Gynecol Laparosc 1: 333–338
111. Spirtos NM, Eisenkop SM, Schlaerth JB, Ballon SC (2002) Laparoscopic radical hysterectomy (type III) with aortic and pelvic lymphadenectomy in patients with stage I cervical cancer: surgical morbidity and intermediate follow-up. Am J Obstet Gynecol 187:340–348
112. Pomel C, Atallah D, Le Bouedec G et al (2003) Laparoscopic radical hysterectomy for invasive cervical cancer: 8-year experience of a pilot study. Gynecol Oncol 91:534–539
113. Ramirez PT, Slomovitz BM, Soliman PT et al (2006) Total laparoscopic radical hysterectomy and lymphadenectomy: the M.D. Anderson Cancer Center experience [see comment]. Gynecol Oncol 102:252–255
114. Xu H, Chen Y, Li Y et al (2007) Complications of laparoscopic radical hysterectomy and lymphadenectomy for invasive cervical cancer: experience based on 317 procedures. Surg Endosc 21:960–964
115. Malzoni M, Malzoni C, Perone C et al (2004) Total laparoscopic radical hysterectomy (type III) and pelvic lymphadenectomy. Eur J Gynaecol Oncol 25: 525–527
116. Vidal O, Garza-Leal JG (1996) Laparoscopy versus laparotomy for radical hysterectomy. J Am Assoc Gynecol Laparosc 3:S53
117. Abu-Rustum NR, Gemignani ML, Moore K et al (2003) Total laparoscopic radical hysterectomy with pelvic

lymphadenectomy using the argon-beam coagulator: pilot data and comparison to laparotomy. Gynecol Oncol 91:402–409 [erratum appears in Gynecol Oncol. 2004 Apr;93(1):275]

118. Zakashansky K, Chuang L, Gretz H et al (2007) A case-controlled study of total laparoscopic radical hysterectomy with pelvic lymphadenectomy versus radical abdominal hysterectomy in a fellowship training program. Int J Gynecol Cancer 17:1075–1082

119. Shafer A, Boggess J, Gehrig PA et al (2007) Type III radical hysterectomy for obsese women with cervical carcinoma: robotic versus open. Gynecol Oncol 104:S

120. Li G, Yan X, Shang H et al (2007) A comparison of laparoscopic radical hysterectomy and pelvic lymphadenectomy and laparotomy in the treatment of Ib-IIa cervical cancer. Gynecol Oncol 105:176–180

121. Kim DH, Moon JS (1998) Laparoscopic radical hysterectomy with pelvic lymphadenectomy for early, invasive cervical carcinoma. J Am Assoc Gynecol Laparosc 5: 411–417

122. Magrina JF, Kho RM, Weaver AL et al (2008) Robotic radical hysterectomy: comparison with laparoscopy and laparotomy. Gynecol Oncol 109:86–91

123. Fanning J, Fenton B, Purohit M (2008) Robotic radical hysterectomy. Am J Obstet Gynecol 198(649):e1–e4

124. Nezhat F, Yadav J, Rahaman J, Grez H, and Cohen C (2008) Analysis of Survival after Laparoscopic Management of Endometrial Cancer. J Min Inv Gynecol 15(2):181–187

Part V
Special Issues in Cancer Management

Minimally Invasive Surgery in Pediatric Oncology

Keith A. Kuenzler, Steven S. Rothenberg

Contents

Introduction

In the 1990s, improvements in miniaturized endoscopes and surgical instruments allowed minimally invasive surgery (MIS) to extend its applications to the treatment of children and even the smallest infants. Over the last decade, there has been an immense interest in the use of MIS in the pediatric population. As experience has increased, so has the complexity of cases from diagnostic and biopsy procedures in older children to difficult reconstruction of newborn anomalies. Recently, the design and availability of devoted MIS operating suites has also facilitated the optimal positioning of patients and video monitors to allow more complex procedures to be accomplished in smaller spaces. These advances along with the widespread use of the Internet and advanced telemedicine technology have allowed the sharing of information on new procedures and technical successes and failures as never before. This has enabled all pediatric surgeons to benefit from the vast experience of MIS experts and to develop protocols and studies using these techniques in the treatment of cancer in children.

A summary of the earliest pediatric minimally invasive oncology experience was presented in 1995, when Dr. George W. Holcomb addressed the 48th Annual Cancer Symposium of the Society of Surgical Oncology [1]. He described 85 children treated at 15 different Children's Cancer Group (CCG) institutions between 1991 and 1993. At that time, the applications of pediatric MIS in cancer were limited to (1) the evaluation of a new mass, (2) staging or determination of resectability, (3) second-look evaluation, (4) investigation into recurrent or metastatic tumor, and (5) evaluation for suspected infection. Paralleling the advances of adult MIS, pediatric procedures have been successfully used for virtually all diagnoses. Not surprisingly, the advances in pediatric MIS have extended to surgical oncology as well. Considering that today's pediatric

F.L. Greene, B.T. Heniford (eds.), *Minimally Invasive Cancer Management*,
DOI 10.1007/978-1-4419-1238-1_23,

surgeons perform a range of procedures from thoracoscopic lung lobectomy and esophageal atresia repair to complicated biliary reconstructions and solid tumor removal, it is evident that there are fewer technical limitations in MIS. As with any new technology in surgery, now that we have shown that most MIS procedures *can* be done, we must rigorously challenge the notion that they *should* be performed, especially in the pediatric cancer patient. In treating children with cancer, it is imperative to ensure enthusiasm for new procedures and the perceived advantages of MIS do not compromise accepted oncologic principles.

This chapter will describe the current applications of MIS in pediatric oncology with regard to diagnosis, staging, tumor resection, and in the supportive care of immunocompromised patients. Additionally, we will discuss the many advantages and specific limitations of MIS techniques as applied to pediatric oncology.

Equipment and Technical Considerations

Patient Position and Port Placement

There are a number of general tenets in pediatric MIS which optimize conditions for successful completion of any procedure. These simple principles are critical especially in the setting of infants and small children, where the workspace can be extremely limited. The video monitor, the target organ, and the surgeon should always be positioned in a straight line if possible to avoid any paradox. This can be greatly facilitated in the devoted MIS operating suite by the numerous flat-screen monitors positioned around the room on ceiling-mounted brackets rather than confined to bulky towers. Additionally, the video screen and operating table should both be at a height which limits neck and shoulder strain, especially for lengthy procedures. This also allows the simulation of a familiar "open surgery" trajectory. In nearly all cases, the camera port should be positioned between the surgeons' right- and left-hand "working" ports. This triangulation of instruments also closely mimics the surgeon's natural position in open techniques and also avoids the awkwardness of working in a different direction to what is displayed onscreen. Additional ports for retraction or assistance should always be introduced if doing so will increase visibility, safety, and/or significantly decrease the anesthetic time.

Access

Most pediatric MIS cases can be accomplished with 3 or 5 mm ports. A 12 mm port may be used if a stapler or endoscopic bag is desired. For abdominal cases, the umbilicus in a child often has a tiny hernia which allows easy entry with the Veress needle. Of course, one may certainly alternatively opt for an open technique trans- or periumbilically. In children, we prefer to use a system of radially expanding laparoscopic ports (Covidien) for larger ports (5 mm or greater) which serve to minimize the fascial opening, limit trocar slippage, and allow fascial collapse when the port is withdrawn. An additional advantage of this system is the ease of upsizing a port site without removing the sheath, which maintains access to the body cavity and further minimizes tissue trauma.

Access for thoracoscopy uses a similar technique with initial insufflation of the pleural space with a Veress needle and then placement of valved trocars in the intercostal spaces. The radially expanding ports provide an advantage here as well as limit injury to the intercostal vessels and nerve, especially in the limited interspace afforded in smaller infants.

Insufflation

In thoracoscopic cases in small children, it is often not possible to get complete single-lung ventilation. In most cases a mainstem intubation of the contralateral side along with CO_2 insufflation of the pleural cavity being accessed gives excellent lung collapse and visualization. A low flow of CO_2(1 l/min) and limited pressures (3–8 mmHg) are tolerated well by the infant or child. For lung or mediastinal biopsies, establishing a low pressure pneumothorax without single-lung ventilation is often enough for visualization. Creating a working space in the posterior thorax or mediastinum is facilitated by positioning the child in a modified prone position to allow gravity to assist in "retracting" the lung. In both thoracic and abdominal cases, leaving one of the insufflation valves on a port slightly open and increasing gas flow can allow a proper workspace, evacuate smoke generated by tissue cautery, and allow a "pop-off" for the pressure of the pneumothorax or pneumoperitoneum if necessary. Most infants and children will tolerate a pneumoperitoneum of 12–15 mmHg, and small increases in insufflation pressure can often have a significant impact on the working space which may avoid the need for conversion to open laparotomy.

Instruments

Most pediatric MIS cases are performed with instruments with shaft diameters of 3 or 5 mm. We prefer instruments of 20 cm working length for infants and 30–36 cm instruments for older children. There are many techniques for effectively achieving hemostasis while limiting collateral thermal damage within a small space, and the type of energy source used depends on the size of the patient and the procedure being performed. The LigaSure instruments, a variation on bipolar technology (Covidien), are very effective and are able to reliably seal arteries of up to 7 mm diameter as well as dividing across solid organs and lung with limited bleeding. Of course, spatula and hook monopolar electrocautery devices, argon beam coagulator, surgical clips, and suture ligatures should also be in the armamentarium of the advanced MIS surgeon.

Thoracic Lesions

The most common thoracoscopic procedure in pediatric oncology is excisional lung biopsy. Excision of suspected metastatic lesions is common, especially with rhabdomyosarcoma, Wilms' tumor, and osteogenic sarcoma (Fig. 23.1a, b). Confirming and characterizing potential infectious infiltrates in immunocompromised patients can also be accomplished with thoracoscopy. Much less frequently in children, MIS may aid in the diagnosis of a primary lung tumor. In a febrile chemotherapy recipient, determining whether a new lesion on CT scan represents a metastatic or infectious process will have a tremendous clinical impact. Prompt thoracoscopic biopsy in such patients allows the oncologist to decide whether an immediate increase or decrease in chemotherapeutics is appropriate, while requiring small wounds in the immunocompromised child. Of course, identifying an infectious cause allows one to focus antibiotic or antifungal therapy, minimizing polypharmacy and limiting side effects. Finally, in some pediatric cancers, resection of pulmonary metastases may result in increased survival rates.

Smith and colleagues [2] reported on the efficacy of thoracoscopy for lung biopsy in pediatric cancers. The authors described 29 thoracoscopic wedge resections for metastases from osteogenic sarcoma, Ewing sarcoma, Wilms' tumor, and other malignancies. Their success rate, defined as an accurate diagnosis with complete resection of the suspicious nodule, was 96.6% (28 of 29). In the same report, the authors described an additional 15 patients who underwent successful MIS biopsies to define infectious infiltrates. For this indication, the 100% diagnostic yield allowed the appropriate therapy to be promptly initiated. In 63 total thoracoscopic cases, there were three morbidities (4.7%) – one diaphragmatic injury and two patients with excessive bleeding with one requiring transfusion.

While lesions on the pleural surfaces can readily be excised by MIS, one obvious limitation of thoracoscopy is the inability to palpate deeper lung lesions surrounded by normal parenchyma or to visualize those less than 1 cm. Several solutions have been proposed. Intraoperative ultrasound during thoracoscopy may be employed to target smaller lesions [3]. Another

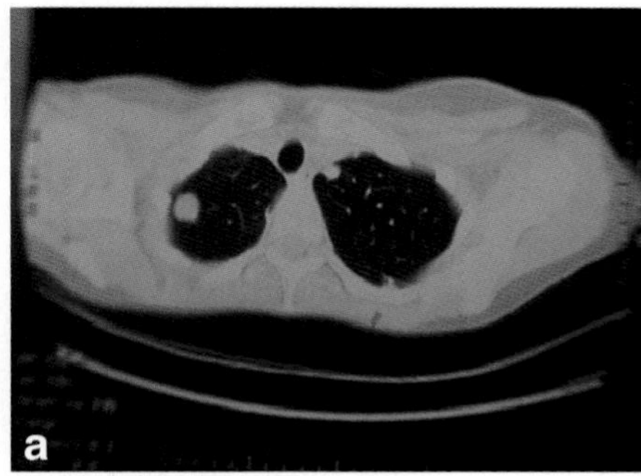

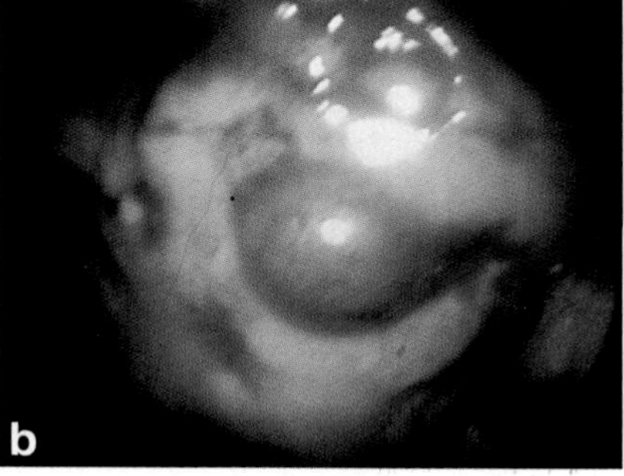

Figure 23.1

(a) CT scan showing a metastatic lesion (Wilm's tumor) in the right upper lobe. (b) The same lesion at thoracoscopic exploration easily visualized on the patients pleura

suggested method is CT-guided needle localization followed by prompt transfer to the operating room for wedge biopsy of the adjacent tissue. A local injection of methylene blue dye may either be added to needle localization or used alone to color the lung surface over the suspicious lesion [4, 5]. An alternative to methylene blue is the "blood patch" technique, in which 1 cc of the patient's blood is injected into the surface of the lung overlying the lesion (Fig. 23.2). Using a blood patch may improve upon the shortcomings of the other methods by avoiding both the potential for wire dislodgement and the occasional spillage of excess methylene blue which makes localizing the lesion nearly impossible. In one author's experience, the blood patch has been used for deep parenchymal lesions with a diagnostic yield of over 95%.

Despite these MIS advances, there remains significant debate specifically regarding the resection of osteosarcoma lung metastases. In these patients, increased survival has been demonstrated with excision of all macroscopic metastases, traditionally by thoracotomy [6]. CT scan appears to underestimate the number of palpable and, thus, removable lesions [7]. Proponents of aggressive metastectomy point out that thoracoscopy does not afford the necessary tactile feedback to locate the small, deep parenchymal lesions.

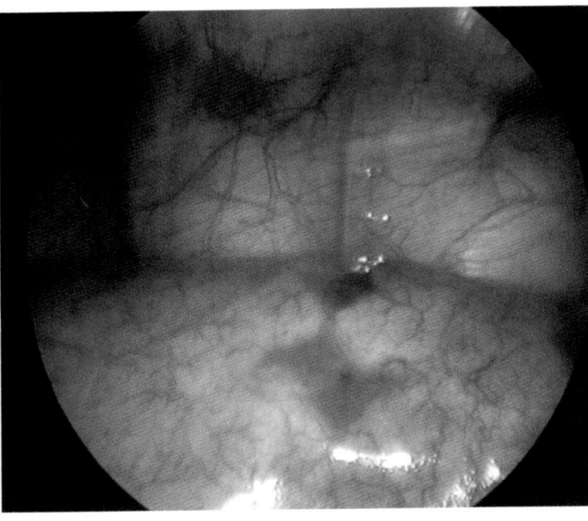

Figure 23.2

Blood patch used to mark the pleura for a deeper smaller lesion not viable on the pleural surface

Other surgeons have argued that the advantages of palpating and removing disease not visible by CT scan are unclear and may not justify the added morbidity of unilateral or bilateral thoracotomies [2].

Another concern related specifically to MIS applications in metastatic osteosarcoma is the potential for port-site recurrence. In 1996, Sartorelli and colleagues [8] published a single case report of chest wall osteosarcoma recurrence at a posterior trocar site, 4 months following the thoracoscopic wedge resection of metachronous disease. The tissue had been extirpated at this location without the use of an endoscopic retrieval bag, and the assumption was that direct contact with the small incision was the cause of tumor cell implantation. Other reports have described excellent results and *no* port-site recurrences with MIS for osteosarcoma metastectomy. The safest course is that all potentially cancerous lesions should either be removed through the lumen of the trocar or placed in a specimen retrieval bag to avoid any risk of port-site contamination.

In a 2003 retrospective review, Sailhamer et al. [9] described the successful resection of pulmonary metastases in six patients with osteosarcoma and one with rhabdomyosarcoma. These patients were "cured" with no apparent disease at the time of the report with short follow-up time. In another retrospective review, five of nine (56%) patients were alive at least 2 years following thoracoscopic resection of osteosarcoma lung metastases [2]. Of the four deaths, three had high-risk features (such as metastases at diagnosis), so it is unclear whether thoracotomy would have significantly improved the survival of these patients. In summary, although there is ample evidence that pulmonary metastectomy improves survival when compared to non-surgical treatments alone, it remains debatable whether resecting non-palpable lesions via open surgery is the factor responsible for the increased survival. Until a randomized, prospective study compares thoracotomy and thoracoscopy for this indication, the controversy will be difficult to resolve.

Children with pulmonary metastases from hepatoblastoma are potentially curable if the lung lesions are resectable in conjunction with complete primary tumor resection. Early results seem to support better outcomes for synchronous metastases and those persistent after induction chemotherapy than for metachronous disease [10]. Thoracoscopy may be applicable for hepatoblastoma metastectomy but has not yet been tested.

Mediastinal Masses

Pediatric *anterior* mediastinal masses usually represent lymphoma, and large lesions often raise concerns for respiratory embarrassment upon general anesthesia induction (Fig. 23.3). Thus, the preferred methods for diagnostic biopsies of large tumor masses are by excision of palpable cervical nodes, thoracentesis with fluid analysis, or anterior mediastinotomy (Chamberlain procedure) under local anesthesia. For smaller, deeper lesions not causing airway compromise, thoracoscopy may be used for tissue diagnosis (Fig. 23.4). After chemotherapy treatment for lymphoma, any remaining suspicious lesions seen on CT scan or metabolically active on PET/CT can be approached thoracoscopically (Fig. 23.5).

The effectiveness of various biopsy techniques were investigated in 2007 by the Children's Oncology Group (COG) [11]. In this report, the diagnostic accuracy for biopsy procedures in patients with Hodgkin lymphoma was analyzed. One hundred sixty-nine cases of Hodgkin lymphoma were reviewed at several institutions. Of those, 148 initial biopsies were performed with "open" technique, the vast majority (133) of these by cervical lymph node excision. Not surprisingly, the success rate for obtaining an appropriate volume of diagnostic material by these methods approached 100%. In this series, only nine initial biopsies were attempted thoracoscopically, and only five yielded an adequate sample, for a 55% success rate. The authors proposed that when MIS is considered for lymphoma biopsy, clear communication between the surgeons and oncologists may help to increase diagnostic accuracy. They did admit that their review had a clearly small thoracoscopy sample size. Additionally, because the report focused on patients *with* the diagnosis of lymphoma (true positives and false negatives), it failed to highlight the benefits of MIS biopsies of suspicious mediastinal lesions which *ruled out* malignancy without a thoracotomy (true negatives). The routine use of intraoperative frozen section may also serve to decrease the false-negative rate.

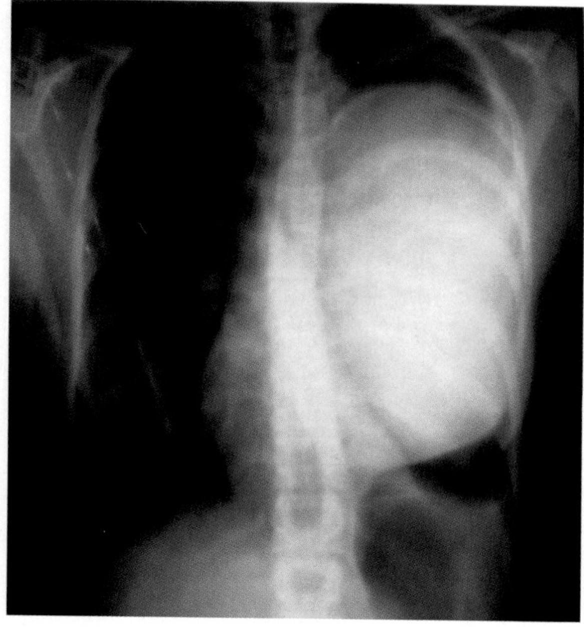

Figure 23.3

A massive anterior mediastinal lymphoma causing tracheal compression, not appropriate for thoracoscopy

Other anterior mediastinal masses may be amenable to MIS excision. Minimally invasive procedures are well described for resection of teratoma, the second most common lesion after lymphoma [12]. Also, thymectomy is readily accomplished thoracoscopically [13]. However, in pediatric age groups, thymectomy is almost always for the treatment of myasthenia gravis, as thymoma is quite unusual. Malignant thymus tumors are exceedingly rare [14].

The overwhelming majority of *posterior* mediastinal masses are neurogenic in origin. Most are malignant (neuroblastoma) (Fig. 23.6), but may be fully differentiated and benign (ganglioneuroma) or may contain elements of each (ganglioneuroblastoma). For a suspected neurogenic tumor, the optimal first-line treatment is gross total resection and tumor analysis. However, survival rates of neuroblastoma patients are predicated to a much greater extent on patient age, tumor histology, and n-myc oncogene expression than microscopic negative margins [15]. In fact, in neurologically intact patients, if tumor invades the neural foramina, the tumor is divided flush with the spine and a positive margin is accepted. Following these oncologic principles, it seems reasonable to expect that MIS will achieve the equivalent outcomes as traditional open surgery.

In a 2006 retrospective analysis, Petty et al. [16] compared thoracoscopy and thoracotomy for neurogenic tumor resections in 17 patients. They found no statistical differences in pathology, outcomes,

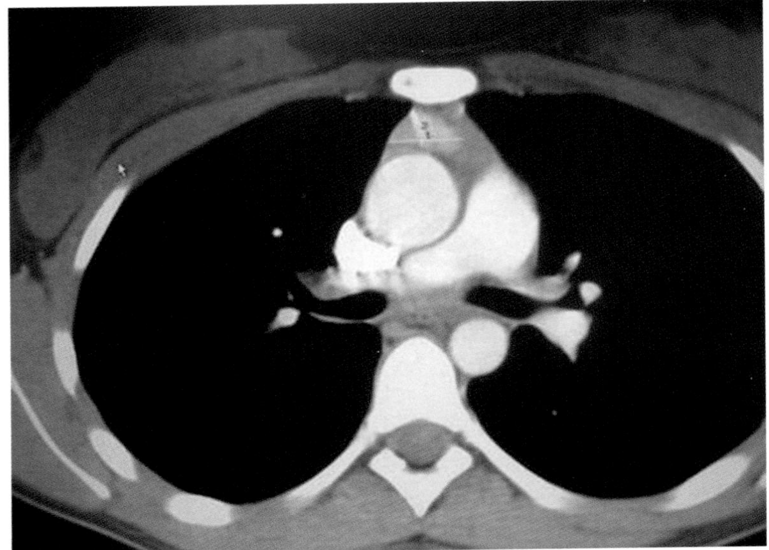

Figure 23.4

CT scan of a mediastinal parathyroid adenoma. A perfect lesion for thoracoscopic resection

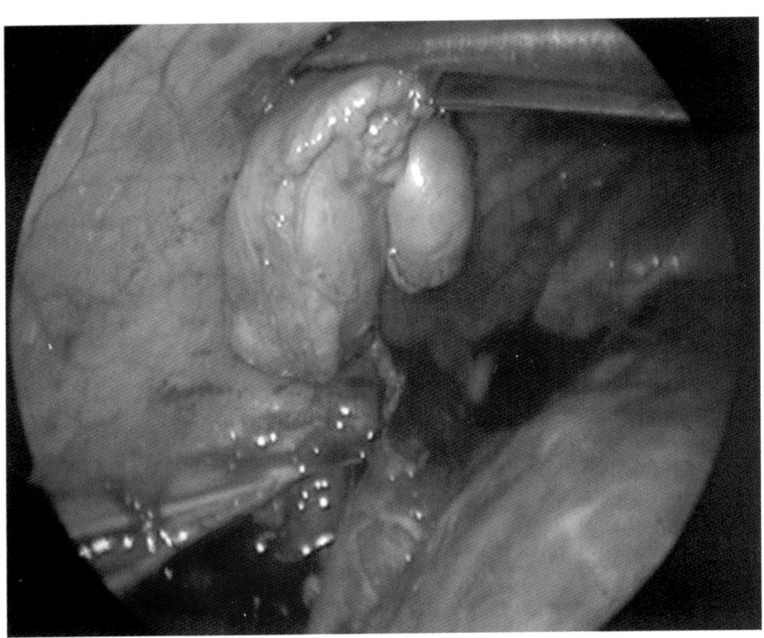

Figure 23.5

Thoracoscopic excisional biopsy of an enlarged anterior mediastinal lymph node following treatment for Hodgkin's lymphoma

or complications. However, the thoracoscopic group recovered more quickly and enjoyed the advantage of a significantly shorter hospital stay. Other institutions have also reported on successful thoracoscopic resections of mediastinal neurogenic tumors [17, 18]. The authors in these series describe equivalent oncologic operations as those achieved with thoracotomy, with the advantages of superior visualization while avoiding the pain and long-term complications associated with posterolateral thoracotomy. In short follow-up, these studies report no failures or port-site recurrences.

Abdominal and Retroperitoneal Lesions

Biopsy

Abdominal masses in children may be approached laparoscopically for biopsy, staging, to determine resectability, for definitive resection, and to evaluation for recurrence. For most pediatric abdominal tumors, obtaining an adequate volume of tissue is often the first step in diagnosis, especially with large, initially unresectable masses. Accomplishing this goal with the

Figure 23.6

Thoracoscopic visualization of a neuroblastoma in a 6 month old

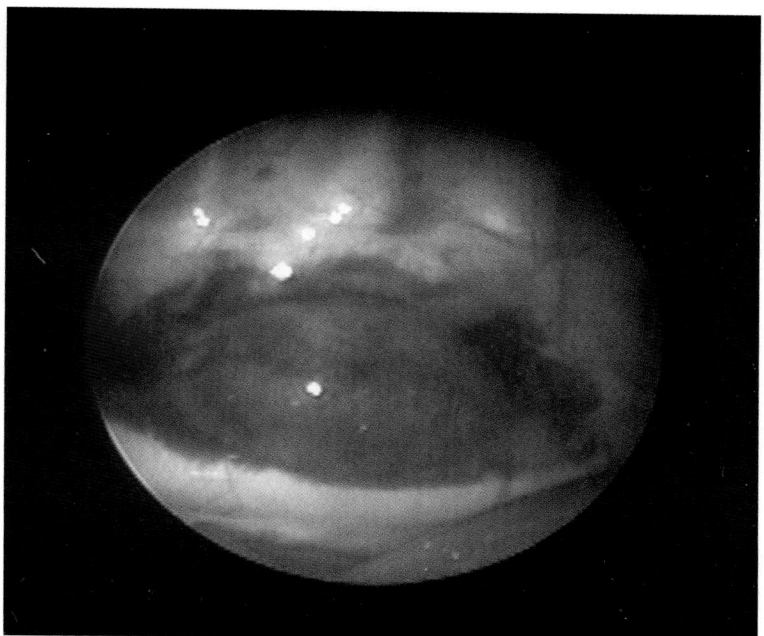

smallest possible wounds helps children rapidly recover and allows prompt initiation of chemotherapy when indicated.

In their retrospective review of 5 years of MIS in pediatric cancer patients, Spurbeck et al. [19] reported on 10 laparoscopic abdominal mass biopsies, all of which yielded appropriate tissue for diagnosis and analysis with very low morbidity rates. These primary tumors included rhabdomyosarcoma, neuroblastoma, hepatoblastoma, lymphoma, and mesothelioma. Sandoval and colleagues [20] described similar techniques and indications for primary biopsy in several patients with advanced stage neuroblastoma and rhabdomyosarcoma. Numerous prospective studies have additionally shown excellent results for solid tumor MIS biopsy [21, 22]. As mentioned previously, it is of the utmost importance that ongoing communication between the surgeon, oncologist, and pathologist ensures that the volume of the biopsy is acceptable, and that it is processed promptly and in the appropriate medium. We usually invite the oncologist to the operating room in such cases to see the laparoscopic views of the primary tumor in situ and then to directly handle the specimen.

As discussed in the section on mediastinal masses, in cases of suspected lymphoma, MIS incisional biopsy may allow prompt initiation of therapy. If the abdominal lymphoma is small or are responsible for local complication (such as intestinal obstruction), it may be appropriate to attempt complete excision. Laparoscopy can also be used to evaluate the completeness of treatment post-chemotherapy (Fig. 23.7a, b). In specific cases of Burkitt's lymphoma, large bulky tumors can be expected to rapidly respond to chemotherapy, and therefore, incisional biopsy should be performed expeditiously [23, 24].

Liver tumors in children are most commonly hepatoblastoma, especially in the first 4–5 years of life. Complete surgical resection provides the greatest chances for cure [25]. For large masses unresectable at diagnosis, neoadjuvant treatment is indicated, as most hepatoblastomas are chemosensitive, and this may increase the likelihood for complete resection later. In these cases, obviously, prompt tissue biopsy is critical to initiate chemotherapy. Laparoscopic wedge resection or tru-cut biopsies are excellent means of obtaining tissue and evaluating the primary tumor without laparotomy. MIS biopsy was demonstrated in a study of adult patients with unresectable liver tumors; patients undergoing laparoscopy were able to be discharged home in an average of 1.5 days versus 5.6 days for patients having open biopsy [26].

Excision

Curative resection of solid abdominal tumors by minimally invasive techniques remains somewhat controversial. Several reports have advocated laparoscopic adrenalectomy as a safe and effective procedure for

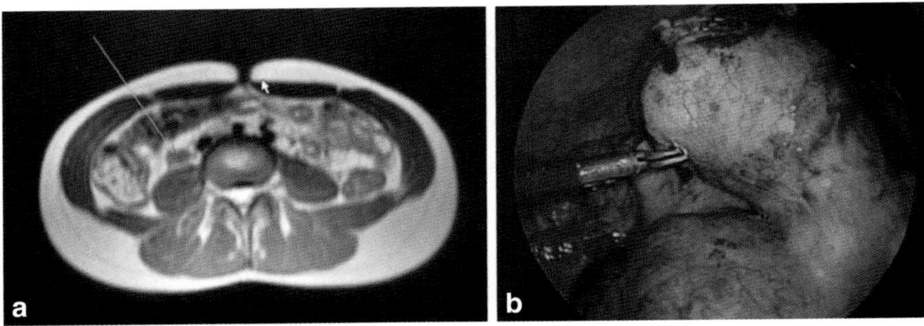

Figure 23.7

(**a**) CT scan showing residual tumor mass after chemotherapy for Burkitt's lymphoma. (**b**) Residual mass as seen at laparoscopy. A complete resection was achieved

neuroblastoma and a variety of tumors in children [9, 20, 27]. Early-stage neuroblastoma originating from the sympathetic chain can also be completely resected laparoscopically and removed using an endoscopic bag to avoid direct contact of tumor with the port sites (Fig. 23.8). Since more advanced cases often preclude microscopic negative margins in open surgery, it is conceivable that gross total resection or debulking procedures for neuroblastoma might be done as effectively laparoscopically, provided that the surgeon has the experience and comfort with advanced MIS techniques in proximity to the major blood vessels

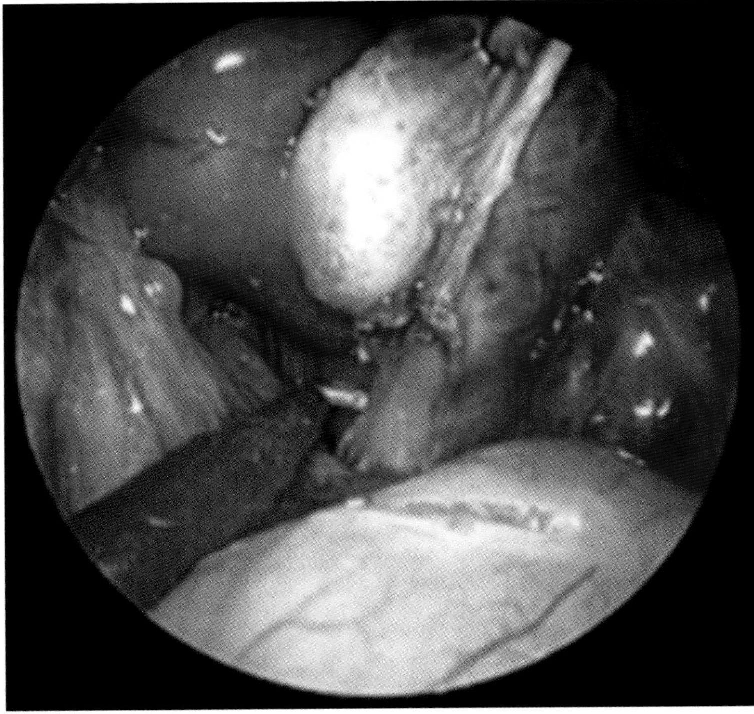

Figure 23.8

Laparoscopic resection of an abdominal neuroblastoma extending up through the esophageal hiatus

in the retroperitoneum. So far, the literature supports MIS for adrenalectomy in early-stage tumors.

In a German prospective study of 301 open and MIS cases performed between 2000 and 2005, of the 139 abdominal tumor resections, only 24 were attempted laparoscopically, and 10 of those cases were converted to open [21]. The authors explained that the usual reason for conversion was poor exposure, even when the operations were performed by surgeons experienced with MIS. They concluded that for resection, pediatric MIS still has a limited role. In another retrospective review published in 2004, Iwanaka et al. [28] described similarly limited indications for biopsy and resection, but did demonstrate significant benefits in MIS patients. In their patients undergoing laparoscopic biopsy for advanced neuroblastoma and in those who had MIS adrenalectomy for early-stage neuroblastoma, there were statistically significant reductions in the times to postoperative feeding when compared with the open groups. There was also a significantly decreased time to the initiation of chemotherapy in the advanced patients who underwent laparoscopic biopsy.

Saad et al. [29] reported six laparoscopic adrenalectomies for neuroblastoma and ganglioneuroblastoma of moderate sizes (2–4 cm). All primary tumors were completely resected and regional lymph nodes were sampled by MIS techniques. These surgeons used an endosurgical specimen bag and morsellated the tumor in situ for removal via the umbilical incision. Five of the six patients were discharged tolerating a regular diet within 48 h of their operation.

For Wilms' tumor, MIS techniques are indicated for staging and evaluation of contralateral kidney involvement (when imaging studies are equivocal or suggest bilateral disease), for biopsies of suspected tumor recurrence, and for thoracoscopic lung biopsy of potential metastases (Fig. 23.9). MIS nephrectomy for Wilms' tumor is not currently supported in the United States, because according to the protocols of the National Wilms' Tumor Study, any violation of the tumor capsule results in an upstage of the tumor (to stage III), with the addition of radiation therapy to a more intensive chemotherapy regimen [30]. Therefore, most pediatric surgeons are not willing to risk capsular violation during either the dissection or removal processes. Because the International Society of Pediatric Oncology (SIOP) protocols call for neoadjuvant therapy in all Wilms' tumor cases, there may be a role for laparoscopic nephrectomy following chemotherapy and reduction in tumor size [31]. Duarte and colleagues [32] reported eight cases of laparoscopic nephrectomy for Wilms' tumor following induction chemotherapy, with no evidence of tumor recurrence in their 5–23 month follow-up.

Pelvic Tumors

Laparoscopy for evaluation and excision of pediatric ovarian masses is well described [33]. Most pediatric surgeons are experienced in laparoscopic ovary-sparing procedures for simple cysts and smaller, benign germ cell neoplasms (Fig. 23.10). For very large masses, and when malignancy is more likely, the role of

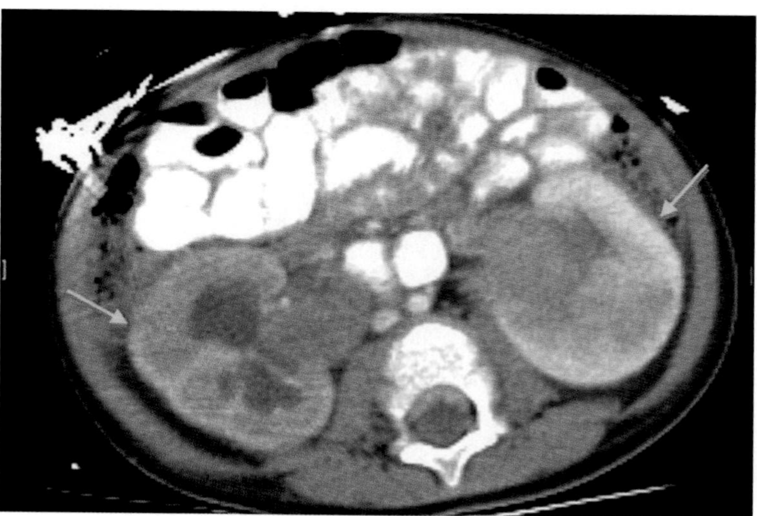

Figure 23.9

CT scan of a large Wilm's tumor, probably not appropriate for laparoscopic resection

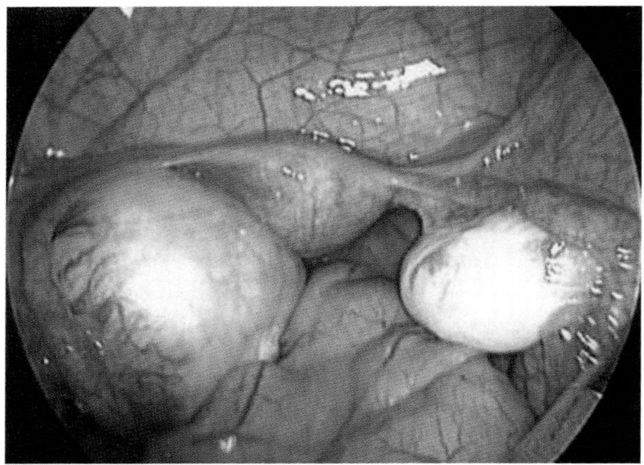

Figure 23.10

An ovarian teratoma as seen at laparoscopic exploration

MIS is less clear. Preoperative serologic tumor markers, including alpha-fetoprotein, beta-hCG, and CA-125, should be evaluated in all girls with an ovarian lesion. Diagnostic imaging which reveals either a simple cyst or a complex mass containing calcifications, in the absence of serologic tumor markers, certainly provides a strong preoperative case for a benign lesion possibly amenable to laparoscopic or laparoscopic-assisted surgery. Depending on their size, ovarian lesions may be removed via a port site or a small Pfannenstiel incision. On the other hand, when imaging or serology raises the question of malignancy, laparoscopy can be used initially to assess the primary tumor and obtain a detailed view of the peritoneal cavity. However, complete staging, including omental examination and possible omentectomy and salpingo-oophorectomy, is probably best accomplished by laparotomy. In addition, to avoid potential peritoneal spread of malignant cells, MIS decompression of the cystic components of large, complex tumors should not be performed in an effort to reduce their size [34].

Sacrococcygeal teratoma (SCT) is the most common solid tumor in newborns, with an incidence of about 1:35,000 births. The vast majority of these tumors are initially benign, but prompt resection is necessary as malignant degeneration has been described. As originally classified by Altman [35], SCT may have a significant presacral pelvic or abdominal component (Fig. 23.8a, b). The arterial supply to these often large tumors may be substantial enough to induce high-output cardiac failure perioperatively or hemorrhage during resection via the standard posterior sacrococcygeal approach. Both mobilization of the presacral portion of the tumor and control of the middle sacral artery may be accomplished laparoscopically [36] (Fig. 23.11a, b). During MIS mobilization of SCT, one has excellent visualization of delicate pelvic structures, and this may prevent injuries to ureters, nerves, rectum, and bladder [33, 37].

MIS Applications in Treating Morbidities of Chemotherapy

We have already described the importance of prompt lung biopsy in the evaluation of infectious lung lesions.

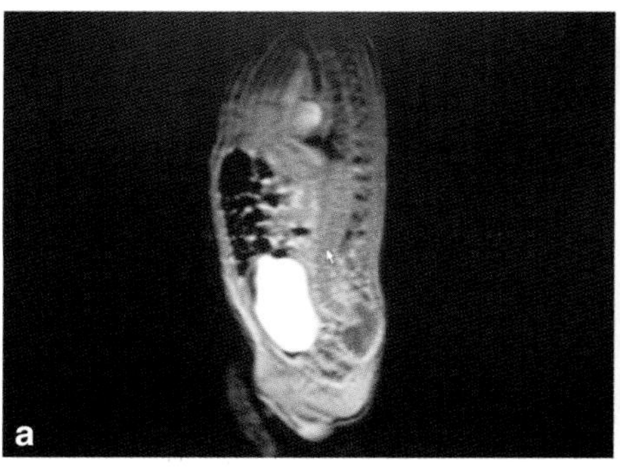

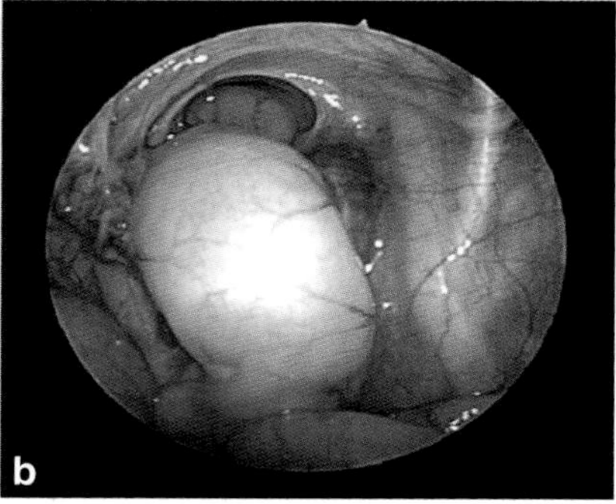

Figure 23.11

(**a**) CT scan of a patient with a recurrent intraabdominal SCT after resection of the primary tumor as a newborn. (**b**) Laparoscopic visualization of the pelvis and tumor in this 8-month-old patient

MIS can also assist in the treatment of malignant pleural effusions. Thoracoscopic surgery can be used to better drain septated effusions, to optimize the position of the thoracostomy tube, and perform mechanical pleurodesis. Furthermore, chronically ill oncology patients frequently suffer from nausea, weight loss, and failure to thrive. Laparoscopic-assisted gastrostomy placement or percutaneous endoscopic gastrostomy insertion offers the means to help maintain nutrition without erosive nasogastric tubes or a large laparotomy wound.

Advantages and Disadvantages of Pediatric MIS

Minimally invasive techniques for biopsy and excision create smaller wounds to heal in patients immunocompromised from chemotherapy and in tissue potentially subject to the damage of radiation therapy. MIS causes less pain, inflammation, and adhesion formation. Patients often resume feeding earlier and are discharged home sooner. Adjuvant treatments may begin earlier in patients who recover from surgery faster. Modern MIS equipment allows for clear, high-definition, magnified views to aid in difficult dissections. Body cavities such as the thoracic spaces and the deep aspects of the pelvis are more easily accessible and visualized than in open surgery. Evaluation of the entire peritoneal cavity may be done with a single 3 mm transumbilical port, enabling diagnosis and accurate staging without laparotomy.

Many of the rare complications associated with pediatric MIS such as umbilical hernia, trocar injuries, and Veress needle complications [38] should continue to decline as our collective "learning curve" is further behind us. Surgeons receive a rich training experience these days in MIS early in general surgery residencies and pediatric surgery fellowships. Improvements in instrumentation such as retractable trocars, bipolar cautery devices, and high-definition images should also help reduce the risks of iatrogenic injuries.

Certainly, there remain limitations of MIS in patients with respiratory insufficiency who are unable to tolerate the CO_2 insufflation, due to restricted tidal volumes or carbon dioxide absorption. Additionally, little is known about the biology of cancer cells exposed to CO_2 pneumoperitoneum. Some in vitro studies show a reduced proliferation rate in various pediatric tumor cell lines [39]. Furthermore, while some animal studies have demonstrated an increased growth and peritoneal implantation rate attributable to CO_2 exposure [40], others support an actual benefit of CO_2 pneumoperitoneum over laparotomy in reducing pulmonary metastasis from adenocarcinoma [41]. Additionally, there is evidence that laparoscopic surgery is associated with a reduction in stress cytokines as compared to laparotomy [42].

Concerns about port-site recurrences after minimally invasive cancer surgery are not unfounded, as this has been described following laparoscopic cholecystectomy (with unsuspected gallbladder cancer), colectomy, esophagectomy, pancreatectomy, and diagnostic laparoscopy for ovarian cancer [43–46]. However, most recent pediatric oncology series report no port-site recurrences thus far [4, 19, 21, 32, 33]. A recent Japanese survey attempted to discover any cases of port-site recurrence among their pediatric MIS cases [47]. Through questionnaires sent to members of the Japanese Society of Pediatric Endosurgeons, the authors found that among 129 MIS biopsies or excisions at 29 different institutions, there were no reported port-site recurrences with follow-up between 5 months and 8 years.

Critics of MIS point out that the techniques and outcomes have not been subjected to proper scientific comparison with traditional open surgery via randomized, prospective trials. In 1996, the Children's Cancer Group (CCG) and the Pediatric Oncology Group (POG) attempted two prospective, randomized studies to compare open surgery to both thoracoscopic and laparoscopic techniques in pediatric cancer. Neither arm accrued sufficient patient enrollment and both were subsequently closed [48]. Some authors have proposed that prospective, randomized trials may not be possible in the current era [49]. Because of preconceived opinions regarding MIS by surgeons, oncologists, and patients, it may be challenging to enroll patients to potentially be randomized to one approach or the other. Individual institutions would likely have inadequate case numbers, but multi-institutional analysis would be complicated by surgeons' variability in techniques and skills [9].

Conclusion

Minimally invasive biopsy, staging, definitive resection, and the management of complications are possible and becoming more widespread for pediatric surgical oncology as our skills and technology advance. In many cases, oncology patients can enjoy numerous advantages of MIS techniques. Since it is of the utmost importance to adhere to the principles of surgical oncology, the role of MIS for certain indications, such as solid tumor excision, is still evolving. Long-term follow-up will be required to ensure that the high standards of pediatric oncologic outcomes are met or exceeded relative to open surgery.

References

1. Holcomb GW 3rd, Tomita SS, Haase GM et al (1995) Minimally invasive surgery in children with cancer. Cancer 76:121–128
2. Smith TJ, Rothenberg SS, Brooks M et al (2002) Thoracoscopic surgery in childhood cancer. J Pediatr Hematol Oncol 24(6):429–435
3. Santambrogio R, Montorsi M, Bianchi P et al (1999) Intraoperative ultrasound during thoracoscopic procedures for solitary pulmonary nodules. Ann Thorac Surg 68: 218–222
4. Waldhausen JHT, Tapper D, Sawin RS (2000) Minimally invasive surgery and clinical decision-making for pediatric malignancy. Surg Endosc 14:250–253
5. Partrick DA, Bensard DD, Teitelbaum DH et al (2002) Successful thoracoscopic lung biopsy in children utilizing preoperative CT-guided localization. J Pediatr Surg 37: 970–973
6. Saenz NC, Conlon KC, Aronson DC et al (1997) The application of minimal access procedures in infants, children, and young adults with pediatric malignancies. J Laparoendosc Adv Surg Tech 7(5):289–294
7. Kayton ML, Huvos AG, Casher J et al (2006) Computed tomographic scan of the chest underestimates the number of metastatic lesions in osteosarcoma. J Pediatr Surg 41:200–206
8. Sartorelli KH, Pertrick D, Meagher DP (1996) Port-site recurrence after thoracoscopic resection of pulmonary metastasis owing to osteogenic sarcoma. J Pediatr Surg 31(10):1443–1444
9. Sailhamer E, Jackson CC, Vogel AM et al (2003) Minimally invasive surgery for pediatric solid neoplasms. Am Surg 69(7):566–568
10. Meyers RL, Katzenstein HM, Malagolowkin MH (2007) Predictive value of staging systems in hepatoblastoma. J Clin Oncol 25:737–738
11. Ehrlich PF, Friedman DL, Schwartz CL et al (2007) Monitoring diagnostic accuracy and complications. A report from the Children's Oncology Group Hodgkin lymphoma study. J Pediatr Surg 42:788–791
12. Esposito C, Lima M, Mattioli G et al (2007) Thoracoscopic surgery in the management of pediatric malignancies: a multicentric survey of the italian society of videosurgery in infancy. Surg Endosc 21:1772–1775
13. Skelly CL, Jackson CC, Wu Y et al (2003) Thoracoscopic thymectomy in children with myasthenia gravis. Am Surg 69(12):1087–1089
14. Kaplinsky C, Mor C, Cohen IJ et al (1992) Childhood malignant thymoma: clinical, therapeutic, and immunohistochemical considerations. Pediatr Hematol Oncol 9: 261–268
15. Grosfeld JL (2006) Neuroblastoma. In: O'Neill JA, Coran AG, Fonkalsrud E et al (eds) Pediatric surgery, 6th edn. Mosby, Philadelphia, PA, pp 467–488
16. Petty JK, Bensard DD, Partrick DA et al (2006) Resection of neurogenic tumors in children: is thoracoscopy superior to thoracotomy? J Am Coll Surg 203(5):699–703
17. Lacreuse I, Valla JS, de Lagausie P (2007) Thoracoscopic resection of neurogenic tumors in children. J Pediatr Surg 42:1725–1728
18. DeCou JM, Schlatter MG, Mitchell DS et al (2005) Primary thoracoscopic gross total resection of neuroblastoma. J Laparoendosc Adv Surg Tech 15(5):470–473
19. Spurbeck WW, Davidoff AM, Lobe TE et al (2004) Minimally invasive surgery in pediatric cancer patients. Ann Surg Oncol 11(3):340–343
20. Sandoval C, Strom K, Stringel G (2004) Laparoscopy in the management of pediatric intraabdominal tumors. JSLS 8:115–118
21. Metzelder ML, Kuebler JF, Shimotakahara A et al (2007) Role of diagnostic and ablative minimally invasive surgery. Cancer 109:2343–2348
22. Warmann S, Fuchs J, Jesch NK et al (2003) A prospective study of minimally invasive techniques in pediatric surgical oncology: preliminary report. Med Pediatr Oncol 40:155–157
23. Gahukamble DB, Khamage AS (1995) Limitations of surgery in intraabdominal Burkitt's lymphoma in children. J Pediatr Surg 30(4):519–522
24. Shamberger RC, Weinstein HJ (1992) The role of surgery in abdominal Burkitt's lymphoma. J Pediatr Surg 27(2): 236–240
25. Meyers RL (2007) Tumors of the liver in children. Surg Oncol 16:195–203
26. Forse RA, Babineau T, Bleday R et al (1993) Laparoscopy/thoracoscopy for staging: I. staging endoscopy in surgical oncology. Semin Surg Oncol 9:51–55
27. Skarsgard ED, Albanese CT (2005) The safety and efficacy of laparoscopic adrenalectomy in children. Arch Surg 140:905–908
28. Iwanaka T, Arai M, Kawashima H et al (2004) Endosurgical procedures for pediatric solid tumors. Pediatr Surg Int 20:39–42
29. Saad DF, Gow KW, Milas Z et al (2005) Laparoscopic adrenalectomy for neuroblastoma in children: a report of 6 cases. J Ped Surg 40:1948–1950
30. Tagge EP, Thomas PB, Othersen HB (2006) Wilms' tumor. In: O'Neill JA, Coran AG, Fonkalsrud E et al (eds) Pediatric surgery, 6th edn. Mosby, Philadelphia, PA, pp 445–463
31. Duarte RJ, Denes FT, Cristofani LM et al (2004) Laparoscopic nephrectomy for Wilm's tumor after chemotherapy: initial experience. J Urol 172:1438–1440
32. Duarte RJ, Denes FT, Cristofani LM et al (2006) Further experience with laparoscopic nephrectomy for Wilms' tumor after chemotherapy. BJU Int 98:155–159

33. Chan KW, Lee KH, Tam YH et al (2007) Minimal invasive surgery in pediatric solid tumors. J Laparoendosc Adv Surg Tech 17(6):817–820
34. Ehrlich PF, Teitelbaum DH, Hirschl RB et al (2007) Excision of large ovarian tumors: combining minimal invasive surgery techniques and cancer surgery – the best of both worlds. J Periatr Surg 42:890–893
35. Altman RP, Randolph JG, Lilly JR (1973) Sacrococcygeal teratoma: American academy of pediatrics surgical section survey. J Pediatr Surg 9:389–398
36. Lukish JR, Powell DM (2004) Laparoscopic ligation of the median sacral artery before resection of a sacrococcygeal teratoma. J Pediatr Surg 39:1288–1290
37. Bax NMA, Van der Zee DC (2004) The laparoscopic approach to sacrococcygeal teratomas. Surg Endosc 18:128–130
38. Chen MK, Schropp KP, Lobe TE (1996) Complications of minimal-access surgery in children. J Pediatr Surg 31: 1161–1165
39. Schmidt AI, Reismann M, Kubler JF et al (2006) Exposure to carbon dioxide and helium reduces in vitro proliferation of pediatric tumor cells. Pediatr Surg Int 22:72–77
40. Shen MY, Huang IP, Chen WS (2008) Influence of pneumoperitoneum on tumor growth and pattern of intra-abdominal tumor spreading: in vivo study of a murine model. Hepatogastroenterology 55(84): 947–951
41. Wildbrett P, Oh A, Carter JJ et al (2002) Increased rates of pulmonary metastases following sham laparotomy compared to CO_2 pneumoperitoneum and the inhibition of metastases utilizing perioperative immunomodulation and a tumor vaccine. Surg Endosc 16: 1162–1169
42. Carter JJ, Whelan RL (2001) The immunologic consequences of laparoscopy in oncology. Surg Oncol Clin North Am 10(3):655–677
43. Paolucci V, Schaeff B, Schneider M et al (1999) Tumor seeding following laparoscopy: international study. World J Surg 23:989–997
44. Lavie O, Cross PA, Beller U et al (1999) Laparoscopic port-site metastasis of an early stage adenocarcinoma of the cervix with negative lymph nodes. Gynecol Oncol 75: 155–157
45. van Dam PA, DeCloedt J, Tjalma WAA et al (1999) Trocar implantation metastasis after laparoscopy in patients with advanced ovarian cancer: can the risk be reduced? Am J Obstet Gynecol 181:536–541
46. Wang PH, Yen MS, Yuan CC et al (1997) Port site metastasis after laparoscopic-assisted vaginal hysterectomy for endometrial cancer – possible mechanisms and prevention. Gynecol Oncol 66:151–155
47. Iwanaka T, Arai M, Yamamoto H et al (2003) No incidence of port-site recurrence after endosurgical procedure for pediatric malignancies. Pediatr Surg Int 19:200–203
48. Erlich PF, Newman KD, Haase GM et al (2002) Lessons learned from a failed multi-institutional randomized controlled study. J Pediatr Surg 37:431–436
49. Cribbs RK, Wulkan ML, Heiss KF et al (2007) Minimally invasive surgery and childhood cancer. Surg Oncol 16:221–228

Endoscopic Diagnosis and Treatment of Breast Diseases

Rashmi P. Pradhan, Jill R. Dietz

Contents

In the last 3 decades breast conservation has shown survival rates comparable to more extensive surgical treatments for breast cancer. Over this period sentinel node has replaced axillary dissection for staging, minimally invasive percutaneous biopsy has replaced excisional biopsy for diagnosis, and the trend continues with the investigation of percutaneous ablative therapies for small breast cancers. Minimally invasive approaches have changed the practice of breast surgery and steered us toward endoscopic techniques, which are the future of breast surgery.

Eighty-five percentage or more of breast cancers arise in the epithelial lining of mammary ducts within the terminal duct lobular unit (TDLU) from morphologically identifiable precursor lesions. Therefore, mammary ductoscopy (MD) potentially can detect breast cancer several years before detection by mammography. The ductoscopic appearances of breast cancer include irregular polypoid growths, ulcerating lesions, elevations, bridging structures, and extrinsic compression. By contrast, the internal surface of a normal duct appears lustrous and smooth, and intraductal papillomas form intraductal solid nodules, being yellow or pink in most cases and red at the site of hemorrhage [1]. Over the last decade, the development of minute endoscopes less than 1 mm in outer diameter has revitalized the field of mammary ductoscopy (MD) [2]. Endoscopy of the breast allows for both visualization of the internal ductal anatomy and sampling for cytological, proteomic, and histological evaluation of the ductal epithelium.

In addition to endoscopic evaluation of the ductal system via mammary ductoscopy, there has been recent interest in using endoscopic techniques for the evaluation of the axilla. This technique, combined with lymphatic mapping, allows for creation of a minimally invasive working space within the axilla, recognition of key axillary anatomic landmarks, and identification of sentinel nodes [3].

F.L. Greene, B.T. Heniford (eds.), *Minimally Invasive Cancer Management*,
DOI 10.1007/978-1-4419-1238-1_24,

In the last few years, endoscopic surgery has also been applied successfully to lumpectomy, breast augmentation, subcutaneous mastectomy for gynecomastia, and axillary dissection [4–7]. Recent literature suggests that skin- and nipple-sparing mastectomy has comparable and acceptable recurrence rates to that of standard mastectomy in select patient groups and hence is oncologically safe [8–12]. Interest has since developed for using endoscopic techniques to perform mastectomies for breast cancer [4]. This chapter will review the indications and techniques for various endoscopic breast procedures.

Mammary Ductoscopy (MD)

MD allows direct visualization of the mammary ducts using fiberoptic micro-endoscopes inserted through the ductal opening on the nipple surface. This has diagnostic and therapeutic implications.

Indications for Mammary Ductoscopy

Pathologic Nipple Discharge (PND)

PND is seen in 5% of women seeking care at a breast clinic and is the most common indication for MD. Patients have unilateral, spontaneous single duct, bloody, or clear nipple discharge. Approximately 10% of PND is caused by an underlying breast cancer [13, 14]. Papilloma is the most common pathological finding in women with PND as seen in about 40–70% of cases.

Margin Assessment During Lumpectomy

One study has shown that the nipple-ward margin in patients undergoing lumpectomy can be better evaluated under direct visualization, decreasing positive margin and re-excision rates [15].

Intraductal Breast Biopsy

Biopsy or excision of small intraductal lesions is possible for diagnostic purposes using the ductoscope. Future directions would include proteomic analysis of ductal tissue as marker for cancer.

Ductoscopy-Directed Duct Excision

This is the therapeutic application of ductoscopy helping guide the extent of lumpectomy for patients with breast cancer. Intraductal lesions can appear as red patches, ductal obstruction, or micro-calcifications. High-resolution ductoscopy is able to detect extensive intraductal disease in a considerable number of women with breast cancer. In selected patients, a combination of both preoperative imaging and intraoperative ductoscopy may help to avoid incomplete resections and re-excisions [13, 16].

Ductoscopy Equipment

Current rigid or flexible ductoscopes (micro-endoscopes) are 0.7–1.2 mm in external diameter and up to 10 cm in length (Solos^{TM} Ductoscope, Solos Endoscopy, Boston, MA). The ductoscope allows for magnification up to 60 times normal size with a focal distance of 1–2 mm. In most MD models, a semi-rigid scope fits into a disposable introducer thus creating a working channel for insufflation, irrigation, and extraction of tissue as well as possible therapeutic intervention. A 100 W xenon light source is used for intraductal observation through the ductoscope and transillumination to assist with directed excision. Specially designed dilators are available to assist in ductal cannulation if needed such as the FirstCyteTM Ultra slim straight 0.010" dilator (comparable to 31 gauge) and tapered dilators. In most cases of PND, Bowman's lacrimal dilators (sizes 0000–1) are sufficient for dilating the discharging duct (Figs. 24.1, 24.2, and 24.3).

Procedure

Patient Analgesia

This procedure can be performed under straight local in an office setting using EMLA cream and a lidocaine nipple block described below. However, it is most often performed in an operative setting combined with either duct excision or lumpectomy where the patient is under monitored anesthesia with sedation or general anesthesia.

Nipple Block

One percentage lidocaine without epinephrine (to avoid nipple necrosis) is injected in the avascular

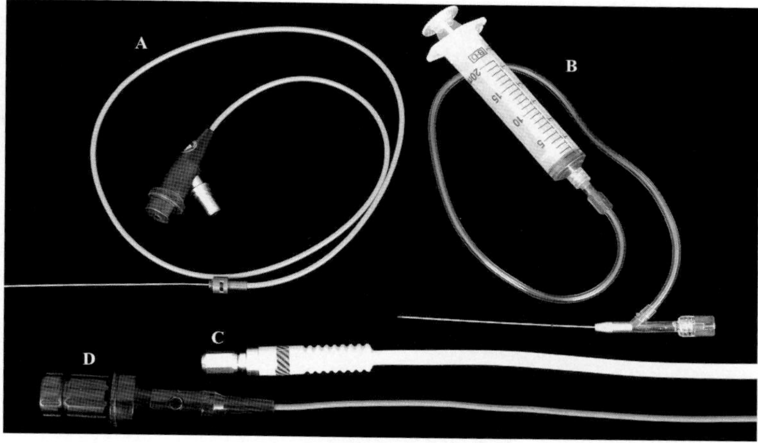

Figure 24.1

Ductoscope with irrigation channel. (**a**) Ductoscope, (**b**) irrigation channel, (**c**) light source, and (**d**) camera (Patricia Shoda, Photographer, Cleveland Clinic Plastic Surgery)

sub-dermal space in a fan-like distribution from the areola edge to (but not into) the base of the nipple.

Ductoscope Preparation

The sterile ductoscope is attached to the draped camera cord and sterile light cord. The sterile disposable cannula is inserted over the scope after priming the catheter with either lidocaine or saline. Air bubbles should be removed carefully from the cannula and 20 cc syringe of irrigant and the tubing as they impair visualization within the ductal system. The scope is focused until a clear rim is seen on the screen or a suture packet is easily legible at 2 mm.

The ductoscope is white-balanced and focused. The scope is oriented by noting the site of entry of the irrigation tubing into the ductoscope based on the face of a clock.

Identification and Cannulation of the Correct Duct

The duct with the pathological nipple discharge is identified and the orifice carefully and serially dilated using Bowman's lacrimal dilators. If the orifice is too tiny to admit a 0000 dilator, then an Ultra slim^{TM} or a 000 Prolene suture could be used. Once the involved duct opening is dilated to a 1 Bowman's dilator, the ductoscope is introduced into the ductal orifice with continuous gentle saline irrigation. Care must be taken to avoid puncturing the wall of the duct which creates a false passage and collapses the true duct lumen making the chances of successful cannulation slim (Fig. 24.4).

The nipple is extended with one hand which straightens the ductal system allowing for easier navigation. The fingers of this hand can gently push the breast tissue and duct in front of the scopes pathway (Fig. 24.5).

Irrigation and Visualization

Saline solution or lidocaine is continuously injected into the duct through the working channel to facilitate the passage of the endoscope and visualize the intraductal space. All branches are traversed and abnormalities noted.

Intraductal Breast Biopsy (IDBB)

The steps for the IDBB examination are as follows: (a) the ductoscope is covered with a metallic tube with a side aperture near the tip and the ductoscope with the metallic tube is inserted into the mammary duct, (b) the metallic tube is advanced along the outside of the ductoscope to the intraductal mass and the mass is entrapped in the tube through a side aperture under observation through the ductoscope, (c) then the metallic tube is turned to cut off the intraductal mass, and (d) afterward, the ductoscope is removed and the tissue piece within the metallic tube is collected by manually applied negative pressure [17].

Ductoscopy-Directed Duct Excision

In cases of pathological nipple discharge or in cases of breast cancer with suspected extensive intraductal

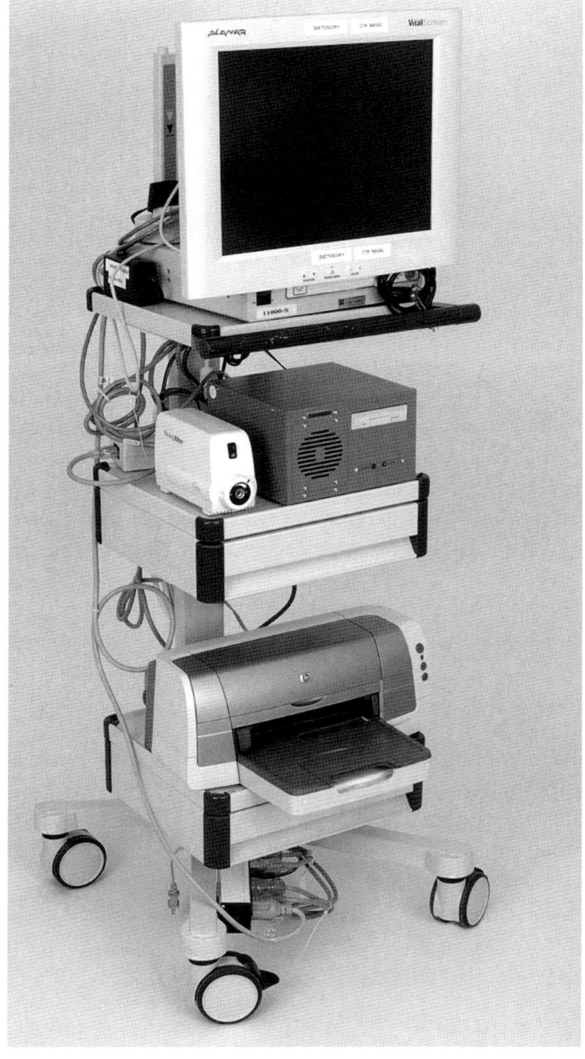

Figure 24.2
Monitor with light source (Patricia Shoda, Photographer, Cleveland Clinic Plastic Surgery)

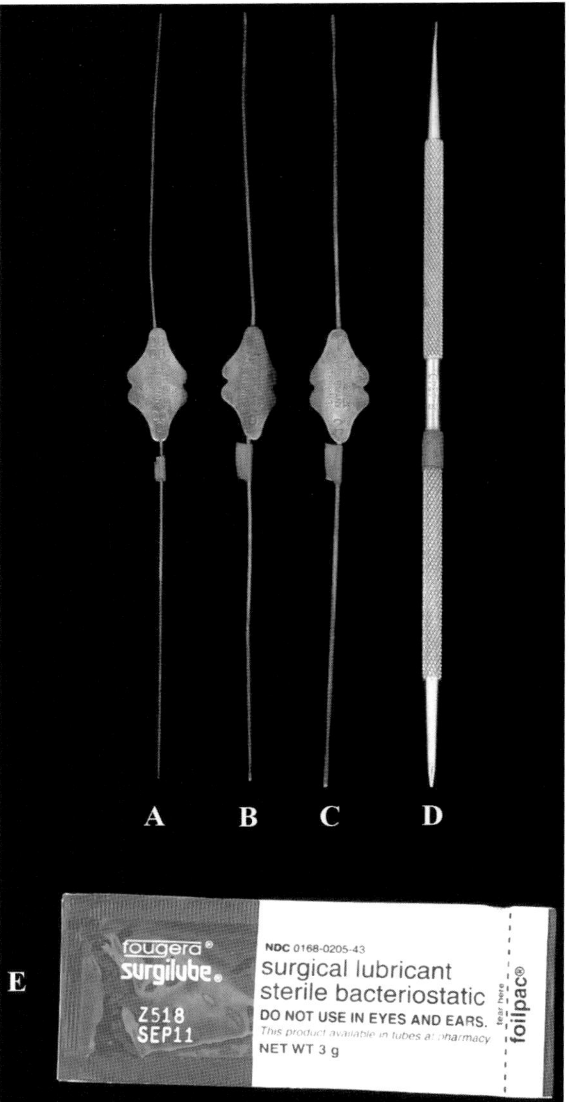

Figure 24.3
Lacrimal dilators. (**a–c**) Lacrimal dilators' size 0000–2 and (**d**) Castroviejo double-ended lacrimal dilator. It has one end as a needle point and the other a medium taper, (**e**) lubricating jelly (Patricia Shoda, Photographer, Cleveland Clinic Plastic Surgery)

component, intraoperative ductoscopy can help direct the amount of tissue to be excised [16, 18]. The intraductal lesion is identified 90% of the time in cases of ductoscopy for PND. An attempt is made to get beyond the intraductal mass as 25% of cases will have deeper additional lesions that require removal [13, 18]. The scope is positioned 1–2 cm past the lesion (or if it is obstructing, just next to the lesion). The scope is held in place by an assistant while a circumareolar incision is made. Dissection back to the base of the nipple in the avascular plane is carried out with cautery on a low setting. The offending duct and scope are encircled with a tie at the base of the nipple. Dissection is carried

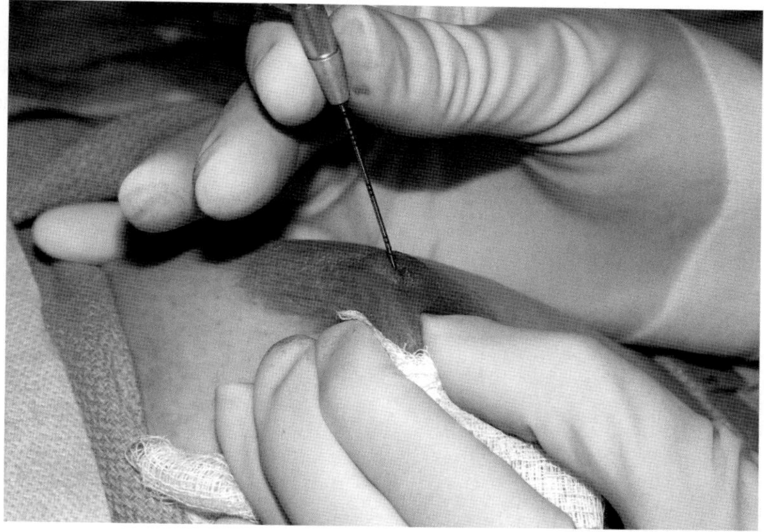

Figure 24.4
Cannulating the duct via the nipple (Patricia Shoda, Photographer, Cleveland Clinic Plastic Surgery)

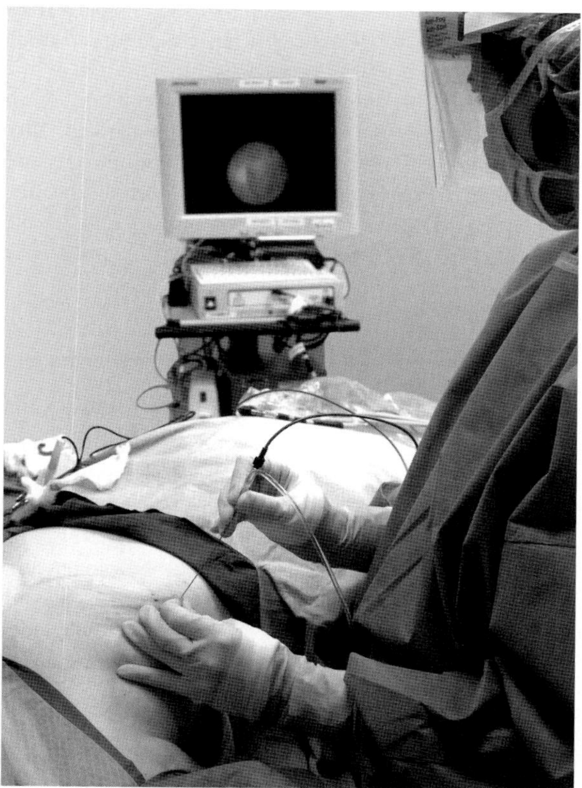

Figure 24.5
Performing ductoscopy (Patricia Shoda, Photographer, Cleveland Clinic Plastic Surgery)

out with cautery anterior to the scope. As the lesion is approached, the OR lights are diverted and room lights dimmed so that transillumination from the light of the ductoscope can assist with the dissection. The lateral planes are dissected on either side of the scope and finally the posterior plane. Once the dissection has gone beyond the lesion and light of the scope, ductoscopy can again be used to visualize the lesion within the specimen and mark the external surface of the specimen for the pathologist. The retrograde dissection is completed while carefully withdrawing the scope so as not to fracture or bend it. The ducts are then tied off at the base of the nipple. If the lesion is visualized within the nipple itself it would necessitate coring out the nipple. If a nipple core is performed, a chromic suture can repair the hole in the nipple and a 5-point star cerclage suture of 3–0 PDS at the inner aspect of the base of the nipple prevents nipple inversion. The wound is then closed in two layers. The specimen is marked at the nipple end and sent to pathology for permanent sectioning.

Cannulating the High-Risk or Cancer Patient

In the absence of pathological nipple discharge the ducts are not dilated and cannulation can be challenging. The same principles are followed for scoping a high-risk or cancer patient; however, more care and experience is needed.

Pathology Considerations

Marking the specimen for the pathologist and describing the visual findings assist in identifying the lesions. Breast lesions as small as 1/100 the size of those detected by mammography and MRI can be found on ductoscopy but missed by routine pathologic sectioning. Serial sectioning every 2–3 mm can help identify these smaller lesions and this may need to be discussed with the pathologist.

Limitations

1. MD only evaluates a portion of the ducts that have been cannulated. The other ducts remain unexamined.
2. Cancers starting in terminal ductal units cannot always be visualized due to size limitations of the ductoscope.
3. False passages occurring early during the procedure could make anatomy difficult to interpret and render further scoping unsuccessful.

Advantages

1. MD allows accurate visualization, analysis, and excision of intraductal abnormalities with a higher yield of proliferative lesions then standard duct excision.
2. Ductoscopy-directed duct excision of abnormalities requires resection of smaller amounts of breast tissue as compared to conventional duct excision for pathological nipple discharge.

Pitfalls and Management

1. Failed cannulation due to small orifice or false tract: In this event, a circumareolar incision is made and dissection carried sharply toward base of nipple. The dilated duct full of discharge or irrigation is usually evident. The duct is isolated, controlled proximally and distally with vicryl suture. A tiny angled opening is made on the duct. The ductoscope is passed into duct to evaluate internal ductal anatomy.
2. If cannulation via the nipple or through the incision is not possible, major duct excision is recommended due to the increased rate of malignancy in patients with failed cannulation [13].
3. If a false passage has been made, irrigation should be stopped as the fluid will exit the opening further collapsing the duct. The ductoscope is withdrawn and an attempt is made to pass beyond the breach. If this fails, discharging duct is found from within the incision as described above.

Future Directions

1. Differential expression of nipple aspirate fluid proteins exists between women with normal and diseased breasts, and proteomic analysis may predict the presence of breast cancer. Thus, it may be possible to use ductoscopy for screening for cancer and precancerous lesions by identifying its earliest molecular evolution [19].
2. Genetic analysis of ductal epithelial cells using techniques such as methylation-specific polymerase chain reaction or fluorescence in situ hybridization may assist in the detection of rare cancer cells, which may improve detection of early cancers [20].
3. Micro-instruments, auto fluorescence, or spectrography-based techniques that can enhance identification of atypical ductal epithelium and laser ductoscopy may help to direct tissue sampling making ductoscopy more of an interventional procedure and probably therapeutic procedure [21].

Endoscopic Axillary Procedures

Sentinel lymph node biopsy has become the standard of care for staging the axilla in a patient with breast cancer due to lower morbidity and acceptable false-negative rates. It provides prognostic information and determines adjuvant therapy [22]. Endoscopic sentinel lymph node biopsies and axillary dissections have been performed successfully with equal accuracy and reliability and have provided a minimally invasive approach for the same.

Indications

Endoscopic technique for evaluation of the axilla in breast cancer patients allows

a. creation of a minimally invasive work space within the axilla;
b. recognition of key axillary anatomic landmarks; and

c. instrument manipulation within the axilla to identify and extract lymph nodes and apply the sentinel node technique [3].

Sentinel Lymph Node Biopsy

Endoscopic sentinel lymph node biopsy is a reliable technique for evaluation of the axilla with a high rate of sentinel node identification and high predictive value for nodal status [6]. As for a standard open sentinel lymph node biopsy, the technique may be performed using isosulfan blue dye peritumoral or subareolar injection preoperatively. Once the axillary space is entered, the blue stained sentinel node is identified and resected using a 5 mm grasping forceps and a pair of monopolar scissors. The sentinel node is sent separately for frozen section or touch prep. When positive level I and II axillary dissection can be carried out as described below.

Axillary Lymph Node Dissection

Endoscopic axillary dissection is beneficial for patients undergoing a skin-sparing mastectomy or a lumpectomy for breast cancer when simultaneous axillary dissection is required. It is minimally invasive, functionally optimal for ipsilateral arm mobilization, and cosmetically appealing [9].

Equipment

A standard laparoscopic 10 mm port is used as the camera port, two 5 mm ports are used for inserting short-arm dissecting (25 cm) and grasping forceps, scissors and a 30° long endoscope is optimal for visualizing the slanting, irregular axillary borders. The light source, camera, video monitor, and CO_2 cylinder are as per standard laparoscopic surgery requirements.

Procedure

Positioning of the Patient

After induction of general anesthesia, patient is placed supine with ipsilateral arm abducted to 90°. Breast, chest wall, axilla prepped and draped in usual sterile fashion. Lateral aspects of pectoralis major and anterior border of latissimus dorsi muscle are delineated with a marking pen (Fig. 24.6).

Establishment of Gas Space in the Axilla

a. *Technique with lipoaspiration*: After induction of general anesthesia, patient is placed supine with arm abducted to 90°. A lipolysis liquid (saline 200–250 ml, distilled water 200–250 ml, lidocaine 800 mg, adrenaline 0.5–1 mg) is injected into the axilla using a lumbar puncture needle. After 20 min

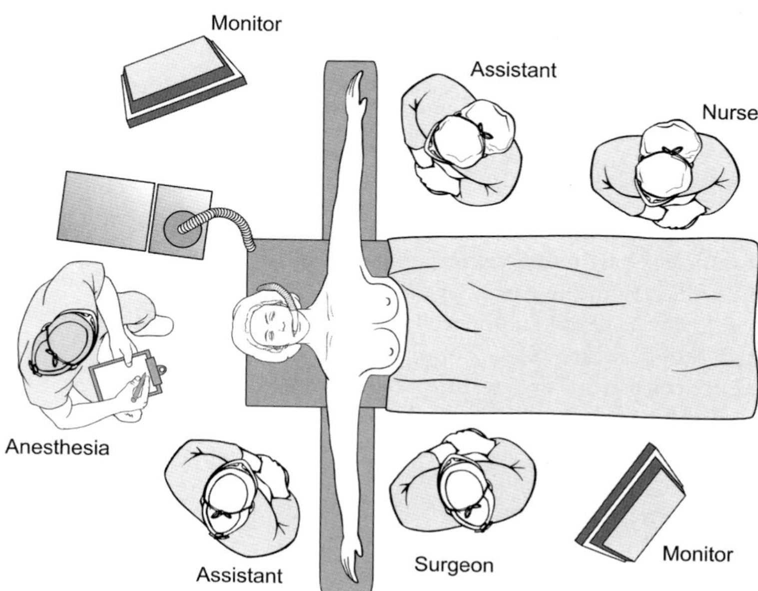

Figure 24.6

Position of patient for endoscopic axillary dissection or endoscopic-assisted mastectomy. Reprinted with permission of The Cleveland Clinic Center for Medical Art and Photography © 2009. All rights reserved

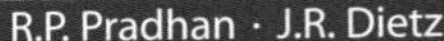

the fat of the axilla is aspirated using a lipo-aspirator through a 10 mm incision located in the midline of axilla and parallel to the level of the nipple, between the lateral border of the pectoralis major and lateral border of latissimus dorsi muscle. Care must be taken in choosing the injection site as this is where the optical trocar will be placed. The incision must be superior enough to avoid flow of liquid over the optics and block vision and also provide good visibility. It should be far enough from the chest wall to allow panoramic view of the axilla and low enough to not miss the first nodes in the lymphatic chain. The clavipectoral fascia is then incised in its inferior portion using a 14 mm Mayo scissors through the 10 mm incision so that further dissection is carried out in the axillary space now freed of fatty tissue [23]. A 10 mm trocar is later introduced through this hole and CO_2 is used to inflate the axilla [7].

b. *Technique with balloon expansion of axilla*: A 1 cm skin incision is made at the superior aspect of the axilla in mid-axillary line and carried to the lateral border of the pectoralis major muscle. The clavipectoral fascia is incised at that level and a tract created into the axilla using blunt finger dissection. A balloon distension device is inserted into the tract and carefully distended under direct endoscopic vision to create a working space. Balloon is then replaced with a blunt-tipped cannula. CO_2 is insufflated to a pressure of 8–12 mmHg. A 30° scope is introduced to visualize axillary contents. Two 5 mm ports are placed at the lateral border of pectoralis major and latissimus dorsi muscles for grasping and dissecting axillary contents mostly at the anterior axillary line [3] (Fig. 24.7).

Control of Gas Pressure in Axillary Space

Excessive gas can cause subcutaneous emphysema and insufficient gas makes visualization of axillary space difficult. Due to the nature of the tissues, an effective seal is not achieved and hence keeping the gas speed high (but between 8 and 12 mmHg) is the only way to ensure consistent CO_2 pressure while limiting the risk of subcutaneous emphysema.

Placement of Trocars

The ideal position for the camera is the crossing point of the middle axially line and the nipple level.

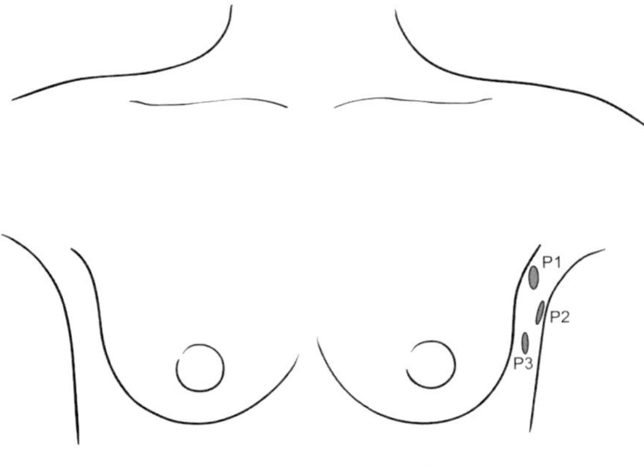

Figure 24.7

Locations of axillary incisions for endoscopic axillary dissection or mastectomy. Reprinted with permission of The Cleveland Clinic Center for Medical Art and Photography © 2009. All rights reserved

Two working trocars (dissecting forceps and scissors) should be placed away from the apex of the axilla preferably at the lateral edge of the pectoralis major anteriorly and the anterior border of latissimus dorsi posteriorly. The distance between the two trocars should not be more than 5 cm as it makes dissection harder.

Procedure for Lymph Node Dissection

1. One of the first structures seen on entering axilla through the 10 mm port with the camera is the intercostobrachial nerve. It spans like a crossbeam in the axillary cavity. The fat and lymphatics around it is peeled off by electrocautery using the grasper and dissecting forceps via the two 5 mm ports. Preservation of intercostobrachial nerve decreases the morbidity such as numbness on medial side of arm, pain, burning, and warmth.
2. The space between the major and minor pectoralis muscles is developed. This dissection helps finding the Rotter's lymph node. The principal axis of dissection is along the inferior border of the axillary vein, anterior to the thoracodorsal neurovascular bundle and lateral to the long thoracic nerve [23].
3. The dissection of the fat and lymphatic tissues starts laterally along the length of the pectoralis major border and then medially along the undersurface of this muscle and cephalad from the medial side

of the thoracoacromial vessels to caudally toward the latissimus dorsi muscle layer by layer using the axillary vein as the guide. The fat and lymphatic tissue is gently dissected off laterally till the latissimus muscle becomes tendinous [24].

4. Extraction of the fatty lymphatic tissues dissected can be done from the medial 5 mm port by enlarging it to 10 mm. A 10 mm port is placed and then a 10–5 mm reducer is placed on the port and a toothed grasper is used to hold the lymphatic tissue, allowing direct visualization of the lymphatic chain as it is being withdrawn [23]. Alternatively the 10 mm incision can be enlarged and the lymphatic tissue removed from there.
5. Management of axillary cavity – The cavity is palpated for enlarged nodes, irrigated, and closed in two layers after placement of a suction drain.

Advantages of Endoscopic Sentinel Lymph Node and Axillary Dissection

1. Once liposuction and CO_2 insufflation is done, the axillary space becomes a reticular structure like spider webs with lymph nodes suspended in it.
2. A more magnified view of the axilla is obtained and operative dissection is clearer with a high rate of sentinel lymph node identification and subsequent axillary level I and II dissection with the number of lymph nodes harvested comparable to open techniques [6, 22, 23, 25].
3. Precise identification and preservation of the intercostobrachial nerve, axillary vein, lateral thoracic vessels, dorsal thoracic nerve, long thoracic nerve, and the medical thoracic nerve [7].

Limitations

1. This technique, while widely used in Japan and China, has been rarely performed in the United States. The learning curve for performing endoscopic sentinel node biopsy and axillary dissection can be considerable.
2. Prolonged duration of endoscopic axillary procedures as compared to open surgery.
3. Even minimal bleeding can cause poor visualization of the operative field.
4. Possible injury to intercostobrachial nerve, thoracodorsal nerve, long thoracic nerve, and medial and lateral pectoral nerves, axillary vein, lateral thoracic vessels is similar to open surgery.

Challenges for Endoscopic Axillary Dissection

1. Axilla is a parenchymatous tissue with no preexisting space in it. A working space has to be created.
2. It is hard to establish a stable CO_2 gas space.
3. It is a highly vascular and complex region populated with nerves and blood vessels.
4. Operative working space is narrow.
5. It is harder to maintain a seal between the skin and trocar as in the abdomen due to laxity of the axillary tissue. Due to the gas leakage then, higher gas flows are required to maintain the pressure.

Endoscopic-Assisted Subcutaneous Mastectomy with Immediate Mammary Prosthesis Reconstruction for Early Breast Cancer

Indications

Endoscopic surgery for the breast was first attempted by plastic surgeons in 1992 and since then it has been used for breast lump excision, augmentation, and mastectomy.

The technique of skin-sparing mastectomy is an oncologically safe one, based on the absence of breast ductal epithelium at the margins of the native skin flaps and a local recurrence rate comparable to non-skin-sparing mastectomy. Skin-sparing mastectomy and immediate breast reconstruction may be considered an excellent alternative treatment to breast conservation for patients with ductal carcinoma in situ and early-stage invasive breast cancer [26, 27].

Interest has developed in minimally invasive options for performing the mastectomy endoscopically since subcutaneous mastectomy in select patients has been documented to be oncologically safe [4].

Equipment

A general laparoscopic 10 mm/30° scope, an endoscopic breast retractor, endoscopic breast dissector, and a 7-in. harmonic scalpel are the instruments used for the procedure. The position of the patient and the axillary incisions are similar to those depicted for endoscopic axillary dissection (Figs. 24.6 and 24.7).

Procedure

A 5 cm skin incision is made along the lowest axillary skin crease. Dissection is continued down to the lateral border of pectoralis major muscle. A sub-pectoral pocket is gently created by an endoscopic breast dissector. The endoscopic breast retractor and 10 mm/30° scope are inserted into the sub-pectoral pocket and further dissection is carried out with the help of the harmonic scalpel under endoscopic vision down to a level 1 cm caudal to the inframammary fold. The sub-pectoral space is used for insertion of the mammary implant later.

A subcutaneous mastectomy is carried out using the harmonic scalpel. The plane between the breast disc and the pectoralis major muscle is opened up via diathermy under direct vision to create a working space. The endoscopic breast retractor is placed into the space to lift up the breast disc. Using the harmonic scalpel, the breast disc is dissected off the pectoralis major muscle up to the clavicle under endoscopic vision. The plane between the skin flap and the breast is opened under direct vision to create a working space for the excision of all the breast tissue endoscopically. This is done by sharp dissection using the harmonic scalpel and scissors in the plane between the subcutaneous tissue under the skin and the breast parenchyma. The skin flaps are of the same thickness as in a routine skin-sparing mastectomy.

In large volume breasts an inferior circumareolar incision is made for easier dissection of the medial lower quadrant of the breast. Excised breast tissue is pulled out through the axillary wound. A level I or II axillary dissection or sentinel lymph node biopsy can be done through the same incision.

A McGhan style expandable implant is used for immediate sub-pectoral reconstruction. Once the prosthesis is placed in the sub-pectoral pocket, normal saline is injected to inflate the prosthesis and check its position and ensure the inframammary line is defined. A subcutaneous pocket is created in the sub-axillary region for the port. A suction drain is left in the axilla. Light supportive dressing is applied to the breast for 48 h to keep prosthesis medially [4].

Advantages

1. Minimizes skin incision and scarring
2. Excellent cosmetic results
3. Reduces blood loss
4. Improves reconstructive and rehabilitative outcome
5. Reduces psychosocial morbidity

Limitations

1. Learning curve associated with endoscopic-assisted surgery and careful endoscopic dissection in the limited axillary space in proximity of neurovascular structures
2. Inability to use technique for tumors greater than 3 cm and central lesions
3. Poor scope visualization in the event of even minimal bleeding

References

1. Escobar P et al (2006) The clinical applications of mammary ductoscopy. Am J Surg 191:211–215
2. Morrow M, Jordan VC (2003) Role of breast epithelial sampling techniques. In: Morrow M (ed) Managing breast cancer risk. BC Decker, London, pp 138–156
3. Tsangaris TN, Brody FJ, Jacobs LK (1999) Endoscopic axillary exploration and sentinel lymphadenectomy. Surg Endosc 13:43–47
4. Ho WS, Ying SY, Chan ACW (2002) Endoscopic assisted subcutaneous mastectomy and axillary dissection with immediate mammary prosthesis reconstruction for early breast cancer. Surg Endosc 16:302–306
5. Yamashita K, Shimizu K (2008) Video assisted breast surgery and sentinel lymph node biopsy guided by three dimensional tomographic lymphography. Surg Endosc 22:392–397
6. Kuhn T et al (2000) Axilloscopy and endoscopic sentinel node detection in breast cancer patients. Surg Endosc 14:573–577
7. Luo C et al (2008) Experience of a large series of masoscopic axillary lymph node dissection. J Surg Oncol 98:89–93
8. Gerber B et al (2003) Skin-sparing mastectomy with conservation of the nipple-areola complex and autologous reconstruction is an oncologically safe procedure. Ann Surg 238:120–127
9. Ward DC, Edwards MH (1983) Early results of subcutaneous mastectomy with immediate silicone prosthetic implant for carcinoma of the breast. Br J Surg 70:651–653
10. Palmer BV, Mannur KR, Ross WB (1992) Subcutaneous mastectomy with immediate reconstruction as treatment for early breast cancer. Br J Surg 79:1309–1311
11. Kroll SS, Ames F, Singletary SE (1991) The ontological risks of skin preservation at mastectomy when combined with immediate reconstruction of the breast. Surg Gynecol Obstet 172:17–20
12. Hinton CP et al (1984) Subcutaneous mastectomy for primary operable breast cancer. Br J Surg 71:469–472
13. Dietz JR et al (2002) Directed duct excision using mammary ductoscopy in patients with pathological nipple discharge. Surgery 132:582–587
14. Dietz JR (2003) Nipple discharge. Prob Gen Surg 20(4): 42–55
15. Dooley WC (2003) Routine operative breast endoscopy during lumpectomy. Ann Surg Oncol 10:38–42

16. Hünerbein M, Raubach M, Gebauer B, Schneider W, Schlag PM (2006) Intraoperative ductoscopy in women undergoing surgery for breast cancer. Surgery 139(6): 833–838
17. Matsunaga T, Kawakami Y, Namba K (2004) Intraductal biopsy for diagnosis and treatment of intraductal lesions of the breast. Cancer 101:2164–2169
18. Dooley WC (2002) Routine operative breast endoscopy for bloody nipple discharge. Ann Surg Oncol 9(9): 920–923
19. Sauter ER et al (2002) Proteomic analysis of nipple aspirate fluid to detect biologic markers of breast cancer. Br J Cancer 86:1440–1443
20. Dooley WC (2005) The future prospect: ductoscopy directed brushing and biopsy. Clin Lab Med 25:845–850
21. Jacobs VR et al (2007) Breast ductoscopy: Technical development from a diagnostic to an interventional procedure and its future perspective. Onkologie 30:545–549
22. Kocher T et al (2006) Significance of endoscopic axillary dissection in invasive breast carcinoma after introduction of the "sentinel lymph node" method. Swiss Surg 3: 121–127
23. Salvat J et al (1996) Endoscopic exploration and lymph node sampling of the axilla; preliminary findings of a randomized pilot study comparing clinical and anatomopathologic results of endoscopic axillary lymph node sampling with traditional surgical treatment. Eur J Obstet Gynecol Reprod Biol 70:165–173
24. Gomatos IP, Filippakis G, Albanopoulos K et al (2006) Complete endoscopic axillary lymph node dissection without liposuction for breast cancer: Initial experience and mid-term outcome. Surg Laparosc Endosc Percutan Tech 16(4):232–236
25. Suzanne F et al (1997) Axillary lymphadenectomy by lipoaspiration and endoscopic picking: apropos of 72 cases. Chirurgie 122:138–142
26. Newman LA et al (1998) Presentation, treatment and outcome of local recurrence after skin-sparing mastectomy and immediate breast reconstruction. Ann Surg Oncol 5: 620–626
27. Slavin SA, Schnitt SJ, Duda RB, Houlihan MJ (1998) Skin-sparing mastectomy and immediate reconstruction: oncologic risks and aesthetic results in patients with early-stage breast cancer. Plast Reconstr Surg 102:49–62

The Applications of Sentinel Lymph Node to Cancer

Anton J. Bilchik, Maria M. Gonzalez,
Alexander Stojadinovic

Contents

Introduction

It is likely that every solid neoplasm drains to an initial lymph node (sentinel lymph node – SLN) before spreading to regional nodes or systemically. Focused evaluation of the SLN as originally described by Morton et al. in 1990 [1] has improved staging accuracy in melanoma and breast cancer and has been applied to other solid neoplasms with the purpose of minimizing the morbidity of lymph node dissections and/or to increase the accuracy of staging. Until the development of this technique, there was significant controversy and difficulty in the selection of patients needing full lymph node dissections in the setting of clinically negative nodes. The incidence of complications, most prominently lymphedema, had to be balanced against the possible additional staging information gleaned by complete nodal evaluation.

Both dyes and radiopharmaceutical tracers have been used for the identification of SLN. In the initial description, isosulfan blue dye [2] was used to intraoperatively map the pathway from a primary cutaneous melanoma to one or more SLNs in the regional lymphatic basin. Pathologic analysis of the SLN accurately reflected the tumor status of the entire regional lymphatic basin.

The technique was then modified to combine isosulfan blue dye with a radiopharmaceutical and was adapted successfully to breast cancer [3]. Since then the SLN concept has been examined in numerous solid neoplasms including gastric and colorectal cancer.

While outside the scope of this chapter, SLN technology has also been utilized in both gynecologic and urologic applications. For gynecology, successful applications of SLN techniques in endometrial [4], cervical [5], and vulvar cancers [6] have been described. Urologic applications have included prostate [7] and bladder [8] cancers. As yet, SLN biopsy has not

F.L. Greene, B.T. Heniford (eds.), *Minimally Invasive Cancer Management*,
DOI 10.1007/978-1-4419-1238-1_25,

gained wide acceptance in the gynecologic and urologic communities and is still primarily done as a part of an experimental protocol.

This chapter reviews current techniques and the application of SLN to skin malignancies, head and neck cancer, breast cancer, lung cancer, and gastrointestinal neoplasms.

Melanoma

SLN Mapping Technique

The standard technique of SLN identification involves the injection of a tracer (most commonly isosulfan blue) to identify the lymphatic drainage pathway from a primary tumor. Although isosulfan blue is safe, anaphylaxis has been reported in up to 1% of patients [9]. Subsequent reports [10] describe the use of radioisotopes such as Technetium-99m bound colloids (^{99m}Tc) for preoperative lymphoscintigraphy and intraoperative localization of the SLN using a gamma probe [11, 12]. The most commonly used radiolabeled colloid in the United States is ^{99m}Tc-sulfur colloid, while ^{99m}Tc-nanocolloid and ^{99m}Tc-antimony sulfide are more commonly used in Europe and Australia, respectively.

The most accurate mapping technique uses a combination of isosulfan blue and a radioisotope, although single modality techniques show excellent results in experienced hands. Using the standard technique, tracer is injected in the location of the primary tumor. Lymphoscintigraphy performed before SNB can demonstrate drainage to unexpected lymph node basins (Fig. 25.1). A gamma counter identifies the SLN and additional nodes and is marked on the skin. An incision is then made to identify the blue node (Fig. 25.2) and/or the most radioactive node. Radioactivity counts of the lymphatic basin are taken and recorded before and after nodal excision including counts of each individual node. It is recommended that all blue nodes and any node that has a count of at least 10% of the radioactivity of the "hottest" node be excised [13]. There is very limited radiation exposure during the procedure; therefore, no special handling of the SLN is required.

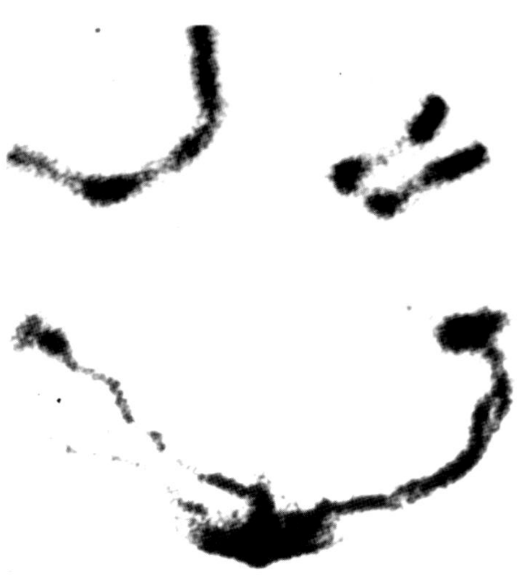

Figure 25.1

Preoperative lymphoscintigraphy of truncal melanoma to both axillae

Surgical Management

The surgical management of lymph nodes in skin cancers, in particular melanoma, has been controversial for many years. Some retrospective studies have demonstrated a survival advantage of routine elective lymph node dissection (ELND) in patients without clinical evidence of regional lymph node metastases [14, 15], while prospective trials have failed to show an overall survival benefit for patients undergoing ELND over wide excision alone [16–19]. There is, however, consensus that SLNB can identify patients with regional lymph node metastases who may benefit from a complete lymphadenectomy, while avoiding the morbidity of complete lymph node dissection for patients without lymph node metastases. It is also practical to examine a smaller number of lymph nodes for micrometastases (MM) using HMB45 and S100. Although SLNB is generally recommended for melanomas greater than 1.0 mm thick [20], the indications have been expanded to include patients with thinner melanomas, especially those with evidence of regression, ulceration, or positive deep margins [2]. SLNB is not recommended in patients with clinically positive nodes and in situations where the clinical management will not be affected. In addition, the technique may be insensitive in patients that have had extensive surgeries such as rotational flaps where the lymphatic pathways have been disrupted. SLNB has become widely adopted for regional lymph node staging in early-stage melanoma. The technique offers a valuable method to accurately evaluate the regional lymph node basin for both prognostication and selecting patients for adjuvant therapy.

Figure 25.2

Blue lymphatic draining to sentinel lymph node in groin

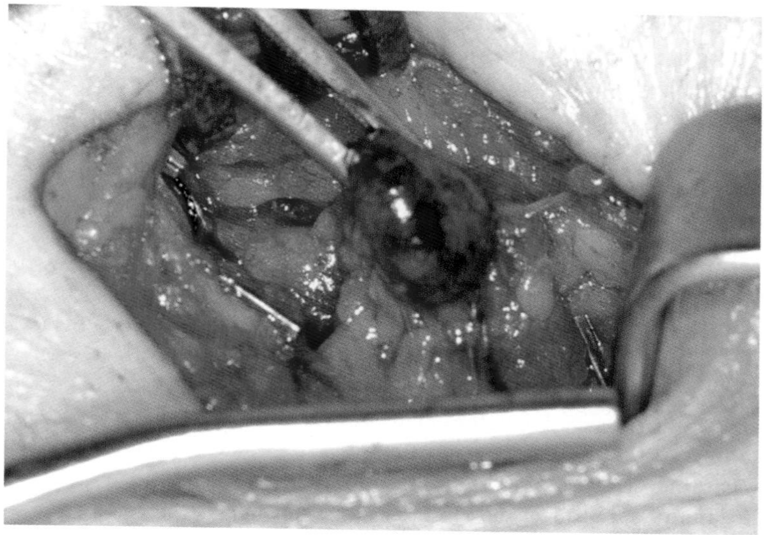

A learning curve for SLNB was confirmed by Morton et al. [21] when the accuracy rate increased from 81 to 96% after the first 58 cases. It is recommended that at least 30 procedures be performed before surgeons reach an acceptable accuracy and sensitivity. Surgeons should monitor their false-negative rate through the learning phase by routinely performing CLND or performing the procedure with surgeons who have completed the learning phase.

In 1994 the Multicenter Selective Lymphadenectomy Trial (MSLT-1) was begun by Morton and colleagues at the John Wayne Cancer Institute to determine the therapeutic benefit of SLNB and the accuracy of the technique on a worldwide basis. Patients with intermediate-thickness (1–4 mm) melanoma were prospectively randomized to wide local excision (WLE) of the primary and observation of the nodal basin or WLE and SLNB. CLND was performed only in regional lymph node basins that had tumor-positive SN by H&E or immunohistochemistry.

The accuracy of SLNB was confirmed with only a 5% false-negative rate and a low minor complication rate of 10% [22]. In 2006 the results were reported in the *New England Journal of Medicine* [23]. Among 1,269 patients with an intermediate-thickness primary melanoma, the 5-year melanoma-specific survival rates were similar in the two groups (87 and 86%, respectively). However, in the WLE group, the presence of metastases in the SLN was the most important prognostic factor; the 5-year survival rate was 72% among patients with tumor-positive SLNs and was 90% among those with tumor-negative SLNs. Among patients with nodal metastases, the 5-year survival rate was higher among those who underwent immediate lymphadenectomy than among those in whom lymphadenectomy was delayed (72% vs. 52%). These data confirm that the staging of intermediate-thickness primary melanomas provides important prognostic information and demonstrates that survival can be prolonged with immediate lymphadenectomy in patients with nodal metastases. Evaluation of the regional node basin by SLNB has therefore become the standard approach for staging the regional lymph nodes.

Currently, Morton et al. have initiated MSLT II, a study to evaluate the therapeutic value of CLND in melanoma patients with evidence of SN metastases (by conventional H&E histopathology, IHC, or RT-PCR) randomized to CLND or observation of the nodal basin. The trial was initiated in January 2005 and should provide insight into the natural history of patients with a tumor-positive SN and the therapeutic benefit of CLND.

Other Skin Cancers

Several small single institution studies have reported the use of SLNB for non-melanoma skin cancers, mostly for Merkel cell and squamous cell skin cancers (SCC) [24–26]. Since these are skin cancers, the rationale for SLNB is similar to melanoma, namely the ability to identify a limited lymph node sample that will be representative of the likelihood of lymphatic spread, and the avoidance of morbidity of a complete lymph node dissection in those in which the

SLN is negative. Both cancers are known to spread through regional lymphatics, Merkel cell frequently and SCC seldomly, and thus all patients with Merkel cell tumors should be considered for SLNB, while only those patients with squamous cell skin cancer with risk factors for metastases (greater than 2 cm in diameter, immunosuppressed patients, or invasion into deeper structures) may benefit from SLNB [26]. The combination technique of isosulfan blue and radiotracer should be preferred due to the variability of lymphatic drainage. The accuracies and identification rates in these small studies have paralleled melanoma suggesting a role for SLNB in non-melanoma skin cancer [24–26]. However, due to the small size and often short follow-up of these case series, definitive conclusions regarding accuracy and identification rates in non-melanoma skin cancer remain unclear. Nevertheless, it would be reasonable to offer the procedure as an alternative to ELND or observation in selected patients in a controlled setting.

Breast Cancer

Axillary lymph node evaluation by complete nodal dissection has been the standard of care in breast cancer for many years. Complete nodal dissection has been viewed as a prognostic indicator and as a mechanism of selecting patients for adjuvant chemotherapy [27, 28]. It is also performed to improve local control and some have suggested an improvement in survival. Unfortunately, ALND is associated with increased morbidity including nerve paresthesias and most significantly lymphedema. SLNB was therefore applied to breast cancer as an alternative to ALND particularly to reduce the morbidity in patients with tumor-free lymph nodes. Because focused analysis can be performed on a limited number of nodes, staging accuracy is also improved and treatment decisions optimized.

SLN Technique

SLNB for breast cancer can be performed using isosulfan blue only, lymphoscintigraphy with intraoperative radiolocalization, or a combination of both. All evaluation methods produce similar identification and false-negative rates in the hands of experienced surgeons [29–32]. The choice of technique should be based on institutional and surgeon experience. If radiocolloid is used, ^{99m}Tc-labeled sulfur colloid should be injected preferably within 6 h of surgery.

Surgical Management

At the time of surgery 2–5 ml of isosulfan blue dye is injected in a peritumoral or peribiopsy location. Subareolar injection has also been used and may be useful in multifocal or nonpalpable disease. Approximately 5 min after injection, an incision is made beneath the axillary hair line. The clavipectoral fascia is divided and the axilla explored for a blue-stained lymphatic channel draining to the SLN. A Geiger counter is used if preoperative lymphoscintigraphy and injection of a radiocolloid has been performed. The SLN is then removed and serial sectioning performed. Both routine H&E staining and immunohistochemistry can be used to identify MM. If metastases are identified, the patient is then taken back for an ALND because of the possibility of other tumor involved lymph nodes.

In breast cancer, SLNBs accuracy is not affected by the type of diagnostic biopsy, the location of the primary breast tumor, type of definitive surgery (breast conservation or mastectomy), or tumor size [33–35]. Initially SLNB was thought to be inaccurate in larger tumors because of obstructed lymphatic pathways but several studies have demonstrated low false-negative rates in large tumors as well [33–35]. SLNB in patients thought to only have ductal carcinoma in situ (DCIS) is also controversial, since by definition, DCIS does not metastasize to lymph nodes. SLNB may only be beneficial in a subset of patients in whom occult invasive disease may have been undetected such as high-grade DCIS or multifocal disease including DCIS [36].

The role of SLNB after neoadjuvant chemotherapy is controversial. While some authors [37] have indicated high concordance rates of SLNB and ALND after chemotherapy, the NSABP B-27 reported a false-negative rate of 11%, substantially higher than routine SLNB [38]. Less is also known as to the prognosis of patients not undergoing ALND after conversion from node-positive to node-negative disease by neoadjuvant therapy. Accordingly, the ASCO 2005 practice guidelines concluded that there is insufficient data to recommend SLNB for patients receiving preoperative systemic chemotherapy [39]. Currently, some surgeons perform SLNB before neoadjuvant chemotherapy which has been established to be accurate [40], with the exception of inflammatory breast cancer, while other surgeons believe that SLNB should be performed in the setting of a protocol after neoadjuvant chemotherapy.

The identification and management of MM found by IHC in the SLN is extremely controversial. Unlike melanoma, routine use of IHC is not recommended in breast cancer since the significance is unknown. Until recently there was no clear definition for MM. In 2002, the American Joint Committee on Cancer (AJCC) sixth edition provided a definition of MM [41] classifying tumor deposits less than 0.2 mm as isolated tumor cells (i) and pN0 while deposits between 0.2 and 2 mm are $pN1_{mi}$. Isolated tumor cells (pN0) that lack the morphologic characteristics of tumor cells are not considered positive and therefore ALND is not recommended in this group. The significance of isolated tumor cells and micrometastatic disease has been the subject of much debate and the clinical trials such as the International Breast Cancer Study Group 23-01 trial [42] and the American College of Surgeons Oncology Group Z0010 trial are evaluating the controversy [43].

Depending on the institution, intraoperative analysis of the SLN with either frozen section or touch preparation is performed. Using such techniques for the reliable identification of SLN metastases would allow completion lymphadenectomy to be performed at the time of the initial surgery, avoiding a second surgery. However insensitive the results of frozen section, touch preparation and cytological smear for intraoperative identification of SLN metastases, have been reported [44] with sensitivities of 59, 57, and 59% respectively. Because of the possibility of missing small metastases and low sensitivity from frozen section, some institutions prefer to perform permanent section followed by ALND for positive SLNs. Intraoperative evaluation is then reserved for patients that have clinically suspicious SLN at the time of surgery. As with melanoma, the experience of the surgeon and institution is associated with accurate identification of the SLN.

Cox et al. [45] at the Moffitt Cancer Center evaluated their own experience using a combination technique with isosulfan blue and radiocolloid and found that 22 cases needed to be performed to achieve failure rates less than 10% and 54 cases to achieve rates lower than 5%. Furthermore surgeons needed to perform six or more procedures per month to continue to maintain accuracy [46]. A multicenter trial of both academic and community surgeons revealed that after 30 cases identification and false-negative rates were 90 and 4.3%, respectively [47].

The morbidity associated with SLNB in breast cancer has been evaluated. Two major prospective randomized trials have shown decreased morbidity with SLNB in breast cancer. The American College of Surgeons Oncology Group Z0010 trial reported a low rate of complications following SLNB [48]. Anaphylaxis to blue dye occurred in 0.1% of subjects. Other complications include wound infection (1.0%), axillary seroma (7.1%), and hematoma (1.4%). At 6 months, 8.6% of patients reported paresthesias, 3.8% decreased upper extremity range of motion, and 6.9% lymphedema. These figures are lower than ALND confirming that SLNB is a safe alternative to ALND. Veronesi et al. [49] compared ALND to SLNB and found that patients with SLNB had better arm mobility and aesthetic appearance, as well as less pain, paresthesias, and lymphedema. With SLNB for early-stage breast cancer validated in several prospective trials, it has become the standard of care in patients with clinically node-negative breast cancer.

Colorectal Cancer

Lymph node evaluation is essential for accurately staging colorectal cancer. Survival has also been shown to be impacted by the number of nodes retrieved [50, 51] possibly secondary to stage migration. The identification of nodal metastases is essential in determining which patients may benefit from chemotherapy. Adjuvant therapy has demonstrated a survival benefit, particularly with the combination of 5-fluorouracil, leucovorin, and oxaliplatin (FOLFOX) [52]. Current guidelines, however, do not support the routine use of adjuvant therapy in stage II colon cancer [53]. Despite this up to 25% of patients with node-negative disease recur possibly because of poor biology or missed MM. It is neither time nor cost-effective to perform a focused analysis on numerous LNs and therefore SLNB was examined in CRC to improve staging accuracy.

SLN Technique

The technique for mapping in colon cancer is performed via the injection of a blue dye either percutaneously or via a colonoscope for laparoscopic colectomy or after minimal mobilization when performed via open laparotomy.

Surgical Management

After resectability of the primary tumor has been determined, 0.5–1 ml of isosulfan blue dye is injected subserosally around the periphery of the tumor (Fig. 25.3). A radiocolloid (1 mCi of 99m-Tc) may also be used as an adjunct to facilitate the detection of the SLN. Typically, the dye reaches the SLN within 30–60 s via the lymphatics, so when performed laparoscopically, the colonoscopy must be performed after the laparoscopic examination of the abdomen. Occasionally gentle dissection of the mesentery is needed to trace the lymphatic path to the blue-stained SLN (Fig. 25.4). If a radiotracer is used, a gamma probe may help direct this dissection (Fig. 25.5). Since the isosulfan blue dye washes out with time and with further pathologic processing, each stained node is marked with a suture or clip. After this marking, all blue nodes should be included in the standard colectomy. The specimen is submitted for a focused pathologic examination of the SLNs, as well as a standard evaluation of all other lymph nodes. If aberrant drainage is noted, the resection boundaries are extended to include the mesenteric areas and blood supply.

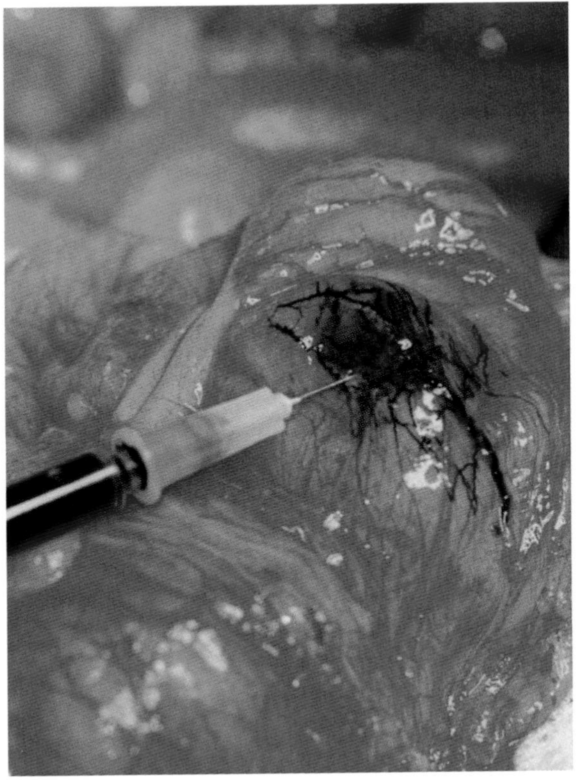

Figure 25.3
Injection of isosulfan blue dye in a primary colon cancer

As an alternate technique, ex vivo SLNB was first described by Wong et al. [54] and has proven to be successful both as a primary lymphatic mapping procedure and as a salvage technique when in vivo mapping fails [55, 56]. In the operating room, the colectomy specimen is immediately taken to a side table and 1–2 ml of isosulfan blue dye is injected subserosally around the tumor using a tuberculin syringe. The dye can be visualized as it progresses from the primary site along the lymphatic channels to the SLN(s) within the mesentery (Fig. 25.6). Again, each SLN is marked with sutures and the specimen is submitted for pathologic review, including a focused examination of the SLNs.

Initial reports of SLNB for colon cancer had high identification and accuracy rates ranging from 70% [57] to 100% [58]. As the technique has developed, most investigators are now able to routinely achieve over 90% success in identifying the SLN and accuracy rates of around 90% [59]. One notable exception is the Cancer and Leukemia Group B (CALGB) trial reported by Bertagnolli et al. [60] which found that despite a 92% success rate in localizing a SLN, accuracy was only 80% and a high false-negative rate of 54% when H&E analysis was used alone. A subsequent analysis of the same patients by IHC increased the sensitivity rate to as high as 88% depending on the definition used for a tumor-positive SLN [61]. In addition, its relatively small number of patients (91) enrolled over a large number of surgeons (25) and centers (13) may have impacted the results. This contrasts to a larger multicenter series reflecting those with more extensive experience which demonstrated an accuracy rates of 95% with an 11% false-negative rate over 408 colon cancer patients and an accuracy rate of 98% and a false-negative rate of 7% over 92 rectal cancer patients [62]. All surgeons in this series had over 30 colon cancer SLNB cases performed as compared to those in the CALGB trial who were only required to be proficient in the SLNB for breast cancer and melanoma.

The AJCC and the UICC stricter definitions for MM were recently applied to two prospective multicenter trials with similar results [63, 64]. Stringent pathologic criteria were also used whereby tumor cells identified by IHC without characteristic tumor morphology were not considered positive. Targeted analysis of the SN using IHC upstaged 11% of patients and isolated

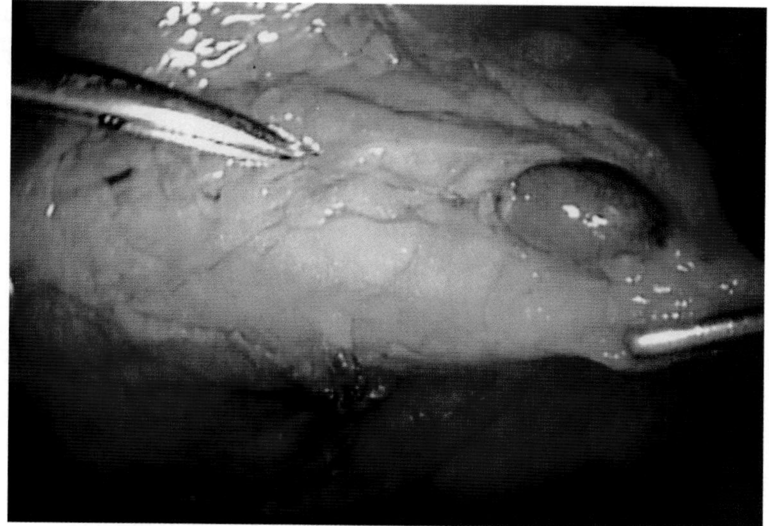

Figure 25.4

Laparoscopic blue node identified during colon resection

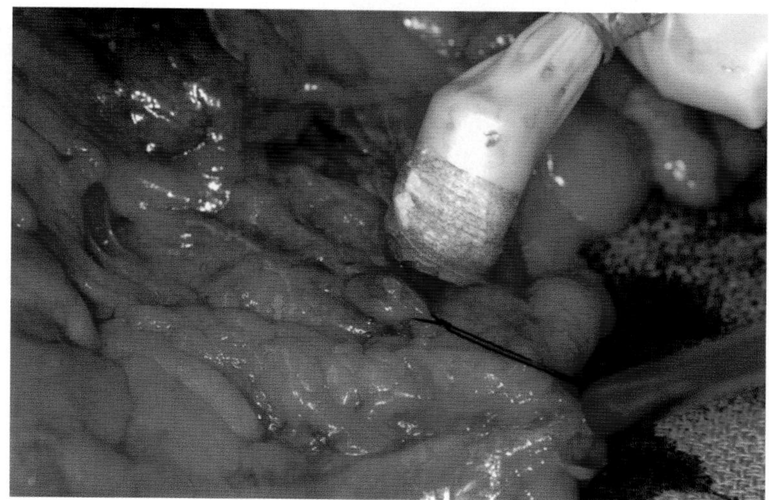

Figure 25.5

Gamma probe used to identify SLN in thickened mesentery in colon cancer

tumor cells/clusters were found in 23% of patients with stage II CC that would not have been detected by conventional methods (Fig. 25.7). Translational molecular studies also identified MM within the SN via qRT [63] and identified potential factors in facilitating these MM using RNA and DNA markers. At a mean follow-up of 25 months there were no recurrences in patients whose SN was negative by H&E/IHC and qRT suggesting that this may represent a low-risk group cured by surgery alone. However, since the follow-up was relatively short and many patients received chemotherapy; it is unclear whether the presence of MM represents a high-risk group.

A larger prospective multicenter trial supported by the NCI (2RO1CA090848) will address whether the presence of MM represents a high-risk group in the absence of chemotherapy. This trial will also integrate primary tumor characteristics and gene signatures to develop a more comprehensive staging system since it is likely that some patients may be at high risk for recurrence regardless of the MM environment.

Rectal cancer SLNB is performed in a similar fashion to colon cancer SLNB. Difficulties can arise from the rectal cancer location being inaccessible without disrupting the mesocolon if the lesion is extraperitoneal. While, the ability to find SLNs has been reported to be as high as 91% [62], concerns have been expressed due to the use of preoperative chemoradiation. Braat et al. [65] reported a sensitivity of 40% in rectal cancer treated with preoperative radiotherapy. This contrasted with the same authors' sensitivity rate of 90% for colon cancers.

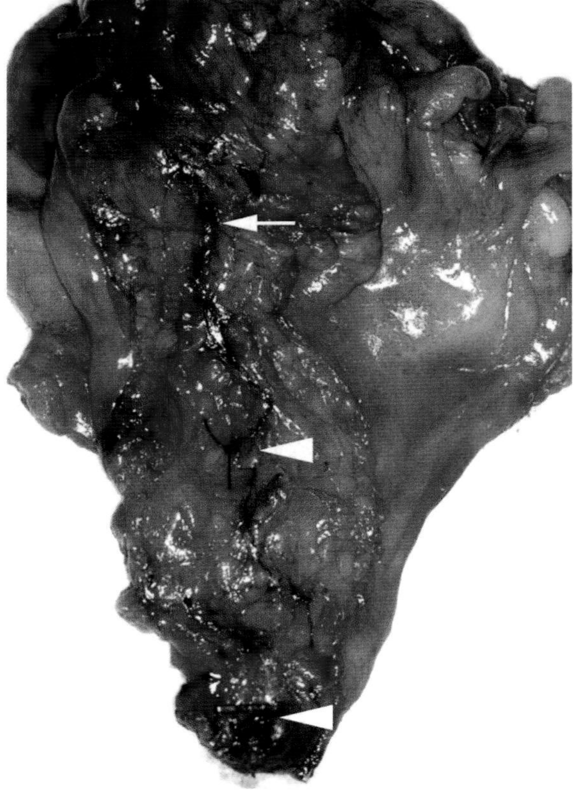

Figure 25.6
Colon cancer specimen: blue lymphatic channel tracking to sentinel node

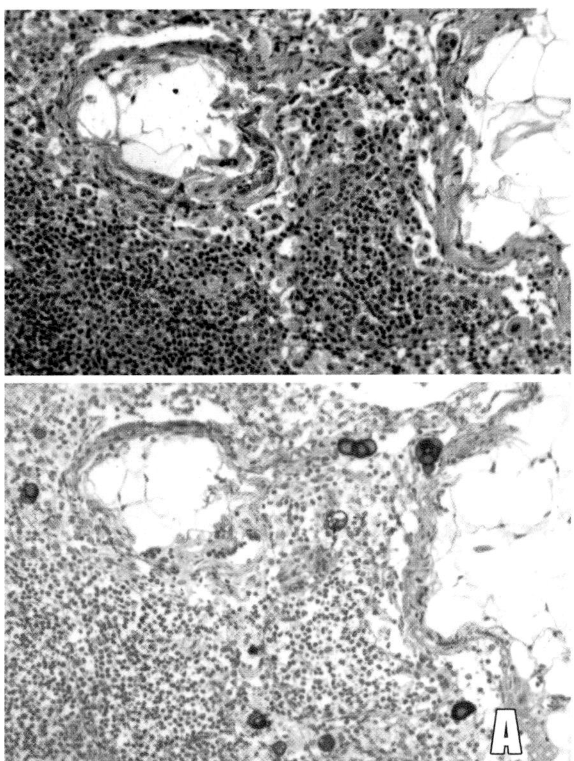

Figure 25.7
Isolated tumor cells identified by cytokeratin IHC in colon cancer node negative by H&E

Overall, while SLNB continues to be a promising technique for the evaluation of the colorectal nodal basins, more work is necessary to standardize the procedure and determine the minimum number of cases needed for proficiency such that accuracy can be assured across surgeons and pathologists. Rectal carcinomas should be approached with more caution, and in no cases should a standard mesenteric resection be forgone in favor of a SLNB alone.

Gastric Cancer

Although progress is being managed in both the diagnosis and the treatment of gastric cancer the mortality remains unacceptably high; perhaps because the majority of patients are diagnosed with advanced disease. The extent of nodal dissection is defined as a major factor in staging and can influence outcome by stage. There continues to be extensive debate on the optimal extent of lymphadenectomy for the surgical treatment of these patients. The role of extended lymph node dissection has been studied in prospective randomized trials showing no overall survival benefit but perhaps benefit to selected subgroups [66–69]. A randomized, controlled trial by Sasako et al. [70] in 523 patients randomly assigned to either D2 lymphadenectomy or D2 lymphadenectomy and para-aortic nodal dissection demonstrated no survival benefit beyond D2 resection. While it is well recognized that a D2 lymphadenectomy extends a survival benefit in patients with node-positive disease; the same benefit is not seen in node-negative disease.

Unfortunately preoperative imaging is insensitive in predicting nodal metastases. Since the incidence of nodal metastases may be less than 15% in superficial gastric cancers (T1), a more radical lymphadenectomy with a higher morbidity may be unnecessary. Advances in laparoscopic surgery have improved quality of life (QOL) with limited lymphadenectomy and gastric preservation particularly in patients with early gastric cancer. Gastric cancers, however, can have unpredictable lymphatic drainage pathways with over 30% of gastric cancers having their first site of metastasis in nodal stations beyond the perigastric area [71]. We therefore applied SLNB to gastric cancer in 1998 [72] to determine whether staging accuracy could be improved thereby guiding the extent of resection (Fig. 25.8).

The use of intraoperative frozen section analysis of the SLN may also have particular relevance during laparoscopic surgery to limit the extent of resection thereby reducing the morbidity of a more extensive lymphadenectomy in those patients with node-negative disease [73, 74]. Recently, the validity of the SN concept has been demonstrated by a number of single institutional studies, and prospective multicenter trials are currently ongoing [73, 75–78]. Theoretically, better function-preserving operations could be applied in cases of early gastric cancer with negative SNs to improve long-term QOL. Since adjuvant chemotherapy after curative resection is typically reserved for those at high risk for recurrence [79], SLNB may also improve the selection of patients for adjuvant therapy.

Sentinel Node Technique

The choice of isosulfan blue dye or radiocolloid is based on surgeon preference, although a combined technique has been reported to reduce technical errors [80]. For those using ^{99m}Tc radiocolloid, the typical technique is injection via an esophagogastroduodenoscopy (EGD) of approximately 0.5 ml of radiocolloid in four quadrants surrounding the tumor corresponding to an approximately 150 MBq dose [81]. Injection can be performed between 2 and 20 h. ^{99m}Tc-tin colloid has been reported as the optimal tracer [80]. For those preferring blue dye, 0.5–1 ml injection of isosulfan blue dye or indocyanine green [82] is injected intra-operatively, after minimal dissection. SLNs are identified via visual inspection and/or use of the gamma probe. Frozen section of the SLN can also be considered particularly during laparoscopic procedures to refine the extent of resection.

Surgical Management

Intraoperatively the SLN basin is identified either at laparoscopically or at laparotomy by tracing the blue channel to the SLNs. If a radiopharmaceutical is used a gamma probe identifies increased radioactivity in the SLNs. After the SLNs are marked by either a suture or a clip they can either be removed as a separate package or en bloc with the rest of the lymphadenectomy.

Reported rates by single institutions of SLN identification are 94–100% and reported sensitivity of SLN assessment exceeds 85% [82, 83]. Prospective multicenter trials are underway internationally in both Japan and Europe and should provide answers as to its usefulness in more general practice. The Gastric Cancer Surgical Study Group of the Japan Clinical Oncology

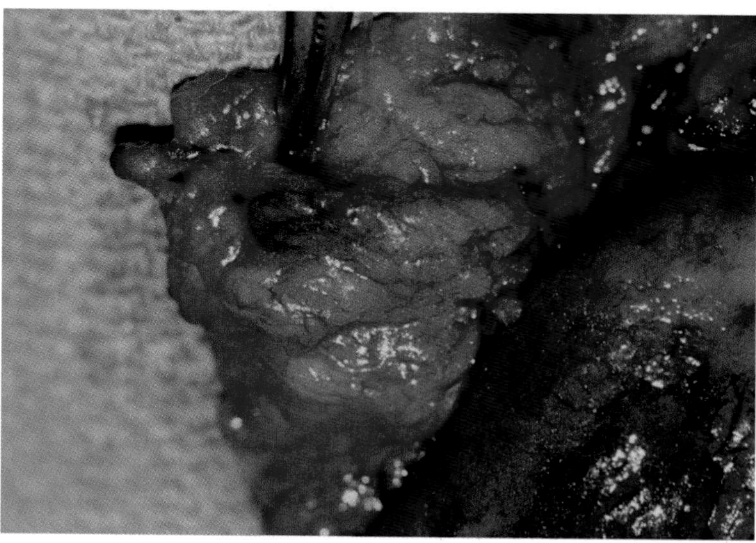

Figure 25.8

Lymphatic mapping of gastric cancer demonstrating blue-stained lymphatic channel draining to SN in an unexpected location

Group (JCOG) initiated a multicenter prospective study of SN mapping by the dye-guided method using subserosal injection of indocyanine green [73, 75–78]. If these results demonstrate low false-negative rates this may be a preferred approach. Simultaneously the Japan Society of Sentinel Node Navigation Surgery (SNNS) is also conducting a multicenter prospective trial of SN mapping using a dual tracer method with isosulfan blue dye and radioactive colloid. The results of these prospective clinical trials will be important in evaluating the role of SLN evaluation in gastric cancer.

Esophageal Cancer

Unlike breast cancer and melanoma the lymphatic pathways in esophageal cancer are extremely complex. Drainage can occur to thoracic, abdominal, or cervical lymph nodes. Similar to gastric cancer a radical lymphadenectomy is associated with increased morbidity but also prolonged survival in certain subsets of patients [84–86]. SLNB offers the ability to identify patients with lymph node metastases who would receive benefit from extended lymphadenectomy. In addition, pathological ultrastaging of the lymph nodes identified as SLNs can determine which patients should receive adjuvant therapy.

Technique

Lymphatic mapping using blue dye alone is generally not feasible in esophageal cancer since real-time observation of the dye would require mobilization of the esophagus which would likely disrupt the lymphatic pathways [87]. Therefore, Kitagawa et al. has described a technique of preoperative endoscopic injection using 2.0 ml Tc-99m tin colloid in four quadrants surrounding the tumor. Preoperative lymphoscintigraphy 3 h after injection can be very useful to identify the SLN basin which may influence the extent of the lymphadenectomy.

Surgical Management

Similar to gastric cancer after minimal dissection the dye-stained lymphatic channel is followed to the SLN and confirmed by a gamma probe. The SLN is marked with a suture or clip and a regional lymphadenectomy performed. Preoperative imaging can sometimes be difficult to interpret due to the close proximity of the primary tumor to the SLN [88].

Feasibility studies report that SLNB can predict the status of the lymphatic basin in 69–100% of patients. These small studies (6–40 patients) evaluated heterogeneous populations with different stages of disease [84, 85, 89]. SLNB for esophageal cancer, while promising, continues to be in its infancy and thus should be performed on protocol. Validation of this technique in prospective clinical trials is needed before this can be considered in standard practice.

Head and Neck Tumors

Regional lymph nodes are the most common site for metastases from primary head and neck tumors. Traditional management has therefore involved a neck dissection which can result in significant morbidity. Radical neck dissections including resection of the internal jugular vein and sternocleidomastoid muscle have largely been replaced by modified neck dissections. Since many patients with early oral and oropharyngeal carcinomas have negative lymph nodes limited neck dissections have been proposed. In these selected cases, negative histologic results of level I lymph nodes have been used to predict the nodal status of the remaining neck (levels II–VI). Since selective nodal analysis has been used for years with acceptable negative predictive values, SLNB as a predictive marker [90–98] has been proposed as a minimally invasive alternative which can decrease morbidity by further limiting the neck dissection. Patients with a positive SLN can then undergo a complete neck dissection. The majority of patients who do not have lymphatic metastases can avoid unnecessary completion neck dissections. Focused pathologic examination of the SLN(s) may also provide for upstaging of patients who might otherwise have had missed metastases.

Surgical Technique

As in esophageal neoplasms the lymphatic drainage pathway is complex with numerous nodal pathways and basins. It is recommended therefore that preoperative lymphoscintigraphy be obtained to identify the SLN and intraoperatively a handheld gamma probe and blue dye be used to locate the SLN [99]. There is a large variation in the amount of radioactive tracer (sulfur colloid) used to detect a SLN; a recent review of 19 studies reported dose variations from 0.037 to 111 MBq [100].

Surgical Management

Since SLNB in head and neck cancers is an evolving technique it requires careful coordination among the surgeon, nuclear medicine physician, and pathologist. This was confirmed by Ross et al. who demonstrated that although SLNB improves the staging of head and neck squamous cell cancer [101–103], it is associated with a steep learning curve [103]. Cote et al. [104] recently reviewed the existing literature on SLNB for early-stage oral and oropharyngeal head and neck squamous cell carcinoma (HNSCC) in clinically negative (N0) necks and identified 43 pertinent published trials and reviews in the English-language literature from 1990 to 2005. High sensitivities >93% were reported for T1 and T2 HNSCC but not for T3 and T4 tumors supporting its use in early HNSCC. A meta-analysis by Paleri et al. [100] reported a 97.7% SLN identification rate with a negative predictive value of 96% [90–93, 105–109].

Furthermore focused analysis of the SLN upstaged approximately 29% of patients (mostly MM) with an approximately 4% false-negative rate [99]. Since the impact of micrometastatic disease is still controversial, the current benefit of SLNB lies in its ability to reduce the need for lymph node dissection by accurate prediction of the tumor status of the remaining nodal basin. Multicenter trials are ongoing in the United States to evaluate its potential utility in early HNSCC. One of the trials sponsored by the American College of Surgeons and the National Cancer Institute (ACOSOG-Z0360) is designed to determine whether a SLN that is H&E negative for tumor accurately predicts the absence of tumor in other cervical lymph nodes in patients with stage I or II squamous cell carcinoma of the oral cavity. The trial will also determine the extent and pattern of disease spread in the nodal bed and the use of IHC to evaluate nodes in these patients. Until these trials are complete it is recommended that SLNB be performed under study protocol only. It is likely, however, that SLNB will have a large impact on patients with early HNSCC by reducing the need for node-negative lymph node dissections [110, 111].

Lung Cancer

Non-small cell lung cancer (NSCLC) is the most common cause of cancer-related deaths in the United States. As in other solid neoplasms, lymphatic metastasis has clear prognostic value [112] and is essential in both staging and selecting patients for adjuvant therapy [113–115]. Although early-stage NSCLC (T1/T2 N0) patients have favorable survival rates, there are high rates of recurrence for (20–50%) which may be explained by understaging or missed MM as a result of incomplete lymphadenectomy. The identification of intra-operative lymphatic drainage pathways has been proposed as a method of improving the selection of the lymphatic basin for dissection thereby limiting the number of unnecessary mediastinal lymphadenectomies and providing the pathologist the opportunity to perform a focused pathologic exam in order to identify MM, which may have a similar prognosis to macrometastases (N1) [116–118].

In the initial report by Little et al. in 1999 [119], the SLN identification rate was only 46% using peritumoral injection of isosulfan blue dye. This may be explained by the difficulty in identifying a blue-stained SLN within anthracotic thoracic lymph nodes. More recent reports have demonstrated improved sensitivity by applying different methods of injection and different radiopharmaceutical tracers [118, 120–122]. Methods for tracer injection include intra-operative, CT-guided preoperative, and transbronchoscopic techniques. The tracers used include isosulfan blue dye alone, ^{99Tc}sulfur or tin colloid alone or in combination with blue dye, indocyanine green, Technetium (Tc)-99 nanocolloid, and magnetite [123–134]. In 2003 two studies were able to identify the SLN ≥95% of the time using a combination of preoperative and intraoperative and/or transbronchoscopic injection of ^{99Tc}nanocolloid [123, 125]. Using the combined blue dye and radiotracer approach, Faries et al. reported in 2004, a 100% SLN identification rate in over 39 patients with primary NSCLC [126]. The largest series of SLND in stage I NSCLC was recently reported [118] in 291 patients. Only six patients had skip metastases. In a second analysis of 64 patients, 53 patients (83%) did not undergo a mediastinal lymph node dissection because of a negative SLN. Local recurrence was only reported in two patients and the 5-year survival rate was 82%. This encouraging data suggests that the procedure is feasible and safe and may improve staging accuracy in stage I NSCLC [118, 120]. However, prospective validation is needed in larger multicenter trials as well as a comparison with standard staging procedures including mediastinoscopy and PET imaging.

Conclusions

SLNB has revolutionized the management of several cancers by improving staging accuracy and reducing the morbidity of unnecessary lymph node dissections. Complete lymph node dissections have largely been replaced by SLNB in breast cancer and melanoma. In other malignancies that metastasize primarily through lymphatic channels SLNB is under investigation largely to improve staging accuracy by focusing pathologic analysis on a limited number of lymph nodes. To the extent that MM disease becomes an important consideration in the prognosis of patients, SLNB also remains an efficient way of identifying a subset of lymph nodes that can be staged in an intensive manner. This improved staging may allow clinicians to better stratify patients for clinical trials who might benefit from adjuvant therapy. Further prospective clinical trials are needed to determine whether SLNB offers a survival benefit.

Acknowledgments The research was performed pursuant to agreement under Research Project Grant No.2RO1 CA90848-05A2 with the National Institutes of Health, Department of Health and Human Services. Supported by funding from the Davidow Charitable Fund (Los Angeles, CA), Mrs. Ruth Weil (Los Angeles, CA), the Sequoia Foundation for achievement in the arts and education, Nancy and Bruce Newberg Charitable Fund, and Mrs. Marguerite Perkins Mautner.

References

1. Morton D, Cagle L, Wong J et al Intraoperative lymphatic mapping and selective lymphadenectomy: technical details of a new procedure for clinical stage I melanoma. Presented at Annual Meeting of the Society Surgical Oncology, Washington, DC, May 1990
2. Morton DL, Wen DR, Wong JH et al (1992) Technical details of intraoperative lymphatic mapping for early stage melanoma. Arch Surg 127:392–399
3. Giuliano AE, Kirgan DM, Guenther JM, Morton DL (1994) Lymphatic mapping and sentinel lymphadenectomy for breast cancer. Ann Surg 220:391–398
4. Niikura H, Okamura C, Utsunomiya H et al (2005) Sentinel lymph node detection in patients with endometrial cancer. Gynecol Oncol 92:669–674
5. Di Stefano AB, Acquaviva G, Garozzo G et al (2005) Lymph node mapping and sentinel node detection in patients with cervical carcinoma: a 2-year experience. Gynecol Oncol 99:671–679
6. Dhar KK, Woolas RP (2005) Lymphatic mapping and sentinel node biopsy in early vulvar cancer. BJOG 112: 696–702
7. Wawroschek F (2003) Prostate lymphoscintigraphy and radio-guided surgery for sentinel node identification in prostate cancer. Urol Int 70:303–310
8. Liedberg F, Chebil G, Davidsson T et al (2006) Intraoperative sentinel node detection improves nodal staging in invasive bladder cancer. J Urol 175:84–88
9. Leong SP, Donegan E, Heffernon W et al (2000) Adverse reactions to isosulfan blue during selective sentinel lymph node dissection in melanoma. Ann Surg Oncol 7:361–366
10. Gershenwald JE, Tseng CH, Thompson W et al (1998) Improved sentinel lymph node localization in patients with primary melanoma with the use of radiolabelled colloid. Surgery 24:203–210
11. Krag DN, Meijer SJ, Weaver DL et al (1994) Minimal access surgery for staging of malignant melanoma. Arch Surg 130:654–658
12. Essner R (1997) The role of lymphoscintigraphy and sentinel node mapping in assessing patient risk in melanoma. Semin Oncol 24:S8–S10
13. McMasters KM, Reintgen DS, Ross MI et al (2001) Sentinel lymph node biopsy for melanoma: how many radioactive nodes should be removed? Ann Surg Oncol 8: 192–197
14. Balch CM, Soong SJ, Murad TM et al (1979) A multifactorial analysis of melanoma. II. Prognostic factors in patients with stage I (localized) melanoma. Surgery 86:343–351
15. Milton GW, Shaw HM, McCarthy WH et al (1982) Prophylactic lymph node dissection in clinical stage I cutaneous malignant melanoma: results of surgical treatment in 1319 patients. Br J Surg 69:108–111
16. Sim FH, Taylor WF, Ivins JC et al (1978) A prospective randomized study of the efficacy of routine elective lymphadenectomy in management of malignant melanoma. Preliminary results. Cancer 41:948–956
17. Veronesi U, Adamus J, Bandiera DC et al (1977) Inefficacy of immediate node dissection in stage 1 melanoma of the limbs. N Engl J Med 297:627–630
18. Veronesi U, Adamus J, Bandiera DC et al (1982) Delayed regional lymph node dissection in stage I melanoma of the skin of the lower extremities. Cancer 49:2420–2430
19. Balch CM, Soong SJ, Bartolucci AA et al (1996) Efficacy of an elective regional lymph node dissection of 1 to 4 mm thick melanomas for patients 60 years of age and younger. Ann Surg 224:255–266
20. Balch CM, Soong SJ, Milton GW et al (1982) A comparison of prognostic factors and surgical results in 1,786 patients with localized (stage I) melanoma treated in Alabama, USA, and New South Wales, Australia. Ann Surg 196(6):677–684
21. Morton DL, Thompson JF, Essner R et al (1999) Validation of the accuracy of intraoperative lymphatic mapping and sentinel lymphadenectomy for early-stage melanoma: a multicenter trial. Multicenter Selective Lymphadenectomy Trial Group. Ann Surg 230:453–465

22. Morton DL, Cochran AJ, Thompson JF et al (2005) Sentinel node biopsy for early-stage melanoma accuracy and morbidity in MSLT-1, an international multicenter trial. Ann Surg 242(3):302–311, discussion 311–3
23. Morton DL, Thompson JF, Cochran AJ, Mozzillo N, Elashoff R, Essner R, Nieweg OE, Roses DF, Hoekstra HJ, Karakousis CP, Reintgen DS, Coventry BJ, Glass EC, Wang HJ, MSLT Group (2006) Sentinel-node biopsy or nodal observation in melanoma. N Engl J Med 355(13):1307–1317 (Erratum in: N Engl J Med. 2006 Nov 2;355(18):1944)
24. Bilchik AJ, Giuliano A, Essner R et al (1998) Universal application of intraoperative lymphatic mapping and sentinel lymphadenectomy in solid neoplasms. Cancer J Sci Am 4:351–358
25. Hill AD, Brady MS, Coit DG (1999) Intraoperative mapping and sentinel lymph node biopsy for Merkel cell carcinoma. Br J Surg 86:518–521
26. Wagner JD, Evdokimov DZ, Weisberger E et al (2004) Sentinel lymph biopsy for high risk non-melanoma cutaneous malignancy. Arch Dermatol 140:75–79
27. Carter CL, Allen C, Henson DE (1989) Relation of tumor size, lymph node status, and survival in 24,740 breast cancer cases. Cancer 63:181–187
28. Fisher ER, Anderson S, Redmond C et al (1993) Pathologic findings from the National Surgical Adjuvant Breast Project Protocol B-06. 10-year pathologic and clinical prognostic discriminants. Cancer 71:2507–2514
29. Giuliano AE, Jones RC, Brennan M et al (1997) Sentinel lymphadenectomy in breast cancer. J Clin Oncol 15: 2345–2350
30. Krag D, Weaver D, Ashikaga T et al (1998) The sentinel node in breast cancer a multicenter validation study. N Engl J Med 339:941–946
31. McMasters KM, Tuttle TM, Carlson DJ et al (2000) Sentinel lymph node biopsy for breast cancer: a suitable alternative to routine axillary dissection in multi-institutional practice when optimal technique is used. J Clin Oncol 18:2560–2566
32. Hsueh EC, Hansen N, Giuliano AE (2000) Intraoperative lymphatic mapping and sentinel lymph node dissection in breast cancer. CA Cancer J Clin 50:279–291
33. Wong SL, Chao C, Edwards MJ et al (2001) Accuracy of sentinel lymph node biopsy for patients with T2 and T3 breast cancers. Am Surg 67:522–526
34. Bedrosian I, Reynolds C, Mick R et al (2000) Accuracy of sentinel lymph node biopsy in patients with large primary breast tumors. Cancer 88:2540–2545
35. Chung MH, Ye W, Giuliano AE (2001) Role for sentinel lymph node dissection in the management of large (> or = 5 cm) invasive breast cancer. Ann Surg Oncol 8:688–692
36. Pendas S, Dauway E, Giuliano R et al (2000) Sentinel node biopsy in ductal carcinoma in situ patients. Ann Surg Oncol 7:15–20
37. Reitsamer R, Peintinger F, Rettenbacher L et al (2003) Sentinel lymph node biopsy in breast cancer patients after neoadjuvant chemotherapy. J Surg Oncol 84:63–67
38. Mamounas EP, Brown A, Anderson S et al (2005) Sentinel node biopsy after neoadjuvant chemotherapy in breast cancer: results from National Surgical Adjuvant Breast and Bowel Project Protocol B-27. J Clin Oncol 23(12):2694–2702 (Erratum in: J Clin Oncol. 2005 Jul 20;23(21):4808)
39. Lyman GH, Giuliano AE, Somerfield MR et al (2005) American Society of Clinical Oncology guideline recommendations for sentinel lymph node biopsy in early-stage breast cancer. J Clin Oncol 23:7703–7720
40. Sabel MS, Schott AF, Kleer CG et al (2003) Sentinel node biopsy prior to neoadjuvant chemotherapy. Am J Surg 186:102–105
41. Singletary SE, Connolly SJ (2006) Breast cancer staging: working with the sixth edition of the AJCC staging manual. CA Cancer J Clin 56:37–47
42. National Cancer Institute. Phase III Randomized Study of Surgical Resection with or Without Axillary Lymph Node Dissection in Women with Clinically Node-Negative Breast Cancer with Sentinel Node Micrometastases. http://www.cancer.gov/clinicaltrials/IBCSG-23-01. Accessed 17 Apr 2006
43. American College of Surgeons Oncology Group. A prognostic study of sentinel node and bone marrow micrometastases in women with clinical T1 or T2 N0 M0 breast cancer. Available on the World Wide Web at: https://www.acosog.org/studies/synopses/Z0010_Synopsis.pdf. Accessed 17 Apr 2006
44. Brogi E, Torres-Matundan E, Tan LK, Cody HS III (2005) The results of frozen section, touch preparation, and cytological smear are comparable for intraoperative examination of sentinel lymph nodes: a study of 133 breast cancer patients. Ann Surg Oncol 12:173–180
45. Cox CE, Furman B, Dupont EL et al (2004) Novel techniques in sentinel lymph node mapping and localization of nonpalpable breast lesions: the Moffitt experience. Ann Surg Oncol 11:222S–226S
46. Cox CE, Salud CJ, Cantor A et al (2001) Learning curves for breast cancer sentinel lymph node mapping based on surgical volume analysis. J Am Coll Surg 193: 593–600
47. Tafra L, Lannin DR, Swanson MS et al (2001) Multicenter trial of sentinel node biopsy for breast cancer using both technetium sulfur colloid and isosulfan blue dye. Ann Surg 233:51–59
48. Wilke LG, McCall LM, Posther KE et al (2006) Surgical complications associated with sentinel lymph node biopsy: results from a prospective international cooperative trial. Ann Surg Oncol 13:491–500
49. Veronesi U, Paganelli G, Viale G et al (2003) A randomized comparison of sentinel-node biopsy with routine axillary dissection in breast cancer. N Engl J Med 349(6):546–553
50. Swanson RS, Compton CC, Stewart AK, Bland KI (2003) The prognosis of T3N0 colon cancer is dependent on the number of lymph nodes examined. Ann Surg Oncol 10:65–71
51. Le Voyer TE, Sigurdson ER, Hanlon AL et al (2003) Colon cancer survival in associated with increasing number of lymph nodes analyzed: a secondary survey of Intergroup trial INT-0089. J Clin Oncol 21:2912–2919
52. André T, Boni C, Mounedji-Boudiaf L et al (2004) Oxaliplatin, fluorouracil, and leucovorin as adjuvant treatment for colon cancer. N Engl J Med 350:2343–2351
53. Benson AB, Schrag D, Somerfield MR et al (2004) American Society of Clinical Oncology recommendations

on adjuvant chemotherapy for stage II colon cancer. J Clin Oncol 22:3408–3419

54. Wong JH, Steineman S, Calderia C et al (2001) Ex vivo sentinel node mapping in carcinoma of the colon and rectum. Ann Aurg 233:515–521
55. Wong JH, Johnson DS, Namiki T et al (2004) Validation of ex vivo lymphatic mapping in hematoxylin-eosin node-negative carcinoma of the colon and rectum. Ann Surg Oncol 11:772–777
56. Tuech JJ, Regenet N, Ollier JC, Rodier JF (2003) Sentinel lymph node mapping in colorectal cancer. Gastroenterol Clin Biol 27(2):204–211
57. Joosten JJ, Strobbe LJ, Wauters CA et al (1999) Intraoperative lymphatic mapping and the sentinel node concept in colorectal carcinoma. Br J Surg 86: 482–486
58. Bilchik AJ, Saha S, Wiese D et al (2001) Molecular staging of early colon cancer on the basis of sentinel node analysis: a multicenter phase II trial. J Clin Oncol 19:1128–1136
59. Stojadinovic A, Allen PJ, Protic M et al (2005) Colon sentinel lymph node mapping: practical surgical applications. J Am Coll Surg 201(2):297–313
60. Bertagnolli M, Miedema B, Redston M et al (2004) Sentinel node staging of resectable colon cancer: results of a multicenter study. Ann Surg 240:624–630
61. Redston M, Compton CC, Miedema BW et al, Leukemia Group B Trial 80001 (2006) Analysis of micrometastatic disease in sentinel lymph nodes from resectable colon cancer: results of Cancer and Leukemia Group B Trial 80001. J Clin Oncol 24(6):878–883
62. Saha S, Seghal R, Patel M et al (2006) A multicenter trial of sentinel lymph node mapping in colorectal cancer: prognostic implications for nodal staging and recurrence. Am J Surg 191:305–310
63. Bilchik AJ, Hoon DSB, Saha S et al (2007) Prognostic impact of micrometastases in colon cancer: interim results of a prospective multicenter trial. Ann Surg 246(4): 568–577
64. Stojadinovic A, Nissan A, Protic M et al (2007) Prospective randomized study comparing sentinel lymph node evaluation with standard pathologic evaluation for the staging of colon carcinoma: results from the United States Military Cancer Institute Clinical Trials Group Study GI-01. Ann Surg 245(6):846–857
65. Braat AE, Oosterhuis JW, Moll FC et al (2005) Sentinel node detection after preoperative short-course radiotherapy in rectal carcinoma is not reliable. Br J Surg 92: 1533–1538
66. Songun I, van de Velde CJ (2009) How does extended lymphadenectomy influence practical care for patients with gastric cancer? Nat Clin Pract Oncol 6(2):66–67
67. Brennan MF (2005) Current status of surgery for gastric cancer: a review. Gastric Cancer 8(2):64–70
68. McCulloch P, Nita ME, Kazi H et al (2004). Extended versus limited lymph nodes dissection technique for adenocarcinoma of the stomach. Cochrane Database Syst Rev 18(4):CD001964
69. Sano T, Sasako M, Yamamoto S et al (2004) Gastric cancer surgery: morbidity and mortality results from a prospective randomized controlled trial comparing D2 and extended para-aortic lymphadenectomy – Japan Clinical Oncology Group study 9501. J Clin Oncol 22(14): 2759–2761
70. Sasako M, Sano T, Yamamoto S et al. Japan Clinical Oncology Group (2008) D2 lymphadenectomy alone or with para-aortic nodal dissection for gastric cancer. N Engl J Med 359(5):453–462
71. Sano T, Katai H, Sasko M et al (2000) Gastric lymphadenectomy and detection of sentinel nodes. Recent Results Cancer Res 157:253–258
72. Bilchik AJ, Giuliano A, Essner R et al (1998) Universal application of intraoperative lymphatic mapping and sentinel lymphadenectomy in solid neoplasms. Cancer J Sci Am 4:351–358
73. Kitagawa Y, Kitano S, Kubota T et al (2005) Minimally invasive surgery for gastric cancer – toward a confluence of two major streams: a review. Gastric Cancer 8(2): 103–110
74. Otani Y, Furukawa T, Kitagawa Y et al (2004) New method of laparoscopy-assisted function-preserving surgery for early gastric cancer: vagus-sparing segmental gastrectomy under sentinel node navigation. J Am Coll Surg 198(6):1026–1031
75. Takeuchi H, Kitagawa Y (2008) Sentinel node navigation surgery for esophageal cancer. Gen Thorac Cardiovasc Surg 56(8):393–396, Epub 2008 Aug 13. Review
76. Kitagawa Y, Saikawa Y, Takeuchi H, Mukai M, Nakahara T, Kubo A, Kitajima M (2006) Sentinel node navigation in early stage gastric cancer – updated data and current status. Scand J Surg 95(4):256–259
77. Kitagawa Y, Kubota T, Kumai K, Otani Y, Saikawa Y, Yoshida M, Nakahara T, Kubo A, Kitajima M (2005) Recent studies of sentinel lymph node. Multicenter prospective clinical trials of SN biopsy for gastric cancer. Gan To Kagaku Ryoho 32(5):695–698
78. Kitagawa Y, Fujii H, Kumai K, Kubota T, Otani Y, Saikawa Y, Yoshida M, Kubo A, Kitajima M (2005) Recent advances in sentinel node navigation for gastric cancer: a paradigm shift of surgical management. J Surg Oncol 90(3): 147–151, discussion 151–152
79. Macdonald JS, Smalley SR, Benedetti J et al (2001) Chemoradiotherapy after surgery compared with surgery alone for adenocarcinoma of the stomach or gastroesophageal junction. N Eng J Med 345:725–730
80. Kitagawa Y, Fujii H, Kumai K et al (2005) Recent advances in sentinel node navigation for gastric cancer: a paradigm shift of surgical management. J Surg Oncol 90:147–152
81. Zulfikaroglu B, Koc M, Ozmen MM et al (2005) Intraoperative lymphatic mapping and sentinel lymph node biopsy using radioactive tracer in gastric cancer. Surgery 138:899–904
82. Kitagawa Y, Fujii H, Mukai M et al (2005) Sentinel lymph node mapping in esophageal and gastric cancer. Cancer Treat Res 127:123–139
83. Park DJ, Lee HJ, Lee HS et al (2006) Sentinel node biopsy for cT1 and cT2a gastric cancer. Eur J Surg Oncol 32:48–54
84. Kitagawa Y, Fujii H, Mukai M et al (2000) The role of the sentinel lymph node in gastrointestinal cancer. Surg Clin North Am 80:799–809
85. Yasuda S, Shimada H, Chino O et al (2003) Sentinel lymph node detection with Tc-99m tin colloids in patients with esophagogastric cancer. Jpn J Clin Oncol 33:68–72

86. Udagawa H, Akiyama H (2001) Surgical treatment of esophageal cancer: Tokyo experience of the three-field technique. Dis Esophagus 14:110–114
87. Kitagawa Y, Fujii H, Mukai M et al (2004) Current status and future prospects of sentinel node navigational surgery for gastrointestinal cancers. Ann Surg Oncol 11:242S–244S
88. Udagawa H (2005) Sentinel node concept in esophageal surgery: an elegant strategy. Ann Thorac Cardiovasc Surg 11:1–3
89. Lamb PJ, Griffen SM, Burt AD et al (2005) Sentinel node biopsy to evaluate the metastatic dissemination of esophageal adenocarcinoma. Br J Surg 92:60–67
90. Alex JC, Sasaki CT, Krag DN, Wenig B, Pyle PB (2000) Sentinel lymph node radiolocalization in head and neck squamous cell carcinoma. Laryngoscope 110:198–203
91. Shoaib T, Soutar DS, Prosser JE et al (1999) A suggested method for sentinel lymph node biopsy in squamous cell carcinoma of the head and neck. Head Neck 21:728–733
92. Stoeckli SJ, Steinert H, Pfaltz M, Schmid S (2001) Sentinel lymph node evaluation in squamous cell carcinoma of the head and neck. Otolaryngol Head Neck Surg 125:221–226
93. Civanto FJ, Gomez C, Duque C et al (2003) Sentinel node biopsy in oral cavity cancer: correlation with PET scan and immunohistochemistry. Head Neck 25:1–9
94. Barzan L, Sulfaro S, Alberti F et al (2002) Gamma probe accuracy in detecting the sentinel node in clinically N0 squamous cell carcinoma of the head and neck. Ann Otol Rhinol Laryngol 111:794–798
95. Mozzillo N, Chiesa F, Botti G et al (2001) Sentinel node biopsy in head and neck cancer. Ann Surg Oncol 8: 103–105
96. Chone CT, Magalhes RS, Etchehebere E, Camargo E, Altemani A, Crespo AN (2008) Predictive value of sentinel node biopsy in head and neck cancer. Acta Otolaryngol 128(8):920–924
97. Civantos F Jr, Zitsch R, Bared A, Amin A (2008) Sentinel node biopsy for squamous cell carcinoma of the head and neck. J Surg Oncol 97(8):683–690
98. Hornstra MT, Alkureishi LW, Ross GL, Shoaib T, Soutar DS (2008) Predictive factors for failure to identify sentinel nodes in head and neck squamous cell carcinoma. Head Neck 30(7):858–862
99. Stoeckli SJ, Pfaltz M, Ross GL, Steinert HC, MacDonald DG, Wittekind C, Soutar DS (2005) The second international conference on sentinel node biopsy in mucosal head and neck cancer. Ann Surg Oncol 12(11):919–924
100. Paleri V, Rees G, Arullendran P, Shoaib T, Krishman S (2005) Sentinel node biopsy in squamous cell cancer of the oral cavity and oral pharynx: a diagnostic meta-analysis. Head Neck 27(9):739–747
101. Ross GL, Soutar DS, Gordon MacDonald D et al (2004) Sentinel node biopsy in head and neck cancer: preliminary results of a multicenter trial. Ann Surg Oncol 11:690–696
102. Ross G, Shoaib T, Soutar D et al (2002) The use of sentinel node biopsy to upstage the clinically N0 Neck in head in neck cancer. Arch Otolaryngol Head Neck Surg 128: 1287–1291
103. Ross GL, Soutar D, MacDonald DG, Shoaib T, Camilleri IG (2004) Improved staging of cervical metastasis in clinically negative patients with head and neck squamous cell carcinoma. Ann Surg Oncol 11:213–218
104. Côté V, Kost K, Payne RJ, Hier MP (2007) Sentinel lymph node biopsy in squamous cell carcinoma of the head and neck: where we stand now, and where we are going. J Otolaryngol 36(6):344–349
105. WernerJ A, Dunne AA, Ramaswamy A et al (2004) The sentinel node concept in head and neck cancer: solution for the controversies in the N0 neck? Head Neck 26:603–611
106. Kovacs AF, Acker P, Berner U, Risse JH (2001) Sentinel lymph node excision. Treatment method of the N0 neck in patients with oral and oropharyngeal carcinoma. HNO 49:646–653
107. Pitman KT, Johnson JT, Brown ML, Myers EN (2002) Sentinel lymph node biopsy in head and neck carcinoma. Laryngoscope 112:2101–2113
108. Shoaib T, Soutar DS, MacDonald DG et al (2001) The accuracy of head and neck carcinoma sentinel lymph node biopsy in the clinically N0 neck. Cancer 91:2077–2083
109. Pastore A, Turetta GD, Tarabini A, Turetta D, Feggi L, Pelucchi S (2002) Sentinel lymph node analysis in squamous cell carcinoma of the oral cavity and oralpharynx. Tumori 88:S58–S60
110. Keski-Säntti H, Kontio R, Leivo I, Törnwall J, Mätzke S, Mäkitie AA, Atula T (2008) Sentinel lymph node biopsy as an alternative to wait and see policy in patients with small T1 oral cavity squamous cell carcinoma. Acta Otolaryngol 128(1):98–102
111. Hart RD, Henry E, Nasser JG, Trites JR, Taylor SM, Bullock M, Barnes D (2007) Sentinel node biopsy in N0 squamous cell carcinoma of the oral cavity and oropharynx in patients previously treated with surgery or radiation therapy: a pilot study. Arch Otolaryngol Head Neck Surg 133(8):806–809
112. Keller SM, Adak S, Wagner H, Johnson DH (2000) Mediastinal lymph node dissection improves survival in patients with stages II and IIIa non-small cell lung cancer. Eastern Cooperative Oncology Group. Ann Thorac Surg 70:358–365
113. Graham AN, Chan KJ, Pastorino U et al (1999) Systemic nodal dissection in the intrathoracic staging of patients with non-small cell lung cancer. J Thorac Cardiovasc Surg 117:246–251
114. Izbicki JR, Passlick B, Pantel K et al (1998) Effectiveness of radical systematic mediastinal lymphadenectomy in patients with respectable non-small cell lung cancer: results of a prospective randomized trial. Ann Surg 227:138–144
115. Wu YL, Huang ZF, Wang SY et al (2002) A randomized trial of systematic nodal dissection in respectable non-small cell lung cancer. Lung Cancer 36:1–6
116. Kubuschok B, Passlick B, Izbicki JR, Thette O, Pantel K (1999) Disseminated tumor cells in lymph nodes as a determinate for survival in surgically resected non-small cell lung cancer. J Clin Oncol 17:19–24
117. Osaki T, Oyama T, Gu CD et al (2002) Prognostic impact of micrometastatic tumor cells in the lymph nodes and bone marrow of patients with completely respectable stage I non-small cell lung cancer. J Clin Oncol 20:2930–2936
118. Muraoka M, Akamine S, Oka T, Tagawa T, Nakamura A, Tsuchiya T, Hayashi T, Nagayasu T (2007) Sentinel node sampling limits lymphadenectomy in stage I non-small cell

lung cancer. Eur J Cardiothorac Surg 32(2):356–361, Epub 2007 May 21

119. Little AG, DeHoyos A, Kirgan DM, Arcomano TR, Murray KD (1999) Intraoperative lymphatic mapping for non-small cell lung cancer: the sentinel node technique. J Thorac Cardiovasc Surg 117:220–224
120. Minamiya Y, Ogawa J (2005) The current status of sentinel lymph node mapping in non-small cell lung cancer. Ann Thorac Cardiovasc Surg 11(2):67–72
121. Ueda K, Suga K, Kaneda Y, Sakano H, Tanaka T, Hayashi M, Li TS, Hamano K (2004) Radioisotope lymph node mapping in nonsmall cell lung cancer: can it be applicable for sentinel node biopsy? Ann Thorac Surg 77(2):426–430
122. Liptay MJ, Masters GA, Winchester DJ, Edelman BL, Garrido BJ, Hirschtritt TR, Perlman RM, Fry WA (2000) Intraoperative radioisotope sentinel lymph node mapping in non-small cell lung cancer. Ann Thorac Surg 70(2): 384–389, discussion 389–90
123. Lardinois D, Brack T, Gaspert A et al (2003) Bronchoscopic radioisotope injection for sentinel lymph-node mapping in potentially respectable non small-cell lung cancer. Eur J Cardiothorac Surg 23:824–827
124. Lipatay MJ, Masters GA, Winchenchester DJ et al (2000) Intraoperative radioisotope sentinel lymph node mapping in non-small cell lung cancer. Ann Thorac Surg 70: 384–389
125. Melfi FM, Chella A, Menconi GF et al (2003) Intraoperative radioguided sentinel lymph node biopsy in non-small cell lung cancer. Eur J Cardthorac Surg 23:214–220
126. Faries MB, Bleicher RJ, Ye X et al (2004) Lymphatic mapping and sentinel lymphadenectomy for primary and metastatic pulmonary malignant neoplasms. Arch Surg 139:870–877
127. Nakagawa T, Minamia Y, Katayose Y et al (2003) A novel method for sentinel node mapping using magnetite in patients with non small cell lung cancer. J Thorac Cardiovasc Surg 126:563–567
128. Nomori H, Horio H, Naruke T et al (2002) Use of technetium-99m tin colloid for sentinel lymph node identification in non-small cell lung cancer. J Thorac Cardiovasc Surg 124:486–492
129. Nomori H, Wantanabe K, Ohtsuka T et al (2004) In vivo identification of sentinel lymph nodes for clinically stage I non-small cell lung cancer for abbreviation of mediastinal lymph node dissection. Lung Cancer 46:49–55
130. Pulte D, Li E, Crawford BK et al (2005) Sentinel lymph node mapping and molecular staging in non-small cell lung carcinoma. Cancer 104:1453–1461
131. Schnidt FE, Woltering EA, Webb WR et al (2002) Sentinel nodal assessment in patients with carcinoma of the lung. Ann Thorac Surg 74:870–874
132. Sugi K, Fukuda M, Nakamura H, Kaneda Y (2003) Comparison of three tracers for detection sentinel lymph nodes in patients with clinical N0 lung cancer. Lung Cancer 39:37–40
133. Tiffet O, Nicholson A, Khaddage A et al (2005) Feasibility of the detection of the sentinel lymph node in peripheral non-small cell lung cancer with radio isotopic and blue dye techniques. Chest 127:443–448
134. Yoshimasu T, Miyoshi S, Oura S et al (2005) Limited mediastinal lymph node dissection for non-small cell lung cancer according to intraoperative histologic examinations. J Thorac Cardiovasc Surg 130:241–242

Future Prospects

Frederick L. Greene, B. Todd Heniford

Contents

In this first decade of the twenty-first century, we have seen the introduction of many innovative techniques for the diagnosis and treatment of cancer. With certainty, the last two decades of the twentieth century will be judged as a milestone in the history of surgery. However, the advances that have been made cannot compare with those that will be possible in the twenty-first century. It has been fortuitous that the 1990s saw the introduction of a valuable tool for general surgeons that has now become inculcated in virtually every specialty dealing with cancer management. Minimal access approaches to patients with malignant disease have created new methods of diagnosis and treatment that will be extended to future methodologies, allowing novel surgical approaches to be performed. In addition, endoscopic management will give way to the creation of avenues for the application of chemotherapy and radiation therapy techniques.

There is no doubt, unfortunately, that the current population growth, especially in developing countries, will be associated with increasing forms of cancer that will challenge physicians and surgeons. In 2009, it was estimated that there will be 1.44 million new cases of cancer in the United States [1]. As our population expands and increases in age, problems relating to malignancy will continue to be on the forefront. In specific sites, increases in esophageal and colorectal cancer will continue. These are disease processes in which minimal access treatment has already gained a stronghold. The increase in hepatic and pancreatic malignancy will also continue to challenge the ingenuity of physicians. While the incidence of certain gastrointestinal malignancies (e.g., gastric carcinoma) remains constant or decreases, it is likely that an increase in pancreatic and hepatobiliary tumors will occur due to ongoing issues of hepatitis and environmental pollutants.

The specific areas where minimal access techniques will continue to be important in cancer management

F.L. Greene, B.T. Heniford (eds.), *Minimally Invasive Cancer Management*,
DOI 10.1007/978-1-4419-1238-1_26,

are diagnosis, ablative therapies, and extirpation of malignancy. In all three areas, the use of minimal access techniques will play a leading role. Current approaches to metastatic and primary disease in the liver, kidney, and other organs include radiofrequency and microwave ablation performed with small probes placed directly into the organ under ultrasound guidance. These and other ablative therapies, such as high-intensity focused ultrasound, will become an even greater force in the future when combined with advanced imaging technologies. We have worked with real-time magnetic resonance imaging under an open magnet, and this appears promising. It is not difficult to see how these techniques could expand the use of ablation procedures for primary and metastatic disease of the adrenal gland, brain, breast, spinal cord, and bone. The obvious problem with these destructive therapies is lack of accurate staging, which is so important when attempting to compare various treatment modalities or to determine the need for additional treatment such as radiation or chemotherapy. The need for accurate staging, which is imperative in any study, has been a passion for the senior author (F.L.G.) for more than a decade; we will be interested to see how the concept of staging is affected by the move to less precise, but noninvasive diagnosis.

Until accurate pathologic staging can be formed totally noninvasively, the diagnostic and staging usefulness of minimal access approaches will become more important as these minimally intrusive ablative procedures and newer chemotherapeutic and radiation techniques are developed. There is no doubt that large, extirpative, debulking procedures, performed so commonly in the twentieth century, will be relegated to history in the twenty-first century. For this change to take place, more aggressive approaches for staging malignancies in the abdomen and thorax must be introduced. Patients having unresectable disease will no longer be taken to the operating room for suboptimal intervention. These patients will be identified by aggressive imaging in concert with laparoscopic or thoracoscopic maneuvers. Once staging has been accomplished, novel therapeutic management will be instituted on a neoadjuvant basis.

One of the most exciting areas for the future of minimal access techniques will be in the extirpation of small cancers that are identified by appropriate surveillance using new imaging modalities, serum markers, or the combination of both with subsequent signal enhancement. Potentially, virtual colonoscopy or advanced helical computed tomography (CT) scanning with three-dimensional (3D) reconstruction of the colon will allow for the identification of small colonic lesions, which then may be resected using a combination of flexible and laparoscopic techniques. The introduction of fully functional, smaller diameter instrumentation, often when combined with flexible endoscopy, will continue to allow for intraluminal resection and the ability to salvage organs such as the esophagus and stomach. Given these advances and the fact that genetic testing will direct physicians to act even prior to the development of a cancer, the functional disorders created by major resection of the gastrointestinal tract may be reduced and lead to an improved quality of life for patients with malignancy or the predisposition for malignancy.

The introduction of these exciting technical innovations will depend on training. There is no doubt that traditional "open" surgical maneuvers will continue to be necessary, and thus will need to be taught at least for the foreseeable future. It is the responsibility of surgical educators, however, to impart confidence and competence in minimally invasive surgery to our residents. For those who have finished their training, adaptability will be an essential attribute. With the rapidity of change that we have seen over the last decade and expect in the future, surgeons will need to acquire new skills in the various modalities of therapy throughout their careers. It will be mandatory to assure that skill acquisition using inanimate training models and virtual reality surgical simulators facilitate surgical continuing medical education and maintenance of competence in minimal access cancer techniques.

The true acceptance of minimal access management of cancer patients will only be achieved by appropriate development of clinical pathways and the continued formulation of clinical trials that will test the appropriateness and value of newer techniques compared with traditional approaches. These studies, in addition to randomized prospective trials, will be large population-based observational studies that will attempt to prove or disprove the value of minimal access procedures. All of the major aspects of health care should be compared including clinical efficacy, patient satisfaction, functional status, and cost-effectiveness.

The benefactor of these new and exciting technical efforts will be the patient. Reduced need for hospital stay and overall reduction of pain and suffering may be the most important outcomes in assessing minimal access cancer management. The ultimate benchmarks of overall outcome and disease-free survival must be studied, especially in relation to traditional cancer management. With earlier identification of cancer and less invasive extirpative techniques, cancer management in the future will be changed forever. Realizing that these technical advances are dependent on the skill and appropriate application by physicians, we must constantly be reminded that technology moves faster than knowledge, which, in turn, moves faster than wisdom.

References

1. Jemal A, Siegel R, Ward E et al (2008) Cancer statistics, 2008. CA Cancer J Clin 58:71–96

Index

Note: The letters 'f' and 't' following locators refer to figures and tables respectively.

A

B

F.L. Greene, B.T. Heniford (eds.), *Minimally Invasive Cancer Management*,
DOI 10.1007/978-1-4419-1238-1,

C

D

E

F

G

H

I

J

K

L

M

N

T

U

9 781441 912374